Editors

Silvia Pastorekova
Juraj Kopacek

Slovak Academy of Sciences
SPECTRUM SLOVAKIA Series
Volume 1

Tumour Hypoxia:
Molecular Mechanisms and Clinical Implications

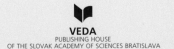

VEDA
PUBLISHING HOUSE
OF THE SLOVAK ACADEMY OF SCIENCES BRATISLAVA

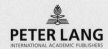

PETER LANG
INTERNATIONAL ACADEMIC PUBLISHERS

Bibliographic Information published by the Deutsche Nationalbibliothek
The Deutsche Nationalbibliothek lists this publication in the Deutsche
Nationalbibliografie;
detailed bibliographic data is available in the internet at http://dnb.d-nb.de.

Editors:
Prof. Silvia Pastorekova, Ph.D., D.Sc.
Juraj Kopacek, Mv.D., Ph.D., D.Sc.

Reviewers:
Prof. Dr. med. Dörthe M. Katschinski
Georg-August Universität Göttingen, Germany
Prof. Jose Lopez-Barneo MD, PhD
Instituto de Biomedicina de Sevilla, Spain

Department of Molecular Medicine
Institute of VirologySlovak Academy of Sciences
Bratislava
Slovak Republic
virusipa@savba.sk
virukopa@savba.sk

The cover layout is composed of an image of migrating cancer cell that shows
red signal representing interaction between carbonic anhydrase IX and
anion exchanger 2 detected by proximity ligation assay (courtesy of Dr. Eliska
Svastova and Dr. Ivan Kosik, Institute of Virology, Slovak Academy
of Sciences, Bratislava).

ISBN 978-3-631-63991-7   ISBN 978-80-224-1261-2
© Peter Lang GmbH   © VEDA, SAS Publishing House
International Academic Publishers   Slovak Academy of Sciences
Frankfurt am Main 2012   Bratislava 2012

Preface

Hypoxia, an insufficient supply of oxygen, typically occurs in a broad range of solid tumours due to aberrant vasculature. It is a key component of tumour microenvironment that affects many biological processes at the molecular, cellular and tissue levels. Adaptive responses to oxygen deficiency shape signal transduction, cell metabolism, proliferation, differentiation, survival, angiogenesis, immunosurveillance etc. and thereby contribute to tumour invasion and metastasis. The presence of tumour hypoxia is significantly associated with poor prognosis and therapy resistance. Therefore, it represents a clinically relevant phenomenon that can be utilised for improvement of existing diagnostic and treatment procedures as well as for the development of new, targeted strategies. This book summarizes the current state of knowledge on hypoxia-regulated pathways and their biological consequences and describes promising approaches to the clinical application of this knowledge. It represents the first concise and complex guide to understanding the basic principles and medical aspects of tumour hypoxia offered by renowned authors, many of whom have made key discoveries in this area.

Assembly of this book was inspired by regular meetings of the experts in the research of hypoxia, who participate in the HypoxiaNet network funded by the EU within the COST action TD0901. These meetings always bring new exciting ideas, build excellent research relationships and invoke vivid scientific collaborations in this area. The book represents the effort in sharing this excitement with newcomers to the field as well as with all those who want to gain better insight into this interesting and important phenomenon.

Silvia Pastorekova
Juraj Kopacek

Contents

Part **III**
Medical aspects of hypoxia

Part I

Molecular pathways regulating responses to hypoxia

Chapter 1

Oxygen sensing by HIF hydroxylases

Norma Masson and Peter J. Ratcliffe[*]

[*]Author for correspondence:
Nuffield Department of Clinical Medicine, Centre for Cellular and Molecular Physiology,
University of Oxford, Henry Wellcome Building for Molecular Physiology, Old Road Campus,
Oxford OX3 7BN, United Kingdom, Tel: +44 (1865) 287 990, Fax: +44 (1865) 287 992,
E-mail: pjr@well.ox.ac.uk

Contents

Key points

— The activity of the hypoxia-inducible factor (HIF) pathway is controlled by oxygen-dependent hydroxylation, a feature conserved in all animals.

— The HIF prolyl hydroxylases (PHD1-3) and asparaginyl hydroxylase (FIH) fulfil the criteria for oxygen sensors.

— The multiple co-factor and co-substrate requirements of the PHD and FIH enzymes suggest a capacity to integrate metabolic and redox signals.

— The PHD enzymes (PHD1-3) contribute non-redundantly to HIF-α regulation, and (like FIH) may also act on other (HIF-independent) cellular substrates.

— The PHD and FIH enzymes belong to the Fe(II) and 2-OG dependent dioxygenase superfamily where other members may also have oxygen-sensing function.

Historical perspectives on oxygen sensing

Interactions between biological pathways and atmospheric oxygen are fundamental to the evolution of modern life forms. Large quantities of energy can be generated from the reduction of molecular oxygen to water. Organisms with the capacity for aerobic respiration obtain this energy through the oxidation of a range of biological substrates. Since molecular oxygen may also be reduced to potentially toxic oxygen radicals, biochemical systems also evolved to eliminate oxygen radicals or repair the associated oxidative damage. To permit survival in the face of varying environmental oxygen concentrations, organisms evolved adaptive systems that regulate oxygen-consuming metabolic pathways and control the activation of oxidant defence systems. However, the very high levels of molecular oxygen that currently characterize the earth's atmosphere generated additional evolutionary opportunities and even more complicated physiological challenges. Increasing levels of atmospheric oxygen, reaching modern day levels approximately 550 million years ago, were associated with, and are believed to have enabled, the rapid evolution of animal life forms in the Cambrian Era (Berner *et al.*, 2007; Canfield *et al.*, 2007). Such organisms utilise oxygen gradients to deliver oxygen to large masses of specialised and co-operating cells. As size and complexity increased, animals became dependent on complex oxygen delivery systems to ensure adequate supplies of oxygen to the respiring tissues. The development of these systems in turn provided capability for extremely high rates of metabolism, for instance to support very rapid movement, but added further to the complexity of maintaining oxygen homeostasis and vulnerability to failure in disease.

In mammals, the lungs, heart, vascular and red blood cell systems are all critically required for adequate oxygen delivery and serious dysfunction in any one system is ultimately fatal. On the other hand the growth of malignant tumours is itself dependent on a vascular oxygen supply, and at least some level of oxygen homeostasis in order to preserve cell viability within the tumour mass.

The co-ordination of these complex homeostatic systems requires robust mechanisms for detecting and responding to changes from the desired matching of oxygen supply to metabolic need. In principle detection systems that 'sense' mismatch might operate at different levels. For instance, inadequate oxygen might be detected either indirectly through the compromise of metabolism, or directly through changes in the availability of oxygen itself.

Anatomical and physiological studies of different organs in the early twentieth century provided ample evidence that oxygen delivery systems were indeed well matched to metabolic needs. For instance, in liver, different metabolic processes were recognised to be organised in zonal patterns that match oxygen demand with oxygen availability across the lobules of the liver. In muscle, August Krogh examined the capillary density of muscles, concluding in his seminal paper of 1919 that 'the number of capillaries per square mm of the striated muscle appears to be a function of metabolism' (Krogh, 1919). A large body of further work showed that capillary density was under dynamic control, increasing over a period of days in response to training or muscle stimulation and declining in the context of disuse (Jozsa *et al.*, 1980; Hudlicka *et al.*, 1982). Theories of causation generally focused on metabolic mediators such as ADP, adenosine, lactate and/or mechanical factors such as capillary flow, stretch or filtration rates (Clark *et al.*, 1939; Fraser *et al.*, 1979; Hudlicka *et al.*, 1982; Dusseau and Hutchins, 1988). Other investigators directly studied the role of altered oxygen delivery in vascular development, particularly that of the retinal circulation, where alterations could readily be observed in response to breathing high or low concentrations of oxygen (partially reviewed in Imre, 1964). Even in these studies, where oxygen delivery rather than metabolic demand was being altered, theories of the sensing process tended to focus on metabolism. Despite clearly recognising the importance of exposure to hyperoxia in retrolental fibroplasias (Ashton, 1957a), Ashton summarised the factors promoting (retinal) neovascularization as follows: (i) active metabolism (ii) lower oxygen resulting in the pre-dominance of anaerobic metabolism (iii) inadequate venous flow causing the retention of anaerobic metabolic products and vasoproliferative factor (Ashton, 1957b). Overall, remarkably little attention was paid to the possibility that at least some of the adaptive responses might be stimulated by reduced oxygen *per se*. In part, this bias appears to have been generated by the plethora of ways in which oxygen can disturb energy metabolism together with the difficulty or impossibility of distinguishing metabolic from hypoxic signals in the complex systems under study.

Very highly dynamic responses such as control of breathing and responses of the pulmonary vasculature to hypoxia offered greater potential for distinguishing metabolic from hypoxic signals. Yet early studies of lung ventilation also emphasised metabolic control. In their seminal work on the regulation of ventilation, Haldane and Priestley noted that 'the respiratory centre is exquisitely sensitive to any rise in the alveolar CO_2 pressure' (Haldane and Priestley, 1905). They also noted that during very vigorous exercise alveolar CO_2 concentration actually fell, a response that they attributed to the further stimulation of breathing by lactic acidosis. A similar effect (i.e. stimulation of breathing that reduced alveolar CO_2 levels) was observed in subjects breathing in a hypobaric atmosphere to simulate altitude (Boycott and Haldane, 1908). This was corrected by the addition of oxygen to the hypobaric atmosphere, indicating that lack of oxygen rather than low pressure was responsible. Haldane postulated that the stimulation of breathing in low oxygen was also due to lactic acidosis generated by anaerobic metabolism, a hypothesis he set out to test, with colleagues from Yale, in the expedition to Pike's Peak, Colorado (4300 m) in the summer of 1911. Their results essentially ruled out the lactic acid hypothesis. Acidosis was not observed. Furthermore, in contrast to a gradual correction of alveolar CO_2 to baseline (that had been the anticipated consequence of renal correction of the postulated lactic acidosis) they noted that alveolar CO_2 levels continued to fall over a period of days at altitude (Douglas *et al.*, 1913). Thus the expedition excluded a key metabolic candidate for the stimulation of respiration by hypoxia and also provided clear evidence for longer term responses, now recognised as the phenomenon of ventilatory acclimatisation. However, though the absence of an obvious metabolic stimulus suggested that hypoxia *per se* might be the mediator, this was still not proven. Importantly, the expedition yielded a further set of data, measurements made in the surrounding mining towns lying at intermediate altitudes by the only female member of the party, Mabel FitzGerald. FitzGerald's data included measurements of blood haemoglobin and revealed a continuous relationship between altitude and haemoglobin, even modest altitude being associated with an increase in haemoglobin level (FitzGerald, 1913). This work provided one of the earliest demonstrations of the extreme sensitivity of physiological responses to mild hypoxia, findings which were again difficult to explain by a system responding to metabolic compromise by hypoxia.

Further work was aimed to define the anatomical as well as physiological basis of these observations. Thus, studies in the 1920's and 30's by Cornelius Heymans, Fernando De Castro and others established the carotid body as the mediator of ventilatory responses to arterial hypoxaemia (Heymans' Nobel lecture and reviewed in De Castro, 2009). In other work, the hormonal control of red cell production, a possibility first suggested by Carnot in 1906 (Carnot and Deflandre, 1906), was finally proven beyond doubt by Erslev's classic plasma transfer experiments, published in 1953 (Erslev, 1953). Organ ablation studies established the kidney as the principle source of erythropoietin, with the liver also contributing particularly in early life (Jacobson *et al.*, 1957; Schooley and Mahlmann, 1972; Wang and Fried, 1972; Fried, 1972). These insights established a feedback loop in which a deficiency in blood oxygen content was somehow sensed, resulting in production of erythropoietin and hence correction by the formation of more red cells.

Thus at least some of the physiological responses underpinning oxygen homeostasis were difficult to link to potential metabolic mediators and by the second half of the twentieth century it was generally agreed that they implied the existence of specific oxygen sensing systems (i.e. one or more direct interfaces with the availability of oxygen with specific functions in control). In the case of erythropoietin, evidence for a specific oxygen sensing mechanism was reinforced by failure of metabolic poisons such as cyanide to mimic the effects of hypoxia (Necas and Thorling, 1972) and by the ability of cobalt poisoning to stimulate erythropoietin and red cell production despite limited effects on metabolism (Berk *et al.*, 1949). Nevertheless, the prevailing view was that such oxygen sensing systems were restricted to specialised cells located at specific sites, for instance the type 1 cells of the carotid body and the erythropoietin producing cells in the kidney and liver, a perspective reinforced by the exquisitely tuned dynamics of these biological circuits.

The hypoxia-inducible factor (HIF) pathway

In the early 1990's analysis of one of these processes, the regulation of erythropoietin, led to a fundamental change in thinking. These studies revealed that rather than being confined to specific erythropoietin producing cells, the oxygen sensing process that regulates the transcription of the erythropoietin gene is present in every cell and is responsible for a vast array of other cellular and systemic processes that contribute to physiological oxygen homeostasis.

Studies of the transcriptional regulation of the erythropoietin gene in erythropoietin-producing hepatoma cells led to the identification of an oxygen regulated control element in DNA lying 3' to the gene (Beck *et al.*, 1991; Semenza *et al.*, 1991; Pugh *et al.*, 1991) and to the definition of hypoxia inducible factor-1 (HIF-1) as a transcription factor binding this sequence and mediating its oxygen regulated function (Semenza and Wang, 1992). Remarkably however, further studies demonstrated that the same DNA control element could confer oxygen regulated behaviour on reporter genes in a wide range of cells that did not produce erythropoietin and were entirely unrelated to the erythropoietin-producing cells in the liver and kidney (Maxwell *et al.*, 1993).

These findings demonstrated the existence of a widespread oxygen sensing system in mammalian cells, implying that it had functions other than the regulation of erythropoietin. The work was quickly followed by the demonstration that HIF itself (which was first identified in hepatoma cells) was also widely expressed (Wang and Semenza, 1993) and by the identification of genes encoding glycolytic enzymes as the first non-erythropoietin HIF target genes (Firth *et al.*, 1994; *Semenza et al.*, 1994). The connection of the dynamic response of erythropoietin production to hypoxia with such a highly conserved and physiologically distinct process as glycolysis, together with the demonstration of a HIF-like protein in invertebrate cells (Nagao *et al.*, 1996) suggested that the system might be extremely prevalent in biology – a finding that has been amply borne out by subsequent work.

It is now established that the HIF system operates directly or indirectly on the expression of hundreds of genes in human cells (Xia *et al.*, 2009; Mole *et al.*, 2009) and is conserved throughout the animal kingdom (Loenarz *et al.*, 2011). The HIF transcriptional complex binds to a core (RCGTG) motif in the hypoxia-response elements of target genes. HIF is a heterodimer of HIF-α and HIF-β subunits, both of which are members of the bHLH PAS domain (basic-Helix-Loop-Helix Per-AHR/ARNT/Sim) subfamily (Wang *et al.*, 1995). There are three isoforms of HIF-α (HIF-1α, HIF-2α, HIF-3α) and HIF-β (also known as aryl hydrocarbon receptor nuclear translocator, Arnt1, Arnt2 and Arnt3), with additional diversity being generated by alternative promoter usage and splicing (Gothie *et al.*, 2000; Makino *et al.*, 2001; Maynard *et al.*, 2003; Pasanen *et al.*, 2010). HIF-β subunits operate in other transcriptional pathways (reviewed in McIntosh *et al.*, 2010), while HIF-α subunits are specific for hypoxia-dependent signalling. Both HIF-1α and HIF-2α are able to form transcriptionally active heterodimers with HIF-β. Though their DNA binding characteristics are closely similar or identical, some transcriptional targets manifest essentially absolute specificity for HIF-1 or HIF-2, whilst some are activated by both complexes (Hu *et al.*, 2003; Raval *et al.*, 2005; Holmquist-Mengelbier *et al.*, 2006). Differences between the transcriptional activation domains of HIF-1α and HIF-2α appear to confer this target gene specificity (Lau *et al.*, 2007; Hu *et al.*, 2007). The role of HIF-3α is less well understood, the best defined function being that of an alternatively spliced form of HIF-3α that inhibits transcription by forming unproductive heterodimers with other HIF-α subunits (Makino *et al.*, 2001; Maynard *et al.*, 2005; Maynard *et al.*, 2007).

Well established HIF transcriptional target genes include erythropoietin, VEGF-A and VEGFR-2, Glut1/3, PDK1, carbonic anhydrase (CA-IX), TGF-α, and, MMP-2, survivin, PDGF-β, and TGF-2. By the induction of these and other targets, HIF regulates erythropoiesis, cellular invasion, immortalisation, pH gradients, vascularisation, energy metabolism and genetic stability (Semenza, 2007). Dysregulation of these processes accounts for many of the major hallmarks of cancer. Since tumour hypoxia is associated with poor prognosis and with resistance to treatment, understanding the nature of the oxygen sensors responsible for regulating HIF and how the pathways are perturbed in disease has been the subject of intense investigation in oncology, as well as other fields of medical research.

Regulation of HIF by O_2-dependent hydroxylation

Following the identification of cDNAs encoding HIF subunits, delineation of the upstream pathways connecting the regulatory HIF-α subunits to the oxygen sensing machinery began with analyses of the oxygen regulatory activity of fusion proteins containing defined sequences derived from HIF-1α and HIF-2α. These studies identified three distinct regions in each HIF-α subunit that could convey oxygen-regulated behaviour on heterologous proteins (Pugh et al., 1997; O'Rourke et al., 1999; Jiang et al., 1997; Huang et al., 1998). Together with pharmacological and genetic analysis of the regulation of HIF-α subunits in cells bearing defects in the ubiquitin-proteasome path way (Salceda and Caro, 1997), the fusion protein analyses also established that HIF-α subunits are regulated by two distinct oxygen-dependent pathways; rapid ubiquitin-dependent proteolysis and reduced transcriptional activity that is independent of changes in protein stability (Figure 1.1).

Protcolytic regulation of HIF-α subunits was shown to be critically dependent upon the von Hippel-Lindau tumour suppressor (pVHL), a component of the pVHL/ElonginB/C (VBC) E3 ligase complex (Maxwell et al., 1999; Ohh et al., 2000; Cockman et al., 2000; Tanimoto et al., 2000). Subsequent analysis of the HIF-α/pVHL interaction demonstrated that an oxygen and iron-dependent modification of HIF-1α was necessary for the interaction and led to the identification of the *trans*-4-hydroxylation at P564 in human HIF-1α as the regulatory modification (Jaakkola et al., 2001; Ivan et al., 2001; Yu et al., 2001). Structural analysis of the HIF-α/pVHL interaction revealed a single conserved hydroxyproline binding pocket in the β-domain of pVHL (Hon et al., 2002; Min et al., 2002) that binds the hydroxylated prolyl residue in the C^4 *exo* conformation through an optimised hydrogen bonding network involving the alcohol group of the hydroxyproline and pVHL residues within the pocket (Illingworth et al., 2010). This network cannot form with proline thereby allowing

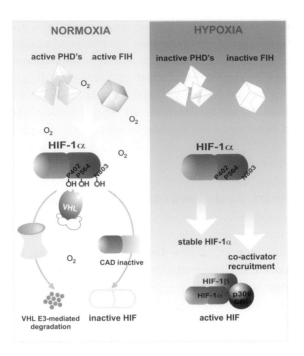

Figure 1.1 _ Oxygen-dependent regulation of HIF-1α by dual pathways: PHD-dependent prolyl hydroxylation leading to pVHL E3 ligase-dependent degradation; and FIH-dependent asparaginyl hydroxylation blocking the transactivation potential of the C-terminal activation domain (CAD).

pVHL to discriminate between non-hydroxylated and hydroxylated HIF-α. A second site of regulatory prolyl hydroxylation that binds to pVHL in a similar manner was subsequently defined in human HIF-1α at P402 (Masson *et al.*, 2001). Hydroxylation of each of these residues acts as a signal for pVHL-dependent proteolytic destruction and together with their surrounding sequences the sites have been termed the N-terminal oxygen dependent degradation domain (NODD) and C-terminal degradation domain (CODD) respectively. Though each site can promote pVHL-dependent proteolytic destruction independently, further work has indicated that in the physiological setting, hydroxylation of P564 precedes that of P402 (Chan *et al.*, 2005; Flashman *et al.*, 2008) and that hydroxylation at both sites is necessary for optimal rates of degradation (Masson *et al.*, 2001).

Structurally informed bio-informatic predictions of candidate prolyl hydroxylases rapidly led to the identification of a highly conserved series of Fe(II) and 2-oxoglutarate (2-OG) dependent dioxygenases that catalyse

HIF prolyl hydroxylation (Epstein *et al.*, 2001; Bruick and McKnight, 2001). The encoding gene family was first recognised in *C. elegans* as a locus at which mutation led to an egg-laying defective phenotype (egl-9), an abnormality now known to arise as a consequence of HIF dysregulation. In mammalian cells, three orthologues were identified termed PHD1, PHD2, PHD3 (prolyl hydroxylase domain containing) or EGLN2, EGLN1, EGLN3 (egg-laying defective-like). All three prolyl hydroxylases contribute to the physiological regulation of HIF, but they differ markedly in their relative abundance, tissue distribution and preference between the two sites of HIF prolyl hydroxylation (Appelhoff *et al.*, 2004). In most cells, PHD2 is by far the most abundant enzyme and hence makes the most important contribution to the regulation of HIF-1α levels (Berra *et al.*, 2003; Takeda *et al.*, 2007; Minamishima *et al.*, 2008). In addition to their catalytic domains PHD1 and PHD2 (but not PHD3) have N-terminal extensions. In particular PHD2 contains an N-terminal MYND (myeloid, Nervy and DEAF-1) type zinc finger domain. Although no function has been ascribed to this sequence in PHD2, the MYND domain is generally believed to be a protein-protein interaction domain that may target proline–rich regions with a 'PXLXP' motif and has been found in a variety of proteins with ubiquitin ligase and/or histone methyltransferase activity (Ansieau and Leutz, 2002; Matthews *et al.*, 2009).

Non-proteolytic regulation of HIF-α involves the regulation of transcriptional activity through hypoxia inducible association of the HIF-α C-terminal activation domain (CAD) with p300/CBP co-activators (Figure 1.1). Mass spectrometric analysis of the HIF-α CAD revealed the regulatory modification to be hydroxylation of a conserved asparagine residue, N803 in human HIF-1α (Lando *et al.*, 2002b). Though the precise mechanism by which hydroxylation of N803 blocks the association with p300/CBP is not yet clear, structural studies of the CH-1 domain of p300 complexed to non-hydroxylated polypeptides encompassing the HIF-1α CAD reveal that the unhydroxylated asparagine residue is within a helix that is buried in a hydrophobic region of the complex, where hydroxylation would be predicted to alter hydrophobic and other interactions (Dames *et al.*, 2002; Freedman *et al.*, 2002).

Hydroxylation was shown to occur on the β-carbon of the target asparagine (McNeill *et al.*, 2002) and to be catalysed by another type of Fe(II) and 2-OG dependent dioxygenase. This molecule, termed FIH (factor inhibiting HIF-1) had been previously identified simply as a protein that inhibited HIF (Mahon *et al.*, 2001). The FIH sequence is quite different to that of the PHDs, being more closely related to the JmjC family (proteins containing a region of homology to the Jumonji family of transcription factors identified as members of the Cupin metalloenzyme superfamily). However closer scrutiny of the FIH JmjC domain exposed signatures present in Fe(II) and 2-OG dependent dioxygenases, prompting the FIH to be tested for the ability to catalyse the HIF asparaginyl hydroxylation and suggesting that the wider JmjC family were also likely to be members of the dioxygenase superfamily (Hewitson et al., 2002; Lando et al., 2002a).

Evolution of the oxygen sensing HIF hydroxylase pathway

Combined bio-informatic and functional studies have indicated that the oxygen sensing HIF hydroxylase system is present in all animals, but probably not other species. The system is represented by a conserved HIF-PHD-VHL triad in the simplest known animal *Trichoplax adhaerans* (Loenarz et al., 2011). Key features include a HIF-α protein with a single site of hydroxylation resembling the C-terminal prolyl hydroxylation site (CODD) in human HIF-α, and a single PHD enzyme that resembles the principal mammalian enzyme PHD2 in possessing the MYND-finger domain at its N-terminus in addition to the C-terminal catalytic domain. Most invertebrate species possess a single HIF-α and PHD gene and the multiple HIF-α and PHD isoforms observed in vertebrate species appear to have been generated by the two genome duplication events in early vertebrate evolution (Taylor and McElwain, 2010; Loenarz et al., 2011). Since the progenitor ODD in primitive animals more closely resembles the CODD than the NODD it has been proposed that the NODD evolved later. Interestingly, studies of HIF-α ODDs reveal that, in all species so far examined, the relative position (i.e. N-terminal versus C-terminal) of the two types of prolyl hydroxylation site is conserved, and the CODD is preferentially hydroxylated over the NODD, suggesting that this arrangement has an important function in oxygen sensing (Loenarz et al., 2011). The origin of the FIH/HIF-CAD couple is less clear and it is not universal, being present in some primitive invertebrate animals such as *Nematostella* and in all vertebrate species, but not *Trichoplax, Drosophila,* or *C.elegans* (Hampton-Smith and Peet, 2009; Loenarz et al., 2011).

Prolyl hydroxylases have also been proposed to have oxygen sensing functions in non-metazoan species. For instance, in the social amoeba, *Dictyostelium,* a prolyl hydroxylase has been identified that regulates a process termed culmination in accordance with environmental oxygen levels. When starved, *Dictyostelium* cells aggregate to form a slug that, in the presence of sufficient oxygen, culminates into a fruiting body bearing aerial spores (West *et al.*, 2010). The oxygen dependent slug to fruit switch is at least in part governed by the activity of a PHD-like prolyl hydroxylase that hydroxylates a target prolyl residue in the *Dictyostelium* protein Skp-1 (van der Wel *et al.*, 2005; West *et al.,* 2010) an orthologue of the Skp-1 protein in SCF-type ubiquitin E3 ligases to which the VBC E3 ligase that targets HIF-α is related. Prolyl hydroxylated Skp-1 is targeted by O-glycosylation, which reduces activity of the Skp-1 protein, which in turn is proposed to reduce the level of one or more hypothetical activators of the slug-to-fruit switch. This contrasts with the animal system in which PHD enzymes hydroxylate HIF and thus control HIF target levels by transcription. Though the involvement of these two types of prolyl hydroxylase in oxygen sensing suggests a link, *Dictyostelium* does not contain a HIF-like molecule, its prolyl hydroxylase does not catalyse hydroxylation of animal HIF molecules and Skp-1 is not a substrate for the animal PHD enzymes (Loenarz *et al.*, 2011). Thus the evolutionary relationship of these oxygen sensing systems, on either side of the protist/animal boundary, is unclear.

Interestingly, conserved HIF target genes such as glycolytic enzymes and metabolic regulators are also regulated by oxygen levels in many non-metazoan species, but by different systems. For instance in yeast, genes encoding different isoforms of cytochrome oxidase are differentially regulated by oxygen, but by an apparently different system involving different transcription factors and a haem-based oxygen sensing process (Kwast *et al.*, 1999; Zhang and Hach, 1999), possibly reflecting convergent evolution of different processes on the regulation of gene expression by oxygen (Fukuda *et al.*, 2007).

Thus, whilst the origins of individual components of the HIF hydroxylase system remain unclear, the assembled functional pathway appears to be unique to animals. It has been proposed that its evolution was important in meeting the greater challenges to oxygen homeostasis that arise from multi-cellular, highly motile life forms that characterize the animal kingdom.

Structural and Mechanistic Properties of the HIF Hydroxylases

Structures determined by X-ray crystallography indicate that the PHDs and FIH contain a conserved enzymatic core that is typical of the Fe(II) and 2-OG dependent dioxygenase superfamily (Lee *et al.*, 2003; Elkins *et al.*, 2003;

McDonough *et al.*, 2006; Chowdhury *et al.*, 2009). Members of this superfamily act on diverse substrates including small molecules, antibiotic precursors and bases in RNA and DNA in addition to proteins (for reviews see Clifton *et al.*, 2006; Loenarz and Schofield, 2008; McDonough *et al.*, 2010). Thus considerable structural and sequence variation occurs outside the core enzymatic domain. In contrast, the enzymatic core structure is highly conserved, featuring eight β-strands that form a "jelly-roll" topology known as the double-stranded β-helix (DSBH) fold motif. One turn of the helix is made by two pairs of anti-parallel strands linked with short turns. Four strands comprise each side of the barrel-shaped DSBH fold where substrates are bound at the active site located at the internal furrow. This furrow contains the conserved sequence His-X-Asp/Glu-Xn-His that forms the canonical metal coordinating motif known as the 2-His-1-carboxylate facial triad (Koehntop *et al.*, 2005; Clifton *et al.*, 2006; McDonough *et al.*, 2006). The catalytic Fe(II) is secured by coordination with the side chains of the two histidines and the side chain of either aspartate or glutamate arranged at the vertices of a triangular face (Figure 1.2). This forms part of an octahedral geometry for the Fe(II) binding ligands, with the remaining three coordination positions occupied by water molecules.

Mechanistic properties have in part been inferred from analyses of the wider Fe(II) and 2-OG dependent dioxygenase family, in some cases supported by direct observations on the PHDs and FIH. These studies indicate an ordered sequential reaction (Figure 1.2) in which 2-OG co-substrate coordinates the active site of the enzyme.Fe(II) complex, displacing two water molecules. 2-OG binding is also stabilized by non-covalent interactions with other residues in the active site, and these residues are found to differ significantly between the PHDs and FIH (Lee *et al.*, 2003; Hewitson *et al.*, 2002; Elkins *et al.*, 2003).

Following formation of the enzyme.Fe(II).2-OG complex, the prime substrate (i.e. the target HIF-α polypeptide) enters the active site causing a conformational change, leading to the release of the remaining water molecule (Clifton *et al.*, 2006; Flashman *et al.*, 2010b). The conformational change is necessary to enable the correct positioning of the HIF-α substrate in the active site. Interestingly, the conformational change observed for PHD2 is significantly larger than that of FIH and other studied Fe(II) and 2-OG dependent dioxygenases and involves the β2β3 loop (Chowdhury *et al.*, 2009), a region in PHD enzymes that also confers substrate specificity (Villar *et al.*, 2007; Flashman *et al.*, 2008).

With HIF-α substrate bound, and resultant coordination at only five positions, the Fe(II) site is now poised to bind and activate O_2 The O_2 mol-

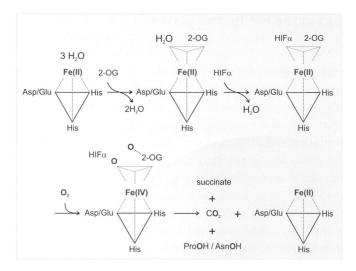

Figure 1.2 _ Proposed order of binding and coordination changes at the active site located in the DSBH fold motif of the PHD and FIH enzymes. Fe(II) is coordinated by the 2-His-1-carboxylate facial triad. The Fe(IV)=O intermediate is used by most Fe(II) and 2OG-dependent dioxygenases and is likely used by PHDs and FIH.

ecule is split, one atom is incorporated into CO_2, as a co-product of oxidative decarboxylation of the 2-OG to form succinate. In most enzymes of this class, the other oxygen atom is incorporated into a highly unstable Fe (IV)=O intermediate (Krebs *et al.*, 2007), a highly active oxidising species that rapidly targets the substrate. The PHDs and FIH likely proceed via the same mechanism (Flashman *et al.*, 2010b). Thus binding of the HIF-α substrate immediately precedes and is necessary for the activation of O_2, a feature proposed to be a mechanistic strategy that protects the enzymes from oxidative damage and self-inactivation.

Additional mechanistic insight has come from stereochemical studies of the PHD2–HIF-α substrate interaction. These demonstrate that the conformation of the target HIF-α prolyl residue is important in binding and catalysis (Loenarz *et al.*, 2009). In the active site of PHD2, the bound prolyl residue adopts a C^4 *endo* conformation, positioning it perfectly for hydroxylation (Loenarz *et al.*, 2009; Chowdhury *et al.*, 2009). In contrast the formation of the 4-hydroxyproline product forces a C^4 *exo* conformation that (as a result of a steric clash with active site residues) drives product release (Loenarz *et al.*, 2009; Chowdhury *et al.*, 2009).

Regulation of the HIF hydroxylases

Although the elucidation of the HIF hydroxylase pathway provides a clear link between the availability of oxygen and transcriptional regulation in animal cells, much remains to be understood about the exact mechanisms by which the pathway is regulated. Understanding how such an apparently simple system achieves the flexibility necessary for physiological homeostasis is the focus of a great deal of on-going work. Amongst other questions, the multiple co-substrate and co-factor requirements of the PHDs and FIH including Fe(II), ascorbate and the tricarboxylic acid cycle intermediate 2-OG as well as molecular oxygen, raises the intriguing possibility that these enzymes might integrate hypoxic, redox and metabolic signals as part of their role in oxygen homeostasis (Figure 1.3). Below we review some of the emerging data on regulation of the HIF hydroxylases by oxygen and other co-substrates/co-factors.

Molecular Oxygen

The obligatory use of molecular oxygen as co-substrate in the catalysis of prolyl and asparaginyl hydroxylation provides a mechanistic basis for the function of the HIF hydroxylases as oxygen sensors. Nevertheless the effective operation of these enzymes as sensors is dependent on two additional criteria; first the rate of HIF hydroxylation must be dependent on the level of oxygen over the physiological operating range, second the rate of HIF hydroxylation must be rate-limiting for the operation of the system as a whole (for instance prolyl hydroxylation must be the rate-limiting step in the overall prolyl hydroxylation-pVHL-degradation pathway). A substantial body of evidence indicates that these criteria are in fact met, at least under most physiological conditions.

Early data obtained using binding to pVHL to measure hydroxylation of HIF-α peptides demonstrated that the reaction was sensitive to changes in the levels of environmental oxygen even in the range 10-20% (Epstein *et al.*, 2001). Consistent with this, formal kinetic studies on purified or partially purified preparations of enzyme gave high values for the Michaelis-Menton constant for oxygen (K_mO_2, the concentration of oxygen required for a half-maximal initial rate of hydroxylation). For PHD1, 2 and 3, similar values of K_mO_2 were obtained, in the range of 230-250 µM (Hirsila *et al.*, 2003), whilst for FIH the value was somewhat lower at 120 µM (Koivunen *et al.*, 2004). However these measurements were obtained using short HIF-α peptides and consistent with the proposal (see above) that it is the assembled enzyme.Fe.2-OG. HIF-α substrate complex that ultimately reacts with oxygen, the length of the HIF-α polypeptide substrate was found to have a large effect on the reaction kinetics and on the apparent K_mO_2; substantially lower values in the range 100 µM being obtained for both the PHD and FIH enzymes using longer HIF-α polypeptide substrates (Koivunen *et al.*, 2006; Ehrismann *et al.*, 2007). These values are not dissimilar from those obtained for other enzymes in this class (Ehrismann *et al.*, 2007). Tissue pO_2 levels are generally well below all the measured K_mO_2 values for both the PHDs and FIH and indeed below those for other enzymes in this family (Vaupel *et al.*, 1991; Hockel *et al.*, 1991). Thus, whilst this qualifies the HIF hydroxylases to function in an oxygen dependent manner across the range of physiological tissue oxygen tensions, it does not support the view that differences in the K_mO_2 from other 2-OG oxygenases (or differences between the K_mO_2 of the PHDs and FIH) are relevant to their specialisation in oxygen sensing. Overall, it is not yet clear if the PHDs or FIH have special features that underpin their role as oxygen sensors or whether they are ordinary 2-OG oxygenases that achieve this function simply through the regulation of HIF-α, which is itself rate-limiting for transcriptional activity of the pathway. Nevertheless some unusual kinetic properties have been described for purified recombinant PHD2 that may be relevant to its function as an oxygen sensor.

First the PHDs, in particular PHD2, have an unusually high affinity for Fe(II), a property that is conserved in *Trichoplax* PHD, and which has also been reported for the oxygen sensing prolyl hydroxylase in *Dictyostelium* (Hirsila *et al.*, 2005; McNeill *et al.*, 2005; Loenarz *et al.*, 2011; van der Wel *et al.*, 2005). Second, in the absence of HIF-α substrate, the PHD2.Fe.2-OG complex is unusually stable even in the presence of oxygen (i.e. uncoupled turnover is low, McNeill *et al.*, 2005). Conceivably, such properties might be important in enabling the enzyme to operate accurately on low levels of endogenous HIF-α substrates and in minimising confounding effects on activity from changes in the availability of Fe(II) (see below). Third, the reaction of the PHD2.Fe.2-OG.HIFαCODD peptide complex with oxygen appears to be unusually slow in comparison with reaction rates of other 2-OG oxygenases (Flashman *et al.*, 2010b). Structural features of PHD2 that could be relevant to these findings and/or the function of PHD2 as an oxygen sensor are the relatively large conformational changes that occur upon substrate binding and the observation that the co-ordinated water molecule that must be displaced to enable oxygen to bind, is stabilized by a hydrogen bond to the enzyme protein (McDonough *et al.*, 2006; Chowdhury *et al.*, 2009).

Despite the existence of multiple oxygen-independent pathways that regulate the activity of HIF proteins through controls of synthesis, activity, or pVHL-independent degradation (Yee Koh et al., 2008; Majmundar et al., 2010), a wealth of data supports the second criterion for a sensing function, that both prolyl hydroxylation and asparaginyl hydroxylation of HIF-α are indeed rate-limiting steps that have major effects on the activity of the pathway under physiological conditions. Genetic and pharmacological manipulation of the PHDs and FIH, and substitutions at any of the three sites of hydroxylation, all have substantive effects on the activity of the HIF pathway and hydroxylations at different sites in HIF-α are regulated so as to be non-redundant.

For instance, for asparaginyl hydroxylation to be non-redundant in the regulation of responses to hypoxia, FIH must have the capacity to hydroxylate HIF-α molecules that have escaped the prolyl hydroxylation-pVHL-degradation pathway. Both indirect evidence, obtained from manipulating FIH levels (Mahon et al., 2001; Stolze et al., 2004; Sakamoto and Seiki, 2009), and direct evidence from monitoring of hydroxylation by mass spectrometry and hydroxy-residue specific antibodies, indicate that this is the case (Tian et al., 2011). These experiments reveal that under physiological conditions in cells, HIF asparaginyl hydroxylation is less sensitive to suppression by hypoxia than HIF prolyl hydroxylation. Similarly, even though each site of prolyl hydroxylation in HIF-α can independently promote pVHL-mediated degradation, hydroxylation at the two sites appears to be co-ordinated in a way that tunes the oxygen sensitive output. Thus hydroxylation at the CODD site generally precedes that at the NODD site, most probably because of competition (Hirsila et al., 2003; Chan et al., 2005; Flashman et al., 2008). However hydroxylation at both sites is necessary for maximal rates of pVHL-mediated degradation (Masson et al., 2001). When tissue culture cells are exposed to moderate hypoxia, HIF-1α builds up in a form that is hydroxylated on CODD, but not NODD, suggesting that at higher oxygen levels hydroxylation of NODD is the major regulatory step governing HIF-1α protein levels (Tian et al., 2011). Interestingly PHD3, which has a strong preference for CODD over NODD (Epstein et al., 2001; Appelhoff et al., 2004) contributes more to the regulation of HIF-2α than HIF-1α (Appelhoff et al., 2004), most probably reflecting a difference in the importance of CODD versus NODD in degradation of the two HIF-α proteins.

Iron, Ascorbate and Oxygen Radicals

Unlike haem enzymes, 2-OG dependent oxygenases co-ordinate the active site Fe(II) atom at just three positions using the 2-histidine-1-carboxylate triad; a feature that results in relatively labile iron binding (Koehntop et al., 2005). Recombinant 2-OG oxygenases often (though not always) purify as apo-enzymes. Addition of Fe(II) is required to restore catalytic activity and the enzymes are readily inactivated, both *in vitro* and *in vivo*, by iron chelators – properties that extend, albeit to varying extents, to the PHDs and FIH (Hirsila et al., 2005; Tian et al, 2011). PHD and FIH activity is also ascorbate-dependent (Hirsila et al., 2003; Ehrismann et al., 2007; Dao et al., 2009), a feature of many, but not all 2-OG dependent oxygenases. It is believed that ascorbate stimulates activity by maintaining the catalytic iron centre in its functional Fe(II) state, though the mechanism is not absolutely clear. One possibility is that ascorbate acts simply to maintain levels of intracellular Fe(II) that are required to assemble the enzyme.Fe complex. However a more specific interaction has been proposed in which ascorbate acts as an alternative substrate to enable the enzyme to complete uncoupled cycles. If activation of the catalytic Fe is not coupled to substrate oxidation, the enzyme is left in an inactive oxidised form. Oxidation of ascorbate then allows the enzyme to complete the catalytic cycle and return to the active Fe(II) state. The latter mechanism is supported by the incomplete ability of other reducing agents to substitute for ascorbate (Flashman et al., 2010a) and by studies of procollagen prolyl hydroxylases, in which the promotion of uncoupled turnover increased oxidation of ascorbate (Jong et al., 1982; Myllyla et al., 1984). However, the mechanisms are not mutually exclusive and modulation of ascorbate and iron levels have partially overlapping effects on PHD and FIH activity in cells.

In vitro measurements of the K_m values for ascorbate have been reported in the range 140-170 µM for the PHDs and 260 µM for FIH using short HIF-α peptides as substrates, compared to approximately 300 µM for procollagen prolyl hydroxylases (Koivunen et al., 2004). These values are well above plasma levels of ascorbate (in the region of 25 µM) but below the millimolar levels that can be accumulated in cells by Na^+-linked active transport and dehydroascorbate reductase activity (Mandl et al., 2009). Whether physiological variation in cellular ascorbate levels plays a role in modulation of the activity of the PHDs and FIH cannot therefore be readily predicted from these measurements, though this is of considerable interest in relation to the proposal that the PHDs and FIH might act as sensors of cellular redox as well as hypoxic stresses. Uncertainties also surrounded the interpretation of *in vitro* measurements of PHD and FIH kinetics with respect to Fe(II). As outlined above, the PHDs, particularly PHD2, bind iron very tightly and apparent K_m values for Fe(II) as low as 0.03 µM have been reported (Hirsila *et al.*, 2005). However, this contrasts with behaviour in cells, where exposure to iron chelators can readily suppress PHD activity. Taken together these observations suggest the existence of a more complex interface between intracellular Fe(II) and enzyme function than has so far been revealed by *in vitro* studies of recombinant PHD.

Tissue culture media are not generally supplemented with iron or ascorbate, which are ordinarily derived in uncertain quantities from added serum. A number of studies have clearly demonstrated that under these conditions (where cellular ascorbate levels can be close to zero) PHD activity is insufficient to completely suppress HIF-α levels even in the presence of oxygen. In cultured cells with an intact prolyl hydroxylase-pVHL-degradation pathway, addition of ascorbate and/or Fe(II) to the culture medium results in complete suppression of normoxic HIF-α expression, demonstrating that PHD activity is restricted by the availability of these substances under normal, fully oxygenated, tissue culture conditions (Knowles *et al.*, 2003). Supplementation with 10 µM ascorbate was found to be sufficient to suppress HIF-α levels in normoxic cells, whereas higher concentrations were required to reduce levels of HIF-α in hypoxic cells (Vissers *et al.*, 2007; Knowles *et al.*, 2003).

Under similar tissue culture conditions, a large number of studies have demonstrated that pro-oxidant chemicals, cytokine stimulation, and genetic manipulations that either enhance oxidant stresses or reduce the cell's antioxidant defences can upregulate HIF-α. Furthermore, in many of these situations, it has been shown that this is due to a restriction in PHD activity and that the upregulation of HIF-α can be corrected by the addition of ascorbate (Gerald *et al.*, 2004; *Page et al.*, 2008; Knowles *et al.*, 2006 Pan *et al.*, 2007; Kaczmarek *et al.*, 2007). These observations have led to the proposal that oxidant stresses might regulate PHD or FIH activity by effects on either the availability of, or requirement for cellular ascorbate.

Consistent with the complexity of the underlying biochemistry, several mechanisms have been proposed for the inactivation of the PHDs and/or FIH by oxidant stress, including reduction in cytosolic Fe(II) levels (Knowles *et al.*, 2003), oxidation of the catalytic Fe in PHD2 (Gerald *et al.*, 2004), auto-hydroxylation of FIH (Chen *et al.*, 2008b; Chen *et al.*, 2008a) and oxidation of protein thiols. (Nytko *et al.*, 2011) The findings raise important questions as to what extent reduced availability of iron and ascorbate and/or redox signals participate in the physiological and pathophysiological regulation of HIF by the PHDs and FIH. Several studies have suggested that such signals are involved, in addition to hypoxia, in the pathophysiology of HIF activation in cancer. Upregulation of HIF-α has been observed in tumour-associated macrophages, even outside hypoxic perinecrotic zones (Talks *et al.*, 2000; Burke *et al.*, 2002). In tissue culture, differentiation and activation of normoxic monocytic cell lines is associated with inhibition of HIF hydroxylases and induction of the HIF pathway, an effect that coincides with a reduction in intracellular levels of chelatable Fe that occurs as part of the differentiation/activation response (Knowles *et al.*, 2006). The upregulation of HIF is corrected by supplementation with iron or ascorbate. Taken together, the findings suggest that physiological iron sequestration by these cells inhibits PHD activity and activates the HIF transcriptional cascade (Knowles *et al.*, 2006).

Both systemic and cellular iron deficiency is common in cancer and cellular ascorbate levels have been inversely correlated with tumour grade in endometrial cancer (Kuiper *et al.*, 2010). A number of recent experimental studies are consistent with the possibility that iron and/or ascorbate deficiency in rapidly growing tumour cells contributes to the activation of HIF. Suppression of iron uptake in breast cancer cells by expression of shRNA directed against transferrin receptor mRNA has been shown to activate HIF and enhance angiogenesis in xenograft and *in vitro* co-culture models (Eckard *et al.*, 2010). In another study both ascorbate and the anti-oxidant N-acetylcysteine were reported to suppress HIF activation and the growth of human lymphoma cells as xenografts (Gao *et al.*, 2007). This effect was reversed by ectopic expression of a stable HIF-1α protein bearing substitutions at the sites of prolyl hydroxylation, suggesting that the anti-tumourigenic action of the antioxidants was due, at least in part, to activation of PHDs and consequent suppression of HIF (Gao *et al.*, 2007). Whether the efficacy of these interventions in model systems might extend to clinical cancer is unclear. The well known claims by Pauling and colleagues that ascorbate could improve the prognosis of cancer (Cameron *et al.*, 1979) were not substantiated by a controlled trial of oral ascorbate supplementation (Creagan *et al.*, 1979; Moertel *et al.*, 1985). Nevertheless, given the new insights into the biology of iron and ascorbate, it seems opportune to reconsider whether there are circumstances in which the clinical behaviour of human cancer may be affected by cellular levels of these substances.

A related but distinct question is whether and under what circumstances does inactivation of the PHDs and FIH by oxygen radicals, as opposed to restricted availability of molecular oxygen, play a role in the reduced hydroxylase activity that signals hypoxia. In chemical terms, such oxidant stresses are generally considered to be increased at high rather than low levels of oxygen availability. However the multiple sites and mechanisms of oxygen radical production that may arise in complex biological systems allow the reverse possibility; that hypoxia generates higher levels of oxygen radicals. Increased oxygen radical production is well established to occur in cells damaged by ischaemia, and has been proposed to contribute to reperfusion injury (Saeed *et al.*, 2005; Abu-Amara *et al.*, 2010). Persistent activation of HIF occurs in cultured cells and animals subject to cycles of intermittent hypoxia and is associated with evidence of increased oxygen radical production. Analysis of this process has indicated that the activation of HIF is in part to be due to reduction in PHD activity (Yuan *et al.*, 2008). Unexpectedly however, such stimulation differentially affects the expression of HIF-α isoforms, with induction of HIF-1α and suppression of HIF-2α reflecting effects on other regulatory pathways (Nanduri *et al.*, 2009).

It has also been proposed that in continuous hypoxia, increased mitochondrial oxygen radical production contributes to or even dominates the mechanistic inactivation of the HIF hydroxylases by hypoxia (Chandel, 2010), the proposed site of oxygen radical production being the ubiquinone (coenzyme Q) oxidation-reduction cycle at complex III (Bell *et al.*, 2007). In support of this, several studies have demonstrated that in tissue culture cells incubated in moderate hypoxia, exposure to mitochondrial inhibitors, which reduce mitochondrial oxygen radical production, reduce the induction of HIF-α (Chandel *et al.*, 1998; Brunelle *et al.*, 2005; Guzy *et al.*, 2005). Thus it has been proposed that in modest hypoxia PHD activity is suppressed by oxygen radicals, whilst in severe hypoxia it is suppressed by lack of molecular oxygen. A problem that has led to uncertainty over this interpretation is that the reduction in mitochondrial oxygen consumption produced by inhibitors will itself have very substantial effects on oxygen gradients in tissue culture cells (Hagen *et al.*, 2003; Doege *et al.*, 2005). Hence their action will increase the availability of molecular oxygen to the PHDs and FIH. Thus it has been difficult to distinguish whether increased PHD activity associated with mitochondrial blockade reflects reduced oxygen radical production or increased availability of molecular oxygen – possibilities that are not mutually exclusive. Nevertheless, from experiments using cells deficient in the cytochrome b component of complex III (which impairs oxygen consumption but retains increased oxygen radical production in hypoxia), it has been deduced that enhanced oxygen radical production in hypoxia itself impairs HIF prolyl hydroxylation (Bell *et al.*, 2007). However, these findings are disputed (Chua *et al.*, 2010).

Nitric oxide

The interaction of hypoxia pathways with gaseous signalling molecules such as nitric oxide, carbon monoxide and hydrogen sulfide has focused interest on the potential for these molecules to regulate HIF hydroxylase activity. The most intensely studied interaction has been that of nitric oxide on the activity of the PHDs, particularly PHD2. A substantial body of data indicates that the effects of nitric oxide on the PHDs are dose dependent and bi-directional. Given the potential for nitric oxide-mediated inhibition of PHDs (like hypoxia) to promote HIF-dependent increases in their expression and hence to cause biphasic temporal changes in total PHD activity, interactions with nitric oxide may be even more complex (Berchner-Pfannschmidt et al., 2007).

At low doses, nitric oxide inhibits the induction of HIF by hypoxia (Sogawa et al., 1998). At least in part, this arises from inhibition of mitochondrial oxygen consumption by the action of nitric oxide on cytochrome aa3 (Taylor and Moncada, 2010). As with other mitochondrial inhibitors, it is proposed that reduction in oxygen consumption reduces oxygen gradients within cells and hence increases the availability of molecular oxygen as substrate for the PHDs. However, it has also been reported that nitric oxide inhibits the induction of HIF by desferrioxamine and cobalt ions (Sandau et al., 2001; Callapina et al., 2005b). In accordance with these findings other possible mechanisms by which nitric oxide might enhance the activity of the PHDs have been suggested, including increasing levels of chelatable iron in cells and interactions with oxygen radicals (Wang et al., 2002; Callapina et al., 2005a; Brune and Zhou, 2007).

At higher concentrations nitric oxide has been shown to inhibit PHD activity and to induce HIF (Metzen et al., 2003b; reviewed in Berchner-Pfannschmidt et al., 2010). That the action of higher concentrations of nitric oxide to induce HIF might be pathophysiologically relevant is supported by the results of over-expression of iNOS in renal tubular (LLC-PK1) cells and of co-culture with an activated macrophage cell line (RAW 264.7), both of which induced HIF in the target cells in a nitric oxide dependent manner (Sandau et al., 2001). Based on X-ray crystal structures of nitric oxide complexed to another 2-OG dioxygenase (Clavaminate synthase), it has been proposed that nitric oxide interacts with the PHDs directly to co-ordinate the catalytic Fe(II), acting as an inhibitory oxygen analogue (Zhang et al., 2002). However competition with oxygen has not been demonstrated and given the large number of potential interfaces between nitric oxide and the HIF pathway, mechanistic extrapolation from *in vitro* studies is subject to considerable uncertainty.

2-oxoglutarate

Finally, because 2-OG is also used as a co-substrate for HIF-α hydroxylation (Figure 1.2) it is also possible that PHD and FIH enzymes respond to
changes in this intermediary metabolite (for review see Boulahbel *et al.*, 2009).
Also known as α-ketoglutarate, 2-OG is a tricarboxylic acid cycle intermediate subject to NAD-linked oxidation by α-ketoglutarate (2-OG) dehydrogenase; a co-substrate/product in (reversible) reductive amination/oxidative
deamidation by glutamate dehydrogenase (the key steps in the synthesis
and breakdown of a range of amino acids), and it is the major amino group
acceptor for transaminases. Intracellular levels of 2-OG are reduced by
nutritional deprivation in a variety of systems. Thus 2-OG would be well
placed to act as a metabolic sensor directing response pathways by the
regulation of HIF hydroxylase activity or that of other 2-OG oxygenases
(Figure 1.3). Interestingly, genetic inactivation of FIH and two other 2-OG oxygenases for which phenotypes have recently been described, Jhdm2a and
FTO, manifest dysregulated energy metabolism (Zhang *et al.*, 2010; Tateishi *et
al.*, 2009; Fischer *et al.*, 2009). However, it is unclear whether and under what

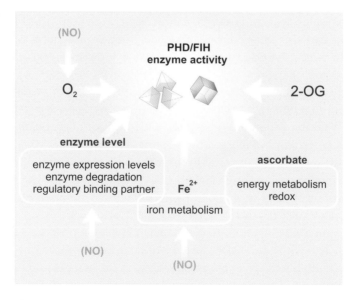

Figure 1.3 _ Primary (depicted in red) and secondary e.g. nitric oxide (NO,
depicted in grey) modulators of PHD and FIH activity.

physiological circumstances cellular 2-OG levels become limiting for 2-OG oxygenase activity.

Nevertheless, pharmacological manipulation by addition of exogenous 2-OG has been demonstrated to down-regulate hypoxic induction of HIF activity in cultured cells and to inhibit angiogenesis and tumour xenograft growth in various *in vivo* models (Matsumoto *et al.*, 2006; Matsumoto *et al.*, 2009). Though this work did not demonstrate that the observed effects were necessarily due to activation of the HIF hydroxylases by increased intracellular 2-OG, such a mechanism has been demonstrated by others using derivatives of 2-OG that were designed to enhance cell permeability (Tennant *et al.*, 2009). In the latter work, addition of cell-permeant 2-OG analogues to tissue culture cells and tumour xenografts was shown not only to promote prolyl hydroxylation and pVHL-dependent degradation of HIF-α, but also to kill hypoxic cells in culture in a manner that was dependent on active PHD2.

Other TCA intermediates and related metabolites may alter PHD and FIH activity by competing with 2-OG for binding to the enzyme.Fe complex (fumarate, succinate) or by product inhibition (succinate) (Koivunen *et al.*, 2007; Hewitson *et al.*, 2007). This process is of particular interest in relation to certain inherited cancer syndromes associated with mutations in particular TCA enzymes. Germline mutations in succinate dehydrogenase (SDH) and fumarate hydratase (FH) are associated with inherited paraganglioma and hereditary leiomyomatosis and papillary renal cancer (HLRCC) respectively (Gottlieb and Tomlinson, 2005). In each syndrome, the defective gene behaves like a classical tumour suppressor, with somatic inactivation of the second allele being required for the associated neoplasia. Affected cells accumulate very high levels of fumarate and succinate which inhibit the activity of 2-OG oxygenases including the HIF hydroxylases, leading to activation of HIF pathways (Selak *et al.*, 2005; Isaacs *et al.*, 2005; Pollard *et al.*, 2005). Consistent with competition with 2-OG, elevation of intracellular 2-OG levels using cell-permeating 2-OG derivatives can reverse the HIF stabilization mediated by succinate or fumarate (Mackenzie *et al.*, 2007). Interestingly, inhibition of 2-OG oxygenases is selective; for instance, fumarate is a particularly effective inhibitor of PHD, but not FIH (Koivunen *et al.*, 2007). Consistent with this, HIF-α accumulates in FH-defective cells in a form which retains hydroxylation on asparagine (O'Flaherty *et al.*, 2010).

Though it has been proposed that activation of HIF plays a role in oncogenesis in FH- and SDH-associated neoplasia, this is unproven (Adam et al., 2011). Effects of retained metabolites on other 2-OG oxygenases, or indeed entirely unrelated oncogenic mechanisms remain possible. Similar considerations apply to certain forms of malignant glioblastoma and leukaemia that are associated with mutations in isocitrate dehydrogenase (IDH) 1 and 2 (Yan *et al.*, 2009; Mardis *et al.*, 2009). The mutant IDH enzymes catalyse the formation of 2-hydroxyglutarate (2-HG) from 2-OG and 2-HG accumulates to high concentrations in affected cells (Dang *et al.*, 2009; Gross *et al.*, 2010). Like fumarate and succinate, 2-HG also binds 2-OG oxygenases competitively with respect to 2-OG (Welford *et al.*, 2003). However, again, the oncogenic significance of this finding is unclear; *R*-2HG, the enantiomer that is produced by mutant IDH is a poor inhibitor of the PHDs and FIH (Xu *et al.*, 2011; Chowdhury *et al.*, 2011).

Enzyme abundance

Since the HIF hydroxylases are not equilibrium enzymes, the rate of HIF hydroxylation at each site is directly related to the abundance of the enzyme(s) catalyzing that hydroxylation. Therefore, regulation of enzyme expression levels represents an important control over the activity of the system (Figure 1.3).

In some studies it has been reported that levels of PHD1 are reduced by hypoxia (Erez *et al.*, 2004). In contrast, PHD2 and PHD3 are strongly inducible by hypoxia, at least in part by the transcriptional activity of HIF itself (Epstein *et al.*, 2001; del Peso *et al.*, 2003; Metzen and Ratcliffe, 2004; Stiehl *et al.*, 2006). Since levels of PHD2 (and induced levels of PHD3) are much higher than those of PHD1 (Appelhoff *et al.*, 2004), total PHD abundance is greatly increased in hypoxia, generating a feedback loop that limits the duration of activation of HIF in response to acute hypoxia. At steady-state this process is also predicted to function as a 'range-finding' process in which increased PHD abundance in hypoxic tissue serves to offset the reduction in activity, thereby extending the operating range.

A number of hormonal, growth factor, apoptotic and cytokine stimuli affect the levels of the PHDs, particularly those of PHD1 and PHD3. Whether these responses are directed at the physiological tuning of the HIF pathway under different circumstances, or are primarily a reflection of the operation of these enzymes in other pathways (either catalytic or non-catalytic) is as yet unclear. PHD1 is inducible in certain cells by oestrogens (Seth *et al.*, 2002). PHD3 is an immediate response gene for a range of physiological stimuli. For example, PHD3 is induced by interferon gamma through a Jak/STAT pathway in endothelial cells (Gerber *et al.*, 2009) and is also a c-Myc responsive gene (Nesbit *et al.*, 2000). PHD3 (otherwise known as

SM-20 in the rat) is downregulated by angiotensin II dependent differentiation of neuronal PC12 cells (Wolf *et al.*, 2004). PHD3 is induced by apoptosis-
promoting stimuli such as p53 activation (Madden *et al.*, 1996) and is induced
by nerve growth factor withdrawal in cells of the sympatho-adrenal line-
age (Lipscomb *et al.*, 1999; Lipscomb *et al.*, 2001; Straub *et al.*, 2003). Expression of the
C-terminus of PHD3, but not the full length protein was found to confer
resistance to cisplatin induced growth arrest (Erez *et al.*, 2002). PHD3 is also
up-regulated in vascular smooth muscle cells by growth agonists such as
PDGF and angiotensin II (Wax *et al.*, 1994), and induced during skeletal muscle differentiation (Lieb *et al.*, 2002; Fu *et al.*, 2007). For PHD2, down-regulation
in response to endothelin-1 has been reported in melanoma cells (Spinella
et al., 2010).

In addition to control of synthesis, the PHDs are also regulated through
changes in protein stability. In humans, two isoforms of PHD1 (denoted
PHD1p43 and PHD1p40) arise from alternative initiation, with PHD1p40
lacking the N-terminal 33 amino acids (Tian *et al.*, 2006). The N-terminal
sequence of PHD1 is proline-rich and contains five PxxP motifs, three of
which are deleted in PHD1p40. PHD1p43 and p40 differ in their stability,
though the physiological significance of this is unclear (Tian *et al.*, 2006).

PHD2 interacts with FKBP38 through its N-terminal region, residues
1-114 (including but extending beyond the MYND domain) being sufficient
for interaction. FKBP38 binding reduces PHD2 levels by promoting proteasomal degradation in a manner which is dependent on the integrity
of the transmembrane domain in FKBP38, but independent of its peptidyl
prolyl *cis/trans* isomerase activity (Barth *et al.*, 2007; Barth *et al.*, 2009). PHD3, and
possibly other PHDs are targeted by Siah (seven in absentia homologue)
ubiquitin E3 ligases. Inactivation of the Siah ligases is associated with
reduced HIF activation and a blunted erythropoietin response to hypoxia
(Nakayama *et al.*, 2004), while blocking of the interaction between Siah and
PHDs reduced tumour growth in a syngeneic mouse model of breast cancer (Moller *et al.*, 2009).

FIH is not regulated by hypoxia and expression levels are in general
more stable than those of the PHDs. However FIH has been reported to
respond to a protein kinase C (PKC) zeta-dependent signalling pathway
through a CDP/Cut binding site in the FIH promoter (Li *et al.*, 2007). Siah-1
ligase has also been implicated in the regulation of FIH protein levels
(Fukuba *et al.*, 2008), as has poly (ADP-ribose) polymerase-1 (Martinez-Romero
et al., 2009).

Enzyme location and protein complexes

Though crystallographic studies of the PHD2 catalytic domain have revealed a homotrimer, it appears that this arrangement is specific to the conditions of crystallization. There is no evidence for the existence of this form in solution and it is likely that PHD2 functions as a monomer (McDonough *et al.*, 2006; Chowdhury *et al.*, 2009). In contrast FIH forms homodimers via a C-terminal α-helical interface and dimerization is absolutely necessary for activity (Lancaster *et al.*, 2004).

Many enzymes function in protein complexes and the physical approximation of an enzyme to its substrate provides another means to regulate the activity of a pathway. Thus, location of the PHDs and FIH within a particular cellular compartment or protein complex could be used to regulate the activity of HIF hydroxylase pathways. Abundant evidence indicates that these enzymes do exist in discrete cellular compartments and protein complexes, though the physiological significance of these findings is still largely unclear.

PHD1 is a nuclear protein containing a classical importin-dependent nuclear localization signal (Metzen *et al.*, 2003a; Steinhoff *et al.*, 2009). PHD2 and PHD3 are distributed between the cytoplasm and the nucleus (Ozer *et al.*, 2005; Rantanen *et al.*, 2008; Steinhoff *et al.*, 2009; Yasumoto *et al.*, 2009), though these patterns have been noted to change in particular circumstances. Increased nuclear PHD2 has been associated with tumour progression (Jokilehto *et al.*, 2006; Jokilehto *et al.*, 2010). PHD3 has been noted to form aggregates in association with a role in promoting apoptosis (Rantanen *et al.*, 2008). FIH is largely localised to the cytoplasm (Stolze *et al.*, 2004; Linke *et al.*, 2004; Zheng *et al.*, 2008), although a number of studies have also identified a nuclear localisation in tumour tissue (Soilleux *et al.*, 2005; Tan *et al.*, 2007) and overexpression of the Notch intracellular domain (an FIH substrate) was found to re-distribute FIH to the nucleus (Zheng *et al.*, 2008).

A large number of interacting proteins have been identified that have been reported to affect enzyme activity of PHDs or FIH or modulate the HIF pathway by non-catalytic mechanisms The DSBH domain of PHD2 interacts non-catalytically with the ING4 tumour suppressor (Ozer *et al.*, 2005), a protein proposed to function in chromatin remodelling. Interestingly PHD2 has also been reported to interact non-catalytically with HIF-α to down-regulate HIF target genes in hypoxia (To and Huang, 2005), though the relationship between these processes has not yet been resolved. Another set of proteins reported to interact with PHD2 are the melanoma antigens (MAGE-11 and MAGE-9), which act to reduce PHD2 catalytic activity through an interaction with sequences lying immediately N-terminal to the catalytic domain (Aprelikova *et al.*, 2009).

Other interactions have been reported to facilitate association with substrates within protein complexes. For instance, the interaction between PHDs and HIF-α has been reported to be assisted by a ubiquitously expressed protein called OS-9 (Baek *et al.*, 2005). However more recent work has identified OS-9 as an ER-resident lectin that functions in ER-associated degradation pathways, making it difficult to understand how the protein might interact with the HIF hydroxylase pathway (Christianson *et al.*, 2008; Alcock and Swanton, 2009; Hosokawa *et al.*, 2009; Brockmeier et al., 2011). More likely to function in this way are proteins termed AKAPs, which act as scaffolding proteins to bring together enzymes involved in cell signalling. It has been reported that perinuclear compartmentalisation by muscle AKAP (mAKAP), provides an optimal arrangement of PHD enzymes, HIF and their respective ligases, positioning them close to the nucleus and enhancing the hypoxic response (Wong *et al.*, 2008).

The adaptor protein Mint3/APBA3 has been identified as an FIH-binding protein that competes with the HIF-1α C-terminal activation domain for interaction with the catalytic site of FIH, and restricts hydroxylation of HIF-1α. In macrophages Mint-3/APBA3 co-operates with the cytoplasmic tail of membrane type 1 matrix metalloproteinase to locate FIH at the perinuclear Golgi apparatus. This is proposed to further limit the ability of FIH to hydroxylate HIF-α by sequestration of FIH away from the cytoplasm, thus allowing HIF-dependent upregulation of glycolysis in activated macrophages (Sakamoto and Seiki, 2009; Sakamoto and Seiki, 2010).

Physiological roles of the different HIF hydroxylases

The HIF prolyl hydroxylases

Studies of genetic inactivation indicate that all three PHD enzymes contribute non-redundantly to the regulation of the HIF system (Appelhoff *et al.*, 2004). However in the majority of tissues and tissue culture cell lines one isoform, PHD2, is by far the most abundant enzyme, often contributing in excess of 90% of total cellular PHD protein. Consistent with this, PHD2 contributes most to the regulation of HIF, particularly to the setting of normoxic levels of HIF-1α (Berra *et al.*, 2003; Takeda *et al.*, 2008; Minamishima *et al.*, 2008). PHD2 inactivation alone is associated with striking, though incomplete, upregulation of HIF-1α protein levels and HIF target gene expression in cultured cells (Berra *et al.*, 2003).

Studies of targeted gene inactivation in the mouse and spontaneously occurring mutation in man both support the critical importance of PHD2 in the regulation of HIF. Constitutive inactivation of PHD2 in the mouse results in embryonic lethality with placental and cardiac defects (Takeda *et al.*, 2006). Although upregulation of HIF was clearly observed in affected placental tissue this was not the case in the heart (Takeda *et al.*, 2006). Whether cardiac dysfunction arises from indirect effects of HIF upregulation or non-HIF pathways affected by PHD2 is unclear. Consistent with upregulation of the HIF pathway by PHD2 inactivation, general conditional inactivation of PHD2 in the adult results in upregulation of erythropoietin, polycythaemia, vascular overgrowth and hepatic steatosis within 10 weeks (Takeda *et al.*, 2007; Minamishima *et al.*, 2008). Endothelial cell specific inactivation of PHD2 is itself sufficient to increase endothelial cell proliferation (Takeda and Fong, 2007). Interestingly, whilst the near-total inactivation of PHD2 in these studies is associated with the development of cardiomyopathy, mice bearing a hypo-morphic PHD2 allele associated with reduced but not absent expression of PHD2 (ranging from 8-85% of mRNA expression in different tissues) did not develop cardiomyopathy and were protected from ischaemia-reperfusion injury to the myocardium (Hyvarinen *et al.*, 2010). This suggests that careful attention to the dose and duration of therapy will be required for the phar-macological approaches to PHD inhibition in heart disease.

Interestingly, recent studies indicate that even heterozygous inactiva-tion of PHD2 has important effects *in vivo*. Thus heterozygous deficiency for PHD2 even when restricted to the endothelial cells was found to restore tumour oxygenation and to reduce metastasis in mice bearing syngeneic tumours which were wild type for PHD2, an effect attributed to vascular normalization arising from altered HIF signalling in the host endothelium (Mazzone *et al.*, 2009). Though these studies demonstrated upregulation of the HIF pathway, particularly HIF-2α in PHD2 heterozygous endothelial cells, it is possible that actions of PHD2 on other pathways may contribute to effects on angiogenesis in tumours. Using shRNAs to silence both PHD2 and HIF-1α in colon cancer (HCT116) cells a PHD2-mediated suppressive effect on tumour angiogenesis was observed that appeared to be independent of HIF and independent of the catalytic function of PHD2 (Chan *et al.*, 2009).

In humans, the importance of PHD2 in regulating hypoxia pathways is supported by the association of heterozygous hypomorphic missense mutations in PHD2 with erythrocytosis (Percy *et al.*, 2006; Ladroue et al., 2012) and by the apparent selection of haplotypes at the PHD2 locus in altitude adapted populations (Simonson et al., 2010; Bigham et al., 2010).

Despite the importance of PHD2, several lines of evidence indicate that PHD1 and PHD3 also contribute significantly to regulation of the HIF pathway both in cell lines and in the intact organism. Studies in cultured cells using siRNA knock-down (Appelhoff et al., 2004) and targeted inactivation in mice indicates that PHD1 and PHD3 contribute more to the regulation of HIF-2α than HIF-1α (Aragones et al., 2008; Takeda et al., 2008). Although, mice with targeted inactivation of either PHD1 or PHD3 are viable and have only mild phenotypes under basal conditions when combined with each other or with inactivation of PHD2 these alleles clearly contribute to the upregulation of HIF and hypoxia pathways. Double 'knockout' of PHD1/3 resulted in moderate erythrocytosis in adult mice due to induction of HIF-2α and erythropoietin production in the liver (Takeda et al., 2008). This activation of the hepatic HIF-2α and erythropoietin production by PHD1/3 double knockout contrasts with the erythrocytosis induced by PHD2 inactivation in adult mice, which was found to occur through upregulation of HIF-1α and erythropoietin production in the kidney (Minamishima et al., 2008). Further analysis of PHD1/2/3 triple knockout mice has confirmed this PHD1/3-dependent reactivation of hepatic erythropoietin production (Minamishima and Kaelin, 2010). Studies of combined PHD3 and PHD2 knockout indicate that inactivation of PHD3 increases the upregulation of HIF and exacerbates both the cardiomyopathy and hepatic steatosis associated with inducible PHD2 inactivation (Minamishima et al., 2009).

An important outstanding question is whether the PHDs have other substrates whose dysregulation contributes to the phenotypes associated with inactivation. PHD1 dependent prolyl hydroxylation of the large subunit of RNA polymerase II (Rbp1) has been proposed to regulate its DNA binding in response to oxidative stress (Mikhaylova et al., 2008). PHD1 was also implicated in hypoxic activation of the NFκB transcription factor through direct negative regulation of IκB kinase-β (IKKβ) (Cummins et al., 2006). Although hydroxylation of IKKβ was proposed, a more recent study has suggested a non-catalytic mode of action for this inhibition (Xue et al., 2010). Analysis of PHD1 knockout mice has revealed an exclusive role for this PHD in promoting HIF-2α dependent oxidative ATP production to reduce ischaemic damage to skeletal muscle following femoral artery occlusion (Aragones et al., 2008). Similar results have been obtained in the liver, with PHD1 knockout mice being protected from hepatic ischaemia. In the heart, PHD1 knockout has been reported to confer protection from ex vivo myocardial ischaemia/reperfusion in a manner that is dependent on HIF-1α (Adluri et al.,

2010). In contrast, PHD1 appears to have a specific role in promoting oxidative death in neurons (Siddiq *et al.*, 2009). Studies of PHD1 knockout mice have also demonstrated suppressed mammary gland proliferation attributable to a PHD1 dependent but HIF independent regulation of cyclin D1 (Zhang *et al.*, 2009). These findings fit with earlier studies in breast carcinoma cells, in which PHD1 mRNA was found to be induced by oestrogen and in which over-expression of PHD1 alone was found to promote oestrogen-independent growth (Seth *et al.*, 2002). However the nature of the proposed non-HIF PHD1 hydroxylation substrate responsible for these effects is not yet clear.

The involvement of PHD3 as an inducible gene in diverse pathways not obviously related to the physiology of HIF signalling has raised the possibility that effects of PHD3 inactivation might also in part be dependent on the disruption of pathways mediated by non-HIF hydroxylation targets. For instance, PHD3 is induced in sympathetic neurons by withdrawal of nerve growth factor and is necessary for the operation of apoptotic pathways that are activated by growth factor withdrawal (Lee *et al.*, 2005). This action of PHD3 is dependent on catalytic activity and though amelioration of the neuronal phenotype by heterozygous inactivation of HIF-2α suggests an interaction with signalling through HIF-2 (Bishop *et al.*, 2008) current evidence suggests that additional PHD3 substrates may be involved. Further study of this pathway indicates that the kinesin KIF1Bβ acts downstream of PHD3, though it has not yet been shown to be a direct PHD3 substrate (Schlisio *et al.*, 2008).

In separate lines of investigation PHD3 has also been shown to have a pro-apoptotic role in tissue culture cells through the O_2-dependent formation of subcellular aggregates (Rantanen *et al.*, 2008). Of potential relevance to this effect is the binding of PHD3 to the TRiC chaperonin complex (Masson *et al.*, 2004). Other work has revealed that PHD3 is important for differentiation of skeletal myoblasts (Lieb *et al.*, 2002; Fu *et al.*, 2007), in part through the direct binding and regulation of the transcription factor myogenin (Fu *et al.*, 2007). More recently, the $β_2$-adrenergic receptor ($β_2$-AR, which is also highly abundant in cardiac and smooth muscle) was identified as a novel substrate for PHD3-dependent prolyl hydroxylation (Xie *et al.*, 2009). Interestingly, hydroxylation of the $β_2$-AR (like HIF-α) appears to target it for destruction in a pVHL-dependent manner (Xie *et al.*, 2009). Pyruvate kinase M2 was also identified as a PHD3 hydroxylation substrate resulting in its enhanced action as a co-activator for HIF-1 (Luo et al, 2011). PHD3 has also been implicated in regulating stability of ATF-4 in an O_2-dependent manner (i.e. although direct hydroxylation remains to be demonstrated, Koditz *et al.*, 2007). How these actions affect the PHD3 knock-out phenotype remain to be understood.

The HIF asparaginyl hydroxylase

In addition to catalysing asparaginyl hydroxylation in the CAD of HIF-α subunits, FIH catalyses hydroxylation of asparaginyl residues positioned in the β-hairpin loops connecting ankyrin repeats (AR) in a wide range of ankyrin repeat domain (ARD) containing proteins. These proteins include p105, IkBα (Cockman *et al.*, 2006), the intracellular domain of Notch receptors (Coleman *et al.*, 2007; Zheng *et al.*, 2008), ASB4 (Ferguson *et al.*, 2007), Tankyrase-2 and Rabankyrin (Cockman *et al.*, 2009a) and MYPT1 (Webb *et al.*, 2009). The target asparaginyl residue is part of the ankyrin consensus and many of these proteins are hydroxylated to varying extents at several sites. Interestingly, when positioned at this site in the AR, other amino acids including aspartyl and histidinyl residues can be hydroxylated by FIH (Yang et al, 2011a, Yang et al, 2011b). Although, given the very high prevalence and (in some cases) high abundance of ARD proteins in the proteome, these modifications are clearly prevalent in biology, their function remains unclear. Hydroxylation increases the thermodynamic stability of at least some ARDs (Yang *et al.*, 2011a) including an artificial consensus ARD (Kelly *et al.*, 2009; Hardy *et al.*, 2009), though not all analyses of the effect of hydroxylation on ARD stability have reported such effects (Devries *et al.*, 2010). In some cases alterations in ARD-protein associations have been observed in association with hydroxylation, but their physiological significance remains unclear (Yang *et al.*, 2011a). Nevertheless FIH-mediated catalysis of ARD-protein hydroxylation is efficient and able to compete with that of the HIF-α CAD suggesting that ARD-proteins constitute a pool of endogenous inhibitors of HIF-α CAD asparaginyl hydroxylation (Coleman *et al.*, 2007; Zheng *et al.*, 2008; Cockman *et al.*, 2009b; Wilkins *et al.*, 2009). Given the oxygen-dependence of ARD-hydroxylation it has been proposed that this competition may therefore tune the HIF-response by regulating the availability of FIH for hydroxylation of HIF-α proteins (Schmierer *et al.*, 2010).

Interestingly, FIH knockout mice are found to exhibit a hypermetabolic phenotype that is largely phenocopied by animals with just a neuron-specific loss of FIH (Zhang *et al.*, 2010). The target(s) for FIH in this neuronal pathway are unclear but are hypothesised to be HIF independent; whether they include ARD-containing proteins is not known (Zhang *et al.*, 2010).

Summary

The identification 10 years ago of the PHD and FIH enzymes as oxygen sensors in human cells has engendered enormous interest in the biochemistry, physiology, and pharmacology of these enzymes, their involvement in disease patho-physiology and their potential for therapeutic manipulation. Though much has been learnt, important uncertainties remain at many levels including the precise biophysical and biochemical properties that underlie their function as oxygen sensors, and how they interact with other physiological stimuli to generate the flexibility necessary for physiological oxygen homeostasis. Other important questions surround the extent to which they are involved in the regulation of biological pathways that are distinct from the HIF system and whether other members of the rapidly expanding family of 2-OG oxygenases also have oxygen-sensing functions in biology.

A c k n o w l e d g e m e n t s _ Work in the authors' laboratory is funded by the Wellcome Trust, the Medical Research Council, BBSRC and the European Union 7th framework.

References

Abu-Amara, M., Yang, S.Y., Tapuria, N., Fuller, B., Davidson, B., and Seifalian, A. (2010). Liver ischemia/reperfusion injury: processes in inflammatory networks–a review. Liver Transpl 16, 1016-1032.

Adam, J., Hatipoglu, E., O'Flaherty, L., Ternette, N., Sahgal, N., Lockstone, H., Baban, D., Nye, E., Stamp, G.W., Wolhuter, K., et al. (2011). Renal cyst formation in Fh1-deficient mice is independent of the Hif/Phd pathway: roles for fumarate in KEAP1 succination and Nrf2 signaling. Cancer Cell 20, 524-537

Adluri RS, Thirunavukkarasu M, Dunna NR, Zhan L, Oriowo B, Takeda K, Sanchez J, Otani H, Maulik G, Fong GH, Maulik N. (2011). Disruption of HIF-Prolyl Hydroxylase-1 (PHD-1-/-) Attenuates Ex Vivo Myocardial Ischemia/Reperfusion Injury through HIF-1alpha Transcription Factor and its Target Genes in Mice. Antioxid Redox Signal 15, 1789-1797.

Ansieau, S., and Leutz, A. (2002). The conserved Mynd domain of BS69 binds cellular and oncoviral proteins through a common PXLXP motif. J Biol Chem 277, 4906-4910.

Alcock, F., and Swanton, E. (2009). Mammalian OS-9 is upregulated in response to endoplasmic reticulum stress and facilitates ubiquitination of misfolded glycoproteins. J Mol Biol 385, 1032-1042.

Ansieau, S., and Leutz, A. (2002). The conserved Mynd domain of BS69 binds cellular and oncoviral proteins through a common PXLXP motif. J Biol Chem 277, 4906-4910.

Appelhoff, R.J., Tian, Y.M., Raval, R.R., Turley, H., Harris, A.L., Pugh, C.W., Ratcliffe, P.J., and Gleadle, J.M. (2004). Differential function of the prolyl hydroxylases PHD1, PHD2 and PHD3 in the regulation of hypoxia-inducible factor. J Biol Chem 279, 38458-38465.

Aprelikova, O., Pandolfi, S., Tackett, S., Ferreira, M., Salnikow, K., Ward, Y., Risinger, J.I., Barrett, J.C., and Niederhuber, J. (2009). Melanoma antigen-11 inhibits the hypoxia-inducible factor prolyl hydroxylase 2 and activates hypoxic response. Cancer Res 69, 616-624.

Aragones, J., Schneider, M., Van Geyte, K., Fraisl, P., Dresselaers, T., Mazzone, M., Dirkx, R., Zacchigna, S., Lemieux, H., Jeoung, N.H., et al. (2008). Deficiency or inhibition of oxygen sensor Phd1 induces hypoxia tolerance by reprogramming basal metabolism. Nat Genet 40, 170-180.

Ashton, N. (1957a). Experimental retrolental fibroplasia. Annu Rev Med 8, 441-454.

Ashton, N. (1957b). Retinal vascularization in health and disease: Proctor Award Lecture of the Association for Research in Ophthalmology. Am J Ophthalmol 44, 7-17.

Baek, J.H., Mahon, P.C., Oh, J., Kelly, B., Krishnamachary, B., Pearson, M., Chan, D.A., Giaccia, A.J., and Semenza, G.L. (2005). OS-9 interacts with hypoxia-inducible factor 1alpha and prolyl hydroxylases to promote oxygen-dependent degradation of HIF-1alpha. Mol Cell 17, 503-512.

Barth, S., Edlich, F., Berchner-Pfannschmidt, U., Gneuss, S., Jahreis, G., Hasgall, P.A., Fandrey, J., Wenger, R.H., and Camenisch, G. (2009). Hypoxia-inducible factor prolyl-4-hydroxylase PHD2 protein abundance depends on integral membrane anchoring of FKBP38. J Biol Chem 284, 23046-23058.

Barth, S., Nesper, J., Hasgall, P.A., Wirthner, R., Nytko, K.J., Edlich, F., Katschinski, D.M., Stiehl, D.P., Wenger, R.H., and Camenisch, G. (2007). The peptidyl prolyl cis/trans isomerase FKBP38 determines hypoxia-inducible transcription factor prolyl-4-hydroxylase PHD2 protein stability. Mol Cell Biol 27, 3758-3768.

Beck, I., Ramirez, S., Weinmann, R., and Caro, J. (1991). Enhancer element at the 3'-flanking region controls transcriptional response to hypoxia in the human erythropoietin gene. J Biol Chem 266, 15563-15566.

Bell, E.L., Klimova, T.A., Eisenbart, J., Moraes, C.T., Murphy, M.P., Budinger, G.R., and Chandel, N.S. (2007). The Qo site of the mitochondrial complex III is required for the transduction of hypoxic signalling via reactive oxygen species production. J Cell Biol 177, 1029-1036.

Berchner-Pfannschmidt, U., Tug, S., Kirsch, M., and Fandrey, J. (2010). Oxygen-sensing under the influence of nitric oxide. Cell Signal 22, 349-356.

Berchner-Pfannschmidt, U., Yamac, H., Trinidad, B., and Fandrey, J. (2007). Nitric oxide modulates oxygen sensing by hypoxia-inducible factor 1-dependent induction of prolyl hydroxylase 2. The J Biol Chem 282, 1788-1796.

Berk, L., Burchenal, J.H., and Castle, W.B. (1949). Erythropoietic effect of cobalt in patients with or without anemia. New Eng J Med 240, 754-761.

Berner, R.A., Vandenbrooks, J.M., and Ward, P.D. (2007). Evolution. Oxygen and evolution. Science 316, 557-558.

Berra, E., Benizri, E., Ginouves, A., Volmat, V., Roux, D., and Pouyssegur, J. (2003). HIF prolyl-hydroxylase 2 is the key oxygen sensor setting low steady-state levels of HIF-1a in normoxia. EMBO J 22, 4082-4090.

Bigham, A., Bauchet, M., Pinto, D., Mao, X., Akey, J.M., Mei, R., Scherer, S.W., Julian, C.G., Wilson, M.J., Lopez Herraez, D., et al. (2010). Identifying signatures of natural selection in Tibetan and Andean populations using dense genome scan data. PLoS Genet 6, e1001116

Bishop, T., Gallagher, D., Pascual, A., Lygate, C.A., de Bono, J.P., Nicholls, L.G., Ortega-Saenz, P., Oster, H., Wijeyekoon, B., Sutherland, A.I., et al. (2008). Abnormal sympathoadrenal development and systemic hypotension in PHD3-/- mice. Mol Cell Biol 28, 3386-3400.

Boulahbel, H., Duran, R.V., and Gottlieb, E. (2009). Prolyl hydroxylases as regulators of cell metabolism. Biochem Soc Trans 37, 291-294.

Boycott, A.E., and Haldane, J.S. (1908). The effects of low atmospheric pressures on respiration. J Physiol 37, 355-377.

Brockmeier, U., Platzek, C., Schneider, K., Patak, P., Bernardini, A., Fandrey, J., and Metzen, E. (2011). The function of hypoxia-inducible factor (HIF) is independent of the endoplasmic reticulum protein OS-9. PLoS One 6, e19151

Bruick, R.K., and McKnight, S.L. (2001). A conserved family of prolyl-4-hydroxylases that modify HIF. Science 294, 1337-1340.

Brune, B., and Zhou, J. (2007). Nitric oxide and superoxide: interference with hypoxic signalling. Cardiovasc Res 75, 275-282.

Brunelle, J.K., Bell, E.L., Quesada, N.M., Vercauteren, K., Tiranti, V., Zeviani, M., Scarpulla, R.C., and Chandel, N.S. (2005). Oxygen sensing requires mitochondrial ROS but not oxidative phosphorylation. Cell Metab 1, 409-414.

Burke, B., Tang, N., Corke, K.P., Tazzyman, D., Ameri, K., Wells, M., and Lewis, C.E. (2002). Expression of HIF-1alpha by human macrophages: implications for the use of macrophages in hypoxia-regulated cancer gene therapy. J Pathol 196, 204-212.

Callapina, M., Zhou, J., Schmid, T., Kohl, R., and Brune, B. (2005a). NO restores HIF-1alpha hydroxylation during hypoxia: role of reactive oxygen species. Free Radic Biol Med 39, 925-936.

Callapina, M., Zhou, J., Schnitzer, S., Metzen, E., Lohr, C., Deitmer, J.W., and Brune, B. (2005b). Nitric oxide reverses desferrioxamine- and hypoxia-evoked HIF-1alpha accumulation–implications for prolyl hydroxylase activity and iron. Exp Cell Res 306, 274-284.

Cameron, E., Pauling, L., and Leibovitz, B. (1979). Ascorbic acid and cancer: a review. Cancer Res 39, 663-681.

Canfield, D.E., Poulton, S.W., and Narbonne, G.M. (2007). Late-Neoproterozoic deep-ocean oxygenation and the rise of animal life. Science 315, 92-95.

Carnot, P., and Deflandre, C. (1906). Sur l'activite hemopoietique des differents organes au cours de la regeneration du sang. Comptes Rendu Academie Science Paris 143, 432-435.

Chan, D.A., Kawahara, T.L., Sutphin, P.D., Chang, H.Y., Chi, J.T., and Giaccia, A.J. (2009). Tumour vasculature is regulated by PHD2-mediated angiogenesis and bone marrow-derived cell recruitment. Cancer Cell 15, 527-538.

Chan, D.A., Sutphin, P.D., Yen, S.E., and Giaccia, A.J. (2005). Coordinate regulation of the oxygen-dependent degradation domains of hypoxia-inducible factor 1 alpha. Mol Cell Biol 25, 6415-6426.

Chandel, N.S., Maltepe, E., Goldwasser, E., Mathieu, C.E., Simon, M.C., and Schumacker, P.T. (1998). Mitochondrial reactive oxygen species trigger hypoxia-induced transcription. Proc Natl Acad Sci USA 95, 11715-11720.

Chandel, N.S.(2010). Mitochondrial regulation of oxygen sensing. Adv Exp Med Biol 661, 339-54.

Chen, Y.H., Comeaux, L.M., Eyles, S.J., and Knapp, M.J. (2008a). Auto-hydroxylation of FIH-1: an Fe(ii), alpha-ketoglutarate-dependent human hypoxia sensor. Chem Commun (Camb), 4768-4770.

Chen, Y.H., Comeaux, L.M., Herbst, R.W., Saban, E., Kennedy, D.C., Maroney, M.J., and Knapp, M.J. (2008b). Coordination changes and auto-hydroxylation of FIH-1: uncoupled O2-activation in a human hypoxia sensor. J Inorg Biochem 102, 2120-2129.

Chowdhury, R., McDonough, M.A., Mecinovic, J., Loenarz, C., Flashman, E., Hewitson, K.S., Domene, C., and Schofield, C.J. (2009). Structural basis for binding of hypoxia-inducible factor to the oxygen-sensing prolyl hydroxylases. Structure 17, 981-989.

Chowdhury, R., Yeoh, KK., Tian, Y-M., Kawamura, A., Hillringhaus, L., Bagg, EA., Rose, N., Leung, IK., Woon, EC., Yang, M., McDonough, MA., Kinh, ON., Clifton, IJ., Klose, RJ., Claridge, TD., Ratcliffe, PJ. and Schofield, CJ. (2011). The oncometabolite 2-hydroxyglutarate inhibits histone lysine demethylases. EMBO Reports 12, 463-469.

Christianson, J.C., Shaler, T.A., Tyler, R.E., and Kopito, R.R. (2008). OS-9 and GRP94 deliver mutant alpha1-antitrypsin to the Hrd1-SEL1L ubiquitin ligase complex for ERAD. Nat Cell Biol 10, 272-282.

Chua, Y.L., Dufour, E., Dassa, E.P., Rustin, P., Jacobs, H.T., Taylor, C.T., and Hagen, T. (2010). Stabilization of hypoxia-inducible factor-1alpha protein in hypoxia occurs independently of mitochondrial reactive oxygen species production. J Biol Chem 285, 31277-31284.

Clark, E., and Clark, EL. (1939). Microscopic observations on the growth of blood capillaries on the living animal. Amer J Anat 64, 251-299.

Clifton, I.J., McDonough, M.A., Ehrismann, D., Kershaw, N.J., Granatino, N., and Schofield, C.J. (2006). Structural studies on 2-oxoglutarate oxygenases and related double-stranded beta-helix fold proteins. J Inorg Biochem 100, 644-669.

Cockman, M.E., Lancaster, D.E., Stolze, I.P., Hewitson, K.S., McDonough, M.A., Coleman, M.L., Coles, C.H., Yu, X., Hay, R.T., Ley, S.C., et al. (2006). Posttranslational hydroxylation of ankyrin repeats in IkappaB proteins by the hypoxia-inducible factor (HIF) asparaginyl hydroxylase, factor inhibiting HIF (FIH). Proc Natl Acad Sci U S A 103, 14767-14772.

Cockman, M.E., Masson, N., Mole, D.R., Jaakkola, P., Chang, G.W., Clifford, S.C.,

Maher, E.R., Pugh, C.W., Ratcliffe, P.J., and Maxwell, P.H. (2000). Hypoxia inducible factor-alpha binding and ubiquitylation by the von Hippel-Lindau tumour suppressor protein. J Biol Chem 275, 25733-25741.

Cockman, M.E., Webb, J.D., Kramer, H.B., Kessler, B.M., and Ratcliffe, P.J. (2009a). Proteomic-based identification of novel factor inhibiting HIF (FIH) substrates indicates widespread hydroxylation of ankyrin repeat domain-containing proteins. Mol Cell Proteomics 8, 535-546.

Cockman, M.E., Webb, J.D., and Ratcliffe, P.J. (2009b). FIH-dependent asparaginyl hydroxylation of ankyrin repeat domain-containing proteins. Ann N Y Acad Sci 1177, 9-18.

Coleman, M.L., McDonough, M.A., Hewitson, K.S., Coles, C., Mecinovic, J., Edelmann, M., Cook, K.M., Cockman, M.E., Lancaster, D.E., Kessler, B.M., et al. (2007). Asparaginyl hydroxylation of the Notch ankyrin repeat domain by factor inhibiting hypoxia-inducible factor. J Biol Chem 282, 24027-24038.

Creagan, E.T., Moertel, C.G., O'Fallon, J.R., Schutt, A.J., O'Connell, M.J., Rubin, J., and Frytak, S. (1979). Failure of high-dose vitamin C (ascorbic acid) therapy to benefit patients with advanced cancer. A controlled trial. N Engl J Med 301, 687-690.

Cummins, E.P., Berra, E., Comerford, K.M., Ginouves, A., Fitzgerald, K.T., Seeballuck, F., Godson, C., Nielsen, J.E., Moynagh, P., Pouyssegur, J., et al. (2006). Prolyl hydroxylase-1 negatively regulates I{kappa}B kinase-beta, giving insight into hypoxia-induced NF{kappa}B activity. Proc Natl Acad Sci USA 103, 18154-18159.

Dames, S.A., Martinez-Yamout, M., Guzman, R.N.D., Dyson, H.J., and Wright, P.E. (2002). Structural basis for hif-1a/CBP recognition in the cellular hypoxic response. Proc Natl Acad Sci USA 99, 5271-5276.

Dang, L., White, D.W., Gross, S., Bennett, B.D., Bittinger, M.A., Driggers, E.M., Fantin, V.R., Jang, H.G., Jin, S., Keenan, M.C., et al. (2009). Cancer-associated IDH1 mutations produce 2-hydroxyglutarate. Nature 462, 739-744.

Dao, J.H., Kurzeja, R.J., Morachis, J.M., Veith, H., Lewis, J., Yu, V., Tegley, C.M., and Tagari, P. (2009). Kinetic characterization and identification of a novel inhibitor of hypoxia-inducible factor prolyl hydroxylase 2 using a time-resolved fluorescence resonance energy transfer-based assay technology. Anal Biochem 384, 213-223.

De Castro, F. (2009). The discovery of sensory nature of the carotid bodies–invited article. Adv Exp Med Biol 648, 1-18.

del Peso, L., Castellanos, M.C., Temes, E., Martin-Puig, S., Cuevas, Y., Olmos, G., and Landazuri, M.O. (2003). The von Hippel Lindau/hypoxia-inducible factor (HIF) pathway regulates the transcription of the HIF-proline hydroxylase genes in response to low oxygen. J Biol Chem 278, 48690-48695.

Devries, I.L., Hampton-Smith, R.J., Mulvihill, M.M., Alverdi, V., Peet, D.J., and Komives, E.A. (2010). Consequences of IkappaB alpha hydroxylation by the factor inhibiting HIF (FIH). FEBS Lett 584, 4725-4730.

Doege, K., Heine, S., Jensen, I., Jelkmann, W., and Metzen, E. (2005). Inhibition of mitochondrial respiration elevates oxygen concentration, but leaves regulation of hypoxia-inducible factor (HIF) intact. Blood, 106:2311-7.

Douglas, C.G., Haldane, J.S., Henderson, Y., Schneider, E.C., Webb, G.B., and Richards, J. (1913). Physiological Observations Made on Pike's Peak, Colorado, with Special Reference to Adaptation to Low Barometric Pressures. Philosophical Transactions of the Royal Society of London Series B, Containing Papers of a Biological Character 203, 185-318.

Dusseau, J.W., and Hutchins, P.M. (1988). Hypoxia-induced angiogenesis in chick chorioallantoic membranes: a role for adenosine. Respir Physiol 71, 33-44.

Eckard, J., Dai, J., Wu, J., Jian, J., Yang, Q., Chen, H., Costa, M., Frenkel, K., and Huang, X. (2010). Effects of cellular iron deficiency on the formation of vascular endothelial growth factor and angiogenesis. Iron deficiency and angiogenesis. Cancer Cell Int 10:28.

Ehrismann, D., Flashman, E., Genn, D.N., Mathioudakis, N., Hewitson, K.S., Ratcliffe, P.J., and Schofield, C.J. (2007). Studies on the activity of the hypoxia-inducible factor hydroxylases using an oxygen consumption assay. Biochem J 401, 227-234.

Elkins, J.M., Hewitson, K.S., McNeill, L.A., Seibel, J.F., Schlemminger, I., Pugh, C.W., Ratcliffe, P.J., and Schofield, C.J. (2003). Structure of factor-inhibiting hypoxia-inducible factor (HIF) reveals mechanism of oxidative modification of HIF-1a. J Biol Chem 278, 1802-1806.

Epstein, A.C.R., Gleadle, J.M., McNeill, L.A., Hewitson, K.S., O'Rourke, J., Mole, D.R., Mukherji, M., Metzen, E., Wilson, M.I., Dhanda, A., et al. (2001). C. elegans EGL-9 and mammalian homologues define a family of dioxygenases that regulate HIF by prolyl hydroxylation. Cell 107, 43-54.

Erez, N., Milyavsky, M., Goldfinger, N., Peles, E., Gudkov, A.V., and Rotter, V. (2002). Falkor, a novel cell growth regulator isolated by a functional genetic screen. Oncogene 21, 6713-6721.

Erez, N., Stambolsky, P., Shats, I., Milyavsky, M., Kachko, T., and Rotter, V. (2004). Hypoxia-dependent regulation of PHD1: cloning and characterization of the human PHD1/EGLN2 gene promoter. FEBS Lett 567, 311-315.

Erslev, A.J. (1953). Humoral regulation of red cell production. Blood 8, 349-357.

Ferguson, J.E., 3rd, Wu, Y., Smith, K., Charles, P., Powers, K., Wang, H., and Patterson, C. (2007). ASB4 is a hydroxylation substrate of FIH and promotes vascular differentiation via an oxygen-dependent mechanism. Mol Cell Biol 27, 6407-6419.

Firth, J.D., Ebert, B.L., Pugh, C.W., and Ratcliffe, P.J. (1994). Oxygen-regulated control elements in the phosphoglycerate kinase 1 and lactate dehydrogenase A genes: similarities with the erythropoietin 3' enhancer. Proc Natl Acad Sci USA 91, 6496-6500.

Fischer, J., Koch, L., Emmerling, C., Vierkotten, J., Peters, T., Bruning, J.C., and Ruther, U. (2009). Inactivation of the Fto gene protects from obesity. Nature 458, 894-898.

FitzGerald, M.P. (1913). The Changes in the Breathing and the Blood at Various High Altitudes. Philosophical Transactions of the Royal Society of London Series B, Containing Papers of a Biological Character 203, 351-371.

Flashman, E., Bagg, E.A., Chowdhury, R., Mecinovic, J., Loenarz, C., McDonough, M.A., Hewitson, K.S., and Schofield, C.J. (2008). Kinetic rationale for selectivity toward N- and C-terminal oxygen-dependent degradation domain substrates mediated by a loop region of hypoxia-inducible factor prolyl hydroxylases. J Biol Chem 283, 3808-3815.

Flashman, E., Davies, S.L., Yeoh, K.K., and Schofield, C.J. (2010a). Investigating the dependence of the hypoxia-inducible factor hydroxylases (factor inhibiting HIF and prolyl hydroxylase domain 2) on ascorbate and other reducing agents. Biochem J 427, 135-142.

Flashman, E., Hoffart, L.M., Hamed, R.B., Bollinger, J.M., Jr., Krebs, C., and Schofield, C.J. (2010b). Evidence for the slow reaction of hypoxia-inducible factor prolyl hydroxylase 2 with oxygen. FEBS J 277, 4089-4099.

Fraser, R.A., Ellis, E.M., and Stalker, A.L. (1979). Experimental angiogenesis in the chorio-allantoic membrane. Bibl Anat, 25-27.

Freedman, S.J., Sun, Z.-Y.J., Poy, F., Kung, A.L., Livingston, D.M., Wagner, G., and Eck, M.J. (2002). Structural basis for recruitment of CBP/p300 by hypoxia-inducible factor-1a. Proc Natl Acad Sci USA 99, 5367-5372.

Fried, W. (1972). The liver as a source of extrarenal erythropoietin production. Blood 40, 671-677.

Fu, J., Menzies, K., Freeman, R.S., and Taubman, M.B. (2007). EGLN3 prolyl hydroxylase regulates skeletal muscle differentiation and myogenin protein stability. J Biol Chem 282, 12410-12418.

Fukuba, H., Takahashi, T., Jin, H.G., Kohriyama, T., and Matsumoto, M. (2008). Abundance of aspargynyl-hydroxylase FIH is regulated by Siah-1 under normoxic conditions. Neurosci Lett 433, 209-214.

Fukuda, R., Zhang, H., Kim, J.W., Shimoda, L., Dang, C.V., and Semenza, G.L. (2007). HIF-1 regulates cytochrome oxidase subunits to optimize efficiency of respiration in hypoxic cells. Cell 129, 111-122.

Gao, P., Zhang, H., Dinavahi, R., Li, F., Xiang, Y., Raman, V., Bhujwalla, Z.M., Felsher, D.W., Cheng, L., Pevsner, J., et al. (2007). HIF-dependent antitumourigenic effect of antioxidants in vivo. Cancer Cell 12, 230-238.

Gerald, D., Berra, E., Frapart, Y.M., Chan, D.A., Giaccia, A.J., Mansuy, D., Pouyssegur, J., Yaniv, M., and Mechta-Grigoriou, F. (2004). JunD reduces tumour angiogenesis by protecting cells from oxidative stress. Cell 118, 781-794.

Gerber, S.A., Yatsula, B., Maier, C.L., Sadler, T.J., Whittaker, L.W., and Pober, J.S. (2009). Interferon-gamma induces prolyl hydroxylase (PHD)3 through a STAT1-dependent mechanism in human endothelial cells. Arterioscler Thromb Vasc Biol 29, 1363-1369.

Gothie, E., Richard, D., Berra, E., Pages, G., and Pouyssegur, J. (2000). Identification of Alternative Spliced Variants of Human Hypoxia-inducible Factor-1a. J Biol Chem 275, 6922-6927.

Gottlieb, E., and Tomlinson, I.P. (2005). Mitochondrial Tumour Suppressors: A genetic and biochemical update. Nat Rev Cancer 5, 857-866.

Gross, S., Cairns, R.A., Minden, M.D., Driggers, E.M., Bittinger, M.A., Jang, H.G., Sasaki, M., Jin, S., Schenkein, D.P., Su, S.M., et al. (2010). Cancer-associated metabolite 2-hydroxyglutarate accumulates in acute myelogenous leukemia with isocitrate dehydrogenase 1 and 2 mutations. J Exp Med 207, 339-344.

Guzy, R.D., Hoyos, B., Robin, E., Chen, H., Liu, L., Mansfield, K.D., Simon, M.C., Hammerling, U., and Schumacker, P.T. (2005). Mitochondrial complex III is required for hypoxia-induced ROS production and cellular oxygen sensing. Cell Metab 1, 401-408.

Hagen, T., Taylor, C.T., Lam, F., and Moncada, S. (2003). Redistribution of intracellular oxygen in hypoxia by nitric oxide: effect on HIF-1a. Science 302, 1975-1978.

Haldane, J.S., and Priestley, J.G. (1905). The regulation of the lung-ventilation. J Physiol 32, 225-266.

Hampton-Smith, R.J., and Peet, D.J. (2009). From polyps to people: a highly familiar response to hypoxia. Ann N Y Acad Sci 1177, 19-29.

Hardy, A.P., Prokes, I., Kelly, L., Campbell, I.D., and Schofield, C.J. (2009). Asparaginyl beta-hydroxylation of proteins containing ankyrin repeat domains influences their stability and function. J Mol Biol 392, 994-1006.

Hewitson, K.S., Lienard, B.M., McDonough, M.A., Clifton, I.J., Butler, D., Soares, A.S., Oldham, N.J., McNeill, L.A., and Schofield, C.J. (2007). Structural and mechanistic studies on the inhibition of the hypoxia-inducible transcription factor hydroxylases by tricarboxylic acid cycle intermediates. J Biol Chem 282, 3293-3301.

Hewitson, K.S., McNeill, L.A., M.V., R., Tian, Y.-M., Bullock, A.N., Welford, R.W., Elkins, J.M., Oldham, N.J., Bhattacharya, S., Gleadle, J.M., et al. (2002). Hypoxia inducible factor (HIF) asparagine hydroxylase is identical to Factor Inhibiting HIF (FIH) and is related to the cupin structural family. J Biol Chem 277, 26351-26355.

Hirsila, M., Koivunen, P., Gunzler, V., Kivirikko, K.I., and Myllyharju, J. (2003). Characterization of the human prolyl 4-hydroxylases that modify the hypoxia-inducible factor HIF. J Biol Chem 278, 30772-30780.

Hirsila, M., Koivunen, P., Xu, L., Seeley, T., Kivirikko, K.I., and Myllyharju, J. (2005). Effect of desferrioxamine and metals on the hydroxylases in the oxygen sensing pathway. FASEB J 19(10):1308-10.

Hockel, M., Schlenger, K., Knoop, C., and Vaupel, P. (1991). Oxygenation of carcinomas of the uterine cervix: evaluation by computerized O2 tension measurements. Cancer Res 51, 6098-6102.

Holmquist-Mengelbier, L., Fredlund, E., Lofstedt, T., Noguera, R., Navarro, S., Nilsson, H., Pietras, A., Vallon-Christersson, J., Borg, A., Gradin, K., et al. (2006). Recruitment of HIF-1a and HIF-2a to common target genes is differentially regulated in neuroblastoma: HIF-2a promotes an aggressive phenotype. Cancer Cell 10, 413-423.

Hon, W.C., Wilson, M.I., Harlos, K., Claridge, T.D., Schofield, C.J., Pugh, C.W., Maxwell, P.H., Ratcliffe, P.J., Stuart, D.I., and Jones, E.Y. (2002). Structural basis for the recognition of hydroxyproline in HIF-1a by pVHL. Nature 417, 975-978.

Hosokawa, N., Kamiya, Y., Kamiya, D., Kato, K., and Nagata, K. (2009). Human OS-9, a lectin required for glycoprotein endoplasmic reticulum-associated degradation, recognizes mannose-trimmed N-glycans. J Biol Chem 284, 17061-17068.

Hu, C.-J., Wang, L.-Y., Chodosh, L.A., Keith, B., and Simon, M.C. (2003). Differential roles of hypoxia-inducible factor 1a (HIF-1a) and HIF-2a in hypoxic gene regulation. Mol Cell Biol 23, 9361-9374.

Hu, C.-J., Sataur, A., Wang, L., Chen, H., and Simon, M.C. (2007). The N-terminal transactivation domain confers target gene specificity of hypoxia-inducible factors HIF-1alpha and HIF-2alpha. Mol Biol Cell 18, 4528-4542.

Huang, L.E., Gu, J., Schau, M., and Bunn, H.F. (1998). Regulation of hypoxia-inducible factor 1a is mediated by an oxygen-dependent domain via the ubiquitin-proteasome pathway. Proc Natl Acad Sci USA 95, 7987-7992.

Hudlicka, O., Dodd, L., Renkin, E.M., and Gray, S.D. (1982). Early changes in fiber profile and capillary density in long-term stimulated muscles. Am J Physiol 243, H528-H535.

Hyvarinen, J., Hassinen, I.E., Sormunen, R., Maki, J.M., Kivirikko, K.I., Koivunen, P., and Myllyharju, J. (2010). Hearts of hypoxia-inducible factor prolyl 4-hydroxylase-2 hypomorphic mice show protection against acute ischemia-reperfusion injury. J Biol Chem. 285(18):13646-57.

Imre, G. (1964). Studies on the Mechanism of Retinal Neovascularization. Role of Lactic Acid. Br J Ophthalmol 48, 75-82.

Illingworth, C.J., Loenarz, C., Schofield, C.J. and Domene, C. (2010). Chemical basis for the selectivity of the von Hippel Lindau tumour suppressor pVHL for prolyl-hydroxylated HIF-1alpha. Biochemistry 49, 6936-44.

Isaacs, J.S., Jung, Y.J., Mole, D.R., Lee, S., Torres-Cabala, C., Merino, M., Trepel, J., Zbar, B., Toro, J., Ratcliffe, P.J., et al. (2005). HIF overexpression correlates with biallelic loss of fumarate hydratase in renal cancer: novel role of fumarate in regulation of HIF stability Cancer Cell 8, 143-153

Ivan, M., Kondo, K., Yang, H., Kim, W., Valiando, J., Ohh, M., Salic, A., Asara, J.M., Lane, W.S., and Kaelin, W.G.J. (2001). HIFa targeted for VHL-mediated destruction by proline hydroxylation: implications for O_2 sensing. Science 292, 464-468.

Jaakkola, P., Mole, D.R., Tian, Y.-M., Wilson, M.I., Gielbert, J., Gaskell, S.J., Kriegsheim, A.v., Hebestreit, H.F., Mukherji, M., Schofield, C.J., et al. (2001). Targeting of HIF-a to the von Hippel-Lindau ubiquitylation complex by O_2-regulated prolyl hydroxylation. Science 292, 468-472.

Jacobson, L.O., Goldwasser, E., Fried, W., and Plzak, L. (1957). Role of the kidney in erythropoiesis. Nature 179, 633-634.

Jiang, B.-H., Zheng, J.Z., Leung, S.W., Roe, R., and Semenza, G.L. (1997). Transactivation and inhibitory domains of hypoxia-inducible factor 1a. Modulation of transcriptional activity by oxygen tension. J Biol Chem 272, 19253-19260.

Jokilehto, T., Hogel, H., Heikkinen, P., Rantanen, K., Elenius, K., Sundstrom, J., and Jaakkola, P.M. (2010). Retention of prolyl hydroxylase PHD2 in the cytoplasm prevents PHD2-induced anchorage-independent carcinoma cell growth. Exp Cell Res 316, 1169-1178.

Jokilehto, T., Rantanen, K., Luukkaa, M., Heikkinen, P., Grenman, R., Minn, H., Kronqvist, P., and Jaakkola, P.M. (2006). Overexpression and nuclear translocation of hypoxia-inducible factor prolyl hydroxylase PHD2 in head and neck squamous cell carcinoma is associated with tumour aggressiveness. Clin Cancer Res 12, 1080-1087.

Jong, L.d., Albracht, S.P.J., and Kemp, A. (1982). Prolyl 4-hydroxylase activity in relation to the oxidation state of enzyme-bound iron. The role of ascorbate in peptidyl proline hydroxylation. Biochim Biophys Acta 704, 326-332.

Jozsa, L., Balint, J., Reffy, A., Jarvinen, M., and Kvist, M. (1980). Capillary density of tenotomized skeletal muscles. II. Observations on human muscles after spontaneous rupture of tendon. Eur J Appl Physiol O 44, 183-188.

Kaczmarek, M., Timofeeva, O.A., Karaczyn, A., Malyguine, A., Kasprzak, K.S., and Salnikow, K. (2007). The role of ascorbate in the modulation of HIF-1alpha protein and HIF-dependent transcription by chromium(VI) and nickel(II). Free Radic Biol Med 42, 1246-1257.

Kelly, L., McDonough, M.A., Coleman, M.L., Ratcliffe, P.J., and Schofield, C.J. (2009). Asparaginyl hydroxylation stabilizes the ankyrin fold. Mol Biosyst 5, 52-58.

Knowles, H.J., Mole, D.R., Ratcliffe, P.J., and Harris, A.L. (2006). Normoxic stabilization of hypoxia-inducible factor-1alpha by modulation of the labile iron pool in differentiating U937 macrophages: effect of natural resistance-associated macrophage protein 1. Cancer Res 66, 2600-2607.

Knowles, H.J., Raval, R.R., Harris, A.L., and Ratcliffe, P.J. (2003). Effect of ascorbate on the activity of hypoxia inducible factor (HIF) in cancer cells. Cancer Res 63, 1764-1768.

Koditz, J., Nesper, J., Wottawa, M., Stiehl, D.P., Camenisch, G., Franke, C., Myllyharju, J., Wenger, R.H., and Katschinski, D.M. (2007). Oxygen-dependent ATF-4 stability is mediated by the PHD3 oxygen sensor. Blood 110, 3610-3617.

Koehntop, K.D., Emerson, J.P., and Que, L., Jr. (2005). The 2-His-1-carboxylate facial triad: a versatile platform for dioxygen activation by mononuclear non-heme iron(II) enzymes. J Biol Inorg Chem 10, 87-93.

Koivunen, P., Hirsila, M., Gunzler, V., Kivirikko, K.I., and Myllyharju, J. (2004). Catalytic properties of the asparaginyl hydroxylase (FIH) in the oxygen sensing pathway are distinct from those of its prolyl-4-hydroxylases. J Biol Chem 279, 9899-9904.

Koivunen, P., Hirsila, M., Kivirikko, K.I., and Myllyharju, J. (2006). The length of peptide substrates has a marked effect on hydroxylation by the hypoxia-inducible factor prolyl 4 hydroxylases. J Biol Chem 281, 28712-28720.

Koivunen, P., Hirsila, M., Remes, A.M., Hassinen, I.E., Kivirikko, K.I., and Myllyharju, J. (2007). Inhibition of hypoxia-inducible factor (HIF) hydroxylases by citric acid cycle intermediates: possible links between cell metabolism and stabilization of HIF. J Biol Chem 282, 4524-4532.

Krebs, C., Galonic Fujimori, D., Walsh, C.T., and Bollinger, J.M., Jr. (2007). Non-heme Fe(IV)-oxo intermediates. Acc Chem Res 40, 484-492.

Krogh, A. (1919). The number and distribution of capillaries in muscles with calculations of the oxygen pressure head necessary for supplying the tissue. J Physiol, London 52, 409-415.

Kuiper, C., Molenaar, I.G., Dachs, G.U., Currie, M.J., Sykes, P.H., and Vissers, M.C. (2010). Low ascorbate levels are associated with increased hypoxia-inducible factor-1 activity and an aggressive tumour phenotype in endometrial cancer. Cancer Res 70, 5749-5758.

Kwast, K.E., Burke, P.V., Staahl, B.T., and Poyton, R.O. (1999). Oxygen sensing in yeast: evidence for the involvement of the respiratory chain in regulating the transcription of a subset of hypoxic genes. Proc Natl Acad Sci USA 96, 5446-5451.

Ladroue, C., Hoogewijs, D., Gad, S., Carcenac, R., Storti, F., Barrois, M., Gimenez-Roqueplo, A.P., Leporrier, M., Casadevall, N., Hermine, O., et al. (2012). Distinct deregulation of the hypoxia inducible factor by PHD2 mutants identified in germline DNA of patients with polycythemia. Haematologica 97, 9-14.

Lancaster, D.E., McNeill, L.A., McDonough, M.A., Aplin, R.T., Hewitson, K.S., Pugh, C.W., Ratcliffe, P.J., and Schofield, C.J. (2004). Disruption of dimerization and substrate phosphorylation inhibit factor inhibiting hypoxia-inducible factor (FIH) activity. Biochem J 383, 429-437.

Lando, D., Peet, D.J., Gorman, J.J., Whelan, D.A., Whitelaw, M.L., and Bruick, R.K. (2002a). FIH-1 is an asparaginyl hydroxylase enzyme that regulates the transcriptional activity of hypoxia-inducible factor. Genes Dev 16, 1466-1471.

Lando, D., Peet, D.J., Whelan, D.A., Gorman, J.J., and Whitelaw, M.L. (2002b). Asparagine hydroxylation of the HIF transactivation domain: a hypoxic switch. Science 295, 858-861.

Lau, K.W., Tian, Y.M., Raval, R.R., Ratcliffe, P.J., and Pugh, C.W. (2007). Target gene selectivity of hypoxia-inducible factor-alpha in renal cancer cells is conveyed by post-DNA-binding mechanisms. Brit J Cancer 96, 1284-1292.

Lee, C., Kim, S.J., Jeong, D.G., Lee, S.I., and Ryu, S.E. (2003). Structure of human FIH-1 reveals a unique active site pocket and interaction sites for HIF-1 and von Hippel-Lindau. J Biol Chem 278, 7558-7563.

Lee, S., Nakamura, E., Yang, H., Wei, W., Linggi, M.S., Sajan, M.P., Farese, R.V., Freeman, R.S., Carter, B.D., Kaelin, W.G., et al. (2005). Neuronal apoptosis linked to EglN3 prolyl hydroxylase and familial pheochromocytoma genes: developmental culling and cancer. Cancer Cell 8, 155-167.

Li, J., Wang, E., Dutta, S., Lau, J.S., Jiang, S.W., Datta, K., and Mukhopadhyay, D. (2007). Protein kinase C-mediated modulation of FIH-1 expression by the homeodomain protein CDP/Cut/Cux. Mol Cell Biol 27, 7345-7353.

Lieb, M.E., Menzies, K., Moschella, M.C., Ni, R., and Taubman, M.B. (2002). Mammalian EGLN genes have distinct patterns of mRNA expression and regulation. Biochem Cell Biol 80, 421-426.

Linke, S., Stojkoski, C., Kewley, R.J., Booker, G.W., Whitelaw, M.L., and Peet, D.J. (2004). Substrate requirements of the oxygen-sensing asparaginyl hydroxylase factor-inhibiting hypoxia-inducible factor. J Biol Chem 279, 14391-14397.

Lipscomb, E.A., Sarmiere, P.D., Crowder, R.J., and Freeman, R.S. (1999). Expression of the SM-20 gene promotes death in nerve growth factor-dependent sympathetic neurons. J Neurochem 73, 429-432.

Lipscomb, E.A., Sarmiere, P.D., and Freeman, R.S. (2001). SM-20 is a novel mitochondrial protein that causes caspase-dependent cell death in nerve growth factor-dependent neurons. J Biol Chem 276, 5085-5092.

Loenarz, C., Coleman, M.L., Boleininger, A., Schierwater, B., Holland, P.W., Ratcliffe, P.J., and Schofield, C.J. (2011). The hypoxia-inducible transcription factor pathway regulates oxygen sensing in the simplest animal, Trichoplax adhaerens. EMBO Reports 12, 63-70.

Loenarz, C., Mecinovic, J., Chowdhury, R., McNeill, L.A., Flashman, E., and Schofield, C.J. (2009). Evidence for a stereoelectronic effect in human oxygen sensing. Angew Chem Int Ed Engl 48, 1784-1787.

Loenarz, C., and Schofield, C.J. (2008). Expanding chemical biology of 2-oxoglutarate oxygenases. Nat Chem Biol 4, 152-156.

Luo, W., Hu, H., Chang, R., Zhong, J., Knabel, M., O'Meally, R., Cole, R.N., Pandey, A., and Semenza, G.L. (2011). Pyruvate kinase M2 is a PHD3-stimulated coactivator for hypoxia-inducible factor 1. Cell 145, 732-744

Mackenzie, E.D., Selak, M.A., Tennant, D.A., Payne, L.J., Crosby, S., Frederiksen, C.M., Watson, D.G., and Gottlieb, E. (2007). Cell permeating {alpha}-ketoglutarate derivatives alleviate pseudo-hypoxia in SDH deficient cells. Mol Cell Biol 27, 3282-3289.

Madden, S.L., Galella, E.A., Riley, D., Bertelsen, A.H., and Beaudry, G.A. (1996). Induction of cell growth regulatory genes by p53. Cancer Res 56, 5384-5390.

Mahon, P.C., Hirota, K., and Semenza, G.L. (2001). FIH-1: a novel protein that interacts with HIF-1a and VHL to mediate repression of HIF-1 transcriptional activity. Genes Dev 15, 2675-2686.

Majmundar, A.J., Wong, W.J., and Simon, M.C. (2010). Hypoxia-inducible factors and the response to hypoxic stress. Mol Cell 40, 294-309.

Makino, Y., Cao, R., Svensson, K., Bertilsson, G., Asman, M., Tanaka, H., Cao, Y., Berkenstam, A., and Poellinger, L. (2001). Inhibitory PAS domain protein is a negative regulator of hypoxia-inducible gene expression. Nature 414, 550-554.

Mandl, J., Szarka, A., and Banhegyi, G. (2009). Vitamin C: update on physiology and pharmacology. Br J Pharmacol 157, 1097-1110.

Mardis, E.R., Ding, L., Dooling, D.J., Larson, D.E., McLellan, M.D., Chen, K., Koboldt, D.C., Fulton, R.S., Delehaunty, K.D., McGrath, S.D., et al. (2009). Recurring mutations found by sequencing an acute myeloid leukemia genome. N Engl J Med 361, 1058-1066.

Martinez-Romero, R., Canuelo, A., Martinez-Lara, E., Javier Oliver, F., Cardenas, S., and Siles, E. (2009). Poly(ADP-ribose) polymerase-1 modulation of in vivo response of brain hypoxia-inducible factor-1 to hypoxia/reoxygenation is mediated by nitric oxide and factor inhibiting HIF. J Neurochem 111, 150-159.

Masson, N., Appelhoff, R.J., Tuckerman, J.R., Tian, Y.M., Demol, H., Puype, M., Vandekerckhove, J., Ratcliffe, P.J., and Pugh, C.W. (2004). The HIF prolyl hydroxylase PHD3 is a potential substrate of the TRiC chaperonin. FEBS Lett 570, 166-170.

Masson, N., Willam, C., Maxwell, P.H., Pugh, C.W., and Ratcliffe, P.J. (2001). Independent function of two destruction domains in hypoxia-inducible factor-a chains activated by prolyl hydroxylation. EMBO J 20, 5197-5206.

Matsumoto, K., Imagawa, S., Obara, N., Suzuki, N., Takahashi, S., Nagasawa, T., and Yamamoto, M. (2006). 2-Oxoglutarate downregulates expression of vascular endothelial growth factor and erythropoietin through decreasing hypoxia-inducible factor-1alpha and inhibits angiogenesis. J Cell Physiol 209, 333-340.

Matsumoto, K., Obara, N., Ema, M., Horie, M., Naka, A., Takahashi, S., and Imagawa, S. (2009). Antitumour effects of 2-oxoglutarate through inhibition of angiogenesis in a murine tumour model. Cancer Sci 100, 1639-1647.

Matthews, J.M., Bhati, M., Lehtomaki, E., Mansfield, R.E., Cubeddu, L., and Mackay, J.P. (2009). It takes two to tango: the structure and function of LIM, RING, PHD and MYND domains. Curr Pharm Des 15, 3681-3696.

Maxwell, P.H., Pugh, C.W., and Ratcliffe, P.J. (1993). Inducible operation of the erythro-poietin 3' enhancer in multiple cell lines: evidence for a widespread oxygen sensing mechanism. Proc Natl Acad Sci USA 90, 2423-2427.

Maxwell, P.H., Wiesener, M.S., Chang, G.W., Clifford, S.C., Vaux, E.C., Cockman, M.E., Wykoff, C.C., Pugh, C.W., Maher, E.R., and Ratcliffe, P.J. (1999). The tumour suppressor protein VHL targets hypoxia-inducible factors for oxygen-dependent proteolysis. Nature 399, 271-275.

Maynard, M.A., Evans, A.J., Hosomi, T., Hara, S., Jewett, M.A., and Ohh, M. (2005). Human HIF-3alpha4 is a dominant-negative regulator of HIF-1 and is down-regulated in renal cell carcinoma. FASEB J 19, 1396-1406.

Maynard, M.A., Evans, A.J., Shi, W., Kim, W.Y., Liu, F.F., and Ohh, M. (2007). Dominant-negative HIF-3 alpha 4 suppresses VHL-null renal cell carcinoma progression. Cell Cycle 6, 2810-2816.

Maynard, M.A., Qi, H., Chung, J., Lee, E.H.L., Kondo, Y., Hara, S., Conaway, R.C., Conaway, J.W., and Ohh, M. (2003). Multiple splice variants of the human HIF-3a locus are targets of the von Hippel-Lindau E3 ubiquitin ligase complex. J Biol Chem 278, 11032-11040.

Mazzone, M., Dettori, D., Leite de Oliveira, R., Loges, S., Schmidt, T., Jonckx, B., Tian, Y.M., Lanahan, A.A., Pollard, P., Ruiz de Almodovar, C., et al. (2009). Heterozygous deficiency of PHD2 restores tumour oxygenation and inhibits metastasis via endothelial normalization. Cell 136, 839-851.

McDonough, M.A., Li, V., Flashman, E., Chowdhury, R., Mohr, C., Lienard, B.M., Zondlo, J., Oldham, N.J., Clifton, I.J., Lewis, J., et al. (2006). Cellular oxygen sensing: Crystal structure of hypoxia-inducible factor prolyl hydroxylase (PHD2). Proc Natl Acad Sci USA 103, 9814-9819.

McDonough, M.A., Loenarz, C., Chowdhury, R., Clifton, I.J., and Schofield, C.J. (2010). Structural studies on human 2-oxoglutarate dependent oxygenases. Curr Opin Struct Biol 20, 659-672.

McIntosh, B.E., Hogenesch, J.B., and Bradfield, C.A. (2010). Mammalian Per-Arnt-Sim proteins in environmental adaptation. Annu Rev Physiol 72, 625-645.

McNeill, L.A., Flashman, E., Buck, M.R., Hewitson, K.S., Clifton, I.J., Jeschke, G., Claridge, T.D., Ehrismann, D., Oldham, N.J., and Schofield, C.J. (2005). Hypoxia-inducible factor prolyl hydroxylase 2 has a high affinity for ferrous iron and 2-oxoglutarate. Mol Biosyst 1, 321-324.

McNeill, L.A., Hewitson, K.S., Claridge, T.D., Seibel, J.F., Horsfall, L.E., and Schofield, C.J. (2002). Hypoxia-inducible factor asparaginyl hydroxylase (FIH-1) catalyses hydroxylation at the beta carbon of asparagine-803. Biochem J 367, 571-575.

Metzen, E., Berchner-Pfannschmidt, U., Stengel, P., Marxsen, J.H., Stolze, I., Klinger, M., Huang, W.Q., Wotzlaw, C., Hellwig-Burgel, T., Jelkmann, W., et al. (2003a). Intracellular localisation of human HIF-1a hydroylases: implications for oxygen sensing. J Cell Sci 116, 1319-1326.

Metzen, E., and Ratcliffe, P.J. (2004). HIF hydroxylation and cellular oxygen sensing. Biol Chem 385, 223-230.

Metzen, E., Zhou, J., Jelkmann, W., Fandrey, J., and Brune, B. (2003b). Nitric oxide impairs normoxic degradation of HIF-1alpha by inhibition of prolyl hydroxylases. Mol Biol Cell 14, 3470-3481.

Mikhaylova, O., Ignacak, M.L., Barankiewicz, T.J., Harbaugh, S.V., Yi, Y., Maxwell, P.H., Schneider, M., Van Geyte, K., Carmeliet, P., Revelo, M.P., et al. (2008). The von Hippel-Lindau tumour suppressor protein and Egl-9-Type proline hydroxylases regulate the large subunit of RNA polymerase II in response to oxidative stress. Mol Cell Biol 28, 2701-2717.

Min, J.-H., Yang, H., Ivan, M., Gertler, F., Kaelin, W.G.J., and Pavletich, N.P. (2002). Structure of an HIF-1a-pVHL complex: hydroxyproline recognition in signalling. Science 296, 1886-1889.

Minamishima, Y.A., and Kaelin, W.G., Jr. (2010). Reactivation of hepatic EPO synthesis in mice after PHD loss. Science 329, 407.

Minamishima, Y.A., Moslehi, J., Bardeesy, N., Cullen, D., Bronson, R.T., and Kaelin, W.G., Jr. (2008). Somatic inactivation of the PHD2 prolyl hydroxylase causes polycythemia and congestive heart failure. Blood 111, 3236-3244.

Minamishima, Y.A., Moslehi, J., Padera, R.F., Bronson, R.T., Liao, R., and Kaelin, W.G., Jr. (2009). A feedback loop involving the Phd3 prolyl hydroxylase tunes the mammalian hypoxic response in vivo. Mol Cell Biol 29, 5729-5741.

Moertel, C.G., Fleming, T.R., Creagan, E.T., Rubin, J., O'Connell, M.J., and Ames, M.M. (1985). High-dose vitamin C versus placebo in the treatment of patients with advanced cancer who have had no prior chemotherapy. A randomized double-blind comparison. N Engl J Med 312, 137-141.

Mole, D.R., Blancher, C., Copley, R.R., Pollard, P.J., Gleadle, J.M., Ragoussis, J., and Ratcliffe, P.J. (2009). Genome-wide association of hypoxia-inducible factor (HIF)-1alpha and HIF-2alpha DNA binding with expression profiling of hypoxia-inducible transcripts. J Biol Chem 284, 16767-16775.

Moller, A., House, C.M., Wong, C.S., Scanlon, D.B., Liu, M.C., Ronai, Z., and Bowtell, D.D. (2009). Inhibition of Siah ubiquitin ligase function. Oncogene 28, 289-296.

Myllyla, R., Majamaa, K., Gunzler, V., Hanauske-Abel, H.M., and Kivirikko, K.I. (1984). Ascorbate is consumed stoichiometrically in the uncoupled reactions catalyzed by prolyl 4-hydroxylase and lysyl hydroxylase. J Biol Chem 259, 5403-5405.

Nagao, M., Ebert, B.L., Ratcliffe, P.J., and Pugh, C.W. (1996). Drosophila melanogaster SL2 cells contain a hypoxically inducible DNA binding complex which recognises mammalian HIF-1 binding sites. FEBS Lett 387, 161-166.

Nakayama, K., Frew, I.J., Hagensen, M., Skals, M., Habelhah, H., Bhoumik, A., Kadoya, T., Erdjument-Bromage, H., Tempst, P., Frappell, P.B., et al. (2004). Siah2 regulates stability of prolyl-hydroxylases, controls HIF1a abundance, and modulates physiological responses to hypoxia. Cell 117, 941-952.

Nanduri, J., Wang, N., Yuan, G., Khan, S.A., Souvannakitti, D., Peng, Y.J., Kumar, G.K., Garcia, J.A., and Prabhakar, N.R. (2009). Intermittent hypoxia degrades HIF-2alpha via calpains resulting in oxidative stress: implications for recurrent apnea-induced morbidities. Proc Natl Acad Sci USA 106, 1199-1204.

Necas, E., and Thorling, E.B. (1972). Unresponsiveness of erythropoietin-producing cells to cyanide. Am J Physiol 222, 1187-1190.

Nesbit, C.E., Tersak, J.M., Grove, L.E., Drzal, A., Choi, H., and Prochownik, E.V. (2000). Genetic dissection of c-myc apoptotic pathways. Oncogene 19, 3200-3212.

Nytko, K.J., Maeda, N., Schlafli, P., Spielmann, P., Wenger, R.H., and Stiehl, D.P. (2011). Vitamin C is dispensable for oxygen sensing in vivo. Blood 117, 5485-5493

O'Flaherty, L., Adam, J., Heather, L.C., Zhdanov, A.V., Chung, Y.L., Miranda, M.X., Croft, J., Olpin, S., Clarke, K., Pugh, C.W., et al. (2010). Dysregulation of hypoxia pathways in fumarate hydratase-deficient cells is independent of defective mitochondrial metabolism. Hum Mol Genet 19, 3844-3851.

O'Rourke, J.F., Tian, Y.-M., Ratcliffe, P.J., and Pugh, C.W. (1999). Oxygen-regulated and transactivating domains in endothelial PAS protein 1: comparison with hypoxia inducible factor-1a. J Biol Chem 274, 2060-2071.

Ohh, M., Park, C.W., Ivan, M., Hoffman, M.A., Kim, T.Y., Huang, L.E., Pavletich, N., Chau, V., and Kaelin, W.G. (2000). Ubiquitination of hypoxia-inducible factor requires direct binding to the beta-domain of the von Hippel-Lindau protein. Nat Cell Biol 2, 423-427.

Ozer, A., Wu, L.C., and Bruick, R.K. (2005). The candidate tumour suppressor ING4 represses activation of the hypoxia inducible factor (HIF). Proc Natl Acad Sci USA 102(21):7481-6.

Page, E.L., Chan, D.A., Giaccia, A.J., Levine, M., and Richard, D.E. (2008). Hypoxia-inducible Factor-1a Stabilization in Nonhypoxia Conditions: Role of Oxidation and Intracellular Ascorbate Depletion. Mol Biol Cell 19, 86-94.

Pan, Y., Mansfield, K.D., Bertozzi, C.C., Rudenko, V., Chan, D.A., Giaccia, A.J., and Simon, M.C. (2007). Multiple factors affecting cellular redox status and energy metabolism modulate hypoxia-inducible factor prolyl hydroxylase activity in vivo and in vitro. Mol Biol Cell 27, 912-925.

Pasanen, A., Heikkila, M., Rautavuoma, K., Hirsila, M., Kivirikko, K.I., and Myllyharju, J. (2010). Hypoxia-inducible factor (HIF)-3alpha is subject to extensive alternative splicing in human tissues and cancer cells and is regulated by HIF-1 but not HIF-2. Int J Biochem Cell Biol 42, 1189-1200.

Percy, M.J., Zhao, Q., Flores, A., Harrison, C., Lappin, T.R., Maxwell, P.H., McMullin, M.F., and Lee, F.S. (2006). A family with erythrocytosis establishes a role for prolyl hydroxylase domain protein 2 in oxygen homeostasis. Proc Natl Acad Sci USA 103, 654-659.

Pollard, P.J., Briere, J.J., Alam, N.A., Barwell, J., Barclay, E., Wortham, N.C., Hunt, T., Mitchell, M., Olpin, S., Moat, S.J., et al. (2005). Accumulation of Krebs cycle intermediates and over-expression of HIF1alpha in tumours which result from germline FH and SDH mutations. Hum Mol Genet 14, 2231-2239.

Pugh, C.W., O'Rourke, J.F., Nagao, M., Gleadle, J.M., and Ratcliffe, P.J. (1997). Activation of hypoxia inducible factor-1; definition of regulatory domains within the a subunit. J Biol Chem 272, 11205-11214.

Pugh, C.W., Tan, C.C., Jones, R.W., and Ratcliffe, P.J. (1991). Functional analysis of an oxygen-regulated transcriptional enhancer lying 3' to the mouse erythropoietin gene. Proc Natl Acad Sci USA 88, 10553-10557.

Rantanen, K., Pursiheimo, J., Hogel, H., Himanen, V., Metzen, E., and Jaakkola, P.M.

(2008). Prolyl Hydroxylase PHD3 Activates Oxygen-dependent Protein Aggregation. Mol Biol Cell 19, 2231-2240.

Raval, R.R., Lau, K.W., Tran, M.G., Sowter, H.M., Mandriota, S.J., Li, J.L., Pugh, C.W., Maxwell, P.H., Harris, A.L., and Ratcliffe, P.J. (2005). Contrasting Properties of Hypoxia-Inducible Factor 1 (HIF-1) and HIF-2 in von Hippel-Lindau-Associated Renal Cell Carcinoma. Mol Cell Biol 25, 5675-5686.

Saeed, S.A., Waqar, M.A., Zubairi, A.J., Bhurgri, H., Khan, A., Gowani, S.A., Waqar, S.N., Choudhary, M.I., Jalil, S., Zaidi, A.H., et al. (2005). Myocardial ischaemia and reperfusion injury: reactive oxygen species and the role of neutrophil. J Coll Physicians Surg Pak 15, 507-514.

Sakamoto, T., and Seiki, M. (2009). Mint3 enhances the activity of hypoxia-inducible factor-1 (HIF-1) in macrophages by suppressing the activity of factor inhibiting HIF-1. J Biol Chem 284, 30350-30359.

Sakamoto, T., and Seiki, M. (2010). A membrane protease regulates energy production in macrophages by activating hypoxia-inducible factor-1 via a non-proteolytic mechanism. J Biol Chem 285, 29951-29964.

Salceda, S., and Caro, J. (1997). Hypoxia-inducible factor 1a (HIF-1a) protein is rapidly degraded by the ubiquitin-proteasome system under normoxic conditions. J Biol Chem 272, 22642-22647.

Sandau, K.B., Fandrey, J., and Brune, B. (2001). Accumulation of HIF-1alpha under the influence of nitric oxide. Blood 97, 1009-1015.

Schlisio, S., Kenchappa, R.S., Vredeveld, L.C., George, R.E., Stewart, R., Greulich, H., Shahriari, K., Nguyen, N.V., Pigny, P., Dahia, P.L., et al. (2008). The kinesin KIF1B-beta acts downstream from EglN3 to induce apoptosis and is a potential 1p36 tumour suppressor. Genes Dev 22, 884-893.

Schmierer, B., Novak, B., and Schofield, C.J. (2010). Hypoxia-dependent sequestration of an oxygen sensor by a widespread structural motif can shape the hypoxic response–a predictive kinetic model. BMC Syst Biol 4, 139.

Schooley, J.C., and Mahlmann, L.J. (1972). Erythropoietin production in the anephric rat. I. Relationship between nephrectomy, time of hypoxic exposure and erythropoietin production. Blood 39, 31 38.

Selak, M.A., Armour, S.M., MacKenzie, E.D., Boulahbel, H., Watson, D.G., Mansfield, K.D., Pan, Y., Simon, M.C., Thompson, C.B., and Gottlieb, E. (2005). Succinate links TCA cycle dysfunction to oncogenesis by inhibiting HIF-alpha prolyl hydroxylase. Cancer Cell 7, 77-85.

Semenza, G.L. (2007). Evaluation of HIF-1 inhibitors as anticancer agents. Drug Discov Today 12, 853-859.

Semenza, G.L., Nejfelt, M.K., Chi, S.M., and Antonarakis, S.E. (1991). Hypoxia-inducible nuclear factors bind to an enhancer element located 3' to the human erythropoietin gene. Proc Natl Acad Sci USA 88, 5680-5684.

Semenza, G.L., Roth, P.H., Fang, H.-M., and Wang, G.L. (1994). Transcriptional regulation of genes encoding glycolytic enzymes by hypoxia-inducible factor 1. J Biol Chem 269, 23757-23763.

Semenza, G.L., and Wang, G.L. (1992). A nuclear factor induced by hypoxia via de novo protein synthesis binds to the human erythropoietin gene enhancer at a site required for transcriptional activation. Mol Cell Biol 12, 5447-5454.

Seth, P., I., K., Porter, D., and Polyak, K. (2002). Novel estrogen and tamoxifen induced genes identified by SAGE (Serial Analysis of Gene Expression). Oncogene 21, 836-843.

Siddiq, A., Aminova, L.R., Troy, C.M., Suh, K., Messer, Z., Semenza, G.L., and Ratan, R.R. (2009). Selective inhibition of hypoxia-inducible factor (HIF) prolyl-hydroxylase 1 mediates neuroprotection against normoxic oxidative death via HIF- and CREB-independent pathways. J Neurosci 29, 8828-8838.

Simonson, T.S., Yang, Y., Huff, C.D., Yun, H., Qin, G., Witherspoon, D.J., Bai, Z., Lorenzo, F.R., Xing, J., Jorde, L.B., et al. (2010). Genetic evidence for high-altitude adaptation in Tibet. Science 329, 72-75.

Sogawa, K., Numayama-Tsuruta, K., Ema, M., Abe, M., Abe, H., and Fujii-Kuriyama, Y. (1998). Inhibition of hypoxia-inducible factor 1 activity by nitric oxide donors in hypoxia. Proc Natl Acad Sci USA 95, 7368-7373.

Soilleux, E.J., Turley, H., Tian, Y.M., Pugh, C.W., Gatter, K.C., and Harris, A.L. (2005). Use of novel monoclonal antibodies to determine the expression and distribution of the hypoxia regulatory factors PHD-1, PHD-2, PHD-3 and FIH in normal and neoplastic human tissues. Histopathology 47, 602-610.

Spinella, F., Rosano, L., Del Duca, M., Di Castro, V., Nicotra, M.R., Natali, P.G., and Bagnato, A. (2010). Endothelin-1 inhibits prolyl hydroxylase domain 2 to activate hypoxia-inducible factor-1 alpha in melanoma cells. PLoS One 5(6), e11241.

Steinhoff, A., Pientka, F.K., Mockel, S., Kettelhake, A., Hartmann, E., Kohler, M., and Depping, R. (2009). Cellular oxygen sensing: Importins and exportins are mediators of intracellular localisation of prolyl-4-hydroxylases PHD1 and PHD2. Biochem Biophys Res Commun 387, 705-711.

Stiehl, D.P., Wirthner, R., Koditz, J., Spielmann, P., Camenisch, G., and Wenger, R.H. (2006). Increased Prolyl 4-Hydroxylase Domain Proteins Compensate for Decreased Oxygen Levels. J Biol Chem 281, 23482-23491.

Stolze, I.P., Tian, Y.M., Appelhoff, R.J., Turley, H., Wykoff, C.C., Gleadle, J.M., and Ratcliffe, P.J. (2004). Genetic analysis of the role of the asparaginyl hydroxylase FIH in regulating HIF transcriptional target genes. J Biol Chem 279, 42719-42725.

Straub, J.A., Lipscomb, E.A., Yoshida, E.S., and Freeman, R.S. (2003). Induction of SM-20 in PC12 cells leads to increased cytochrome c levels, accumulation of cytochrome c in the cytosol, and caspase-dependent cell death. J Neurochem 85, 318-328.

Takeda, K., Aguila, H.L., Parikh, N.S., Li, X., Lamothe, K., Duan, L.J., Takeda, H., Lee, F.S., and Fong, G.H. (2008). Regulation of adult erythropoiesis by prolyl hydroxylase domain proteins. Blood 111, 3229-3235.

Takeda, K., Cowan, A., and Fong, G.H. (2007). Essential role for prolyl hydroxylase domain protein 2 in oxygen homeostasis of the adult vascular system. Circulation 116, 774-781.

Takeda, K., and Fong, G.H. (2007). Prolyl hydroxylase domain 2 protein suppresses hypoxia-induced endothelial cell proliferation. Hypertension 49, 178-184.

Takeda, K., Ho, V., Takeda, H., Duan, L.J., Nagy, A., and Fong, G.H. (2006). Placental but not Heart Defect Is Associated with Elevated HIF{alpha} Levels in Mice Lacking Prolyl Hydroxylase Domain Protein 2. Mol Cell Biol. 22, 8336-46.

Talks, K., Turley, H., Gatter, K.C., Maxwell, P.H., Pugh, C.W., Ratcliffe, P.J., and Harris, A.L. (2000). The expression and distribution of the hypoxia-inducible factors HIF-1alpha and HIF-2alpha in normal human tissues, cancers, and tumour-associated macrophages. Am J Pathol 157, 411-421.

Tan, E.Y., Campo, L., Han, C., Turley, H., Pezzella, F., Gatter, K.C., Harris, A.L., and Fox, S.B. (2007). Cytoplasmic location of factor-inhibiting hypoxia-inducible factor is associated with an enhanced hypoxic response and a shorter survival in invasive breast cancer. Breast Cancer Res 9, R89.

Tanimoto, K., Makino, Y., Pereira, T., and Poellinger, L. (2000). Mechanism of regulation of the hypoxia-inducible factor-1a by the von Hippel-Lindau tumour suppressor protein. EMBO J 19, 4298-4309.

Tateishi, K., Okada, Y., Kallin, E.M., and Zhang, Y. (2009). Role of Jhdm2a in regulating metabolic gene expression and obesity resistance. Nature 458, 757-761.

Taylor, C.T., and McElwain, J.C. (2010). Ancient atmospheres and the evolution of oxygen sensing via the hypoxia-inducible factor in metazoans. Physiology (Bethesda) 25, 272-279.

Taylor, C.T., and Moncada, S. (2010). Nitric oxide, cytochrome C oxidase, and the cellular response to hypoxia. Arterioscler Thromb Vasc Biol 30, 643-647.

Tennant, D.A., Frezza, C., MacKenzie, E.D., Nguyen, Q.D., Zheng, L., Selak, M.A., Roberts, D.L., Dive, C., Watson, D.G., Aboagye, E.O., et al. (2009). Reactivating HIF prolyl hydroxylases under hypoxia results in metabolic catastrophe and cell death. Oncogene 28, 4009-4021.

Tian, Y., Yeoh, KK., Lee, MK., Ericsson, T., Kessler, BM., Kramer, HB., Edelmann, MJ., William, C., Pugh, CW., Schofield, CJ. and Ratcliffe, PJ. (2011). Differential sensitivity of HIF hydroxylation sites to hypoxia and hydroxylase inhibitors. J Biol Chem 286, 13041-13051.

Tian, Y.M., Mole, D.R., Ratcliffe, P.J., and Gleadle, J.M. (2006). Characterization of different isoforms of the HIF prolyl hydroxylase PHD1 generated by alternative initiation. Biochem J 397, 179-186.

To, K.K., and Huang, L.E. (2005). Suppression of hypoxia-inducible factor 1alpha (HIF-1alpha) transcriptional activity by the HIF prolyl hydroxylase EGLN1. J Biol Chem 280, 38102-38107.

van der Wel, H., Ercan, A., and West, C.M. (2005). The Skp1 prolyl hydroxylase of dictyostelium is related to the HIFa-class of animal prolyl 4-hydroxylases. J Biol Chem. 280(15):14645-55.

Vaupel, P., Schlenger, K., Knoop, C., and Hockel, M. (1991). Oxygenation of human tumours: evaluation of tissue oxygen distribution in breast cancers by computerized O2 tension measurements. Cancer Res 51, 3316-3322.

Villar, D., Vara-Vega, A., Landazuri, M.O., and Del Peso, L. (2007). Identification of a region on hypoxia-inducible-factor prolyl 4-hydroxylases that determines their specificity for the oxygen degradation domains. Biochem J 408, 231-240.

Vissers, M.C., Gunningham, S.P., Morrison, M.J., Dachs, G.U., and Currie, M.J. (2007).

Modulation of hypoxia-inducible factor-1 alpha in cultured primary cells by intra-cellular ascorbate. Free Radic Biol Med 42, 765-772.

Wang, F., and Fried, W. (1972). Renal and extrarenal erythropoietin production in male and female rats of various ages. J Lab Clin Med 79, 181-186.

Wang, F., Sekine, H., Kikuchi, Y., Takasaki, C., Miura, C., Heiwa, O., Shuin, T., Fujii-Kuriyama, Y., and Sogawa, K. (2002). HIF-1a-prolyl hydroxylase: molecular target of nitric oxide in the hypoxic signal transduction pathway. Biochem Biophys Res Commun 295, 657-662.

Wang, G.L., Jiang, B.-H., Rue, E.A., and Semenza, G.L. (1995). Hypoxia-inducible factor 1 is a basic-helix-loop-helix-PAS heterodimer regulated by cellular O_2 tension. Proc Natl Acad Sci USA 92, 5510-5514.

Wang, G.L., and Semenza, G.L. (1993). General involvement of hypoxia-inducible factor 1 in transcriptional response to hypoxia. Proc Natl Acad Sci USA 90, 4304-4308.

Wax, S.D., Rosenfield, C.L., and Taubman, M.B. (1994). Identification of a novel growth factor-responsive gene in vascular smooth muscle cells. J Biol Chem 269, 13041-13047.

Webb, J.D., Murányi, A., Pugh, C.W., Ratcliffe, P.J., and Coleman, M.L. (2009). MYPT1, the targeting subunit of smooth muscle myosin phosphatase, is a substrate for the asparaginyl hydroxylase factor inhibiting hypoxia inducible factor (FIH). Biochem J 420, 327-333.

Welford, R.W.D., Schlemminger, I., McNeill, L.A., Hewitson, K.S., and Schofield, C.J. (2003). The selectivity and inhibition of AlkB. J Biol Chem 278, 10157-10161.

West, C.M., Wang, Z.A., and van der Wel, H. (2010). A cytoplasmic prolyl hydroxylation and glycosylation pathway modifies Skp1 and regulates O2-dependent development in Dictyostelium. Biochim Biophys Acta 1800, 160-171.

Wilkins, S.E., Hyvarinen, J., Chicher, J., Gorman, J.J., Peet, D.J., Bilton, R.L., and Koivunen, P. (2009). Differences in hydroxylation and binding of Notch and HIF-1alpha demonstrate substrate selectivity for factor inhibiting HIF-1 (FIH-1). Int J Biochem Cell Biol 41, 1563-1571.

Wolf, G., Schroeder, R., and Stahl, R.A. (2004). Angiotensin II induces hypoxia-inducible factor-1 alpha in PC 12 cells through a posttranscriptional mechanism: role of AT2 receptors. Am J Nephrol 24, 415-421.

Wong, W., Goehring, A.S., Kapiloff, M.S., Langeberg, L.K., and Scott, J.D. (2008). mAKAP compartmentalizes oxygen-dependent control of HIF-1alpha. Sci Signal 1, ra18.

Xia, X., Lemieux, M.E., Li, W., Carroll, J.S., Brown, M., Liu, X.S., and Kung, A.L. (2009). Integrative analysis of HIF binding and transactivation reveals its role in maintaining histone methylation homeostasis. Proc Natl Acad Sci USA 106, 4260-4265.

Xie, L., Xiao, K., Whalen, E.J., Forrester, M.T., Freeman, R.S., Fong, G., Gygi, S.P., Lefkowitz, R.J., and Stamler, J.S. (2009). Oxygen-regulated beta(2)-adrenergic receptor hydroxylation by EGLN3 and ubiquitylation by pVHL. Sci Signal 2, ra33.

Xu, W., Yang, H, Liu, Y, Yang, Y, Wang, P, Kim, S-H, Ito, S, Yang, C, Wang, P, Xiao M-T, Liu, L, Jiang, W, Liu, J, Zhang, J, Wang, B, Frye, S, Zhang, Y, Xu, Y, Lei, Q, Guan, K, Zhao, S, Xiong, Y. (2011). Oncometabolite 2-Hydroxyglutarate Is a Competitive Inhibitor of α-Ketoglutarate-Dependent Dioxygenases. Cancer Cell 19, 17-30.

Xue, J., Li, X., Jiao, S., Wei, Y., Wu, G., and Fang, J. (2010). Prolyl hydroxylase-3 is down-regulated in colorectal cancer cells and inhibits IKKbeta independent of hydroxylase activity. Gastroenterology 138, 606-615.

Yan, H., Parsons, D.W., Jin, G., McLendon, R., Rasheed, B.A., Yuan, W., Kos, I., Batinic-Haberle, I., Jones, S., Riggins, G.J., et al. (2009). IDH1 and IDH2 mutations in gliomas. N Engl J Med 360, 765-773.

Yang, M., Ge, W., Chowdhury, R., Claridge, T.D., Kramer, H.B., Schmierer, B., McDonough, M.A., Gong, L., Kessler, B.M., Ratcliffe, P.J., et al. (2011a). Asparagine and aspartate hydroxylation of the cytoskeletal ankyrin family is catalysed by factor inhibiting hypoxia-inducible factor (FIH). J Biol Chem 286, 7648-7660.

Yang M, Chowdhury, R., Ge W, Hamed R.B., McDonough M.A., Claridge T.D., Kessler B.M., Cockman M.E., Ratcliffe P.J., and Schofield C.J. (2011b). Factor-Inhibiting Hypoxia-Inducible Factor (FIH) Catalyses the Posttranslational Hydroxylation of Histidinyl Residues within Ankyrin Repeat Domains. FEBS J 278, 1086-1097

Yasumoto, K., Kowata, Y., Yoshida, A., Torii, S., and Sogawa, K. (2009). Role of the intracellular localization of HIF-prolyl hydroxylases. Biochim Biophys Acta 1793, 792-797.

Yee Koh, M., Spivak-Kroizman, T.R., and Powis, G. (2008). HIF-1 regulation: not so easy come, easy go. Trends Biochem Sci 33, 526-534.

Yu, F., White, S.B., Zhao, Q., and Lee, F.S. (2001). HIF-1a binding to VHL is regulated by stimulus-sensitive proline hydroxylation. Proc Natl Acad Sci USA 98, 9630-9635.

Yuan, G., Nanduri, J., Khan, S., Semenza, G.L., and Prabhakar, N.R. (2008). Induction of HIF-1alpha expression by intermittent hypoxia: involvement of NADPH oxidase, Ca2+ signalling, prolyl hydroxylases, and mTOR. J Cell Physiol 217, 674-685.

Zhang, L., and Hach, A. (1999). Molecular mechanism of heme signalling in yeast: the transcriptional activator Hap1 serves as the key mediator. Cell Mol Life Sci 56, 415-426.

Zhang, N., Fu, Z., Linke, S., Chicher, J., Gorman, J.J., Visk, D., Haddad, G.G., Poellinger, L., Peet, D.J., Powell, F., et al. (2010). The asparaginyl hydroxylase factor inhibiting HIF-1alpha is an essential regulator of metabolism. Cell Metab 11, 364-378.

Zhang, Q., Gu, J., Li, L., Liu, J., Luo, B., Cheung, H.W., Boehm, J.S., Ni, M., Geisen, C., Root, D.E., et al. (2009). Control of cyclin D1 and breast tumourigenesis by the EglN2 prolyl hydroxylase. Cancer Cell 16, 413-424.

Zhang, Z., Ren, J.-S., Harlos, K., McKinnon, C.H., Clifton, I.J., and Schofield, C.J. (2002). Crystal structure of a clavaminate synthase-Fe(II)-2-oxoglutarate-substrate-NO complex: evidence for metal centred rearrangements. FEBS Lett 517, 7-12.

Zheng, X., Linke, S., Dias, J.M., Zheng, X., Gradin, K., Wallis, T.P., Hamilton, B.R., Gustafsson, M., Ruas, J.L., Wilkins, S., et al. (2008). Interaction with factor inhibiting HIF-1 defines an additional mode of cross-coupling between the Notch and hypoxia signalling pathways. Proc Natl Acad Sci USA 105, 3368-3373.

Chapter 2

VHL Inactivation

Thomas M. F. Connor and Patrick H. Maxwell[*]

[*]Author for correspondence:
Department of Medicine, University College London, London WC1E 6JJ, UK,
Tel: +4420 7679 6351; Fax: +4420 7679 6211; E-mail: p.maxwell@ucl.ac.uk

Contents

Key points

— Von Hippel-Lindau (VHL) disease is a dominantly inherited familial cancer syndrome caused by mutations in the *VHL* tumour suppressor gene.

— Germline mutations that inactivate *VHL* cause a very high lifetime risk of tumours including haemangioblastoma, clear cell renal cancers (CCRCC), and phaeochromocytoma. *VHL* mutations are also common in sporadic CCRCC and haemangioblastoma.

— The *VHL* gene product has multiple functions, the best characterized of which is the ubiquitination of hypoxia-inducible factor alpha (HIF-α). Recognition by VHL requires modification of the HIF-α subunit by oxygen-dependent prolyl hydroxylase (PHD) family members.

— Loss of VHL leads to constitutive activation of HIF target genes, which probably plays a causative role in CCRCC and haemangioblastoma. This is supported by a correlation between the effect of an individual mutation on VHL's ability to regulate HIF and the risk of CCRCC or haemangioblastoma.

Introduction

A major challenge at the end of the 20th century was to understand how Hypoxia Inducible Factor responded to oxygen tension. The answer came indirectly, from the study of a rare familial cancer syndrome, von Hippel-Lindau (VHL) disease. This is a dominantly inherited condition caused by mutations in the *VHL* tumour suppressor gene. Clinical features of VHL-associated tumours led to the recognition that VHL is a critical negative regulator of mRNAs that are induced by low oxygen (Iliopoulos et al., 1996; Lonergan et al., 1998). In 1999, VHL was shown to target HIFα subunits for oxygen-dependent proteolysis (Maxwell et al., 1999). Further research rapidly revealed that VHL was the substrate recognition component of an ubiquitin protein ligase complex that is responsible for the oxygen-dependent degradation of HIF.

VHL is a small, highly conserved gene that gives rise to a ubiquitously expressed mRNA. It forms an important component of a molecular pathway used by metazoans to sense and respond to changes in oxygen. The protein encoded by *VHL* interacts with numerous protein partners. The best understood of these is the interaction with the alpha subunits of the HIF heterodimer. VHL also forms distinct multi-protein complexes with roles in transcriptional regulation, and which interact with the microtubule cytoskeleton and extracellular matrix components (Frew and Krek, 2008).

Loss of VHL leads to increased expression of HIF target genes, many of which play important roles in cancer biology. HIF activation is considered to play a critical role in both hereditary and sporadic *VHL*-defective CCRCC and haemangioblastoma. *VHL* mutations are very rare in other cancers, although many solid tumours show HIF activation in hypoxic regions (Zhong et al., 1999). HIF accumulates in these regions as a result of impaired hydroxylation, rather than VHL loss, and is predicted to have major effects on tumour behaviour. HIF activity is also affected by diverse signalling pathways that are activated in cancer.

The relationship between genotype and phenotype in kindreds with classical VHL disease has provided insight into the role of different VHL functions in tumour development. More recently, hypomorphic *VHL* mutations and mutations in *PHD2* and *HIF2A* have been linked with erythrocytosis. Importantly these individuals do not appear to have an increased risk of cancer, and provide insight into the physiological effects of HIF activation in humans.

Von Hippel-Lindau disease

Von Hippel-Lindau (VHL) disease (MIM 193300) is a dominantly inherited familial cancer syndrome caused by mutations in the *VHL* tumour suppressor gene. It was named after Eugene von Hippel, who described angiomas in the eye in 1904, and Arvid Lindau, who described angiomas of the cerebellum and spine in 1927. The incidence of VHL disease is approximately 1 per 36000 live births, with similar prevalence in both genders and across all ethnic backgrounds (Maher, 2004; Maher et al., 1991). Most patients with VHL disease have a positive family history, but de novo *VHL* mutations and mosaisicm are not uncommon. Genetic testing and active screening for clinical manifestations is now started in childhood and has greatly improved the prognosis for patients with VHL disease (Nordstrom-O'Brien et al., 2010).

The most frequent manifestations of VHL disease are retinal and central nervous system haemangioblastomas, renal cell carcinomas, and phaeochromocytomas. These are commonly multiple and develop at a younger age than similar sporadic tumours in the general population. Patients may also develop non-secreting neuroendocrine tumours of the pancreas, endolymphatic sac tumours (which can result in deafness), epididymal papillary cystadenoma (men) and cysts of the uterine broad ligament (women) (Gruber et al., 1980; Kaelin, 2007; Maher, 2004; Neumann et al., 1991). In addition to tumours, patients develop multiple cysts of the kidney and other organs including the pancreas (Hough et al., 1994; Lubensky et al., 1998; Maher, 2004; Maher et al., 1990). All the clinical manifestations of VHL disease involve somatic inactivation of the wild-type *VHL* allele, in accordance with Knudson's 'two-hit' mechanism of tumour suppression (Knudson, 1971).

The morbidity of VHL disease depends on the particular organ system involved. For example, retinal haemangioblastomas can result in retinal detachment or blindness (Webster et al., 1999). Previously, mortality was usually due to either metastasis of RCC or complications of CNS haemangioblastomas (Filling-Katz et al., 1991; Maher et al., 1990; Neumann et al., 1992). Following the introduction of systematic screening for tumour development, life expectancy of VHL patients has greatly improved.

Haemangioblastomas are the commonest manifestations of VHL disease, occurring in up to 80% of patients. They develop earlier than in the general population, with diagnosis almost 20 years earlier than in sporadic cerebellar haemangioblastomas (Wanebo et al., 2003). They are located most commonly in the cerebellum and retina (Maher et al., 1990; Melmon and Rosen, 1964; Weil et al., 2003). These lesions are typically cystic tumours of endothelial cells and lipid-filled stromal cells embedded in capillary networks (Kanno et al., 1994) (Richard et al., 1998). It is now clear that the stromal cells drive the neoplastic process by paracrine release of angiogenic factors, as a direct consequence of loss of VHL function (Wizigmann-Voos et al., 1995). Interestingly, these tumours fluctuate between phases of growth and quiescence, which may be synchronised in patients with numerous tumours (Jagannathan et al., 2008; Wanebo et al., 2003). They are rarely malignant, but enlargement or bleeding within the CNS can result in neurological damage and death (Pavesi et al., 2008).

VHL patients have a 70% risk of developing CCRCC by 60 years of age (Maher et al., 1991; Maher et al., 1990; Whaley et al., 1994). The average age of onset is 44 years, compared to 62 years for sporadic CCRCC in the general population. Renal cysts are also common in VHL patients, and show a higher rate of malignant transformation than the simple cysts seen in the general population (Kaelin, 2004). *VHL*-defective CCRCC is very vascular, due again to the overproduction of angiogenic factors, including VEGF (Berse et al., 1992; Sato et al., 1994; Takahashi et al., 1994).

Phaeochromocytomas are neoplastic intra- or extra-adrenal gland lesions that appear histologically as an expansion of large chromaffin positive cells, derived from neural crest cells (Lee et al., 2005). 7-18% of VHL patients are afflicted with phaeochromocytomas, with a mean age of onset of 29.9 years (Bryant et al., 2003; Crossey et al., 1994; Garcia et al., 1997). Untreated phaeochromocytomas can result in severe, episodic hypertension with subsequent heart disease, stroke, or malignant hypertension. *VHL* is one of a number of genes associated with familial phaeochromocytoma (see below). In contrast to sporadic haemangioblastoma and CCRCC, which are associated with biallelic *VHL* inactivation, this is unusual in sporadic phaeochromocytoma (Kaelin, 2007).

In addition to the association with VHL disease, *VHL* mutations are also associated with congenital polycythemia (also known as Familial Erythrocytosis-2; MIM 263400). In this condition, polycythemia (erythrocytosis) is inherited in an autosomal recessive fashion with either homozygous or compound heterozygous alleles (Ang et al., 2002b; Pastore et al., 2003; Semenza, 2009). This is in contrast to classical VHL disease which is inherited in an autosomal dominant fashion. Erythrocytosis is associated with missense mutations at the C-terminus of the protein, which are thought to have only a minor effect on VHL's ability to regulate HIF. Most mutations have been documented only as isolated case reports, except for several hundred

patients with the R200W mutation, first described in the Chuvash Republic (Sergeyeva et al., 1997). Patients with congenital erythrocytosis manifest
increased red blood cell counts, increased frequency of vertebral haemangiomas, varicose veins, and elevated serum VEGF concentrations, as well
as premature mortality related to cerebrovascular events and peripheral
thrombosis, but do not develop tumours. Occasional patients with classical
VHL disease develop polycythaemia when a CCRCC, haemangioblastoma,
or phaeochromocytoma produces significant amounts of erythropoietin
(Gordeuk et al., 2004).

Clinical Management

Diagnosis of von Hippel-Lindau disease is based on clinical criteria or
genetic testing (Lonser et al., 2003; Melmon and Rosen, 1964). Patients with a family
history, and a CNS (excluding retinal) haemangioblastoma, phaeochromocytoma, or CCRCC are diagnosed with the disease. Those with no relevant
family history must have either two or more CNS haemangioblastoma, or
one haemangioblastoma of the CNS or retina and a visceral tumour (with
exception of epididymal and renal cysts which are common in the general
population).

Mutation analysis is recommended to make a definitive diagnosis (Hes et
al., 2001). Screening for germline *VHL* mutations in individuals with apparently sporadic cerebral and retinal haemangioblastoma should be considered since these are rare in the general population (Cascon et al., 2009; Fukino
et al., 2000; Hes et al., 2000; Neumann et al., 1989; Neumann et al., 2002). Direct sequencing is the gold standard for detecting small germline *VHL* mutations (Klein
et al., 2001). "Mutation negative" patients should be screened with techniques
capable of identifying deletions, such as multiplex ligation-dependent probe
amplification (MLPA), quantitative southern blotting, and fluorescent in
situ hybridization (FISH) (Hes et al., 2007).

Screening for clinical manifestations in individuals who are known to
carry a *VHL* mutation should begin in infancy. The VHL Handbook provides guidelines for screening (http://www.vhl.org/handbook/vhlhb4.php). Early
treatment reduces both morbidity and mortality (Choyke et al., 1995; Lonser et
al., 2003). Similarly, anyone at risk of inheriting a *VHL* mutation who has not
had genetic testing performed should undergo regular clinical screening
to identify tumours before they result in avoidable harm.

Genotype-phenotype correlations in VHL disease

Autosomal dominant VHL disease has a pleiotropic phenotype. Early reports noted that in different kindreds, there were differing patterns of inheritance of haemangioblastoma, phaeochromocytoma, and CCRCC; implying that different mutant alleles at the *VHL* locus were associated with distinct tumour suppressor capabilities (Glenn et al., 1991). There are now more than 350 distinct mutations in the *VHL* gene that have been linked to familial VHL disease (Nordstrom-O'Brien et al., 2010). The clinical phenotype is categorised on the basis of incidence of haemangioblastoma, CCRCC and phaeochromocytoma, as shown in Table 2.1. Striking aspects of the phenotype-genotype relationship are that loss-of-function alleles carry a low risk of phaeochromocytoma (Type 1 disease), while some specific missense mutations predispose to phaeochromocytoma without other manifestations (Type 2C disease). Significantly, mutations associated with Type 2C disease do not alter the ability of VHL to regulate HIF (Clifford et al., 2001).

Table 2.1 _ Classification of VHL kindreds on the basis of tumour risk.

Category	Risk of phaeochromocytoma	Risk of haemangioblastoma	Risk of renal cell carcinoma
1	Low	High	High
2A	High	High	Low
2B	High	High	High
2C	Yes	No	No

High risk: tumour type observed in over 50% of affected individuals. Low risk: tumour type observed in less than 5% of affected individuals. Yes: tumour type observed in all affected individuals. No: tumour type not observed in affected individuals.

Von Hippel-Lindau syndrome (*VHL*) gene

The *VHL* gene is located at 3p25 in 1993, has three exons and gives rise to a 4.5kB mRNA with a long 3' untranslated region (Iliopoulos et al., 1995; Latif et al., 1993; Renbaum et al., 1996). An alternative splice variant lacking exon 2 has been described, but this does not function as a tumour suppressor (Gnarra et al., 1994). The *VHL* promoter contains binding sites for several transcription factors, including nuclear respiratory factor 1, Pax, and TCF4 (Giles et al., 2006; Kuzmin et al., 1995). Promoter hypermethylation in CCRCC has been shown to result in *VHL* inactivation in the absence of coding mutations (Herman et al., 1994; Kim and Kaelin, 2004).

The *VHL* gene encodes two proteins as a result of alternative, in-frame translation initiation codons (Blankenship et al., 1999; Iliopoulos et al., 1998; Schoenfeld et al., 1998). These two proteins migrate with an apparent molecular weight of 24-30 kDa and 19 kDa, and share most biological functions. The longer form contains 213 amino acids, including an N-terminal pentameric acidic repeat domain. The short form consists of amino acid residues 54-213 and lacks this acidic domain. Almost all disease-causing mutations map to the region shared by both isoforms, implying that this region mediates the tumour suppressor actions (Kaelin, 2007).

The VHL protein is distributed throughout the cell and can shuttle between the nucleus and cytoplasm (Bonicalzi et al., 2001; Corless et al., 1997; Duan et al., 1995a; Groulx et al., 2000; Groulx and Lee, 2002; Iliopoulos et al., 1995; Lee et al., 1999; Los et al., 1996; Ye et al., 1998). Most of the protein is cytoplasmic in steady state conditions, but some can be found in mitochondria or in association with the endoplasmic reticulum (Schoenfeld et al., 2001; Shiao et al., 2000). More of the short isoform is nuclear, while more of the long isoform is associated with microtubules in the cytoplasm (Hergovich et al., 2003; Iliopoulos et al., 1998). VHL is predominantly nuclear at low density and cytoplasmic at high density (Lee et al., 1996). Additionally, upon transcriptional arrest or low pH, VHL accumulates in the nucleus (Lee et al., 1999; Mekhail et al., 2004; Mekhail et al., 2005). Manipulation of various nuclear import and export sequences fused to VHL has shown that the specific subcellular localisation can affect tumour suppressor properties (Lewis and Roberts, 2003).

VHL undergoes a variety of posttranslational modifications, particularly on three lysines at residues 159, 171, and 196. Various groups have shown that covalent modification of these residues can affect tumour suppressor function in vivo. Neddylation at lysine 159 is reported to be necessary for fibronectin matrix assembly and suppression of tumour development (Russell and Ohh, 2008; Stickle et al., 2004). VHL can be SUMOylated on lysine 171 by the SUMO E3 ligase PIASy (Cai et al., 2010), leading to increased protein stability and nuclear redistribution. By contrast, ubiquitination of lysine 171 and 196, leads to increased cytoplasmic localisation (Cai and Robertson, 2010). In addition, the N-terminal region of the long isoform is phosphorylated by casein kinase, but the functional consequence of this is not understood (Lolkema et al., 2005).

The protein forms a molten globule under physiological conditions (Sutovsky and Gazit, 2004). Mutational analysis together with X-ray crystallographic and biochemical data determined that the VHL protein contains two functional domains, termed alpha and beta (Stebbins et al., 1999). The beta domain (residues 63-154) consists of a seven-stranded beta sheet and an alpha helix. This region is largely hydrophobic and acts as a substrate-docking site for HIFα (Hon et al., 2002). The alpha domain (residues 155-192) consists of three alpha helices and is required for binding elongin C (Kibel et al., 1995), which results in the formation of a multiprotein E3 ubiquitin ligase complex. This complex may also promote proper folding and stability of VHL, as elongin C provides an alpha helix that together with the three VHL alpha domain helices completes a folded leaf, four helix cluster (Stebbins et al., 1999).

Mutation of the *VHL* gene is detected in nearly all VHL families and, importantly, the great majority (~90%) of non-familial CCRCC (Nickerson et al., 2008). *VHL* functions as a classical tumour suppressor gene. Thus tumour tissue shows inactivation of the remaining normal *VHL* allele in patients with VHL disease, either through mutation, deletion or methylation. Importantly, reintroduction of a *VHL* gene suppresses CCRCC tumour xenografts (Iliopoulos et al., 1995). The fact that it suppresses growth of fully transformed cells implies a 'gatekeeper' rather than a 'caretaker' role in the renal epithelium. It is notable that mutations in *VHL* are rare in all other tumours apart from CCRCC and haemangioblastoma. This suggests that in other cancers, *VHL* loss-of-function would not confer a selective advantage.

Regulation of Hypoxia-Inducible Factor by VHL

The *VHL* gene product has multiple roles, but the best characterized is the proteolytic degradation of the alpha subunit of HIF (Maxwell et al., 1999). The HIF pathway has attracted considerable attention in cancer biology because HIF acts as a master transcriptional regulator of over 100 genes that generally promote adaptation to low O_2 conditions (hypoxia). It is well known that many solid tumours contain regions of hypoxia, and that the degree of hypoxia correlates with poor prognosis (Bertout et al., 2008). In VHL-defective tumours, the HIF transcriptional programme is constitutively activated.

HIF is a highly conserved, sequence-specific DNA binding transcription factor. The active form is a heterodimer composed of a constitutively expressed Aryl Hydrocarbon Receptor Nuclear Translocator (ARNT) beta subunit and one of three alpha subunits (collectively HIFα). When oxygen levels are low, or when VHL function is compromised, HIFα becomes stabilized and is able to heterodimerise with ARNT. The active transcription factor directly activates genes containing hypoxia response elements (HREs), as well as interacting with other transcriptional control complexes, and influencing the expression of other transcription factors and signalling pathways. Many HIF target genes are implicated in tumour progression; for example those encoding angiogenic growth factors.

The VHL protein exists as a complex with elongin B, elongin C, Cul2 and Rbx1 (Duan et al., 1995b; Kamura et al., 1999a; Kamura et al., 1999b; Kibel et al., 1995; Lonergan et al., 1998). The overall enzyme complex has extensive sequence and structural similarities to the Skp1-Cdc53/Cul2-F box class of ubiquitin ligases. Elongin C has similarities to Skp1 and VHL acts like an F box protein (Kamura et al., 1999b; Stebbins et al., 1999). The VHL protein interacts directly with the oxygen-dependent destruction domain of the HIF alpha subunit. This leads to ubiquitination and targeting of the HIF alpha subunit by the 26S proteaseome (Figure 2.2).

The VHL/HIF alpha interaction is crucially dependent on levels of oxygen. This is because VHL only recognises HIF alpha subunits that have been hydroxylated on specific prolyl residues: Pro402 or Pro564 of HIF1α (Hon et al., 2002; Ivan et al., 2001; Jaakkola et al., 2001; Masson et al., 2001; Min et al., 2002; Yu et al., 2001). The hydroxylation reaction requires molecular oxygen and 2-oxoglutarate, and when oxygen levels are low HIF alpha subunits rapidly accumulate and form an active transcriptional complex. Hydroxylation is carried out by three prolyl hydroxylase (PHD) enzymes encoded by the genes *EGLN1, EGLN2,* and *EGLN3* (Bruick and McKnight, 2001; Epstein et al., 2001). These enzymes belong to the extended family of 2-oxoglutarate-dependent dioxygenases, which includes the prolyl hydroxylases that modify procollagen. The HIF–PHD–VHL system is highly conserved in evolution, being present in *C. elegans* (Maxwell et al., 2001).

PHD2 is the dominant HIF prolyl hydroxylase under normal conditions, although PHD1 and PHD3 play a role in specific settings, especially in the case of prolonged hypoxia which strongly induces expression of PHD3 (Appelhoff et al., 2004; Aprelikova et al., 2004; Berra et al., 2003; Marxsen et al., 2004). The K_m for the PHDs is such that prolyl hydroxylation is sensitive to oxygen availability across the physiologically relevant range (Hirsila et al., 2003; McNeill et al., 2002).

The rate of HIF hydroxylation is influenced by other parameters relevant to cancer biology besides oxygen tension. Of note, perturbations in the Krebs cycle, for example due to mutations in fumarate hydratase

(FH) and succinate dehydrogenase (SDH), can impact on HIF regulation by increasing the level of metabolic intermediates (eg fumarate and succinate) that act as PHD inhibitors. PHD activity also requires the cofactors ascorbate and reduced iron (Fe^{2+}). It has also been shown that supplementing prostate cancer cells with ascorbate can decrease HIF activity (Knowles et al., 2003). Several studies indicate that reactive oxygen species (ROS) generated in mitochondria under low oxygen conditions contribute to decreased PHD activity in hypoxia (Guzy et al., 2005; Guzy and Schumacker, 2006; Hamanaka and Chandel, 2009; Mansfield et al., 2005). In addition, activation of signalling pathways can increase ROS production with consequent HIF stabilization (Gerald et al., 2004). PHD activity is also influenced by nitric oxide (NO) (Selak et al., 2005).

In cells lacking VHL, HIF alpha subunits are stable even in the presence of oxygen. CCRCC cells that lack VHL consequently have an activated HIF system in normoxia, resulting in a high constitutive level of expression of angiogenic growth factor and glycolytic enzymes. These characteristics are corrected by reintroduction of VHL. As far as we are aware, VHL is required for inactivation of HIF in normoxia in all mammalian cell types where this has been tested.

In addition to direct effects on HRE-containing HIF-target genes, VHL has numerous other effects via stabilising HIF, including altering the activity of c-Myc (Gordan et al., 2007; Koshiji et al., 2004; Mack et al., 2005), PGC1β (Zhang et al., 2007), OCT4 (Covello et al., 2006), and Notch (Gustafsson et al., 2005), as well as the transcriptional repressors Snail, TCF3, ZFHX1A and ZFHX1B (Evans et al., 2007; Krishnamachary et al., 2006). As a consequence, VHL influences cell cycle progression, mitochondrial biogenesis, stem cell behaviour, and epithelial-to-mesenchymal transition.

HIF-independent functions of VHL

Although the best-characterized function of VHL is the regulation of HIF, it is now clear that VHL has a number of other actions that may contribute to its function as a tumour suppressor. Reported HIF-independent functions of VHL include diverse effects on transcriptional regulation as well as on the extracellular matrix and microtubule cytoskeleton Figure 2.1).

In addition to HIF-associated E3 ligase activity, VHL targets the large subunit of RNA polymerase (Rbp1) for non-degradative ubiquitination

(Kuznetsova et al., 2003). Binding of VHL to Rbp1 in response to oxidative stress requires previous proline hydroxylation of the substrate, similar to the requirement for recognition of HIFα (Mikhaylova et al., 2008). Atypical protein kinase C (aPKC) is also ubiquitinated by VHL (Okuda et al., 2001). This may play a role in the up-regulation of the JunB transcription factor, which is hypothesised to mediate VHL associated phaeochromocytoma (see below).

Loss of *VHL* function is reported to increase activation of NF-κB, via decreased inhibitory phosphorylation of the NF-κB agonist CARD9 by casein kinase II (CKII) (Yang et al., 2007). This may help explain the resistance of CCRCC to apoptosis-inducing therapies and provide another point of attack for the treatment of VHL-defective cancers (Frew and Krek, 2008). VHL is reported to associate with and stabilize p53 by suppressing nuclear export and Mdm2-mediated ubiquitination (Roe et al., 2006). Moreover, this interaction results in an increase in p53 transcriptional activity under genotoxic stress and p53-mediated cell cycle arrest and apoptosis. VHL has also been linked to the p400 chromatin remodelling factor (Young et al., 2008). Acute deletion of *vhlh* in floxed MEFs resulted in a senescent-like phenotype that was independent of p53 and HIF, but dependent on Rb and p400.

VHL also plays a role in extracellular matrix assembly that contributes to its suppressor function (Kurban et al., 2008; Ohh et al., 1998; Stickle et al., 2004). VHL binds directly to fibronectin and collagen IV, and VHL-deficient cells fail to correctly form the collagen IV and fibronectin extracellular matrix, a defect that may facilitate neoangiogenesis and invasion of tumour cells (Grosfeld et al., 2007; Kurban et al., 2008; Ohh et al., 1998). These interactions with VHL probably occur in the endoplasmic reticulum (Kurban et al., 2008), and contribute to the normal delivery of these proteins to the cell surface, where they mediate cell-matrix and cell-cell interactions and participate in signal transduction.

VHL is reported to associate with microtubules in vitro and in vivo and promotes microtubule stability (Hergovich et al., 2003; Lolkema et al., 2004; Thoma et al., 2010). The association of VHL and microtubules is indirect and is at least partly mediated by the interaction of VHL with subunits of kinesin-2 microtubule motors, an interaction that causes the transport of VHL to the cell periphery along microtubules (Lolkema et al., 2007; Mans et al., 2008). This association is independent of E3 ubiquitin ligase activity and is compromised by Type 2A but not 2B *VHL* mutations.

VHL also plays a role in the maintenance of the structure of the primary cilium (Esteban et al., 2006a; Thoma et al., 2007a), a microtubule-based cellular sensory organelle that inhibits uncontrolled epithelial cell proliferation and cyst formation in the kidney (Eley et al., 2005). VHL contributes to the

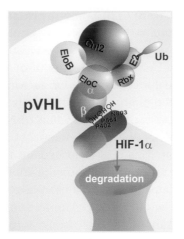

Figure 2.1 _ pVHL as a component of VCB E3 ubiquitin ligase complex regulating stability of HIF-1α. Cul2 - cullin 2, EloB/C – elongin B/C, Ub- ubiquitin, α/β – domains of pVHL.

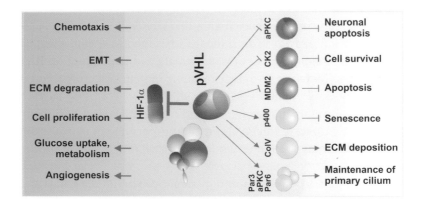

Figure 2.2 _ HIF-dependent and HIF-independent roles of pVHL in cellular processes linked to tumour phenotype. An arrow represents a stimulatory or activating effect a blunted arrow represents an inhibitory effect.

stability of the microtubule skeleton that forms the ciliary axoneme (Thoma et al., 2007a), a function that is abrogated by a subclass of naturally occurring *VHL* mutations (Hergovich et al., 2003; Thoma et al., 2007b). These functions are mediated, at least in part, by inhibition of tubulin guanosine triphosphatase activity (Thoma et al., 2010).

Understanding the extent to which these different functions contribute to tumour suppression in the normal renal epithelium is a considerable challenge. This is complicated by the fact that tumour evolution clearly requires additional events besides loss of VHL function, with dysregulation of other signalling pathways or cellular processes. In primary cells, for example, the cilium-maintaining function of VHL is revealed only when glycogen synthase kinase 3β (GSK-3β) is inactivated (Thoma et al., 2007a). PTEN is a tumour suppressor that acts to limit the activity of the phosphatidylinositol 3-kinase signalling pathway and thus Akt activity. Kidney cysts that arise in patients with inherited *VHL* mutations show glycogen synthase kinase 3β (GSK-3β) inactivation and cilia loss, likely in response to activation of the protein kinases Akt (Frew and Krek, 2008). The potential importance of other signalling pathways and cellular processes that cooperate with *VHL* mutation to allow malignant progression is illustrated by the findings of combining tissue-specific deletion of *vhlh* and *pten* in the mouse (Chen et al., 2010).

VHL and haemangioblastoma

Haemangioblastomas are highly vascular tumours. They are primarily comprised of stromal cells, which may be a form of developmentally arrested angioblast (Vortmeyer et al., 2003). Isolation of these cells from the surrounding blood vessels by microdissection indicates that they represent the neoplastic component, as they exhibit loss of heterozygosity for *VHL* (Chan et al., 1999). Following biallelic *VHL* inactivation, these cells show upregulation of HIF target genes, including VEGF, which is presumed to drive proliferation of the endothelial component of the tumour. These tumours are classified as benign, as they do not metastasize, but they do cause morbidity and mortality through mass effects (see above).

The mutations in *VHL* that are associated with haemangioma development (Type 1, 2A, and 2B disease) all show defective HIF regulation (Kaelin, 2007). This explains why haemangioblastomas frequently overproduce HIF-responsive growth factors, such as VEGF, PDGF, and TGFα (Bohling et al., 1996; Krieg et al., 1998; Reifenberger et al., 1995; Wizigmann-Voos et al., 1995).

VHL and clear cell renal cancer

Individuals from VHL kindreds have an approximately 70% lifetime risk of developing CCRCC. In addition to these relatively rare individuals, bialleleic inactivation of VHL occurs in the great majority of sporadic CCRCC, which is the commonest form of renal cancer (Nickerson et al., 2008). The study of *VHL -/-* CCRCC cell lines, and sublines complemented with a wild-type *VHL* gene, has provided a very powerful system for understanding the functions of VHL, and new insights into CCRCC biology.

CCRCC were believed to originate from the proximal renal tubule. However, premalignant multicellular lesions in VHL patients are almost always in the distal renal tubule, suggesting that the tumours may actually arise in this part of the nephron (Mandriota et al., 2002). Loss of VHL function results in HIF activation and loss of several important characteristics associated with the distal nephron, including expression of E cadherin and Tamm Horsfall protein (Esteban et al., 2006b; Mandriota et al., 2002).

Considerable understanding of VHL function has come from comparison of CCRCC cell lines that are defective for *VHL* with derivatives that have had *VHL* reintroduced. VHL status does not affect cell proliferation or apoptosis under standard culture conditions, although it may effectively suppress growth in xenograft assays (Kaelin, 2007). VHL is required under specific *in vitro* conditions, including cell cycle exit upon serum withdrawal (Pause, Lee et al. 1998) and inhibition of growth at high density (Baba et al., 2003; Schoenfeld et al., 2001). VHL can modulate renal cell apoptosis. Thus loss of VHL can sensitise CCRCC to UV-induced apoptosis, but protect them from apoptosis induced by TNF. The former correlates with a failure to induce p21 and p27 in response to UV damage, possibly acting via BIM(EL) (Guo et al., 2009; Schoenfeld et al., 2000). The latter appears to be multifactorial and may involve NF-κB and the TRAIL receptor DR5 (Mahajan et al., 2008; Qi and Ohh, 2003). VHL loss results in features consistent with an epithelial to mesenchymal transition (Esteban et al., 2006b; Harten et al., 2009; Pantuck et al., 2010). Thus restoration of VHL function promotes epithelial characteristics, and this is more marked when cells are grown under low serum conditions or as three dimensional spheroids (Davidowitz et al., 2001; Lieubeau-Teillet et al., 1998).

VHL mutations linked to CCRCC (Type 1 and 2B) show complete loss of the ability to regulate HIF consistent with HIF activation being critical in tumourigenesis. The low or absent risk of CCRCC seen with Type 2A, Type 2C and Chuvash polycythaemia mutations is plausibly related to the fact that all of these are associated with at least partial ability to regulate HIF (Knauth et al., 2006). Although the mechanism by which HIF activation leads to tumour formation is not fully understood, it does explain why these tumours usually overproduce a wide range of angiogenic growth factors, such as VEGF, PDGF B, and TGFβ (Brown et al., 1993; Takahashi et al., 1994; Wiesener et al., 2001). In these tumours, HIF activation occurs as a very early genetic event, and resultant overproduction of angiogenic factors may minimise the evolutionary pressure on CCRCC to develop resistance to the withdrawal of vascular survival factors (Kaelin, 2007). This may explain why targeted therapies that block the VEGF pathway have clinical activity as single agents in kidney cancer (see below).

A pathogenic role for HIF-1α, as opposed to HIF-1α, in *VHL -/-* CCRCC is supported by several lines of evidence. First, studies of early lesions in VHL kidneys show evidence of a progressive switch from HIF-1α to HIF-2α activation (Mandriota et al., 2002; Raval et al., 2005), with HIF-2α being associated with increased dysplasia, cellular atypia, and expression of Cyclin D1 (Mandriota et al., 2002). Second, *VHL -/-* CCRCC express either HIF-1α and HIF-2α or HIF-2α exclusively, but not HIF-1α alone (Maxwell et al., 1999; Turner et al., 2002), and HIF-1α is genetically inactivated in some tumours (Dalgliesh et al., 2010; Morris et al., 2009). Third, suppression of *VHL -/-* CCRCC growth can be overcome by HIF-2α but not HIF-1α (Kondo et al., 2003; Kondo et al., 2002; Raval et al., 2005). Fourth, inhibition of HIF-2α prevents the ability of *VHL -/-* CCRCC cells to form tumours in nude mice (Kondo et al., 2003; Zimmer et al., 2004).

Studies of other familial cancer syndromes have revealed other genes that are essential for normal renal epithelial homeostasis, with some intriguing links to HIF regulation. Activating *c-Met* mutations are linked to a subset of familial papillary renal cell carcinomas (Linehan and Zbar, 2004; Schmidt et al., 1997). C-MET is a receptor for hepatocyte growth factor that has been shown to be a transcriptional target of HIF and is upregulated by hypoxia in a wide range of cancers. Another subset of familial papillary renal cancers is caused by inactivating mutations in fumarate hydratase (FH). FH loss leads to the accumulation of fumarate, which can inhibit HIF prolyl hydroxylase activity and promote HIF accumulation (Isaacs et al., 2005). Early-onset renal tumours have also been found in individuals with mutations in another tricarboxylic acid cycle enzyme, succinate dehydrogenase subunit B (*SDHB*) (Ricketts et al., 2008; Vanharanta et al., 2004). Tumours harbouring *SDH* mutations exhibit elevated HIF protein levels and associated hypoxia-inducible transcripts (see below) (Gimenez-Roqueplo et al., 2001). Lastly, germline mutations in the tuberous sclerosis genes, *TSC1* and *TSC2*, are associated with early-onset renal tumours (Crino et al., 2006). The products of *TSC1* and *TSC2* form a complex that inhibits mTOR activity; consequent loss of function may result in activation of mTORC1 and increased translation of *HIF-1α* (Brugarolas et al., 2003; Linehan et al., 2010b).

VHL and phaeochromocytoma

Phaeochromocytomas are adrenal tumours that are comprised of chromaffin cells, which are derived from sympathetic neuronal progenitor cells. Germline mutations in *VHL*, neurofibromatosis type 1 (*NF1*), the Receptor for Glial-derived neurotrophic factor (*c-RET*), and succinate dehydrogenase subunit genes (*SDHB, SDHC, SDHD*) are the most frequent cause of familial phaeochromocytoma.

VHL mutations associated with a high risk of phaeochromocytoma (Type 2 disease) are relatively conservative missense mutations. Deletions or disruptive mutations carry a low risk, implying that complete loss of function is incompatible with phaeochromocytoma development. Mutations associated with Type 2C disease, such as L188V, appear not to impair the ability to regulate HIF (Clifford et al., 2001; Hoffman et al., 2001). In addition, bialleleic *VHL* inactivation is very rare in sporadic phaeochromocytomas, while common in sporadic haemangioblastomas or CCRCC. This suggests that phaeochromocytoma development in VHL disease is due to the loss of a critical VHL function unrelated to HIF, and that this has to occur during development. Notably, the other genes linked to familial phaeochromocytoma are also rarely implicated in these tumours when not mutated in the germline and appear to be mutually exclusive with one another and with *VHL* mutations (Bryant et al., 2003; Maher and Eng, 2002).

A model that potentially unifies all of the familial paraganglioma genes was recently proposed, centering on the role of PHD3 in apoptosis during sympathetic neural development (Lee et al., 2005). Primitive sympatho-adrenal precursor cells compete for survival factors such as nerve growth factor (NGF) during development, with the losers undergoing c-Jun–dependent apoptosis (Estus et al., 1994; Ham et al., 1995; Xia et al., 1995). PHD3 is transcriptionally activated by c-Jun following NGF withdrawal and is both necessary and sufficient for neuronal apoptosis in this setting (Lee et al., 2005).

VHL mutations, including the L188V mutant associated with phaeochromocytoma, were shown to promote neuronal survival through up-regulation of JunB, which antagonises c-Jun (Lee et al., 2005). The other genes linked to familial phaeochromocytoma influence this pathway; in the case of mutations in SDH subunits by increasing succinate levels which reduces PHD3 activity (Isaacs et al., 2005), or through the effect of c-RET on TRK signalling (Dechant, 2002). Presumably, cells that have escaped developmental apoptosis lead to tumours later in life.

It remains to be determined, however, why deletions and highly disruptive mutations in *VHL* are associated with a low risk of phaeochromocytoma. This may relate to the complex relationship between VHL status and PHD3 expression. VHL promotes PHD3 accumulation by downregulating JunB, while inhibiting HIF-mediated upregulation of PHD3 (Appelhoff et al., 2004; Aprelikova et al., 2004; Cioffi et al., 2003; Marxsen et al., 2004). It appears that the net effect of different *VHL* mutations on PHD3 levels may determine the risk of phaeochromocytoma. Consistent with this idea, PHD3 protein concentrations appear to be much higher in *VHL* −/− cells transfected with Type 1 *VHL* mutants than in cells expressing *VHL* mutants associated with clinical Type 2 disease (Lee et al., 2005).

Familial erythrocytosis

In addition to the association with VHL disease, the *VHL* gene has more recently been associated with congenital erythrocytosis syndromes. These cases provide a clear link between the VHL-HIF pathway and systems-level response to hypoxia, showing that it plays an important role in determining a number of physiological characteristics in humans, including red blood cell production, respiratory rate and pulmonary vascular tone.

The first erythrocytosis-associated mutation in the oxygen sensing pathway was reported in a large cohort of patients from the Chuvash region of the former Soviet Union, in association with an autosomal recessive hereditary erythrocytosis syndrome originally described by Polyakova in 1974 (Ang et al., 2002a). This condition was initially thought to be restricted to the Chuvash Republic, with a frequency of approximately 1 in 10,000 amongst a population of 1 million. It has subsequently been found in patients from Ischia, North America, Germany, Turkey, and Bangladesh. The mutation responsible is a 598 C>T transition in exon 3 of the *VHL* gene and affected individuals are homozygous. This mutation results in an amino acid change of arginine to tryptophan at residue 200 in the VHL protein (R200W).

The R200W mutation impairs VHL's ability to degradation of HIF under normoxic conditions, with increased expression of some HIF-regulated genes (Ang et al., 2002b; Perrotta et al., 2006). The prevalence and magnitude of altered gene transcription of HIF-regulated genes in different cell types as a result of this mutation have still not been clearly established. In addition to the 598C>T mutation, other *VHL* gene mutations have also been reported to be associated with congenital erythrocytosis (Cario et al., 2005; Pastore et al., 2003). In general, these mutations are distinct from those associated with classical VHL disease, and result in a more modest partial loss of function.

An important question is why these *VHL* mutations cause erythrocytosis without the classical tumour syndrome. One possibility is that they have an insufficient effect on HIF levels, with initiation of CCRCC and haemangioblastoma requiring a greater degree of HIF activation. Alternatively, these mutations may preserve some specific function of VHL other than the ubiquitination of HIFα.

In addition to erythrocytosis caused by mutations in *VHL*, two other types of familial erythrocytosis are caused by mutations in the oxygen-sensing pathway, affecting *PHD2* and *HIF2A*. By contrast with *VHL*-associated erythrocytosis, these mutations behave in an autosomal dominant fashion. The first *PHD2* mutation to be described, P317R, results in a loss of function of the enzyme with respect to hydroxylation of both HIF-1α and HIF-2α (Percy et al., 2006). Subsequent mutations have also been shown to have substantial effects on the catalytic domain of the protein (Al-Sheikh et al., 2008; Ladroue et al., 2008; Percy et al., 2007). The erythrocytosis is likely caused by PHD2 haploinsufficiency, implying that the precise level of PHD2 protein is critical for normal EPO regulation in humans (Lee and Percy, 2010).

Mutations in *HIF2A* cause autosomal dominant erythrocytosis via partial gain of function (Gale et al., 2008; Percy et al., 2008b). Thus the G537W mutant impairs PHD2-mediated hydroxylation and subsequent recognition of the hydroxylated HIF-2α by VHL, resulting in normoxic stabilization of HIF-2α (Furlow et al., 2009). The disease-associated mutations in *HIF2A* described thus far are concentrated in a small region located C-terminal to the primary hydroxylacceptor proline residue (Pro-531) (Furlow et al., 2009). These findings are consistent with HIF-2α playing a critical role in the control of red cell mass, through direct effects on EPO regulation (Lee and Percy, 2010).

In patients with classical VHL disease the HIF pathway functions normally in cells throughout the body [An interesting exception are neutrophils, which exhibit a hypoxia-like phenotype in VHL patients, implying that these cells are sensitive to loss of one copy of *VHL* (Walmsley et al., 2006)].

Somatic inactivation of the remaining wild-type allele then results in constitutive HIF activation, but only in that cell and its descendents. In contrast
patients with hereditary erythrocytosis have subtle activation of the HIF
pathway that probably occurs in all cells. Consequently they provide a powerful experiment of nature for determining the effects of the VHL-PHD-HIF
pathway on physiological parameters (Gale et al., 2008; Martini et al., 2008; Percy
et al., 2008a; Smith et al., 2006; Smith et al., 2008).

Pulmonary hypertension has been observed in individual erythrocyto-
sis-causing mutations in *HIF-2A* gene (Gale et al., 2008). Patients with Chuvash
polycythaemia exhibit disordered vascular physiology, showing a higher
incidence of vertebral haemangiomas, varicose veins, lower blood pressures, and elevated serum VEGF concentrations (Gordeuk and Prchal, 2006).
These patients show an exaggerated physiological response to hypoxia,
characterized by abnormalities in respiratory and pulmonary vascular
regulation (Smith et al., 2008). This response is similar to that seen in association with acclimatisation to the hypoxia of altitude and supported by studies of the Chuvash knock-in mouse (see below).

Genetic studies in mice

Given the critical role of *VHL* in the oxygen-sensing pathway, it is not surprising that germline inactivation of *vhlh* in mice is lethal to the embryo.
Understanding the role of *vhlh* in particular cells and tissues has required
more sophisticated approaches, which have provided insight into the role
of *vhlh* in tumourigenesis, erythrocytosis, and development. The different
roles of HIF-1α and HIF-2α in these processes are being determined using
a multiple conditional knockout approach. Importantly, although *VHL* is
considered to have multiple biological functions that do not involve the
HIF pathway, organ pathologies in *vhlh* knockout mice can generally be
reversed by inactivation of *hif-1α* or *hif-2α*.

Germ line inactivation of *vhlh* results in death of the embryo in mid-
gestation. Development of the embryo and placenta appear normal until
embryonic day 9.5. After this time the placenta shows evidence of abnormal
vascularisation, which is subsequently lethal (Gnarra et al., 1997). Germline
inactivation of *phd2* results in a similar, although not identical, phenotype,
suggesting that the *vhlh* -/- phenotype is mediated by HIF (Takeda et al., 2006).
Vhlh also plays a key role in the development of many other tissues, includ-

ing neuro-epithelial progenitor cells and chondrocytes (Kapitsinou and Haase, 2008; Pfander et al., 2004).

Inactivation of just one *vhlh* allele (+/-) results in the development of cavernous liver haemangiomas, a rare manifestation of VHL disease in humans (Haase et al., 2001). This phenotype is strongly dependent on the genetic background of heterozygous mice, suggesting the importance of polymorphic differences in modifier genes (Ma et al., 2003). The mechanism behind this phenotype involves somatic inactivation of the remaining wild-type *vhlh* allele, HIF activation and an increase in HIF-dependent vascular growth factors. Indeed the liver pathology is phenocopied by hepatocyte-specific inactivation of *vhlh* using either Albumin-Cre or PEPCK-Cre transgenes (Peyssonnaux et al., 2007; Rankin et al., 2007).

Renal cysts are a much more common finding in human VHL disease than liver haemangiomas, however they are found at extremely low frequency in *vhlh* +/- mice (Haase et al., 2001; Kleymenova et al., 2004). Moreover, CCRCC, CNS heamangioblastomas, and retinal angiomas were not observed at all. Treatment with streptozotocin did not result in increased susceptibility to renal carcinogenesis, although it did increase the incidence of haemangiomas and heamangiosarcomas in the liver and other organs such as the uterus and ovaries (Kleymenova et al., 2004).

The development of CCRCC has been studied using cell-specific deletion of *vhlh* in adult renal tissues. Mice with bialelic *vhlh* inactivation in the renal epithelium driven by a PEPCK-Cre transgene developed cysts at a very low frequency, and do not develop CCRCC (Rankin et al., 2006). Renal cysts were also seen in the *vhlh/hif-1α* double knockout, but not in the *vhlh/arnt* double knockout, implying that HIF-2α was required for cyst development (Rankin et al., 2006). Renal tumours were not found either when an inducible B-actin promoter-driven Cre was used to generate mice that lacked *vhlh* in a mosaic pattern (Ma et al., 2003).

The absence of renal tumourigenesis in these models is consistent with the development of CCRCC requiring additional genetic events and suggests that there may be important differences in renal tumourigenesis between rodents and humans. Further insight into this comes from studies of conditional inactivation of *fh1* in the mouse kidney, using the Ksp-Cadherin promoter (Pollard et al., 2007). The experiment was undertaken because germline *FH* mutations in humans are associated with Hereditary Leiomatosis and Renal Cancer (HLRCC), in which individuals are predisposed to developing papillary renal tumours (see above). In the mouse, *fh1* inactivation in the renal epithelium results in multiple clonal renal cysts that are much more frequent than those seen when *vhlh* is inactivated. As predicted, the cysts in mice with *fh1* deletion show stabilization of HIFα and up-regulation of HIF-target genes. But the fact that *vhlh* loss results in constitutive HIF activation with only occasional cysts suggests that cyst formation in *fh1* defective mice is mediated by other effects apart from HIF activation.

VHL has been inactivated in multiple other cell types in the mouse, resulting in HIF activation and a range of interesting phenotypes (Kapitsinou and Haase, 2008). In some instances major effects on cellular growth and differentiation are observed. For example, there is a marked pro-apoptotic effect when *vhlh* is inactivated in thymocytes and this is mediated via action of HIF-1α (Biju et al., 2004). Some particularly interesting insights have come from examining the physiological effects of *vhlh* inactivation. For example, deletion of *vhlh* in adult pancreatic β-cells via two independent strategies was shown to impair normal glucose homeostasis, by preventing mitochondrial coupling of glucose uptake to insulin release (Cantley et al., 2009).

To date there has been more success in modelling VHL-related erythrocytosis in mice than classical VHL disease. *Vhlh* +/- mice show normal erythrocytosis, consistent with the fact that complete loss of one *VHL* allele in humans does not significantly alter red cell production. Mice have been generated that are homozygous for the equivalent of the R200W mutation, the most common cause of VHL-associated erythrocytosis in humans (see above). These *vhlh*[R/R] animals survive to adulthood and do show erythrocytosis. *Vhlh*[R/R] mice show up-regulation of HIF-2α in ES cells, and suggest that enhanced expression of key HIF-2α genes promote splenic erythropoesis, with resultant polycythaemia (Hickey et al., 2007). Moreover, physiological studies of these animals have shown evidence of pulmonary vasoconstriction and enhanced normoxic ventilation, similar to that seen in human patients with this mutation (Hickey et al., 2010). Superimposing decreased HIF-2α activity resulted in partial protection against pulmonary vascular remodelling, haemorrhage and oedema.

Using tissue-specific deletion, there is now evidence that inactivation of *phd2* causes near maximal renal, but not hepatic, EPO production and polycythaemia (Takeda et al., 2008). Conditional deletion of all three PHDs in the adult mouse has been shown to be necessary to efficiently activate hepatic Epo production (Minamishima and Kaelin, 2010).

Therapeutic intervention in VHL-defective tumours

Of the many processes influenced by inactivation of VHL, most therapeutic interest in the cancer field has focused on angiogenesis. Stabilization of HIF increases the expression of a number of secreted growth factors, including VEGF, which are critical to the angiogenic phenotype. Growth factors activate receptor tyrosine kinases, leading to a cascade of intracellular signalling events and endothelial cell activation.

Since December 2005 the FDA has approved six therapeutic agents for the treatment of metastatic CCRCC that are believed to block certain consequences of VHL loss-of-function (Linehan et al., 2010a). These targeted therapies have different mechanisms of action and can be divided into three groups.

1. Monoclonal antibodies, such as bevacizumab, which bind VEGF.
2. Small molecules that inhibit the VEGF receptor, such as sorafenib, sunitinib, and axitinib. It should be noted that these also inhibit other kinases that may contribute to their efficacy.
3. mTOR inhibitors, such as temsirolimus and everolimus. Among many other effects, these decrease the activity of HIF-2α and angiogenic signalling in VHL defective cells.

Research is now focussed on the optimal time to start treatment and potential combination therapy, and there are a large number of targeted agents in early clinical studies.

There is considerable interest in small molecules that would decrease HIF activity. Selective antagonism of HIF-2α would be particularly attractive in CCRCC or haemangioblastoma. Although beyond the scope of this chapter, there is also considerable interest in HIF activators to promote survival in a hypoxic environment, such as that seen after a myocardial infarct or cerebrovascular accident (Kaelin, 2007). Such agents are also being investigated for the treatment of anaemia due to relative EPO deficiency, such as that seen in chronic kidney failure (Safran et al., 2006).

Conclusions

The last century has seen significant advancements in our understanding of the molecular pathways by which oxygen levels influence cancer biology. It is well known that tumour hypoxia is often associated with resistance to therapy and poor prognosis. Moreover, increased levels of HIF within tumours are also associated with poor outcomes. A key question has been whether tumour hypoxia and HIF were simply markers of aggressive tumours, or whether they actually had a causal role in promoting malignant behaviour. The study of VHL disease, together with xenograft studies proves that in the renal epithelium, HIF plays a pivotal role in tumour development. Nevertheless we still have much to learn about what other events are involved and which consequences of HIF activation are critical.

A c k n o w l e d g m e n t s _ Work in the author's laboratory has been funded by the British Heart Foundation, Cancer Research UK, the Medical Research Council, the St Peter's Trust, the Wellcome Trust, and the European Commission Framework 7 integrating project METOXIA.

References

Al-Sheikh, M., Moradkhani, K., Lopez, M., Wajcman, H. and Prehu, C. (2008) Disturbance in the HIF-1alpha pathway associated with erythrocytosis: further evidences brought by frameshift and nonsense mutations in the prolyl hydroxylase domain protein 2 (PHD2) gene. Blood Cells Mol Dis, 40, 160-165.

Ang, S.O., Chen, H., Gordeuk, V.R., Sergueeva, A.I., Polyakova, L.A., Miasnikova, G.Y., Kralovics, R., Stockton, D.W. and Prchal, J.T. (2002a) Endemic polycythemia in Russia: mutation in the VHL gene. Blood Cells Mol Dis, 28, 57-62.

Ang, S.O., Chen, H., Hirota, K., Gordeuk, V.R., Jelinek, J., Guan, Y., Liu, E., Sergueeva, A.I., Miasnikova, G.Y., Mole, D., Maxwell, P.H., Stockton, D.W., Semenza, G.L. and Prchal, J.T. (2002b) Disruption of oxygen homeostasis underlies congenital Chuvash polycythemia. Nat Genet, 32, 614-621.

Appelhoff, R.J., Tian, Y.M., Raval, R.R., Turley, H., Harris, A.L., Pugh, C.W., Ratcliffe, P.J. and Gleadle, J.M. (2004) Differential function of the prolyl hydroxylases PHD1, PHD2, and PHD3 in the regulation of hypoxia-inducible factor. J Biol Chem, 279, 38458-38465.

Aprelikova, O., Chandramouli, G.V.R., Wood, M., Vasselli, J.R., Riss, J., Maranchie, J.K., Linehan, W.M. and Barrett, J.C. (2004) Regulation of HIF prolyl hydroxylases by hypoxia-inducible factors. J Cell Biochem, 92, 491-501.

Baba, M., Hirai, S., Yamada-Okabe, H., Hamada, K., Tabuchi, H., Kobayashi, K., Kondo, K., Yoshida, M., Yamashita, A., Kishida, T., Nakaigawa, N., Nagashima, Y., Kubota, Y., Yao, M. and Ohno, S. (2003) Loss of von Hippel-Lindau protein causes cell density dependent deregulation of CyclinD1 expression through hypoxia-inducible factor. Oncogene, 22, 2728-2738.

Berra, E., Benizri, E., Ginouves, A., Volmat, V., Roux, D. and Pouyssegur, J. (2003) HIF prolyl-hydroxylase 2 is the key oxygen sensor setting low steady-state levels of HIF-1alpha in normoxia. Embo J, 22, 4082-4090.

Berse, B., Brown, L.F., Van de Water, L., Dvorak, H.F. and Senger, D.R. (1992) Vascular permeability factor (vascular endothelial growth factor) gene is expressed differentially in normal tissues, macrophages, and tumours. Mol Biol Cell, 3, 211-220.

Bertout, J.A., Patel, S.A. and Simon, M.C. (2008) The impact of O2 availability on human cancer. Nat Rev Cancer, 8, 967-975.

Biju, M.P., Neumann, A.K., Bensinger, S.J., Johnson, R.S., Turka, L.A. and Haase, V.H. (2004) Vhlh gene deletion induces Hif-1-mediated cell death in thymocytes. Mol Cell Biol, 24, 9038-9047.

Blankenship, C., Naglich, J.G., Whaley, J.M., Seizinger, B. and Kley, N. (1999) Alternate choice of initiation codon produces a biologically active product of the von Hippel Lindau gene with tumour suppressor activity. Oncogene, 18, 1529-1535.

Bohling, T., Hatva, E., Kujala, M., Claesson-Welsh, L., Alitalo, K. and Haltia, M. (1996) Expression of growth factors and growth factor receptors in capillary hemangioblastoma. J Neuropathol Exp Neurol, 55, 522-527.

Bonicalzi, M.E., Groulx, I., de Paulsen, N. and Lee, S. (2001) Role of exon 2-encoded beta -domain of the von Hippel-Lindau tumour suppressor protein. J Biol Chem, 276, 1407-1416.

Brown, L.F., Berse, B., Jackman, R.W., Tognazzi, K., Manseau, E.J., Dvorak, H.F. and Senger, D.R. (1993) Increased expression of vascular permeability factor (vascular endothelial growth factor) and its receptors in kidney and bladder carcinomas. Am J Pathol, 143, 1255-1262.

Brugarolas, J.B., Vazquez, F., Reddy, A., Sellers, W.R. and Kaelin, W.G. (2003) TSC2 regulates VEGF through mTOR-dependent and -independent pathways. Cancer Cell, 4, 147-158.

Bruick, R.K. and McKnight, S.L. (2001) A conserved family of prolyl-4-hydroxylases that modify HIF. Science, 294, 1337-1340.

Bryant, J., Farmer, J., Kessler, L.J., Townsend, R.R. and Nathanson, K.L. (2003) Pheochromocytoma: the expanding genetic differential diagnosis. J Natl Cancer Inst, 95, 1196-1204.

Cai, Q. and Robertson, E.S. (2010) Ubiquitin/SUMO modification regulates VHL protein stability and nucleocytoplasmic localization. PLoS One, 5 e12636.

Cai, Q., Verma, S.C., Kumar, P., Ma, M. and Robertson, E.S. (2010) Hypoxia inactivates the VHL tumour suppressor through PIASy-mediated SUMO modification. PLoS One, 5, e9720.

Cantley, J., Selman, C., Shukla, D., Abramov, A.Y., Forstreuter, F., Esteban, M.A., Claret, M., Lingard, S.J., Clements, M., Harten, S.K., Asare-Anane, H., Batterham, R.L.,

Herrera, P.L., Persaud, S.J., Duchen, M.R., Maxwell, P.H. and Withers, D.J. (2009) Deletion of the von Hippel-Lindau gene in pancreatic beta cells impairs glucose homeostasis in mice. J Clin Invest, 119, 125-135.

Cario, H., Schwarz, K., Jorch, N., Kyank, U., Petrides, P.E., Schneider, D.T., Uhle, R., Debatin, K.M. and Kohne, E. (2005) Mutations in the von Hippel-Lindau (VHL) tumour suppressor gene and VHL-haplotype analysis in patients with presumable congenital erythrocytosis. Haematologica, 90, 19-24.

Cascon, A., Pita, G., Burnichon, N., Landa, I., Lopez-Jimenez, E., Montero-Conde, C., Leskela, S., Leandro-Garcia, L.J., Leton, R., Rodriguez-Antona, C., Diaz, J.A., Lopez-Vidriero, E., Gonzalez-Neira, A., Velasco, A., Matias-Guiu, X., Gimenez-Roqueplo, A.P. and Robledo, M. (2009) Genetics of pheochromocytoma and paraganglioma in Spanish patients. J Clin Endocrinol Metab, 94, 1701-1705.

Chan, C.C., Vortmeyer, A.O., Chew, E.Y., Green, W.R., Matteson, D.M., Shen, D.F., Linehan, W.M., Lubensky, I.A. and Zhuang, Z. (1999) VHL gene deletion and enhanced VEGF gene expression detected in the stromal cells of retinal angioma. Arch Ophthalmol, 117, 625-630.

Chen, S., Sanford, C.A., Sun, J., Choi, V., Van Dyke, T., Samulski, R.J. and Rathmell, W.K. (2010) VHL and PTEN loss coordinate to promote mouse liver vascular lesions. Angiogenesis, 13, 59-69.

Choyke, P.L., Glenn, G.M., Walther, M.M., Patronas, N.J., Linehan, W.M. and Zbar, B. (1995) von Hippel-Lindau disease: genetic, clinical, and imaging features. Radiology, 194, 629-642.

Cioffi, C.L., Liu, X.Q., Kosinski, P.A., Garay, M. and Bowen, B.R. (2003) Differential regulation of HIF-1 alpha prolyl-4-hydroxylase genes by hypoxia in human cardiovascular cells. 303, 947-953.

Clifford, S.C., Cockman, M.E., Smallwood, A.C., Mole, D.R., Woodward, E.R., Maxwell, P.H., Ratcliffe, P.J. and Maher, E.R. (2001) Contrasting effects on HIF-1alpha regulation by disease-causing pVHL mutations correlate with patterns of tumourigenesis in von Hippel-Lindau disease. Hum Mol Genet, 10, 1029-1038.

Corless, C.L., Kibel, A.S., Iliopoulos, O. and Kaelin, W.G. (1997) Immunostaining of the von Hippel-Lindau gene product in normal and neoplastic human tissues. Hum Pathol, 28, 459-464.

Covello, K.L., Kehler, J., Yu, H., Gordan, J.D., Arsham, A.M., Hu, C.-J., Labosky, P.A., Simon, M.C. and Keith, B. (2006) HIF-2alpha regulates Oct-4: effects of hypoxia on stem cell function, embryonic development, and tumour growth. Genes Dev, 20, 557-570.

Crino, P.B., Nathanson, K.L. and Henske, E.P. (2006) The tuberous sclerosis complex. N Engl J Med, 355, 1345-1356.

Crossey, P.A., Richards, F.M., Foster, K., Green, J.S., Prowse, A., Latif, F., Lerman, M.I., Zbar, B., Affara, N.A. and Ferguson-Smith, M.A. (1994) Identification of intragenic mutations in the von Hippel-Lindau disease tumour suppressor gene and correlation with disease phenotype. Hum Mol Genet, 3, 1303-1308.

Dalgliesh, G.L., Furge, K., Greenman, C., Chen, L., Bignell, G., Butler, A., Davies, H., Edkins, S., Hardy, C., Latimer, C., Teague, J., Andrews, J., Barthorpe, S., Beare, D.,

Buck, G., Campbell, P.J., Forbes, S., Jia, M., Jones, D., Knott, H., Kok, C.Y., Lau, K.W., Leroy, C., Lin, M.L., McBride, D.J., Maddison, M., Maguire, S., McLay, K., Menzies, A., Mironenko, T., Mulderrig, L., Mudie, L., O'Meara, S., Pleasance, E., Rajasingham, A., Shepherd, R., Smith, R., Stebbings, L., Stephens, P., Tang, G., Tarpey, P.S., Turrell, K., Dykema, K.J., Khoo, S.K., Petillo, D., Wondergem, B., Anema, J., Kahnoski, R.J., Teh, B.T., Stratton, M.R. and Futreal, P.A. (2010) Systematic sequencing of renal carcinoma reveals inactivation of histone modifying genes. Nature, 463, 360-363.

Davidowitz, E.J., Schoenfeld, A.R. and Burk, R.D. (2001) VHL induces renal cell differentiation and growth arrest through integration of cell-cell and cell-extracellular matrix signalling. Mol Cell Biol, 21, 865-874.

Dechant, G. (2002) Chat in the trophic web: NGF activates Ret by inter-RTK signalling. Neuron, 33, 156-158.

Duan, D.R., Humphrey, J.S., Chen, D.Y., Weng, Y., Sukegawa, J., Lee, S., Gnarra, J.R., Linehan, W.M. and Klausner, R.D. (1995a) Characterization of the VHL tumour suppressor gene product: localization, complex formation, and the effect of natural inactivating mutations. Proc Natl Acad Sci U S A, 92, 6459-6463.

Duan, D.R., Pause, A., Burgess, W.H., Aso, T., Chen, D.Y., Garrett, K.P., Conaway, R.C., Conaway, J.W., Linehan, W.M. and Klausner, R.D. (1995b) Inhibition of transcription elongation by the VHL tumour suppressor protein. Science, 269, 1402-1406.

Eley, L., Yates, L.M. and Goodship, J.A. (2005) Cilia and disease. Curr Opin Genet Dev, 15, 308-314.

Epstein, A.C., Gleadle, J.M., McNeill, L.A., Hewitson, K.S., O'Rourke, J., Mole, D.R., Mukherji, M., Metzen, E., Wilson, M.I., Dhanda, A., Tian, Y.M., Masson, N., Hamilton, D.L., Jaakkola, P., Barstead, R., Hodgkin, J., Maxwell, P.H., Pugh, C.W., Schofield, C.J. and Ratcliffe, P.J. (2001) C. elegans EGL-9 and mammalian homologs define a family of dioxygenases that regulate HIF by prolyl hydroxylation. Cell, 107, 43-54.

Esteban, M.A., Harten, S.K., Tran, M.G. and Maxwell, P.H. (2006a) Formation of primary cilia in the renal epithelium is regulated by the von Hippel-Lindau tumour suppressor protein. J Am Soc Nephrol, 17, 1801-1806.

Esteban, M.A., Tran, M.G.B., Harten, S.K., Hill, P., Castellanos, M.C., Chandra, A., Raval, R., O'Brien, T.S. and Maxwell, P.H. (2006b) Regulation of E-cadherin expression by VHL and hypoxia-inducible factor. Cancer Res, 66, 3567-3575.

Estus, S., Zaks, W.J., Freeman, R.S., Gruda, M., Bravo, R. and Johnson, E.M. (1994) Altered gene expression in neurons during programmed cell death: identification of c-jun as necessary for neuronal apoptosis. J Cell Biol, 127, 1717-1727.

Evans, A.J., Russell, R.C., Roche, O., Burry, T.N., Fish, J.E., Chow, V.W.K., Kim, W.Y., Saravanan, A., Maynard, M.A., Gervais, M.L., Sufan, R.I., Roberts, A.M., Wilson, L.A., Betten, M., Vandewalle, C., Berx, G., Marsden, P.A., Irwin, M.S., Teh, B.T., Jewett, M.A.S. and Ohh, M. (2007) VHL promotes E2 box-dependent E-cadherin transcription by HIF-mediated regulation of SIP1 and snail. Mol Cell Biol, 27, 157-169.

Filling-Katz, M.R., Choyke, P.L., Oldfield, E., Charnas, L., Patronas, N.J., Glenn, G.M., Gorin, M.B., Morgan, J.K., Linehan, W.M., Seizinger, B.R. and et al. (1991) Central nervous system involvement in Von Hippel-Lindau disease. Neurology, 41, 41-46.

Frew, I.J. and Krek, W. (2008) pVHL: a multipurpose adaptor protein. Sci Signal, 1, pe30.

Fukino, K., Teramoto, A., Adachi, K., Takahashi, H. and Emi, M. (2000) A family with hydrocephalus as a complication of cerebellar hemangioblastoma: identification of Pro157Leu mutation in the VHL gene. J Hum Genet, 45, 47-51.

Furlow, P.W., Percy, M.J., Sutherland, S., Bierl, C., McMullin, M.F., Master, S.R., Lappin, T.R.J. and Lee, F.S. (2009) Erythrocytosis-associated HIF-2alpha mutations demonstrate a critical role for residues C-terminal to the hydroxylacceptor proline. J Biol Chem, 284, 9050-9058.

Gale, D.P., Harten, S.K., Reid, C.D.L., Tuddenham, E.G.D. and Maxwell, P.H. (2008) Autosomal dominant erythrocytosis and pulmonary arterial hypertension associated with an activating HIF2 alpha mutation. Blood, 112, 919-921.

Garcia, A., Matias-Guiu, X., Cabezas, R., Chico, A., Prat, J., Baiget, M. and De Leiva, A. (1997) Molecular diagnosis of von Hippel-Lindau disease in a kindred with a predominance of familial phaeochromocytoma. Clin Endocrinol (Oxf), 46, 359-363.

Gerald, D., Berra, E., Frapart, Y.M., Chan, D.A., Giaccia, A.J., Mansuy, D., Pouyssegur, J., Yaniv, M. and Mechta-Grigoriou, F. (2004) JunD reduces tumour angiogenesis by protecting cells from oxidative stress. Cell, 118, 781-794.

Giles, R.H., Lolkema, M.P., Snijckers, C.M., Belderbos, M., van der Groep, P., Mans, D.A., van Beest, M., van Noort, M., Goldschmeding, R., van Diest, P.J., Clevers, H. and Voest, E.E. (2006) Interplay between VHL/HIF1alpha and Wnt/beta-catenin pathways during colorectal tumourigenesis. Oncogene, 25, 3065-3070.

Gimenez-Roqueplo, A.P., Favier, J., Rustin, P., Mourad, J.J., Plouin, P.F., Corvol, P., Rotig, A. and Jeunemaitre, X. (2001) The R22X mutation of the SDHD gene in hereditary paraganglioma abolishes the enzymatic activity of complex II in the mitochondrial respiratory chain and activates the hypoxia pathway. Am J Hum Genet, 69, 1186-1197.

Glenn, G.M., Daniel, L.N., Choyke, P., Linehan, W.M., Oldfield, E., Gorin, M.B., Hosoe, S., Latif, F., Weiss, G., Walther, M. and et al. (1991) Von Hippel-Lindau (VHL) disease: distinct phenotypes suggest more than one mutant allele at the VHL locus. Hum Genet, 87, 207-210.

Gnarra, J.R., Tory, K., Weng, Y., Schmidt, L., Wei, M.H., Li, H., Latif, F., Liu, S., Chen, F. and Duh, F.M. (1994) Mutations of the VHL tumour suppressor gene in renal carcinoma. Nat Genet, 7, 85-90.

Gnarra, J.R., Ward, J.M., Porter, F.D., Wagner, J.R., Devor, D.E., Grinberg, A., Emmert-Buck, M.R., Westphal, H., Klausner, R.D. and Linehan, W.M. (1997) Defective placental vasculogenesis causes embryonic lethality in VHL-deficient mice. Proc Natl Acad Sci U S A, 94, 9102-9107.

Gordan, J.D., Bertout, J.A., Hu, C.-J., Diehl, J.A. and Simon, M.C. (2007) HIF-2alpha promotes hypoxic cell proliferation by enhancing c-myc transcriptional activity. Cancer Cell, 11, 335-347.

Gordeuk, V.R. and Prchal, J.T. (2006) Vascular complications in Chuvash polycythemia. Semin Thromb Hemost, 32, 289-294.

Gordeuk, V.R., Sergueeva, A.I., Miasnikova, G.Y., Okhotin, D., Voloshin, Y., Choyke,

P.L., Butman, J.A., Jedlickova, K., Prchal, J.T. and Polyakova, L.A. (2004) Congenital disorder of oxygen sensing: association of the homozygous Chuvash polycythemia VHL mutation with thrombosis and vascular abnormalities but not tumours. Blood, 103, 3924-3932.

Grosfeld, A., Stolze, I.P., Cockman, M.E., Pugh, C.W., Edelmann, M., Kessler, B., Bullock, A.N., Ratcliffe, P.J. and Masson, N. (2007) Interaction of hydroxylated collagen IV with the von hippel-lindau tumour suppressor. J Biol Chem, 282, 13264-13269.

Groulx, I., Bonicalzi, M.E. and Lee, S. (2000) Ran-mediated nuclear export of the von Hippel-Lindau tumour suppressor protein occurs independently of its assembly with cullin-2. J Biol Chem, 275, 8991-9000.

Groulx, I. and Lee, S. (2002) Oxygen-dependent ubiquitination and degradation of hypoxia-inducible factor requires nuclear-cytoplasmic trafficking of the von Hippel-Lindau tumour suppressor protein. Mol Cell Biol, 22, 5319-5336.

Gruber, M.B., Healey, G.B., Toguri, A.G. and Warren, M.M. (1980) Papillary cystadenoma of epididymis: component of von Hippel-Lindau syndrome. Urology, 16, 305-306.

Guo, Y., Schoell, M.C. and Freeman, R.S. (2009) The von Hippel-Lindau protein sensitizes renal carcinoma cells to apoptotic stimuli through stabilization of BIM(EL). Oncogene, 28, 1864-1874.

Gustafsson, M.V., Zheng, X., Pereira, T., Gradin, K., Jin, S., Lundkvist, J., Ruas, J.L., Poellinger, L., Lendahl, U. and Bondesson, M. (2005) Hypoxia requires notch signalling to maintain the undifferentiated cell state. Dev Cell, 9, 617-628.

Guzy, R.D., Hoyos, B., Robin, E., Chen, H., Liu, L., Mansfield, K.D., Simon, M.C., Hammerling, U. and Schumacker, P.T. (2005) Mitochondrial complex III is required for hypoxia-induced ROS production and cellular oxygen sensing Exp Physiol. 1, 401-408.

Guzy, R.D. and Schumacker, P.T. (2006) Oxygen sensing by mitochondria at complex III: the paradox of increased reactive oxygen species during hypoxia. 91, 807-819.

Haase, V.H., Glickman, J.N., Socolovsky, M. and Jaenisch, R. (2001) Vascular tumours in livers with targeted inactivation of the von Hippel-Lindau tumour suppressor. Proc Natl Acad Sci U S A, 98, 1583-1588.

Ham, J., Babij, C., Whitfield, J., Pfarr, C.M., Lallemand, D., Yaniv, M. and Rubin, L.L. (1995) A c-Jun dominant negative mutant protects sympathetic neurons against programmed cell death. Neuron, 14, 927-939.

Hamanaka, R.B. and Chandel, N.S. (2009) Mitochondrial reactive oxygen species regulate hypoxic signalling. Curr Opin Cell Biol, 21, 894-899.

Harten, S.K., Shukla, D., Barod, R., Hergovich, A., Balda, M.S., Matter, K., Esteban, M.A. and Maxwell, P.H. (2009) Regulation of renal epithelial tight junctions by the von Hippel-Lindau tumour suppressor gene involves occludin and claudin 1 and is independent of E-cadherin. Mol Biol Cell, 20, 1089-1101.

Hergovich, A., Lisztwan, J., Barry, R., Ballschmieter, P. and Krek, W. (2003) Regulation of microtubule stability by the von Hippel-Lindau tumour suppressor protein pVHL. Nat Cell Biol, 5, 64-70.

Herman, J.G., Latif, F., Weng, Y., Lerman, M.I., Zbar, B., Liu, S., Samid, D., Duan, D.S.,

Gnarra, J.R. and Linehan, W.M. (1994) Silencing of the VHL tumour-suppressor gene by DNA methylation in renal carcinoma. Proc Natl Acad Sci U S A, 91, 9700-9704.

Hes, F.J., Lips, C.J. and van der Luijt, R.B. (2001) Molecular genetic aspects of Von Hippel-Lindau (VHL) disease and criteria for DNA analysis in subjects at risk. Neth J Med, 59, 235-243.

Hes, F.J., McKee, S., Taphoorn, M.J., Rehal, P., van Der Luijt, R.B., McMahon, R., van Der Smagt, J.J., Dow, D., Zewald, R.A., Whittaker, J., Lips, C.J., MacDonald, F., Pearson, P.L. and Maher, E.R. (2000) Cryptic von Hippel-Lindau disease: germline mutations in patients with haemangioblastoma only. J Med Genet, 37, 939-943.

Hes, F.J., van der Luijt, R.B., Janssen, A.L.W., Zewald, R.A., de Jong, G.J., Lenders, J.W., Links, T.P., Luyten, G.P.M., Sijmons, R.H., Eussen, H.J., Halley, D.J.J., Lips, C.J.M., Pearson, P.L., van den Ouweland, A.M.W. and Majoor-Krakauer, D.F. (2007) Frequency of Von Hippel-Lindau germline mutations in classic and non-classic Von Hippel-Lindau disease identified by DNA sequencing, Southern blot analysis and multiplex ligation-dependent probe amplification. Clin Genet, 72, 122-129.

Hickey, M.M., Lam, J.C., Bezman, N.A., Rathmell, W.K. and Simon, M.C. (2007) von Hippel-Lindau mutation in mice recapitulates Chuvash polycythemia via hypoxia-inducible factor-2alpha signalling and splenic erythropoiesis. J Clin Invest, 117, 3879-3889.

Hickey, M.M., Richardson, T., Wang, T., Mosqueira, M., Arguiri, E., Yu, H., Yu, Q.C., Solomides, C.C., Morrisey, E.E., Khurana, T.S., Christofidou-Solomidou, M. and Simon, M.C. (2010) The von Hippel-Lindau Chuvash mutation promotes pulmonary hypertension and fibrosis in mice. J Clin Invest, 120, 827-839.

Hirsila, M., Koivunen, P., Gunzler, V., Kivirikko, K.I. and Myllyharju, J. (2003) Characterization of the human prolyl 4-hydroxylases that modify the hypoxia-inducible factor. J Biol Chem, 278, 30772-30780.

Hoffman, M.A., Ohh, M., Yang, H., Klco, J.M., Ivan, M. and Kaelin, W.G. (2001) von Hippel-Lindau protein mutants linked to type 2C VHL disease preserve the ability to downregulate HIF. Hum Mol Genet, 10, 1019-1027.

Hon, W.-C., Wilson, M.I., Harlos, K., Claridge, T.D.W., Schofield, C.J., Pugh, C.W., Maxwell, P.H., Ratcliffe, P.J., Stuart, D.I. and Jones, E.Y. (2002) Structural basis for the recognition of hydroxyproline in HIF-1 alpha by pVHL. Nature, 417, 975-978.

Hough, D.M., Stephens, D.H., Johnson, C.D. and Binkovitz, L.A. (1994) Pancreatic lesions in von Hippel-Lindau disease: prevalence, clinical significance, and CT findings. AJR Am J Roentgenol, 162, 1091-1094.

Iliopoulos, O., Kibel, A., Gray, S. and Kaelin, W.G. (1995) Tumour suppression by the human von Hippel-Lindau gene product. Nat Med, 1, 822-826.

Iliopoulos, O., Levy, A.P., Jiang, C., Kaelin, W.G. and Goldberg, M.A. (1996) Negative regulation of hypoxia-inducible genes by the von Hippel-Lindau protein. Proc Natl Acad Sci U S A, 93, 10595-10599.

Iliopoulos, O., Ohh, M. and Kaelin, W.G. (1998) pVHL19 is a biologically active product of the von Hippel-Lindau gene arising from internal translation initiation. Proc Natl Acad Sci U S A, 95, 11661-11666.

Isaacs, J.S., Jung, Y.J., Mole, D.R., Lee, S., Torres-Cabala, C., Chung, Y.L., Merino, M.,

Trepel, J., Zbar, B., Toro, J., Ratcliffe, P.J., Linehan, W.M. and Neckers, L. (2005) HIF overexpression correlates with biallelic loss of fumarate hydratase in renal cancer: novel role of fumarate in regulation of HIF stability. Cancer Cell, 8, 143-153.

Ivan, M., Kondo, K., Yang, H., Kim, W., Valiando, J., Ohh, M., Salic, A., Asara, J.M., Lane, W.S. and Kaelin , W.G. (2001) HIFalpha targeted for VHL-mediated destruction by proline hydroxylation: implications for O2 sensing. Science, 292, 464-468.

Jaakkola, P., Mole, D.R., Tian, Y.M., Wilson, M.I., Gielbert, J., Gaskell, S.J., Kriegsheim, A., Hebestreit, H.F., Mukherji, M., Schofield, C.J., Maxwell, P.H., Pugh, C.W. and Ratcliffe, P.J. (2001) Targeting of HIF-alpha to the von Hippel-Lindau ubiquitylation complex by O2-regulated prolyl hydroxylation. Science, 292, 468-472.

Jagannathan, J., Lonser, R.R., Smith, R., DeVroom, H.L. and Oldfield, E.H. (2008) Surgical management of cerebellar hemangioblastomas in patients with von Hippel-Lindau disease. J Neurosurg, 108, 210-222.

Kaelin, W.G. (2007) Von Hippel-Lindau disease. Annu Rev Pathol, 2, 145-173.

Kaelin, W.G., Jr. (2004) The von Hippel-Lindau tumour suppressor gene and kidney cancer. Clin Cancer Res, 10, 6290S-6295S.

Kamura, T., Conrad, M.N., Yan, Q., Conaway, R.C. and Conaway, J.W. (1999a) The Rbx1 subunit of SCF and VHL E3 ubiquitin ligase activates Rub1 modification of cullins Cdc53 and Cul2. Genes Dev, 13, 2928-2933.

Kamura, T., Koepp, D.M., Conrad, M.N., Skowyra, D., Moreland, R.J., Iliopoulos, O., Lane, W.S., Kaelin, W.G., Elledge, S.J., Conaway, R.C., Harper, J.W. and Conaway, J.W. (1999b) Rbx1, a component of the VHL tumour suppressor complex and SCF ubiquitin ligase. Science, 284, 657-661.

Kanno, H., Kondo, K., Ito, S., Yamamoto, I., Fujii, S., Torigoe, S., Sakai, N., Hosaka, M., Shuin, T. and Yao, M. (1994) Somatic mutations of the von Hippel-Lindau tumour suppressor gene in sporadic central nervous system hemangioblastomas. Cancer Res, 54, 4845-4847.

Kapitsinou, P.P. and Haase, V.H. (2008) The VHL tumour suppressor and HIF: insights from genetic studies in mice. Cell Death Differ, 15, 650-659.

Kibel, A., Iliopoulos, O., DeCaprio, J.A. and Kaelin, W.G. (1995) Binding of the von Hippel-Lindau tumour suppressor protein to Elongin B and C. Science, 269, 1444-1446.

Kim, W.Y. and Kaelin, W.G. (2004) Role of VHL gene mutation in human cancer. J Clin Oncol, 22, 4991-5004.

Klein, B., Weirich, G. and Brauch, H. (2001) DHPLC-based germline mutation screening in the analysis of the VHL tumour suppressor gene: usefulness and limitations. Hum Genet, 108, 376-384.

Kleymenova, E., Everitt, J.I., Pluta, L., Portis, M., Gnarra, J.R. and Walker, C.L. (2004) Susceptibility to vascular neoplasms but no increased susceptibility to renal carcinogenesis in Vhl knockout mice. Carcinogenesis, 25, 309-315.

Knauth, K., Bex, C., Jemth, P. and Buchberger, A. (2006) Renal cell carcinoma risk in type 2 von Hippel-Lindau disease correlates with defects in pVHL stability and HIF-1alpha interactions. Oncogene, 25, 370-377.

Knowles, H.J., Raval, R.R., Harris, A.L. and Ratcliffe, P.J. (2003) Effect of ascorbate on the activity of hypoxia-inducible factor in cancer cells. Cancer Res, 63, 1764-1768.

Knudson, A.G., Jr. (1971) Mutation and cancer: statistical study of retinoblastoma. Proc Natl Acad Sci U S A, 68, 820-823.

Kondo, K., Kim, W.Y., Lechpammer, M. and Kaelin, W.G. (2003) Inhibition of HIF2alpha is sufficient to suppress pVHL-defective tumour growth. PLoS Biol, 1, E83.

Kondo, K., Klco, J., Nakamura, E., Lechpammer, M. and Kaelin, W.G. (2002) Inhibition of HIF is necessary for tumour suppression by the von Hippel-Lindau protein. Cancer Cell, 1, 237-246.

Koshiji, M., Kageyama, Y., Pete, E.A., Horikawa, I., Barrett, J.C. and Huang, L.E. (2004) HIF-1alpha induces cell cycle arrest by functionally counteracting Myc. Embo J, 23, 1949-1956.

Krieg, M., Marti, H.H. and Plate, K.H. (1998) Coexpression of erythropoietin and vascular endothelial growth factor in nervous system tumours associated with von Hippel-Lindau tumour suppressor gene loss of function. Blood, 92, 3388-3393.

Krishnamachary, B., Zagzag, D., Nagasawa, H., Rainey, K., Okuyama, H., Baek, J.H. and Semenza, G.L. (2006) Hypoxia-inducible factor-1-dependent repression of E-cadherin in von Hippel-Lindau tumour suppressor-null renal cell carcinoma mediated by TCF3, ZFHX1A, and ZFHX1B. Cancer Res, 66, 2725-2731.

Kurban, G., Duplan, E., Ramlal, N., Hudon, V., Sado, Y., Ninomiya, Y. and Pause, A. (2008) Collagen matrix assembly is driven by the interaction of von Hippel-Lindau tumour suppressor protein with hydroxylated collagen IV alpha 2. Oncogene, 27, 1004-1012.

Kuzmin, I., Duh, F.M., Latif, F., Geil, L., Zbar, B. and Lerman, M.I. (1995) Identification of the promoter of the human von Hippel-Lindau disease tumour suppressor gene. Oncogene, 10, 2185-2194.

Kuznetsova, A.V., Meller, J., Schnell, P.O., Nash, J.A., Ignacak, M.L., Sanchez, Y., Conaway, J.W., Conaway, R.C. and Czyzyk-Krzeska, M.F. (2003) von Hippel-Lindau protein binds hyperphosphorylated large subunit of RNA polymerase II through a proline hydroxylation motif and targets it for ubiquitination. Proc Natl Acad Sci U S A, 100, 2706-2711.

Ladroue, C., Carcenac, R., Leporrier, M., Gad, S., Le Hello, C., Galateau-Salle, F., Feunteun, J., Pouyssegur, J., Richard, S. and Gardie, B. (2008) PHD2 mutation and congenital erythrocytosis with paraganglioma. N Engl J Med, 359, 2685-2692.

Latif, F., Tory, K., Gnarra, J., Yao, M., Duh, F.M., Orcutt, M.L., Stackhouse, T., Kuzmin, I., Modi, W. and Geil, L. (1993) Identification of the von Hippel-Lindau disease tumour suppressor gene. Science, 260, 1317-1320.

Lee, F.S. and Percy, M.J. (2010) The HIF Pathway and Erythrocytosis. Annu Rev Pathol.

Lee, S., Chen, D.Y., Humphrey, J.S., Gnarra, J.R., Linehan, W.M. and Klausner, R.D. (1996) Nuclear/cytoplasmic localization of the von Hippel-Lindau tumour suppressor gene product is determined by cell density. Proc Natl Acad Sci U S A, 93, 1770-1775.

Lee, S., Nakamura, E., Yang, H., Wei, W., Linggi, M.S., Sajan, M.P., Farese, R.V., Freeman, R.S., Carter, B.D., Kaelin, W.G. and Schlisio, S. (2005) Neuronal apoptosis linked to EglN3 prolyl hydroxylase and familial pheochromocytoma genes: developmental culling and cancer. Cancer Cell, 8, 155-167.

Lee, S., Neumann, M., Stearman, R., Stauber, R., Pause, A., Pavlakis, G.N. and Klausner, R.D. (1999) Transcription-dependent nuclear-cytoplasmic trafficking is required for the function of the von Hippel-Lindau tumour suppressor protein. Mol Cell Biol, 19, 1486-1497.

Lewis, M.D. and Roberts, B.J. (2003) Role of nuclear and cytoplasmic localization in the tumour-suppressor activity of the von Hippel-Lindau protein. Oncogene, 22, 3992-3997.

Lieubeau-Teillet, B., Rak, J., Jothy, S., Iliopoulos, O., Kaelin, W. and Kerbel, R.S. (1998) von Hippel-Lindau gene-mediated growth suppression and induction of differentiation in renal cell carcinoma cells grown as multicellular tumour spheroids. Cancer Res, 58, 4957-4962.

Linehan, W.M., Bratslavsky, G., Pinto, P.A., Schmidt, L.S., Neckers, L., Bottaro, D.P. and Srinivasan, R. (2010a) Molecular diagnosis and therapy of kidney cancer. Annu Rev Med, 61, 329-343.

Linehan, W.M., Srinivasan, R. and Schmidt, L.S. (2010b) The genetic basis of kidney cancer: a metabolic disease. Nat Rev Urol, 7, 277-285.

Linehan, W.M. and Zbar, B. (2004) Focus on kidney cancer. Cancer Cell, 6, 223-228.

Lolkema, M.P., Gervais, M.L., Snijckers, C.M., Hill, R.P., Giles, R.H., Voest, E.E. and Ohh, M. (2005) Tumour suppression by the von Hippel-Lindau protein requires phosphorylation of the acidic domain. J Biol Chem, 280, 22205-22211.

Lolkema, M.P., Mans, D.A., Snijckers, C.M., van Noort, M., van Beest, M., Voest, E.E. and Giles, R.H. (2007) The von Hippel-Lindau tumour suppressor interacts with microtubules through kinesin-2. FEBS Lett, 581, 4571-4576.

Lolkema, M.P., Mehra, N., Jorna, A.S., van Beest, M., Giles, R.H. and Voest, E.E. (2004) The von Hippel-Lindau tumour suppressor protein influences microtubule dynamics at the cell periphery. Exp Cell Res, 301, 139-146.

Lonergan, K.M., Iliopoulos, O., Ohh, M., Kamura, T., Conaway, R.C., Conaway, J.W. and Kaelin, W.G. (1998) Regulation of hypoxia-inducible mRNAs by the von Hippel-Lindau tumour suppressor protein requires binding to complexes containing elongins B/C and Cul2. Mol Cell Biol, 18, 732-741.

Lonser, R.R., Glenn, G.M., Walther, M., Chew, E.Y., Libutti, S.K., Linehan, W.M. and Oldfield, E.H. (2003) von Hippel-Lindau disease. Lancet, 361, 2059-2067.

Los, M., Jansen, G.H., Kaelin, W.G., Lips, C.J., Blijham, G.H. and Voest, E.E. (1996) Expression pattern of the von Hippel-Lindau protein in human tissues. Lab Invest, 75, 231-238.

Lubensky, I.A., Pack, S., Ault, D., Vortmeyer, A.O., Libutti, S.K., Choyke, P.L., Walther, M.M., Linehan, W.M. and Zhuang, Z. (1998) Multiple neuroendocrine tumours of the pancreas in von Hippel-Lindau disease patients: histopathological and molecular genetic analysis. Am J Pathol, 153, 223-231.

Ma, W., Tessarollo, L., Hong, S.-B., Baba, M., Southon, E., Back, T.C., Spence, S., Lobe, C.G., Sharma, N., Maher, G.W., Pack, S., Vortmeyer, A.O., Guo, C., Zbar, B. and Schmidt, L.S. (2003) Hepatic vascular tumours, angiectasis in multiple organs, and impaired spermatogenesis in mice with conditional inactivation of the VHL gene. Cancer Res, 63, 5320-5328.

Mack, F.A., Patel, J.H., Biju, M.P., Haase, V.H. and Simon, M.C. (2005) Decreased growth of Vhl-/- fibrosarcomas is associated with elevated levels of cyclin kinase inhibitors p21 and p27. Mol Cell Biol, 25, 4565-4578.

Mahajan, S., Dammai, V., Hsu, T. and Kraft, A.S. (2008) Hypoxia-inducible factor-2alpha regulates the expression of TRAIL receptor DR5 in renal cancer cells. Carcinogenesis, 29, 1734-1741.

Maher, E.R. (2004) Von Hippel-Lindau disease. Curr Mol Med, 4, 833-842.

Maher, E.R. and Eng, C. (2002) The pressure rises: update on the genetics of phaeochromocytoma. Hum Mol Genet, 11, 2347-2354.

Maher, E.R., Iselius, L., Yates, J.R., Littler, M., Benjamin, C., Harris, R., Sampson, J., Williams, A., Ferguson-Smith, M.A. and Morton, N. (1991) Von Hippel-Lindau disease: a genetic study. J Med Genet, 28, 443-447.

Maher, E.R., Yates, J.R., Harries, R., Benjamin, C., Harris, R., Moore, A.T. and Ferguson-Smith, M.A. (1990) Clinical features and natural history of von Hippel-Lindau disease. Q J Med, 77, 1151-1163.

Mandriota, S.J., Turner, K.J., Davies, D.R., Murray, P.G., Morgan, N.V., Sowter, H.M., Wykoff, C.C., Maher, E.R., Harris, A.L., Ratcliffe, P.J. and Maxwell, P.H. (2002) HIF activation identifies early lesions in VHL kidneys: evidence for site-specific tumour suppressor function in the nephron. Cancer Cell, 1, 459-468.

Mans, D.A., Lolkema, M.P., van Beest, M., Daenen, L.G., Voest, E.E. and Giles, R.H. (2008) Mobility of the von Hippel-Lindau tumour suppressor protein is regulated by kinesin-2. Exp Cell Res, 314, 1229-1236.

Mansfield, K.D., Guzy, R.D., Pan, Y., Young, R.M., Cash, T.P., Schumacker, P.T. and Simon, M.C. (2005) Mitochondrial dysfunction resulting from loss of cytochrome c impairs cellular oxygen sensing and hypoxic HIF-alpha activation. 1, 393-399.

Martini, M., Teofili, L., Cenci, T., Giona, F., Torti, L., Rea, M., Foà, R., Leone, G. and Larocca, L.M. (2008) A novel heterozygous HIF2AM535I mutation reinforces the role of oxygen sensing pathway disturbances in the pathogenesis of familial erythrocytosis. Haematologica, 93, 1068-1071.

Marxsen, J.H., Stengel, P., Doege, K., Heikkinen, P., Jokilehto, T., Wagner, T., Jelkmann, W., Jaakkola, P. and Metzen, E. (2004) Hypoxia-inducible factor-1 (HIF-1) promotes its degradation by induction of HIF-alpha-prolyl-4-hydroxylases. Biochem J, 381, 761-767.

Masson, N., Willam, C., Maxwell, P.H., Pugh, C.W. and Ratcliffe, P.J. (2001) Independent function of two destruction domains in hypoxia-inducible factor-alpha chains activated by prolyl hydroxylation. EMBO J, 20, 5197-5206.

Maxwell, P.H., Pugh, C.W. and Ratcliffe, P.J. (2001) The pVHL-hIF-1 system. A key mediator of oxygen homeostasis. Adv Exp Med Biol, 502, 365-376.

Maxwell, P.H., Wiesener, M.S., Chang, G.W., Clifford, S.C., Vaux, E.C., Cockman, M.E., Wykoff, C.C., Pugh, C.W., Maher, E.R. and Ratcliffe, P.J. (1999) The tumour suppressor protein VHL targets hypoxia-inducible factors for oxygen-dependent proteolysis. Nature, 399, 271-275.

McNeill, L.A., Hewitson, K.S., Gleadle, J.M., Horsfall, L.E., Oldham, N.J., Maxwell, P.H., Pugh, C.W., Ratcliffe, P.J. and Schofield, C.J. (2002) The use of dioxygen by HIF prolyl hydroxylase (PHD1). Bioorg Med Chem Lett, 12, 1547-1550.

Mekhail, K., Gunaratnam, L., Bonicalzi, M.-E. and Lee, S. (2004) HIF activation by pH-dependent nucleolar sequestration of VHL. Nat Cell Biol, 6, 642-647.

Mekhail, K., Khacho, M., Carrigan, A., Hache, R.R.J., Gunaratnam, L. and Lee, S. (2005) Regulation of ubiquitin ligase dynamics by the nucleolus. J Cell Biol, 170, 733-744.

Melmon, K.L. and Rosen, S.W. (1964) Lindau's Disease. Review of the literature and study of a large kindred. Am J Med, 36, 595-617.

Mikhaylova, O., Ignacak, M.L., Barankiewicz, T.J., Harbaugh, S.V., Yi, Y., Maxwell, P.H., Schneider, M., Van Geyte, K., Carmeliet, P., Revelo, M.P., Wyder, M., Greis, K.D., Meller, J. and Czyzyk-Krzeska, M.F. (2008) The von Hippel-Lindau tumour suppressor protein and Egl-9-Type proline hydroxylases regulate the large subunit of RNA polymerase II in response to oxidative stress. Mol Cell Biol, 28, 2701-2717.

Min, J.-H., Yang, H., Ivan, M., Gertler, F., Kaelin, W.G. and Pavletich, N.P. (2002) Structure of an HIF-1alpha -pVHL complex: hydroxyproline recognition in signalling. Science, 296, 1886-1889.

Minamishima, Y.A. and Kaelin, W.G., Jr. (2010) Reactivation of hepatic EPO synthesis in mice after PHD loss. Science, 329, 407.

Morris, M.R., Hughes, D.J., Tian, Y.M., Ricketts, C.J., Lau, K.W., Gentle, D., Shuib, S., Serrano-Fernandez, P., Lubinski, J., Wiesener, M.S., Pugh, C.W., Latif, F., Ratcliffe, P.J. and Maher, E.R. (2009) Mutation analysis of hypoxia-inducible factors HIF1A and HIF2A in renal cell carcinoma. Anticancer Res, 29, 4337-4343.

Neumann, H.P., Dinkel, E., Brambs, H., Wimmer, B., Friedburg, H., Volk, B., Sigmund, G., Riegler, P., Haag, K. and Schollmeyer, P. (1991) Pancreatic lesions in the von Hippel-Lindau syndrome. Gastroenterology, 101, 465-471.

Neumann, H.P., Eggert, H.R., Scheremet, R., Schumacher, M., Mohadjer, M., Wakhloo, A.K., Volk, B., Hettmannsperger, U., Riegler, P. and Schollmeyer, P. (1992) Central nervous system lesions in von Hippel-Lindau syndrome. J Neurol Neurosurg Psychiatry, 55, 898-901.

Neumann, H.P., Eggert, H.R., Weigel, K., Friedburg, H., Wiestler, O.D. and Schollmeyer, P. (1989) Hemangioblastomas of the central nervous system. A 10-year study with special reference to von Hippel-Lindau syndrome. J Neurosurg, 70, 24-30.

Neumann, H.P.H., Bausch, B., McWhinney, S.R., Bender, B.U., Gimm, O., Franke, G., Schipper, J., Klisch, J., Altehoefer, C., Zerres, K., Januszewicz, A., Eng, C., Smith, W.M., Munk, R., Manz, T., Glaesker, S., Apel, T.W., Treier, M., Reineke, M., Walz, M.K., Hoang-Vu, C., Brauckhoff, M., Klein-Franke, A., Klose, P., Schmidt, H., Maier-Woelfle, M., Peczkowska, M., Szmigielski, C., Eng, C. and (2002) Germ-line mutations in nonsyndromic pheochromocytoma. N Engl J Med, 346, 1459-1466.

Nickerson, M.L., Jaeger, E., Shi, Y., Durocher, J.A., Mahurkar, S., Zaridze, D., Matveev, V., Janout, V., Kollarova, H., Bencko, V., Navratilova, M., Szeszenia-Dabrowska, N., Mates, D., Mukeria, A., Holcatova, I., Schmidt, L.S., Toro, J.R., Karami, S., Hung, R., Gerard, G.F., Linehan, W.M., Merino, M., Zbar, B., Boffetta, P., Brennan, P., Rothman, N., Chow, W.H., Waldman, F.M. and Moore, L.E. (2008) Improved identification of von Hippel-Lindau gene alterations in clear cell renal tumours. Clin Cancer Res, 14, 4726-4734.

Nordstrom-O'Brien, M., van der Luijt, R.B., van Rooijen, E., van den Ouweland, A.M.,

Majoor-Krakauer, D.F., Lolkema, M.P., van Brussel, A., Voest, E.E. and Giles, R.H. (2010) Genetic analysis of von Hippel-Lindau disease. Hum Mutat, 31, 521-537.

Ohh, M., Yauch, R.L., Lonergan, K.M., Whaley, J.M., Stemmer-Rachamimov, A.O., Louis, D.N., Gavin, B.J., Kley, N., Kaelin, W.G. and Iliopoulos, O. (1998) The von Hippel-Lindau tumour suppressor protein is required for proper assembly of an extracellular fibronectin matrix. Mol Cell, 1, 959-968.

Okuda, H., Saitoh, K., Hirai, S., Iwai, K., Takaki, Y., Baba, M., Minato, N., Ohno, S. and Shuin, T. (2001) The von Hippel-Lindau tumour suppressor protein mediates ubiquitination of activated atypical protein kinase C. J Biol Chem, 276, 43611-43617.

Pantuck, A.J., An, J., Liu, H. and Rettig, M.B. (2010) NF-kappaB-dependent plasticity of the epithelial to mesenchymal transition induced by Von Hippel-Lindau inactivation in renal cell carcinomas. Cancer Res, 70, 752-761.

Pastore, Y.D., Jelinek, J., Ang, S., Guan, Y., Liu, E., Jedlickova, K., Krishnamurti, L. and Prchal, J.T. (2003) Mutations in the VHL gene in sporadic apparently congenital polycythemia. Blood, 101, 1591-1595.

Pavesi, G., Feletti, A., Berlucchi, S., Opocher, G., Martella, M., Murgia, A. and Scienza, R. (2008) Neurosurgical treatment of von Hippel-Lindau-associated hemangioblastomas: benefits, risks and outcome. J Neurosurg Sci, 52, 29-36.

Percy, M.J., Beer, P.A., Campbell, G., Dekker, A.W., Green, A.R., Oscier, D., Rainey, M.G., van Wijk, R., Wood, M., Lappin, T.R.J., McMullin, M.F. and Lee, F.S. (2008a) Novel exon 12 mutations in the HIF2A gene associated with erythrocytosis. Blood, 111, 5400-5402.

Percy, M.J., Furlow, P.W., Beer, P.A., Lappin, T.R.J., McMullin, M.F. and Lee, F.S. (2007) A novel erythrocytosis-associated PHD2 mutation suggests the location of a HIF binding groove. Blood, 110, 2193-2196.

Percy, M.J., Furlow, P.W., Lucas, G.S., Li, X., Lappin, T.R.J., McMullin, M.F. and Lee, F.S. (2008b) A gain-of-function mutation in the HIF2A gene in familial erythrocytosis. N Engl J Med, 358, 162-168.

Percy, M.J., Zhao, Q., Flores, A., Harrison, C., Lappin, T.R.J., Maxwell, P.H., McMullin, M.F. and Lee, F.S. (2006) A family with erythrocytosis establishes a role for prolyl hydroxylase domain protein 2 in oxygen homeostasis. Proc Natl Acad Sci U S A, 103, 654-659.

Perrotta, S., Nobili, B., Ferraro, M., Migliaccio, C., Borriello, A., Cucciolla, V., Martinelli, V., Rossi, F., Punzo, F., Cirillo, P., Parisi, G., Zappia, V., Rotoli, B. and Della Ragione, F. (2006) Von Hippel-Lindau-dependent polycythemia is endemic on the island of Ischia: identification of a novel cluster. Blood, 107, 514-519.

Peyssonnaux, C., Zinkernagel, A.S., Schuepbach, R.A., Rankin, E., Vaulont, S., Haase, V.H., Nizet, V. and Johnson, R.S. (2007) Regulation of iron homeostasis by the hypoxia-inducible transcription factors (HIFs). J Clin Invest, 117, 1926-1932.

Pfander, D., Kobayashi, T., Knight, M.C., Zelzer, E., Chan, D.A., Olsen, B.R., Giaccia, A.J., Johnson, R.S., Haase, V.H. and Schipani, E. (2004) Deletion of Vhlh in chondrocytes reduces cell proliferation and increases matrix deposition during growth plate development. Development, 131, 2497-2508.

Pollard, P.J., Spencer-Dene, B., Shukla, D., Howarth, K., Nye, E., El-Bahrawy, M., Deheragoda, M., Joannou, M., McDonald, S., Martin, A., Igarashi, P., Varsani-Brown, S., Rosewell, I., Poulsom, R., Maxwell, P., Stamp, G.W. and Tomlinson, I.P.M. (2007) Targeted inactivation of fh1 causes proliferative renal cyst development and activation of the hypoxia pathway. Cancer Cell, 11, 311-319.

Qi, H. and Ohh, M. (2003) The von Hippel-Lindau tumour suppressor protein sensitizes renal cell carcinoma cells to tumour necrosis factor-induced cytotoxicity by suppressing the nuclear factor-kappaB-dependent antiapoptotic pathway. Cancer Res, 63, 7076-7080.

Rankin, E.B., Biju, M.P., Liu, Q., Unger, T.L., Rha, J., Johnson, R.S., Simon, M.C., Keith, B. and Haase, V.H. (2007) Hypoxia-inducible factor-2 (HIF-2) regulates hepatic erythropoietin in vivo. J Clin Invest, 117, 1068-1077.

Rankin, E.B., Tomaszewski, J.E. and Haase, V.H. (2006) Renal cyst development in mice with conditional inactivation of the von Hippel-Lindau tumour suppressor. Cancer Res, 66, 2576-2583.

Raval, R.R., Lau, K.W., Tran, M.G.B., Sowter, H.M., Mandriota, S.J., Li, J.-L., Pugh, C.W., Maxwell, P.H., Harris, A.L. and Ratcliffe, P.J. (2005) Contrasting properties of hypoxia-inducible factor 1 (HIF-1) and HIF-2 in von Hippel-Lindau-associated renal cell carcinoma. Mol Cell Biol, 25, 5675-5686.

Reifenberger, G., Reifenberger, J., Bilzer, T., Wechsler, W. and Collins, V.P. (1995) Coexpression of transforming growth factor-alpha and epidermal growth factor receptor in capillary hemangioblastomas of the central nervous system. Am J Pathol, 147, 245-250.

Renbaum, P., Duh, F.M., Latif, F., Zbar, B., Lerman, M.I. and Kuzmin, I. (1996) Isolation and characterization of the full-length 3' untranslated region of the human von Hippel-Lindau tumour suppressor gene. Hum Genet, 98, 666-671.

Richard, S., Campello, C., Taillandier, L., Parker, F. and Resche, F. (1998) Haemangioblastoma of the central nervous system in von Hippel-Lindau disease. French VHL Study Group. J Intern Med, 243, 547-553.

Ricketts, C., Woodward, E.R., Killick, P., Morris, M.R., Astuti, D., Latif, F. and Maher, E.R. (2008) Germline SDHB mutations and familial renal cell carcinoma. J Natl Cancer Inst, 100, 1260-1262.

Roe, J.-S., Kim, H., Lee, S.-M., Kim, S.-T., Cho, E.-J. and Youn, H.-D. (2006) p53 stabilization and transactivation by a von Hippel-Lindau protein. Mol Cell, 22, 395-405.

Russell, R.C. and Ohh, M. (2008) NEDD8 acts as a 'molecular switch' defining the functional selectivity of VHL. EMBO Rep, 9, 486-491.

Safran, M., Kim, W.Y., O'Connell, F., Flippin, L., Gunzler, V., Horner, J.W., Depinho, R.A. and Kaelin, W.G., Jr. (2006) Mouse model for noninvasive imaging of HIF prolyl hydroxylase activity: assessment of an oral agent that stimulates erythropoietin production. Proc Natl Acad Sci U S A, 103, 105-110.

Sato, K., Terada, K., Sugiyama, T., Takahashi, S., Saito, M., Moriyama, M., Kakinuma, H., Suzuki, Y., Kato, M. and Kato, T. (1994) Frequent overexpression of vascular endothelial growth factor gene in human renal cell carcinoma. Tohoku J Exp Med, 173, 355-360.

Schmidt, L., Duh, F.M., Chen, F., Kishida, T., Glenn, G., Choyke, P., Scherer, S.W.,

Zhuang, Z., Lubensky, I., Dean, M., Allikmets, R., Chidambaram, A., Bergerheim, U.R., Feltis, J.T., Casadevall, C., Zamarron, A., Bernues, M., Richard, S., Lips, C.J., Walther, M.M., Tsui, L.C., Geil, L., Orcutt, M.L., Stackhouse, T., Lipan, J., Slife, L., Brauch, H., Decker, J., Niehans, G., Hughson, M.D., Moch, H., Storkel, S., Lerman, M.I., Linehan, W.M. and Zbar, B. (1997) Germline and somatic mutations in the tyrosine kinase domain of the MET proto-oncogene in papillary renal carcinomas. Nat Genet, 16, 68-73.

Schoenfeld, A., Davidowitz, E.J. and Burk, R.D. (1998) A second major native von Hippel-Lindau gene product, initiated from an internal translation start site, functions as a tumour suppressor. Proc Natl Acad Sci U S A, 95, 8817-8822.

Schoenfeld, A.R., Davidowitz, E.J. and Burk, R.D. (2001) Endoplasmic reticulum/cytosolic localization of von Hippel-Lindau gene products is mediated by a 64-amino acid region. Int J Cancer, 91, 457-467.

Schoenfeld, A.R., Parris, T., Eisenberger, A., Davidowitz, E.J., De Leon, M., Talasazan, F., Devarajan, P. and Burk, R.D. (2000) The von Hippel-Lindau tumour suppressor gene protects cells from UV-mediated apoptosis. Oncogene, 19, 5851-5857.

Selak, M.A., Armour, S.M., MacKenzie, E.D., Boulahbel, H., Watson, D.G., Mansfield, K.D., Pan, Y., Simon, M.C., Thompson, C.B. and Gottlieb, E. (2005) Succinate links TCA cycle dysfunction to oncogenesis by inhibiting HIF-alpha prolyl hydroxylase. Cancer Cell, 7, 77-85.

Semenza, G.L. (2009) Involvement of oxygen-sensing pathways in physiologic and pathologic erythropoiesis. Blood, 114, 2015-2019.

Sergeyeva, A., Gordeuk, V.R., Tokarev, Y.N., Sokol, L., Prchal, J.F. and Prchal, J.T. (1997) Congenital polycythemia in Chuvashia. Blood, 89, 2148-2154.

Shiao, Y.H., Resau, J.H., Nagashima, K., Anderson, L.M. and Ramakrishna, G. (2000) The von Hippel-Lindau tumour suppressor targets to mitochondria. Cancer Res, 60, 2816-2819.

Smith, T.G., Brooks, J.T., Balanos, G.M., Lappin, T.R., Layton, D.M., Leedham, D.L., Liu, C., Maxwell, P.H., McMullin, M.F., McNamara, C.J., Percy, M.J., Pugh, C.W., Ratcliffe, P.J., Talbot, N.P., Treacy, M. and Robbins, P.A. (2006) Mutation of von Hippel-Lindau tumour suppressor and human cardiopulmonary physiology. PLoS Med, 3.

Smith, T.G., Brooks, J.T., Balanos, G.M., Lappin, T.R., Layton, D.M., Leedham, D.L., Liu, C., Maxwell, P.H., McMullin, M.F., McNamara, C.J., Percy, M.J., Pugh, C.W., Ratcliffe, P.J., Talbot, N.P., Treacy, M. and Robbins, P.A. (2008) Mutation of the von Hippel-Lindau gene alters human cardiopulmonary physiology. Adv Exp Med Biol, 605, 51-56.

Stebbins, C.E., Kaelin, W.G. and Pavletich, N.P. (1999) Structure of the VHL-ElonginC-ElonginB complex: implications for VHL tumour suppressor function. Science, 284, 455-461.

Stickle, N.H., Chung, J., Klco, J.M., Hill, R.P., Kaelin, W.G. and Ohh, M. (2004) pVHL modification by NEDD8 is required for fibronectin matrix assembly and suppression of tumour development. Mol Cell Biol, 24, 3251-3261.

Sutovsky, H. and Gazit, E. (2004) The von Hippel-Lindau tumour suppressor protein is a molten globule under native conditions: implications for its physiological activities. J Biol Chem, 279, 17190-17196.

Takahashi, A., Sasaki, H., Kim, S.J., Tobisu, K., Kakizoe, T., Tsukamoto, T., Kumamoto, Y., Sugimura, T. and Terada, M. (1994) Markedly increased amounts of messenger RNAs for vascular endothelial growth factor and placenta growth factor in renal cell carcinoma associated with angiogenesis. Cancer Res, 54, 4233-4237.

Takeda, K., Aguila, H.L., Parikh, N.S., Li, X., Lamothe, K., Duan, L.-J., Takeda, H., Lee, F.S. and Fong, G.-H. (2008) Regulation of adult erythropoiesis by prolyl hydroxylase domain proteins. Blood, 111, 3229-3235.

Takeda, K., Ho, V.C., Takeda, H., Duan, L.-J., Nagy, A. and Fong, G.-H. (2006) Placental but not heart defects are associated with elevated hypoxia-inducible factor alpha levels in mice lacking prolyl hydroxylase domain protein 2. Mol Cell Biol, 26, 8336-8346.

Thoma, C.R., Frew, I.J., Hoerner, C.R., Montani, M., Moch, H. and Krek, W. (2007a) pVHL and GSK3beta are components of a primary cilium-maintenance signalling network. Nat Cell Biol, 9, 588-595.

Thoma, C.R., Frew, I.J. and Krek, W. (2007b) The VHL tumour suppressor: riding tandem with GSK3beta in primary cilium maintenance. Cell Cycle, 6, 1809-1813.

Thoma, C.R., Matov, A., Gutbrodt, K.L., Hoerner, C.R., Smole, Z., Krek, W. and Danuser, G. (2010) Quantitative image analysis identifies pVHL as a key regulator of microtubule dynamic instability. J Cell Biol, 190, 991-1003.

Turner, K.J., Moore, J.W., Jones, A., Taylor, C.F., Cuthbert-Heavens, D., Han, C., Leek, R.D., Gatter, K.C., Maxwell, P.H., Ratcliffe, P.J., Cranston, D. and Harris, A.L. (2002) Expression of hypoxia-inducible factors in human renal cancer: relationship to angiogenesis and to the von Hippel-Lindau gene mutation. Cancer Res, 62, 2957-2961.

Vanharanta, S., Buchta, M., McWhinney, S.R., Virta, S.K., Peczkowska, M., Morrison, C.D., Lehtonen, R., Januszewicz, A., Jarvinen, H., Juhola, M., Mecklin, J.P., Pukkala, E., Herva, R., Kiuru, M., Nupponen, N.N., Aaltonen, L.A., Neumann, H.P. and Eng, C. (2004) Early-onset renal cell carcinoma as a novel extraparaganglial component of SDHB-associated heritable paraganglioma. Am J Hum Genet, 74, 153-159.

Vortmeyer, A.O., Frank, S., Jeong, S.-Y., Yuan, K., Ikejiri, B., Lee, Y.-S., Bhowmick, D., Lonser, R.R., Smith, R., Rodgers, G., Oldfield, E.H. and Zhuang, Z. (2003) Developmental arrest of angioblastic lineage initiates tumourigenesis in von Hippel-Lindau disease. Cancer Res, 63, 7051-7055.

Walmsley, S.R., Cowburn, A.S., Clatworthy, M.R., Morrell, N.W., Roper, E.C., Singleton, V., Maxwell, P., Whyte, M.K. and Chilvers, E.R. (2006) Neutrophils from patients with heterozygous germline mutations in the von Hippel Lindau protein (pVHL) display delayed apoptosis and enhanced bacterial phagocytosis. Blood, 108, 3176-3178.

Wanebo, J.E., Lonser, R.R., Glenn, G.M. and Oldfield, E.H. (2003) The natural history of hemangioblastomas of the central nervous system in patients with von Hippel-Lindau disease. J Neurosurg, 98, 82-94.

Webster, A.R., Maher, E.R. and Moore, A.T. (1999) Clinical characteristics of ocular angiomatosis in von Hippel-Lindau disease and correlation with germline mutation. Arch Ophthalmol, 117, 371-378.

Weil, R.J., Lonser, R.R., DeVroom, H.L., Wanebo, J.E. and Oldfield, E.H. (2003) Surgical management of brainstem hemangioblastomas in patients with von Hippel-Lindau disease. J Neurosurg, 98, 95-105.

Whaley, J.M., Naglich, J., Gelbert, L., Hsia, Y.E., Lamiell, J.M., Green, J.S., Collins, D., Neumann, H.P., Laidlaw, J., Li, F.P. and et al. (1994) Germ-line mutations in the von Hippel-Lindau tumour-suppressor gene are similar to somatic von Hippel-Lindau aberrations in sporadic renal cell carcinoma. Am J Hum Genet, 55, 1092-1102.

Wiesener, M.S., Munchenhagen, P.M., Berger, I., Morgan, N.V., Roigas, J., Schwiertz, A., Jurgensen, J.S., Gruber, G., Maxwell, P.H., Loning, S.A., Frei, U., Maher, E.R., Grone, H.J. and Eckardt, K.U. (2001) Constitutive activation of hypoxia-inducible genes related to overexpression of hypoxia-inducible factor-1alpha in clear cell renal carcinomas. Cancer Res, 61, 5215-5222.

Wizigmann-Voos, S., Breier, G., Risau, W. and Plate, K.H. (1995) Up-regulation of vascular endothelial growth factor and its receptors in von Hippel-Lindau disease-associated and sporadic hemangioblastomas. Cancer Res, 55, 1358-1364.

Xia, Z., Dickens, M., Raingeaud, J., Davis, R.J. and Greenberg, M.E. (1995) Opposing effects of ERK and JNK-p38 MAP kinases on apoptosis. Science, 270, 1326-1331.

Yang, H., Minamishima, Y.A., Yan, Q., Schlisio, S., Ebert, B.L., Zhang, X., Zhang, L., Kim, W.Y., Olumi, A.F. and Kaelin, W.G. (2007) pVHL acts as an adaptor to promote the inhibitory phosphorylation of the NF-kappaB agonist Card9 by CK2. Mol Cell, 28, 15-27.

Ye, Y., Vasavada, S., Kuzmin, I., Stackhouse, T., Zbar, B. and Williams, B.R. (1998) Subcellular localization of the von Hippel-Lindau disease gene product is cell cycle-dependent. Int J Cancer, 78, 62-69.

Young, A.P., Schlisio, S., Minamishima, Y.A., Zhang, Q., Li, L., Grisanzio, C., Signoretti, S. and Kaelin, W.G. (2008) VHL loss actuates a HIF-independent senescence programme mediated by Rb and p400. Nat Cell Biol, 10, 361-369.

Yu, F., White, S.B., Zhao, Q. and Lee, F.S. (2001) HIF-1alpha binding to VHL is regulated by stimulus-sensitive proline hydroxylation. Proc Natl Acad Sci U S A, 98, 9630-9635.

Zhang, H., Gao, P., Fukuda, R., Kumar, G., Krishnamachary, B., Zeller, K.I., Dang, C.V. and Semenza, G.L. (2007) HIF-1 inhibits mitochondrial biogenesis and cellular respiration in VHL-deficient renal cell carcinoma by repression of C-MYC activity. Cancer Cell, 11, 407-420.

Zhong, H., De Marzo, A.M., Laughner, E., Lim, M., Hilton, D.A., Zagzag, D., Buechler, P., Isaacs, W.B., Semenza, G.L. and Simons, J.W. (1999) Overexpression of hypoxia-inducible factor 1alpha in common human cancers and their metastases. Cancer Res, 59, 5830-5835.

Zimmer, M., Doucette, D., Siddiqui, N. and Iliopoulos, O. (2004) Inhibition of hypoxia-inducible factor is sufficient for growth suppression of VHL-/- tumours. Mol Cancer Res, 2, 89-95.

Chapter 3

Oncogenic activation of HIF pathway

Carine Michiels[*]

[*]Author for correspondence:
URBC, NARILIS, University of Namur, 61 rue de Bruxelles, 5000 Namur, Belgium,
Phone: +32-81-724131, Fax: +32-81-724135, E-mail : carine.michiels@fundp.ac.be

Contents

Key points

— HIF is activated in tumour by hypoxia as well as by oncogene activation or tumour suppressor inactivation.

— HIF activation sustains tumour cell survival, metabolism, angiogenesis and metastasis.

— Oncogene activation or tumour suppressor inactivation may affect HIF-α synthesis, HIF-α stabilization and/or HIF activity.

— There is a very complex interplay between the different regulators of HIF pathway, that may all be influenced by oncogenic mutations.

Introduction

HIF activation has been shown to occur in many solid tumours, thereby promoting tumour growth, angiogenesis and metastasis. It results not only from the development of hypoxic areas within the tumour but also from oncogenic activation of several pathways within cancer cells that interfere with the many regulators involved in modulating HIF activity. This implicates regulation of the synthesis and degradation of the alpha subunits but also of the activity of the dimer HIF transcription factor. This review aims to describe this complex regulatory network.

The HIF pathway has been identified as a critical pathway in regulating homeostasis of multicellular organisms in response to reduced oxygen availability. The most simple system comprises one transcription factor named Hypoxia-Inducible Factor (HIF), one oxygen-sensitive prolyl hydroxylase (PHD), one oxygen-sensitive asparagine hydroxylase (Factor Inhibiting HIF, FIH) and one pVHL-like protein. The complexity of this pathway increased with the adaptation of metazoans to higher atmospheric oxygen concentration (Taylor and McElwain, 2010). Human cells possess three HIFα isoforms, three PHDs, one FIH and one pVHL (Kaelin and Ratcliffe, 2008; Semenza, 2010). HIF is a heterodimeric protein consisting of a constitutively expressed β subunit (also named ARNT) and an oxygen-regulated α subunit (Wang et al., 1995). Under normoxic conditions, the α subunit is hydroxylated on two proline residues by PHDs, the activity of which depends on oxygen availability. Hydroxylated HIFα is recognized by pVHL, a component of an E3 ubiquitin ligase complex, targeting HIFα for proteasomal degradation. In addition, the hydroxylation of HIFα by FIH blocks the interaction of the transcription factor with the co-activators p300/CBP. Under hypoxia, neither PHDs, nor FIH is active. HIF-α, no longer modified, accumulates and translocates into the nucleus where it dimerizes with HIF-β to form an active transcription factor (Semenza, 2003; Wenger, 2002). HIFs regulate the transcription of more than a hundred genes involved in cell and tissue adaptation to hypoxia. In addition, to provide adaptive responses, the HIF pathway has also been co-opted by cancer cells to favor their survival under high proliferative rate, immune pressure and unfavorable microenvironment (Semenza, 2010). HIF-α overexpression is associated with increased patient mortality (Zhong et al., 1999) and has been shown to promote tumour progression. This is particularly true for HIF-2α (Franovic et al., 2009; Rankin et al., 2008). HIF-α levels are increased in many human cancers as the result of intratumoural hypoxia but also from oncogenic alterations. This review is aimed to describe the oncogenic activation of the HIF pathway.

As mentioned earlier, the regulation of HIF transcriptional activity is very complex since it depends on several regulatory steps involving hydroxylases. It also includes kinases, interactions with other proteins, as well as regulation of the transcription of *HIF1A* gene and of its transduction (Semenza, 2010). All of these steps may be affected by gain and/or loss-of-function mutation in oncogenes or in tumour suppressors that are known to influence cell transformation but that may also activate the HIF pathway even in normoxic conditions.

Oncogenic activation of HIFα mRNA and protein synthesis

In many tissues and cells, hypoxia does not lead to an increased HIF-1α mRNA expression. However, *HIF1A* gene transcription has been shown to be enhanced in normoxia by several cytokines or hormones (Bonello et al., 2007; van Uden et al., 2008) in different cell types in a NF-κB dependent manner (Figure 3.1). This has also been evidenced in vivo using IKK-beta deficient mice (Rius et al., 2008).

NF-κB plays an important role in cancer initiation and progression by promoting an inflammatory microenvironment and angiogenesis in solid tumours (Karin, 2008). More recently, oncogenic activation of NF-κB has also been found to lead to apoptosis inhibition: this is notably the case for mutations in CARD11, a component of the signalling complex between the B-cell receptor and IKKs, in non Hodgkin's lymphomas, for genetic hits that stabilize the kinase NIK in multiple myeloma, leading to constitutive activation of NF-κB and for NF-κB activation by unconventional IKK family members like IKKβ and TBK1 downstream of mutant K-ras in epithelial cancers (Staudt, 2010). In addition to lead to a direct inhibition of apoptosis, oncogenic NF-κB activation may also increase *HIF1A* gene transcription, leading to HIF-1α accumulation and increased HIF-1 activity.

The rate of HIF-1α mRNA translation is also regulated. Overall protein synthesis is reduced in hypoxic cells, with the aim of sparing ATP. This inhibition is due to eiF2α phosphorylation and inhibition of mTOR, two components of the cap-dependent translation (van den Beucken et al., 2006). Despite this overall inhibition, several mRNA are preferentially translated under hypoxia, this is notably the case for HIF-1α and HIF-2α mRNA and for mRNA of HIF target genes such as VEGF, ensuring the synthesis of the proteins required for the adaptation of cells to hypoxic conditions.

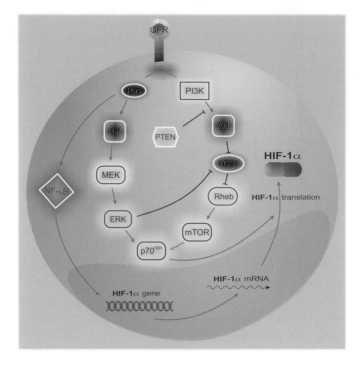

Figure 3.1 _ Oncogenic pathways regulating HIFα synthesis. Gain-of-function activation of oncogenes is represented in red and loss-of-function inactivation of tumour suppressors in yellow.

ERK: extracellular regulated kinase; GFR: growth factor receptor; HIF: hypoxia-inducible factor; MEK: mitogen-activated protein kinase/extracellular signal-regulated kinase kinase; mTOR: mammalian target of rapamycin; NF-kB: nuclear factor kappa-light-chain-enhancer of activated B cells; PI3K: phosphatidyl inositol 3-kinase; PTEN: phosphatase and tensin homolog; Rheb: Ras homolog enriched in brain; TCS2: tuberous sclerosis complex 2.

The PI3K-AKT-mTOR pathway as well as the ras-MAP kinase pathway, activated downstream from several growth factor receptors, in addition to promoting cell cycle initiation, also results in an increased HIF-1α mRNA translation and hence an increased HIF-1α protein level, under normoxic conditions (Figure 3.1). This has been demonstrated for several growth factors as well as cytokines, in different cell types (Bardos and Ashcroft, 2005; Fukuda et al., 2002; Laughner et al., 2001) as well as for oncogenic mutation of growth factor receptors e.g. HER2 (Li et al., 2005) or MET (Costa et al., 2010), parallel to HIF activation and to elevated HIF-target gene expression. Akt and ERK both inhibit TCS2 (tuberous sclerosis complex 2) by phosphorylation; TCS2 is an inhibitor of Rheb which is an activator of mTOR. TCS2 phosphorylation thus leads to mTOR and translation activation. In addition to growth factor receptors themselves, several components of the PI3K-AKT-mTOR and the ras-MAP kinase pathways are bona fide oncogenes (Hanahan and Weinberg, 2000; Hay, 2005; Vogelstein and Kinzler, 2004). Their gain-of-function mutation would thus participate in HIF-1 activation. Moreover, it has recently been reported that AKT activation could also lead to increase of HIF-1α protein translation in a mTOR-independent way (Pore et al., 2006) or via FOXO1 inhibition (Alam et al., 2009). Conversely PTEN, the lipid phosphatase that inhibits the AKT activation downstream of PI3K activation is a tumour suppressor. PTEN loss-of-function mutations are frequently found in melanomas, glioblastomas and prostate cancers (Sansal and Sellers, 2004) and have been shown to lead to HIF-1 target gene overexpression (Tian et al., 2010). In addition to regulating HIF-1α synthesis, PI3K-AKT and ERK pathways also influence HIF-1α stability and activity (Bardos and Ashcroft, 2005) (see below). Therefore, the connection between growth factor-mediated or oncogenic cell activation and HIF signalling is very intricate.

Oncogenic inhibition of HIF-α degradation

HIFα protein expression level is tightly controlled through synthesis but more importantly through degradation (Semenza, 2010; Yee Koh et al., 2008). HIF-α accumulation during hypoxia results mainly from inhibition of its oxygen-dependent degradation by the PHD-pVHL pathway. However, recent data describes new pVHL- and/or oxygen-independent mechanisms for regulating HIF-α stability (Figure 3.2). This is notably the case for the role of RACK1 versus HSP90 (Liu and Semenza, 2007).

Von Hippel-Lindau disease, which is characterized by a high frequency of clear cell renal carcinomas, hemangioblastomas and pheochromocytomas, is the most well known oncogenic mutation affecting the HIF pathway. It is caused by inactivating mutations of the VHL tumour suppressor gene. One of the most documented substrates of this E3 ubiquitine ligase is HIFα. The disruption of this HIF-α degradation pathway leads to HIFα accumulation, VEGF overexpression and the development of highly vascularized tumours (Kaelin, 2007) (for further details, see Maxwell, featured in this book).

This central degradation pathway for HIF-α is also affected by other oncogenic mutations that influence PHD activity. Many metabolic abnormalities in cancer cells increase HIF activity (Chiche et al., 2010; Semenza, 2010) (for further details, see Wenger, featured in this book). Competitive antagonists of α-ketoglutarate but also Krebs cycle metabolites inhibit PHDs, resulting in elevated HIF-α protein level. Two distinct hereditary cancer syndromes caused by mutations in genes encoding Krebs cycle enzymes, succinate dehydrogenase and fumarate hydratase, are associated with HIF upregulation resulting from the accumulation of succinate or fumarate that inhibits the PHDs (Pollard et al., 2007; Ratcliffe, 2007). In addition, the PHDs utilize oxygen and α-ketoglutarate as substrates in an enzymatic reaction to hydroxylate HIF-α. The PHDs contain Fe(II) in their catalytic centre and seem to be sensitive to ROS (reactive oxygen species) (Acker et al., 2006; Chandel, 2010). JunD KO mice show an elevated ROS level, PHD inhibition, activated HIF and increased incidence of tumours (Toullec et al., 2010).

pVHL activity is also modulated by the Wnt signalling pathway. Wnt/β-catenin signalling is usually referred as an oncogenic pathway that promotes tumour progression (Lucero et al., 2010). For example, aberrant activation of β-catenin has been shown to promote cell proliferation and initiate colorectal tumourigenesis while mutations in APC gene are clearly associated with colon cancer. Mutations in β-catenin, which abrogate its regulation by APC, or in axin, another regulator of this pathway, are observed in a variety of different cancers (Hu and Li, 2010). Wnt signalling supports the formation and the maintenance of cancer stem cells (Wend et al., 2010) but also "normal" stem cells in a HIF-1α-dependent manner (Mazumdar et al., 2010). In addition to regulation of proliferation, differentiation and epithelial to mesenchymal transition through the interaction of β–catenin with the TCF/LEF transcription factor, β-catenin also acts as a molecular switch for other transcription factors (Thevenod and Chakraborty, 2010) amongst which is HIF-1. β-catenin-HIF-1α interaction occurs at the promoter region of HIF-1 target genes and analyses indicate that β-catenin can enhance HIF-1-mediated transcription (Kaidi et al., 2007). On the other hand, VHL expression is positively regulated by TCF4 activation and turning off TCF4 leads to an increased HIF-1α protein level and VEGF expression (Giles et al., 2006). More studies are thus necessary to understand the delicate interplay between the Wnt/β-catenin pathway and the HIF pathway.

p53 is a well known tumour suppressor that functions as a transcription factor to induce apoptotic target genes to eliminate developing tumour cells. Moreover, pro-apoptotic transcriptionally independent activity (Yee and Vousden, 2005) and influence on mitochondrial toward glycolytic shift in cancer cells have also been demonstrated for p53 protein (Vousden and Ryan,

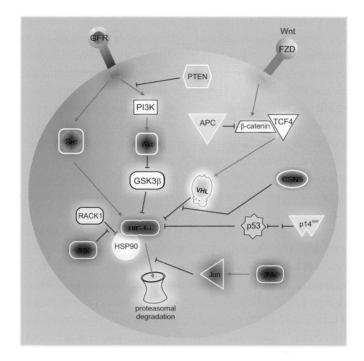

Figure 3.2 _ Oncogenic pathways regulating HIF-α degradation. Gain-of-function activation of oncogenes is represented in red and loss-of-function inactivation of tumour suppressors in yellow.

APC: adenomatous polyposis coli; CSN5: fifth component of the constitutive photomorphogenic-9 (COP9) signalosome; FZD: frizzled; GFR: growth factor receptor; GSK3β: glycogene synthase kinase-3β; HIF: hypoxia-inducible factor; HSP90: heat shock protein 90; JNK: Jun N-terminal kinase; p14ARF: p14 alternate reading frame product of the CDKN2A locus; PI3K: phosphatidyl inositol 3-kinase; PTEN: phosphatase and tensin homolog; pVHL : protein von Hippel-Lindau; RACK1: a receptor for activated protein kinase C; TCF4: Transcription factor 4; Wnt: Wg (wingless) and Int.

2009). In addition, p53 influences HIF-1α stability and activity: a complex interaction network exists between the two proteins. It seems that, under severe hypoxia, p53 would target HIF-1α for proteasome degradation while, under mild hypoxia, p53 competes with HIF-1α for the recruitment of p300/ CBP coactivators (Fels and Koumenis, 2005; Hubert et al., 2006), in any case leading to HIF activity downregulation. In addition to protect cancer cell from apoptosis, p53 loss-of-function mutation would thus favor HIF-1 activation and cell survival (for further details, see Vojtesek, featured in this book).

Jab1/CSN5 was first identified as a c-Jun coactivator and subsequently discovered to be the fifth component of the constitutive photomorphogenic-9 (COP9) signalosome (CSN) complex. Jab1/CSN5 plays an essential role in positively regulating cellular proliferation by functionally inactivating several key negative regulatory proteins and tumour suppressors through their degradation, deneddylation and subcellular localisation. Jab1/CSN5 overexpression has been identified in a number of tumour types and has been implicated in the initiation and progression of several types of cancer (Shackleford and Claret, 2010). Jab1 directly interacts with HIF-1-α and regulates its stability by competing both with pVHL (Bemis et al., 2004) and with p53 (Bae et al., 2002; Larsen et al., 2005), thus inhibiting their pro-degradation interaction with the α subunit.

Glycogen synthase kinase 3 (GSK3) is phosphorylated and inactivated by AKT downstream from growth factor receptor activation, hence also downstream from oncogenic activation of AKT or inactivation of PTEN. GSK3β activation under prolonged hypoxia decreased HIF-1α protein level (Mottet et al., 2003). Similarly, GSK3β overexpression results in PHD- and pVHL-independent HIF-1α ubiquitination and proteasomal degradation via HIF-1α phosphorylation (Flugel et al., 2007). Oncogenic activation of AKT or inactivation of PTEN, through the inhibition of this kinase, thus represents yet another way to regulate, i.e. increase, HIF-1α protein stability (Dimova et al., 2009).

As mentioned above, the Ras-MAP kinase pathway is one of the most well characterized oncogenic pathways (Keshet and Seger, 2010). One of these kinase cascades includes JNK leading to the activation of the AP-1 transcription factor, a dimeric factor made of different subunits. Amongst them c-jun is the most frequent one and is clearly an oncogene (Shaulian, 2010). Both JNK and c-Jun have been reported to enhance HIF-1α stability by preventing its degradation. Oncogenic activation of these proteins is thus susceptible to enhance HIF activity. c-Jun associates with HIF-1α via its oxygen-dependent degradation domain, thus masking the site for ubiquitination, protecting HIF-1α from proteasome degradation (Yu et al., 2009). On the other hand, JNK1 positively modulates the protective role of the chaperones Hsp70/Hsp90 in stabilizing newly synthesized HIF-1α (Zhang et al., 2010). Hsp90 competes with RACK1 for binding the PAS-A domain of HIF-1α and RACK1 activity needed for pVHL-independent degradation of the α subunit (Liu et al., 2007).

The SRC family kinases are a family of tyrosine kinases downstream from growth factor receptor activation. Src, the oldest oncogene, displays transforming activity through proliferation activation (Aleshin and Finn, 2010).

Recently, it has been shown that, in addition to this well described activity, Src also increases HIF-1α protein level, through a yet unknown pathway, leading to higher target gene expression (Takacova et al., 2010).

Oncogenic activation of HIF activity

Once stabilized, HIF-α migrates into the nucleus where it dimerizes with ARNT. HIF-1α nuclear translocation is regulated by its phosphorylation by p42/p44 MAPK on two serine residues located near HIF-1α NLS (Mylonis et al., 2008). Previous results had shown that HIF-1α phosphorylation by p42/p44 MAPK increased its transcriptional activity without affecting HIF-1α stability (Minet et al., 2000; Richard et al., 1999). Oncogenic activation of the MAP kinase pathway thus contributes to HIF activation through several ways including increased HIF-α protein synthesis, stability and activity (Figure 3.3). When translocated into the nucleus, the α subunit of HIF then dimerizes with ARNT. Fatyol et al (Fatyol and Szalay, 2001) evidenced that p14^{ARF} (alternative reading frame product of the INKA4 locus) can directly inhibit HIF-1 by sequestering the α-subunit into the nucleolus, hence inhibiting HIF-1 activity. p14^{ARF} is a tumour suppressor gene whose locus is frequently mutated or deleted in human cancers (Agrawal et al., 2006). Its deletion thus relieves an inhibitory effect on HIF activation. Moreover, p14^{ARF} binds to and inhibits Mdm2, the E3 ubiquitine ligase for p53, resulting in p53 stabilization (Yee and Vousden, 2005). Consequently, deletion of p14^{ARF} also increases p53 degradation, again releasing HIF-1 from an inhibitory pathway.

HIF activity is regulated in an oxygen-dependent manner via FIH. FIH has been identified as a protein interacting with the carboxy-terminal transactivation domain of HIF-1α. Under normoxic conditions, FIH hydroxylates an asparagine residue, which blocks the interaction of the coactivator p300/CBP with HIF-1α (Lando et al., 2002). As PHDs, FIH is no longer active under hypoxic conditions allowing HIF-1 to be transcriptionally active.

c-Myc overexpression is estimated to occur in more than 70 % of human tumours, mainly due to genomic amplification and chromosomal rearrangement. In normal cells, c-Myc is a classical immediate early gene, induced upon growth factor simulation and promoting cell proliferation. Under condition of normal c-Myc expression, HIF-1α and HIF-2α exhibit opposing effect of c-Myc function. HIF-1α, through its PAS domain, directly

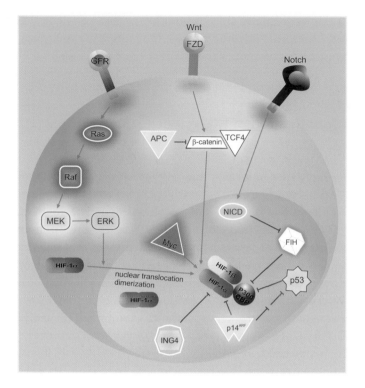

Figure 3.3 _ Oncogenic pathways regulating HIF activity. Gain-of-function activation of oncogenes is represented in red and loss-of-function inactivation of
tumour suppressors in yellow.

APC: adenomatous polyposis coli; CBP: CREB binding protein; ERK: extracellular regulated kinase; FIH: factor inhibiting HIF; FZD: frizzled; GFR: growth
factor receptor; HIF: hypoxia-inducible factor; ING4: inhibitor of growth protein
4; MEK: mitogen-activated protein kinase/extracellular signal- regulated kinase
kinase; NICD: Notch intracellular domain; p14[ARF]: p14 alternate reading frame
product of the CDKN2A locus; TCF4: Transcription factor 4; Wnt: Wg (wingless)
and Int.

interacts with Sp1, to displace c-Myc from the target gene promoter for
gene repression (Koshiji et al., 2004).

On the other hand, HIF-2α promotes hypoxic cell proliferation by
enhancing c-Myc transcriptional activity (Gordan et al., 2007). However, when
dysregulated c-myc is overexpressed in cancer cells, HIF-1α and c-Myc
cooperate to induce the expression of genes such as VEGF and glycolytic
enzymes (Kim et al., 2007), thus driving the aerobic glycolysis (Warburg effect)

of cancer cells (Dang et al., 2008; Gordan et al., 2007) but also the genetic instability observed under hypoxia (Yoo et al., 2009).

More recently, a reverse interaction has been identified that shows that, under normoxic conditions, oncogenic c-Myc is required for constitutive high HIF-1α protein level and activity, thereby influencing VEGF secretion and angiogenic activity of multiple myeloma cells (Podar and Anderson, 2010). c-Myc level and activity is also regulated by p53 as well as by β-catenin, both of which also affect HIF-1α protein level and/or HIF activity, thus rendering the interplay very complex (Yeung et al., 2008).

Notch comprises a signalling pathway that regulates cell proliferation and differentiation. Signalling is initiated when the Jagged or Delta family ligand binds a Notch receptor, triggering a two-step receptor proteolysis event, resulting in the release of the Notch intracellular domain (NICD). NICD migrates into the nucleus and activates the transcription of target genes (Fortini, 2009). There is increasing evidence that this pathway is dysregulated in a variety of malignancies: it could be either oncogenic or tumour suppressive depending on the tissue and organ site in which it is expressed (Yin et al., 2010). Notch pathway is activated under hypoxia and HIF-1α mediates NICD stabilization but reverse cross-talk is also observed (Mazumdar et al., 2009). Notch activation potentiates the recruitment of HIF-1α to target gene promoters (Sahlgren et al., 2008). This may occur through direct interaction between NICD and FIH 1. Since the affinity of FIH-1 for NICD is higher than for HIF-1α, this suggests that NICD sequesters FIH-1 away from HIF-1α, thus de repressing HIF-1 function (Zheng et al., 2008).

A final regulator of HIF-1 activity newly identified is ING4. ING4 is a member of the growth inhibitor family, which regulates G2/M to G1 transition and has tumour suppressor-like functions (Unoki et al., 2009). A direct interaction between HIF-1α and ING4 has been demonstrated, that inhibits HIF-1 activity (Colla et al., 2007; Ozer et al., 2005). This inhibitory effect may involve pVHL recruitment but the exact mechanism underlying HIF-1 inhibition is not yet understood.

Conclusion

In addition to hypoxia, a number of cancer-associated mutations promote HIF-α accumulation and HIF activity. The consequences of HIF activation in tumour cells downstream from oncogenic mutation, in addition to its activation by the decreased oxygen availability in some areas of solid tumours, is evidenced by a large body of evidence showing that HIF activity participates in human cancer progression. It indeed regulates the expression of numerous genes with key roles in cancer cell survival and metabolism but also in angiogenesis and metastasis. Furthermore, it favors cancer cell survival to chemo- and radiotherapies, identifying this factor, but also the pathways leading to its activation, as pharmacological targets for developing new antitumour therapeutic strategies.

References

Acker T, Fandrey J, Acker H. (2006). The good, the bad and the ugly in oxygen-sensing: ROS, cytochromes and prolyl-hydroxylases. Cardiovasc Res 71: 195-207.

Agrawal A, Yang J, Murphy RF, Agrawal DK. (2006). Regulation of the p14ARF-Mdm2-p53 pathway: an overview in breast cancer. Exp Mol Pathol 81: 115-22.

Alam H, Weck J, Maizels E, Park Y, Lee EJ, Ashcroft M, Hunzicker-Dunn M. (2009). Role of the phosphatidylinositol-3-kinase and extracellular regulated kinase pathways in the induction of hypoxia-inducible factor (HIF)-1 activity and the HIF-1 target vascular endothelial growth factor in ovarian granulosa cells in response to follicle-stimulating hormone. Endocrinology 150: 915-28.

Aleshin A, Finn RS. (2010). SRC: a century of science brought to the clinic. Neoplasia 12: 599-607.

Bae MK, Ahn MY, Jeong JW, Bae MH, Lee YM, Bae SK, Park JW, Kim KR, Kim KW. (2002). Jab1 interacts directly with HIF-1alpha and regulates its stability. J Biol Chem 277: 9-12.

Bardos JI, Ashcroft M. (2005). Negative and positive regulation of HIF-1: a complex network. Biochim Biophys Acta 1755: 107-20.

Bemis L, Chan DA, Finkielstein CV, Qi L, Sutphin PD, Chen X, Stenmark K, Giaccia AJ, Zundel W. (2004). Distinct aerobic and hypoxic mechanisms of HIF-alpha regulation by CSN5. Genes Dev 18: 739-44.

Bonello S, Zahringer C, BelAiba RS, Djordjevic T, Hess J, Michiels C, Kietzmann T, Gorlach A. (2007). Reactive oxygen species activate the HIF-1alpha promoter via a functional NFkappaB site. Arterioscler Thromb Vasc Biol 27: 755-61.

Chandel NS. (2010). Mitochondrial regulation of oxygen sensing. Adv Exp Med Biol 661: 339-54.

Chiche J, Brahimi-Horn MC, Pouyssegur J. (2010). Tumour hypoxia induces a metabolic shift causing acidosis: a common feature in cancer. J Cell Mol Med 14: 771-94.

Colla S, Tagliaferri S, Morandi F, Lunghi P, Donofrio G, Martorana D, Mancini C, Lazzaretti M, Mazzera L, Ravanetti L, Bonomini S, Ferrari L, Miranda C, Ladetto M,

Neri TM, Neri A, Greco A, Mangoni M, Bonati A, Rizzoli V, Giuliani N. (2007). The new tumour-suppressor gene inhibitor of growth family member 4 (ING4) regulates the production of proangiogenic molecules by myeloma cells and suppresses hypoxia-inducible factor-1 alpha (HIF-1alpha) activity: involvement in myeloma-induced angiogenesis. Blood 110: 4464-75.

Costa B, Dettori D, Lorenzato A, Bardella C, Coltella N, Martino C, Cammarata C, Carmeliet P, Olivero M, Di Renzo MF. (2010). Fumarase tumour suppressor gene and MET oncogene cooperate in upholding transformation and tumourigenesis. FASEB J 24: 2680-8.

Dang CV, Kim JW, Gao P, Yustein J. (2008). The interplay between MYC and HIF in cancer. Nat Rev Cancer 8: 51-6.

Dimova EY, Michiels C, Kietzmann T. (2009). Kinases as upstream regulators of the HIF system: their emerging potential as anti-cancer drug targets. Curr Pharm Des 15: 3867-77.

Fatyol K, Szalay AA. (2001). The p14ARF tumour suppressor protein facilitates nucleolar sequestration of hypoxia-inducible factor-1alpha (HIF-1alpha) and inhibits HIF-1-mediated transcription. J Biol Chem 276: 28421-9.

Fels DR, Koumenis C. (2005). HIF-1alpha and p53: the ODD couple? Trends Biochem Sci 30: 426-9.

Flugel D, Gorlach A, Michiels C, Kietzmann T. (2007). Glycogen synthase kinase 3 phosphorylates hypoxia-inducible factor 1alpha and mediates its destabilization in a VHL-independent manner. Mol Cell Biol 27: 3253-65.

Fortini ME. (2009). Notch signalling: the core pathway and its posttranslational regulation. Dev Cell 16: 633-47.

Franovic A, Holterman CE, Payette J, Lee S. (2009). Human cancers converge at the HIF-2alpha oncogenic axis. Proc Natl Acad Sci U S A 106: 21306-11.

Fukuda R, Hirota K, Fan F, Jung YD, Ellis LM, Semenza GL. (2002). Insulin-like growth factor 1 induces hypoxia-inducible factor 1-mediated vascular endothelial growth factor expression, which is dependent on MAP kinase and phosphatidylinositol 3-kinase signalling in colon cancer cells. J Biol Chem 277: 38205-11.

Giles RH, Lolkema MP, Snijckers CM, Belderbos M, van der Groep P, Mans DA, van Beest M, van Noort M, Goldschmeding R, van Diest PJ, Clevers H, Voest EE. (2006). Interplay between VHL/HIF1alpha and Wnt/beta-catenin pathways during colorectal tumourigenesis. Oncogene 25: 3065-70.

Gordan JD, Bertout JA, Hu CJ, Diehl JA, Simon MC. (2007). HIF-2alpha promotes hypoxic cell proliferation by enhancing c-myc transcriptional activity. Cancer Cell 11: 335-47.

Gordan JD, Thompson CB, Simon MC. (2007). HIF and c-Myc: sibling rivals for control of cancer cell metabolism and proliferation. Cancer Cell 12: 108-13.

Hanahan D, Weinberg RA. (2000). The hallmarks of cancer. Cell 100: 57-70.

Hay N. (2005). The Akt-mTOR tango and its relevance to cancer. Cancer Cell 8: 179-83.

Hu T, Li C. (2010). Convergence between Wnt-beta-catenin and EGFR signalling in cancer. Mol Cancer 9: 236.

Hubert A, Paris S, Piret JP, Ninane N, Raes M, Michiels C. (2006). Casein kinase 2 inhibition decreases hypoxia-inducible factor-1 activity under hypoxia through elevated p53 protein level. J Cell Sci 119: 3351-62.

Kaelin WG. (2007). Von Hippel-Lindau disease. Annu Rev Pathol 2: 145-73.

Kaelin WG, Jr., Ratcliffe PJ. (2008). Oxygen sensing by metazoans: the central role of the HIF hydroxylase pathway. Mol Cell 30: 393-402.

Kaidi A, Williams AC, Paraskeva C. (2007). Interaction between beta-catenin and HIF-1 promotes cellular adaptation to hypoxia. Nat Cell Biol 9: 210-7.

Karin M. (2008). The IkappaB kinase – a bridge between inflammation and cancer. Cell Res 18: 334-42.

Keshet Y, Seger R. (2010). The MAP kinase signalling cascades: a system of hundreds of components regulates a diverse array of physiological functions. Methods Mol Biol 661: 3-38.

Kim JW, Gao P, Liu YC, Semenza GL, Dang CV. (2007). Hypoxia-inducible factor 1 and dysregulated c-Myc cooperatively induce vascular endothelial growth factor and metabolic switches hexokinase 2 and pyruvate dehydrogenase kinase 1. Mol Cell Biol 27: 7381-93.

Koshiji M, Kageyama Y, Pete EA, Horikawa I, Barrett JC, Huang LE. (2004). HIF-1alpha induces cell cycle arrest by functionally counteracting Myc. EMBO J 23: 1949-56.

Lando D, Peet DJ, Gorman JJ, Whelan DA, Whitelaw ML, Bruick RK. (2002). FIH-1 is an asparaginyl hydroxylase enzyme that regulates the transcriptional activity of hypoxia-inducible factor. Genes Dev 16: 1466-71.

Larsen M, Hog A, Lund EL, Kristjansen PE. (2005). Interactions between HIF-1 and Jab1: balancing apoptosis and adaptation. Outline of a working hypothesis. Adv Exp Med Biol 566: 203-11.

Laughner E, Taghavi P, Chiles K, Mahon PC, Semenza GL. (2001). HER2 (neu) signalling increases the rate of hypoxia-inducible factor 1alpha (HIF-1alpha) synthesis: novel mechanism for HIF-1-mediated vascular endothelial growth factor expression. Mol Cell Biol 21: 3995-4004.

Li YM, Zhou BP, Deng J, Pan Y, Hay N, Hung MC. (2005). A hypoxia-independent hypoxia-inducible factor-1 activation pathway induced by phosphatidylinositol-3 kinase/Akt in HER2 overexpressing cells. Cancer Res 65: 3257-63.

Liu YV, Baek JH, Zhang H, Diez R, Cole RN, Semenza GL. (2007). RACK1 competes with HSP90 for binding to HIF-1alpha and is required for O(2)-independent and HSP90 inhibitor-induced degradation of HIF-1alpha. Mol Cell 25: 207-17.

Liu YV, Semenza GL. (2007). RACK1 vs. HSP90: competition for HIF-1 alpha degradation vs. stabilization. Cell Cycle 6: 656-9.

Lucero OM, Dawson DW, Moon RT, Chien AJ. (2010). A re-evaluation of the "oncogenic" nature of Wnt/beta-catenin signalling in melanoma and other cancers. Curr Oncol Rep 12: 314-8.

Mazumdar J, Dondeti V, Simon MC. (2009). Hypoxia-inducible factors in stem cells and cancer. J Cell Mol Med 13: 4319-28.

Mazumdar J, O'Brien WT, Johnson RS, LaManna JC, Chavez JC, Klein PS, Simon MC. (2010). O2 regulates stem cells through Wnt/beta-catenin signalling. Nat Cell Biol 12: 1007-13.

Minet E, Arnould T, Michel G, Roland I, Mottet D, Raes M, Remacle J, Michiels C. (2000). ERK activation upon hypoxia: involvement in HIF-1 activation. FEBS Lett 468: 53-8.

Mottet D, Dumont V, Deccache Y, Demazy C, Ninane N, Raes M, Michiels C. (2003). Regulation of hypoxia-inducible factor-1alpha protein level during hypoxic conditions by the phosphatidylinositol 3-kinase/Akt/glycogen synthase kinase 3beta pathway in HepG2 cells. J Biol Chem 278: 31277-85.

Mylonis I, Chachami G, Paraskeva E, Simos G. (2008). Atypical CRM1-dependent nuclear export signal mediates regulation of hypoxia-inducible factor-1alpha by MAPK. J Biol Chem 283: 27620-7.

Ozer A, Wu LC, Bruick RK. (2005). The candidate tumour suppressor ING4 represses activation of the hypoxia inducible factor (HIF). Proc Natl Acad Sci U S A 102: 7481-6.

Podar K, Anderson KC. (2010). A therapeutic role for targeting c-Myc/Hif-1-dependent signalling pathways. Cell Cycle 9: 1722-8.

Pollard PJ, Spencer-Dene B, Shukla D, Howarth K, Nye E, El-Bahrawy M, Deheragoda M, Joannou M, McDonald S, Martin A, Igarashi P, Varsani-Brown S, Rosewell I, Poulsom R, Maxwell P, Stamp GW, Tomlinson IP. (2007). Targeted inactivation of fh1 causes proliferative renal cyst development and activation of the hypoxia pathway. Cancer Cell 11: 311-9.

Pore N, Jiang Z, Shu HK, Bernhard E, Kao GD, Maity A. (2006). Akt1 activation can augment hypoxia-inducible factor-1alpha expression by increasing protein translation through a mammalian target of rapamycin-independent pathway. Mol Cancer Res 4: 471-9.

Rankin EB, Rha J, Unger TL, Wu CH, Shutt HP, Johnson RS, Simon MC, Keith B, Haase VH. (2008). Hypoxia-inducible factor-2 regulates vascular tumourigenesis in mice. Oncogene 27: 5354-8.

Ratcliffe PJ. (2007). Fumarate hydratase deficiency and cancer: activation of hypoxia signalling? Cancer Cell 11: 303-5.

Richard DE, Berra E, Gothie E, Roux D, Pouyssegur J. (1999). p42/p44 mitogen-activated protein kinases phosphorylate hypoxia-inducible factor 1alpha (HIF-1alpha) and enhance the transcriptional activity of HIF-1. J Biol Chem 274: 32631-7.

Rius J, Guma M, Schachtrup C, Akassoglou K, Zinkernagel AS, Nizet V, Johnson RS, Haddad GG, Karin M. (2008). NF-kappaB links innate immunity to the hypoxic response through transcriptional regulation of HIF-1alpha. Nature 453: 807-11.

Sahlgren C, Gustafsson MV, Jin S, Poellinger L, Lendahl U. (2008). Notch signalling mediates hypoxia-induced tumour cell migration and invasion. Proc Natl Acad Sci U S A 105: 6392-7.

Sansal I, Sellers WR. (2004). The biology and clinical relevance of the PTEN tumour suppressor pathway. J Clin Oncol 22: 2954-63.

Semenza GL. (2003). Targeting HIF-1 for cancer therapy. Nat Rev Cancer 3: 721-32.

Semenza GL. (2010). Defining the role of hypoxia-inducible factor 1 in cancer biology and therapeutics. Oncogene 29: 625-34.

Semenza GL. (2010). HIF-1: upstream and downstream of cancer metabolism. Curr Opin Genet Dev 20: 51-6.

Semenza GL. (2010). Oxygen homeostasis. Wiley Interdiscip Rev Syst Biol Med 2: 336-61.

Shackleford TJ, Claret FX. (2010). JAB1/CSN5: a new player in cell cycle control and cancer. Cell Div 5: 26.

Shaulian E. (2010). AP-1–The Jun proteins: Oncogenes or tumour suppressors in disguise? Cell Signal 22: 894-9.

Staudt LM. (2010). Oncogenic activation of NF-kappaB. Cold Spring Harb Perspect Biol 2: a000109.

Takacova M, Holotnakova T, Barathova M, Pastorekova S, Kopacek J, Pastorek J. (2010). Src induces expression of carbonic anhydrase IX via hypoxia-inducible factor 1. Oncol Rep 23: 869-74.

Taylor CT, McElwain JC. (2010). Ancient atmospheres and the evolution of oxygen sensing via the hypoxia-inducible factor in metazoans. Physiology (Bethesda) 25: 272-9.

Thevenod F, Chakraborty PK. (2010). The role of Wnt/beta-catenin signalling in renal carcinogenesis: lessons from cadmium toxicity studies. Curr Mol Med 10: 387-404.

Tian T, Nan KJ, Wang SH, Liang X, Lu CX, Guo H, Wang WJ, Ruan ZP. (2010). PTEN regulates angiogenesis and VEGF expression through phosphatase-dependent and -independent mechanisms in HepG2 cells. Carcinogenesis 31: 1211-9.

Toullec A, Gerald D, Despouy G, Bourachot B, Cardon M, Lefort S, Richardson M, Rigaill G, Parrini MC, Lucchesi C, Bellanger D, Stern MH, Dubois T, Sastre-Garau X, Delattre O, Vincent-Salomon A, Mechta-Grigoriou F. (2010). Oxidative stress promotes myofibroblast differentiation and tumour spreading. EMBO Mol Med 2: 211-30.

Unoki M, Kumamoto K, Takenoshita S, Harris CC. (2009). Reviewing the current classification of inhibitor of growth family proteins. Cancer Sci 100: 1173-9.

van den Beucken T, Koritzinsky M, Wouters BG. (2006). Translational control of gene expression during hypoxia. Cancer Biol Ther 5: 749-55.

van Uden P, Kenneth NS, Rocha S. (2008). Regulation of hypoxia-inducible factor-1alpha by NF-kappaB. Biochem J 412: 477-84.

Vogelstein B, Kinzler KW. (2004). Cancer genes and the pathways they control. Nat Med 10: 789-99.

Vousden KH, Ryan KM. (2009). p53 and metabolism. Nat Rev Cancer 9: 691-700.

Wang GL, Jiang BH, Rue EA, Semenza GL. (1995). Hypoxia-inducible factor 1 is a basic-helix-loop-helix-PAS heterodimer regulated by cellular O2 tension. Proc Natl Acad Sci U S A 92: 5510-4.

Wend P, Holland JD, Ziebold U, Birchmeier W. (2010). Wnt signalling in stem and cancer stem cells. Semin Cell Dev Biol 21: 855-63.

Wenger RH. (2002). Cellular adaptation to hypoxia: O2-sensing protein hydroxylases, hypoxia-inducible transcription factors, and O2-regulated gene expression. FASEB J 16: 1151-62.

Yee Koh M, Spivak-Kroizman TR, Powis G. (2008). HIF-1 regulation: not so easy come, easy go. Trends Biochem Sci 33: 526-34.

Yee KS, Vousden KH. (2005). Complicating the complexity of p53. Carcinogenesis 26: 1317-22.

Yeung SJ, Pan J, Lee MH. (2008). Roles of p53, MYC and HIF-1 in regulating glycolysis – the seventh hallmark of cancer. Cell Mol Life Sci 65: 3981-99.

Yin L, Velazquez OC, Liu ZJ. (2010). Notch signalling: emerging molecular targets for cancer therapy. Biochem Pharmacol 80: 690-701.

Yoo YG, Hayashi M, Christensen J, Huang LE. (2009). An essential role of the HIF-1alpha-c-Myc axis in malignant progression. Ann N Y Acad Sci 1177: 198-204.

Yu B, Miao ZH, Jiang Y, Li MH, Yang N, Li T, Ding J. (2009). c-Jun protects hypoxia-inducible factor-1alpha from degradation via its oxygen-dependent degradation domain in a nontranscriptional manner. Cancer Res 69: 7704-12.

Zhang D, Li J, Costa M, Gao J, Huang C. (2010). JNK1 mediates degradation HIF-1alpha by a VHL-independent mechanism that involves the chaperones Hsp90/Hsp70. Cancer Res 70: 813-23.

Zheng X, Linke S, Dias JM, Gradin K, Wallis TP, Hamilton BR, Gustafsson M, Ruas JL, Wilkins S, Bilton RL, Brismar K, Whitelaw ML, Pereira T, Gorman JJ, Ericson J, Peet DJ, Lendahl U, Poellinger L. (2008). Interaction with factor inhibiting HIF-1 defines an additional mode of cross-coupling between the Notch and hypoxia signalling pathways. Proc Natl Acad Sci U S A 105: 3368-73.

Zhong H, De Marzo AM, Laughner E, Lim M, Hilton DA, Zagzag D, Buechler P, Isaacs WB, Semenza GL, Simons JW. (1999). Overexpression of hypoxia-inducible factor 1alpha in common human cancers and their metastases. Cancer Res 59: 5830-5.

Chapter 4

PHD oxygen sensor function and antioxidants

Katarzyna J. Nytko, Daniel P. Stiehl, Roland H. Wenger[*]

[*]Author for correspondence:
Institute of Physiology and Zürich Center for Integrative Human Physiology ZIHP,
University of Zürich, Winterthurerstrasse 190, CH-8057 Zürich, Switzerland
E-mail: roland.wenger@access.uzh.ch

Contents

Key points

— Like the collagen prolyl-4-hydroxylases, oxygen-sensing HIF prolyl-4-hydroxylases (PHDs) require vitamin C for their enzymatic activity.

— Vitamin C deficiency leads to scurvy, raising the question whether it also affects oxygen sensing.

— There is evidence that antioxidants are essential to PHD function, but not necessarily vitamin C.

— Consequently, antioxidants play an important role in HIF-dependent physiological and pathophysiological processes.

— Detailed knowledge of antioxidant function will be necessary for the design of therapies of hypoxia-related diseases such as cancer.

Introduction

Antioxidants and reactive oxygen species (ROS) are powerful modulators of many cellular and systemic pathways involved in physiological and pathophysiological processes of the human body. ROS are continuously generated in living cells and normally excessive production of ROS is antagonized by a number of antioxidative mechanisms. Through evolution cells acquired mechanisms to fight the destructive effects of ROS on DNA, proteins and lipids by developing systems that either enzymatically remove ROS (superoxide dismutase, catalase, glutathione peroxidase etc.) or act as direct acceptors of unpaired electrons from ROS, thereby "scavenging" their harmful effects (carotenoids, vitamins C and E, glutathione etc.). Many diseases including cancer, atherosclerosis or inflammatory disorders are accompanied by an imbalanced antioxidative defense, resulting in severe damage to intra- and extracellular compartments ultimately promoting cell death or transformation.

Besides their rather unspecific protective effects, many antioxidants serve as co-factors or reducing agents for numerous metal-containing cellular enzymes necessary for their designated function. As such, many enzymes require vitamin C for optimal activity, with collagen prolyl-4-hydroxylases (C-P4Hs) being the first described (Tuderman et al., 1977). Vitamin C further functions as a co-factor of other iron(II)-dependent dioxygenases as well as copper(I)-dependent monooxygenases involved in dopamine and tyrosine metabolism, carnitine synthesis, DNA repair, oxygen sensing and many others (Linster and Van Schaftingen, 2007; Mandl et al., 2009).

Ascorbate as a co-factor for prolyl-4-hydroxylases

Ascorbic acid is a water-soluble vitamin that can be found in cells either in the reduced form (ascorbate), as free radical (semidehydroascorbate) or fully oxidized as dehydroascorbate (DHA). At physiological pH, the most abundant form of ascorbic acid is ascorbate (Corti et al., 2010). Ascorbate and DHA are transported into cells by sodium-dependent transporters (SVCT) and glucose transporters (GLUT), respectively (Corti et al., 2010). Intracellular DHA can be reduced to ascorbate by enzymatic and non-enzymatic processes, mostly utilizing glutathione-dependent pathways. Interestingly, primates, guinea pigs and some species of bats and paseriform birds lost the ability to synthesize vitamin C due to a mutation of L-gulono-1,4-lactone oxidase (Gulo) which catalyses the final step of ascorbate synthesis (Linster and Van Schaftingen, 2007; Nishikimi et al., 1988). Other vertebrates *de novo* synthesize ascorbate from D-glucuronate in the liver (mammals) or in the kidney (fish, amphibians and reptiles) (Linster and Van Schaftingen, 2007). Since ascorbate is an essential co-factor of C-P4Hs which hydroxylate proline residue to stabilize the collagen triple helix structure, persistent ascorbate deficiency results in disassembly of connective tissue structures, a common symptom of the nowadays rare disease scurvy. Scurvy is further characterized by apathy, weakness, bleeding gums and external and internal hemorrhages, which in severe cases often led to death (Baron, 2009). The disease occurred endemically amongst sailors at sea having no access to fresh food for a long period of time, and was first described by the French explorer Jacques Cartier in the 16th century (Martini, 2002). More than 200 years later the Scottish physician James Lind discovered that lemon juice can prevent the symptoms of the disease and seamen were subsequently provided with extracts of citrus fruits to treat scurvy (Lind, 1753). Until the discovery of vitamin C in 1932 by the later Nobel laureate Albert Szent-Györgyi, the reason for scurvy remained enigmatic and it took another 35 years until it finally could be established that vitamin C is actually required for full activity of C-P4Hs (Hutton et al., 1967; Li and Schellhorn, 2007). As ascorbate is present in almost all types of diets worldwide, the appearance of scurvy is very rare nowadays.

HIF prolyl-4-hydroxylases (PHDs) belong to the same class of enzymes as C-P4H, namely 2-oxoglutarate and non-heme iron(II)-dependent dioxygenases (EC 1.14.11.2). The prime substrate for C-P4H are prolyl residues within the collagen molecule while two specific prolines of the oxygen susceptible α-subunits of hypoxia-inducible factors (HIFs) are targeted by PHDs (Epstein et al., 2001; Ivan et al., 2001; Jaakkola et al., 2001). So far three isoforms of oxygen sensing PHDs have been described in humans, namely PHD1, PHD2 and PHD3. These proteins are encoded by the human *EGLN2*, *EGLN1* and *EGLN3* genes, respectively. The proteins differ in size, intracellular localization and tissue distribution (Metzen et al., 2003; Stiehl et al., 2006; Wenger et al., 2009). Under experimental *in vitro* conditions, preferences of each PHD isoform for the two target proline substrates within the HIF-α molecule have been observed (Appelhoff et al., 2004; Chan et al., 2005). A new putative prolyl-4-hydroxylase was identified in the endoplasmic reticulum which, when overexpressed, can suppress HIF activity, too (Koivunen et al., 2007; Oehme et al., 2002). However, further studies must be performed to elucidate the physiological function of this isoform. Moreover, an asparaginyl hydroxylase termed factor inhibiting HIF (FIH), hydroxylates a C-terminal Asn-residue of HIF-α subunits in an oxygen-dependent manner, thereby regulating co-factor recruitment and HIF's transcriptional activity (Hewitson et al., 2002).

Structurally, C-P4Hs form α2β2 tetramers whereas soluble PHD2 was preferentially found as α-monomers (McDonough et al., 2006; Myllyharju, 2008). PHD3 can form homo and hetero complexes with other PHDs, and PHD1 and PHD2 can form homo-dimers (Nakayama et al., 2007). Interestingly, PHD1-3 share 42-59% sequence identity but only little similarity with the primary structure of C-P4H, though critical residues involved in the binding of iron(II) and 2-oxoglutarate are conserved between the two subclasses (Myllyharju, 2008). Both, C-P4Hs and PHDs require oxygen, 2-oxoglutarate, iron (II) and/or ascorbate for *in vitro* activity, however they differ in *Km* values for these compounds (Hirsilä et al., 2003). Interestingly, the *Km* value of ascorbate for C-P4H is higher (300-370 µM) than for PHDs (140-180 µM), suggesting different dependency of these enzymes on ascorbate supplementation (Nagel et al., 2010). In contrast to 2-oxoglutarate and iron(II), which are tightly bound to PHDs, ascorbate did not co-purify with PHD2, indicating a rather labile and transient interaction between the enzyme and ascorbate (McNeill, Flashman et al. 2005). The actual role of ascorbate in the reaction catalyzed by PHDs is still a matter for debate: it has been postulated for C-P4Hs that ascorbate reduces ferryl iron(IV) intermediates to the active ferrous form. However, a similar function in the reaction cycle catalyzed by PHDs still awaits formal proof (de Jong et al., 1982; Kaelin and Ratcliffe, 2008). It has been shown for C-P4H that ascorbate is not consumed stoichiometrically during proline hydroxylation, and the enzymes can perform a number of reaction cycles without ascorbate (Myllyharju, 2008). Yet, in the absence of a proline hydroxy-acceptor substrate, C-P4H can catalyze uncoupled reactions characterized by decarboxylation of 2-oxoglutarate to succinate where ascorbate is then consumed stoichiometrically and serves as an alternative oxygen acceptor (Myllylä, Majamaa et al. 1984; Myllyharju 2008).

Among the factors that stabilize HIF-1α protein levels via ROS generation are angiotensin II and thrombin. Angiotensin II–induced generation of ROS (hydrogen peroxide) decreases intracellular ascorbate levels and thus leads to HIF-1α stabilization. Interestingly, ascorbate prevented ROS-induced HIF-1α under normoxic but not hypoxic conditions (Page et al., 2008). The role of ascorbate in modulation of HIF-1α protein levels has also been investigated in primary umbilical vein endothelial cells and in skin fibroblasts (Vissers et al., 2007). Addition of ascorbate to normoxic, hypoxic and cobalt chloride treated primary umbilical vein endothelial cells and skin fibroblasts cells decreased HIF-1α protein levels. As concluded in this study, normoxic cells showed stabilization of HIF-1α protein explained by the lack of ascorbate in the culture medium. However, the medium was supplemented with 20% FCS which might also be a source of ascorbate.

Ascorbate–independent prolyl-4-hydroxylase function

Reducing equivalents for functional HIF-α hydroxylation do not seem to be limited to ascorbate as other antioxidants (e.g. reduced glutathione and DTT) independently support PHD activity *in vitro* and *in vivo* (Flashman et al., 2010, Nytko et al., 2011). Studies on the role of ascorbate and other reducing agents on PHD2 activity *in vitro* revealed that ascorbate can be substituted by its structural analogues if they contain the ene-diol portion conferring reducing properties (Flashman et al., 2010). Furthermore, reduced glutathione (GSH) and dithiothreitol (DTT) at high concentrations could partially replace ascorbate in *in vitro* hydroxylation reactions catalysed by PHDs (Flashman et al., 2010). GSH further enhanced hydroxylation of an artificial consensus ankyrin peptide by FIH, which indicates its activating function also for other hydroxylases involved in oxygen sensing (Flashman et al., 2010).

To study the importance of vitamin C functions *in vivo*, a genetically modified mouse model incapable of synthesizing ascorbate has been generated. Animals with a bi-allelic disruption of the *Gulo* gene (Gulo$^{-/-}$) developed scurvy-like symptoms after 5 weeks of ascorbate withdrawal, evidenced by loss of body weight, internal hemorrhages, and disruption of elastic laminae building vessel walls (Maeda et al., 2000). When Gulo$^{-/-}$ mice were kept on an ascorbate-free diet for more than 6 weeks, the animals die from aortic rupture, pointing out the absolute requirement for vitamin C (Maeda et al., 2000). Partially contradictory to this finding, vitamin C-deficient Gulo$^{-/-}$ mice with a different genetic background still showed ascorbate-independent skin collagen and proline hydroxylation, indicating that *in vivo* other factors might at least partially compensate for the lack of ascorbate (Parsons et al., 2006). Notably, administration of glutathione ester to ascorbate-deficient guinea pigs could delay scurvy symptoms, further supporting the *in vivo* redundancy of intracellular antioxidants in the process of collagen hydroxylation (Martensson et al., 1993). Interestingly, neutrophils known to generate high levels of ROS to execute their pro-inflammatory function had defective apoptosis and increased HIF-1α levels when isolated from ascorbate depleted Gulo$^{-/-}$ mice (Vissers and Wilkie, 2007). Such observations may provide evidence for cell-type specific requirements of ascorbate in maintaining basal HIF activity, which is probably interlinked with the specific ROS burden in distinct cell types.

Whether ascorbate deficiency has an effect on other prolyl-4-hydroxylases *in vivo* at the systemic level is largely unknown. Recent work from our group showed that the physiological response of ascorbate depleted Gulo$^{-/-}$ mice to oxygen deprivation was essentially normal when compared to vitamin C supplemented animals as evidenced by similar erythropoietin transcript and protein induction (Nytko et al., 2011). In line with this finding, ascorbate was also shown to be dispensable for carnitine synthesis *in vivo* (Furusawa et al., 2008). Viewed as a whole, this data strongly points towards the non-essential role of ascorbate for functional HIF-α prolyl-4-hydroxylation at cellular and systemic levels and the possibility of other antioxidants compensating for its lack.

Regulation of PHD activity by redox factors

Interestingly, the β subunits of C-P4H have protein disulfide isomerase (PDI) activity which is required for the stable formation of the tetrameric enzyme (Kivirikko and Myllyharju, 1998). Since PHDs are active in the monomeric form (McDonough et al., 2006), a similar redox-sensitive mechanism is unlikely to exist for PHDs. We noted that recombinant PHD proteins purified from bacterial expression systems generally have low specific activity, with PHD3 being notoriously inactive, indicating the requirement of structural modulators absent in bacteria. In support of this notion, TriC and Morg1 chaperons have been described to interact and stimulate the activity of PHD3 and overexpression of the bacterial GroEL/ES chaperon enhanced the activity of the enzyme from bacterial preparations (Fedulova et al., 2007; Hopfer et al., 2006; Masson et al., 2004). However, it is unclear if these complex partners of PHD3 actively affect the protein structure by interference with intramolecular disulfide bonds.

For other antioxidants, e.g. the polyphenolic green tea ingredients gallic acid or its derivative n-propyl gallate, contradictory effects to ascorbate and glutathione on PHD acticity have been reported: Gallate, but not n-propyl gallate was claimed to inhibit PHDs *in vitro* while both compounds were stabilizing HIF-1α protein in rat heart muscle cells (Tsukiyama et al., 2006). Based on structural predictions of PHD2, inhibitory effects of gallate were attributed to the displacement of enzyme bound 2-oxoglutarate by gallate's carboxy moiety forming an ionic bond with Arg383, while its phenolate oxygen atoms chelate active centre bound iron(II) (Tsukiyama et al., 2006). However, data from our group using purified human PHD isoenzymes showed that either of these compounds was efficiently inhibiting all three PHDs in a dose-dependent manner *in vitro* (Nytko et al., 2007). The contradictory outcome of these experiments is likely explained by the use of crude cell extracts as enzyme source for *in vitro* HIF-α hydroxylation by Tsukiyama et al. We have shown previously that crude cell extracts catalyse non-PHD related turnover of 2-oxoglutarate to succinate and as such are inappropriate to determine specific PHD activity (Wirthner et al., 2007). Similarly, the plant-derived flavonoid quercetin has been shown to inhibit the activity of PHD2 *in vitro* probably involving chelating active site bound iron(II) (Dao et al., 2009; Jeon et al., 2007). Other flavonoids, such as baicalein, luteolin and fisetin, increased HIF-1α protein levels in HeLa cells but only weakly induced HIF transcriptional activity (Triantafyllou et al., 2008). Despite an assumed role in HIF-α protein stabilization, these compounds paradoxically blunted deferoxamine (DFX) induced HIF transcriptional activity, probably by interfering with MAPK-dependent activation of the HIF pathway (Triantafyllou et al., 2008). In a screen for small molecule inhibitors of PHD2, bicalein was independently identified as a potent inhibitor of PHD2 *in vitro* but also reduced asparaginyl hydroxylation of HIF-1α by FIH (Cho et al., 2008). Inhibitory effects of bicalein on PHD activity could be abrogated by an excess of 2-oxoglutarate and iron(II), suggesting a competitive mechanism. Spectroscopic measurements provided indirect evidence for binding of bicalein to PHD2, which was specific for the iron(II) containing enzyme (Cho et al., 2008).

Clearly, the variety of opposite effects reported for antioxidants on the PHDs' hydroxylation activity was caused by the different modes of activatory or inhibitory action (Figure 4.1). One common inhibitory mechanism involves chelation of metal co-factors required for PHD enzymatic activity, another mechanism might be the scavenging of some short-lived transition states of oxygen generated during the hydroxylation reaction cycle (Nytko et al., 2007). Moreover, phenolic antioxidants might contribute to the generation of reactive oxygen species such as hydrogen peroxide in cell culture models, subsequently inhibiting the cellular oxygen sensing pathway (Halliwell and Gutteridge, 2007).

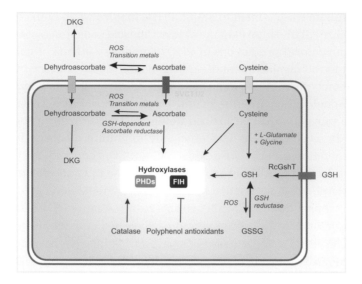

Figure 4.1 _ Crosstalk between different antioxidants affecting the activity of HIF prolyl and asparaginyl hydroxylases. ROS, reactive oxygen species; PHDs, prolyl-4-hydroxylase domain proteins; FIH, factor inhibiting HIF; DKG, diketogulonate; GSH, glutathione; GSSG, oxidized glutathione dimer; GLUT, glucose transporter; SVCT, sodium-dependent vitamin C transporter; ASC, alanine, serine, cysteine preferring transport system; RcGshT, rat canalicular GSH transporter. Bold arrows indicate the preferred direction of the reaction.

Ascorbate and transition metals

Historically, cobalt(II) was described as a factor inducing erythropoiesis with medical applications in the treatment of anemia (Goldberg et al., 1988; Nagel et al., 2010; Wolf and Levy, 1954). However, mechanisms by which cobalt and other metals exert their inhibitory function on cellular oxygen sensing remained speculative. In vitro characterization of PHD isoenzymes confirmed that transition metals are potent inhibitors of PHD activity (Hirsilä et al., 2003). Given that PHD enzymes are iron(II)-dependent dioxygenases, it is tempting to speculate that transition metals act via replacement of ferrous iron in the catalytic center of the enzyme as proposed for soluble nickel compounds (Davidson et al., 2006). Moreover, chromium(VI), nickel(II) and cobalt(II) have been proposed to regulate HIF-1α protein levels by depletion of intracellular ascorbate in lung cells while neither soluble nickel(II) nor cobalt(II) changed intra-cellular iron levels (Kaczmarek et al., 2007; Salnikow et al., 2004). Mechanistically, these metals are capable of catalyzing the oxidation of ascorbate to DHA, which can be enzymatically reverted to ascorbate within the cell or irreversibly oxidized to diketogulonate. Of note, in vitro oxidation of ascorbate by air is mainly catalyzed by copper(II) but oxidation is substantially slower by nickel(II) or cobalt(II) with a rate comparable to soluble iron(II), which does not inhibit PHD activity at all (Nytko et al., 2007). While this finding explains the PHD inhibiting effects observed for cupric copper (Martin et al., 2005; Nytko et al., 2007), the "ascorbate depletion" hypothesis by simple metal catalyzed oxidation should be marked with a touch of skepticism. Alternatively, nickel and cobalt could induce oxidative stress within the cell, as defined by the reduction of glutathione and malondialdehyde levels, thereby exhausting the intracellular ascorbate pool, instead of directly catalyzing ascorbate oxidation. Indeed, cobalt has been shown to induce oxidative stress in endothelial cells, which contributed to HIF-1α stabilization and was prevented by ascorbate treatment (Qiao et al., 2009). The increase in intracellular ROS and HIF-1α stabilization upon exposure to cobalt chloride in skeletal muscle cells was prevented by ascorbate treatment (Ciafre et al., 2007). Of note, cobalt chloride was found to robustly carbonylate recombinant PHD2 enzyme in vitro even in the complete absence of ascorbate, suggesting a direct redox interaction of the metal with iron-containing PHD enzymes (Nytko et al., 2011). Moreover, direct binding of cobalt to HIF-1α and subsequent inhibition of HIF-1α protein degradation by the pVHL ubiquitin ligase complex has been described, adding another layer of metal-dependent interference with the oxygen sensing pathway (Yuan et al., 2003). However, since 6xHis-HIF-2α proteins were used in the above experiments, the binding of the cobalt to 6His-tagged HIF-2α could contribute to the observed effect. Overall, in comparison to C-P4H and FIH, most transition metals were less effective inhibitors of PHDs, with PHD2 being particularly resistant to metal-induced regulation (Hirsilä et al., 2003).

Ascorbate and nitric oxide

It has been shown that nitric oxide can contribute to behavioural and developmental responses to hypoxia in *D. melanogaster* (Wingrove and O'Farrell, 1999). Moreover, as iNOS and eNOS (inducible and endothelial NO synthase, respectively) are direct HIF target genes (Coulet et al., 2003; Melillo et al., 1997;

Palmer et al., 1998). NO signalling could provide an additional feedback loop to oxygen sensing via regulating PHD activity (Kaelin and Ratcliffe, 2008). However, a clear picture of how NO affects oxygen signalling has been blurred by numerous opposing reports showing either increase (Kimura et al., 2001) or decrease in HIF-1α protein levels and transcriptional activity upon NO treatment (Huang et al., 1999). A recent report offers an elegant explanation for this dilemma, providing evidence for bi-modal effects of NO on HIF-1α protein accumulation. First, NO administration inhibits PHD activity leading to a rapid induction of HIF-1α protein. With some delay, the cellular hydroxylation capacity increases by HIF-dependent *de novo* synthesis of PHD2 (and likely PHD3) protein, ultimately reducing HIF-1α levels and counteracting the initial NO response (Berchner-Pfannschmidt et al., 2007). A similar model of bi-phasic responses to the notoriously instable ROS intermediates might likewise explain the many controversial results reported for this molecule group with respect to oxygen signalling pathways (Figure 4.2). Adding more complexity, ascorbate has been shown to decrease the levels of HIF-1α protein in HUVECs cells induced by treatment with a NO donor (Muellner et al., 2010). Another study showed that NO-induced HIF-1α accumulates independently of PHD activity, proposing cysteine and not ysteine nitrosylation of HIF-1α interfering with pVHL recruitment and asparagine hydroxylation to be responsible for its stabilization (Park et al., 2008). Adding even more complexity, ascorbate can stimulate NO release from intrinsic S-nitroso groups of the glypican-1 core protein (Mandl et al., 2009). Although this mechanism was primarily shown to play a role in NO-catalysed degradation of heparin sulphates, one could speculate about a similar role for ascorbate-induced NO generation in oxygen sensing (Mandl et al., 2009).

Expression of HIF-1α is affected by stress-activated pathways

Apart from the obvious role of antioxidants in the reaction catalyzed by PHDs and thus stability of HIF-1α protein, antioxidants have also been associated with the regulation of HIF expression. Transcript levels of HIF-1α were shown to be increased by reactive oxygen species involving activation of NF-κB signalling (Bonello et al., 2007). Both hydrogen peroxide and thrombin (shown previously to induce ROS production) also induced HIF-1α mRNA levels, an effect that was blunted in the presence of N-acetyl-cysteine (Belaiba et al., 2007; Bonello et al., 2007). Supporting these findings, the ubiquitous HIF-1α

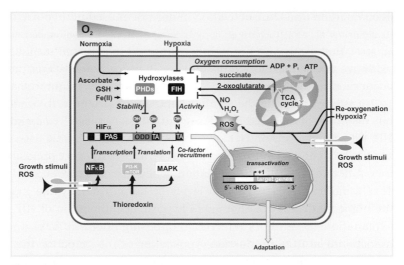

Figure 4.2 _ Regulation of HIF transcription, translation, protein stability and transactivation by reactive oxygen species and antioxidants. PHDs, prolyl-4-hydroxylase domain proteins; FIH, factor inhibiting HIF; HIF, hypoxia inducible factor; ROS, reactive oxygen species; NO, nitric oxide; GSH, glutathione; MAPK, mitogen activated protein kinase; NF-κB, nuclear factor kappa light enhancer of activated B cells; mTOR, mammalian target of rapamycin; PI3-K, phosphatidylinositol 3-kinase; PAS, Per/Arnt/Sim; ODD, oxygen dependent degradation; TA, transactivation domain; TCA, tricarboxylic acid.

promoter contains a functional NF-κB binding site, suggesting a role of this factor in the regulation of HIF-1α transcription (Bonello et al., 2007; Frede et al., 2006). Moreover, silencing of the antioxidant defense enzyme manganese superoxide dismutase (Mn-SOD) increased both HIF-1α mRNA and protein levels following intracellular ROS levels under normoxic and hypoxic conditions (Sasabe et al., 2010). *In vivo* studies using mice lacking IκB kinase (IKK)-β confirmed that basal NF-κB activity is linked with HIF-1α protein accumulation in the liver and brain of hypoxic animals (Rius et al., 2008).

Given the delicate balance of HIF-α production and proteasomal degradation, also regulated translation of HIF-α subunits has been suggested to affect the activity of the oxygen sensing pathway (Semenza, 2002; Yee Koh et al., 2008). Interestingly, the NO-donor NOC18 has been shown to increase the abundance of HIF-1α independent of its stability, which has been explained by concomitant activation of the protein translation regulatory mTOR/p70S6/eIF-4E pathway by NOC18 (Kasuno et al., 2004). Several other laboratories reported a role for PI3K and MAPK pathways in fine-tuning HIF-α accumulation and transactivation under normoxic and hypoxic conditions (Laughner et al., 2001; Richard et al., 1999; Sang et al., 2003; Stiehl et al., 2002; Zhong et al., 2000). Both pathways are tightly connected to external stimuli including oxidative stress, therefore a misbalance in redox homeostasis, particularly occurring during hypoxia followed by reoxygenation, might well affect HIF-1α translation. Among the small cellular redox proteins, thioredoxin (Trx) has also been implicated in HIF regulation, as reduced Trx could enhance HIF-1α protein levels and transcriptional activity (Huang et al., 1996; Welsh et al., 2002). It has later been resolved that Trx1 and Trx2 exert opposing regulatory functions on HIF-1α translation: while forced expression of cytosolic Trx1 enhanced HIF-1α protein levels in human embryonic kidney cells, the mitochondrial Trx2 attenuated hypoxic accumulation of HIF-1α. As an explanation, the authors referred to opposing effects of Trx1 and Trx2 on mitochondrial ROS production. Application of the mitochondria targeting antioxidant MitoQ indeed abolished reduced HIF-1α accumulation in cells with exogenous Trx2 expression (Zhou et al., 2007).

Sirtuin 1 (Sirt1), a redox-sensitive deacetylase, physically interacts specifically with HIF-2α and increases transcription of HIF-2 dependent target genes such as *Epo* in cells and mice (Dioum et al., 2009). While the actual acetylating event remains enigmatic, the same study reported on hypoxically induced acetylation of endogenous HIF-2α which was detectable in the presence of deacetylase inhibitors only. Extending these observations, deacetylation of human HIF-1α at Lys674 by SIRT1 led to impaired interaction of HIF-1α with p300 and consequently reduced HIF transcriptional activity (Lim et al., 2010). Interestingly, the plant derived polyphenolic antioxidant resveratrol has been described a potent regulator of sirtuin activity and hence could influence oxygen sensing *via* the HIF pathway (Howitz et al., 2003). To further strengthen the importance of acetylation in oxygen signalling, SIRT6 has been shown to function as a co-repressor of HIF-1α in the control of expression of several genes involved in glucose homeostasis (Zhong et al., 2010).

Oxidative stress and antioxidants in systemic oxygen sensing and disease

Following the instant response to cellular hypoxia and acute reprogramming of cell metabolism, HIFs also mediate middle- and long-term adaptive responses at the systemic level. HIF-1α protein stabilization by ROS has been discussed in the process of hypoxia-induced pulmonary vascular leakage, which causes pulmonary edema as described in mountain sickness and acute respiratory distress syndrome (ARDS) (Irwin et al., 2009). Cultured bovine pulmonary artery endothelial cell monolayers exposed to 3% O_2 for 24 hours showed increased permeability as measured by FITC-labeled albumin diffusion (Irwin et al., 2009). An antioxidative cocktail containing ascorbic acid, glutathione and α-tocopherol reduced the permeability when added to the cell monolayer, along with decreased hydrogen peroxide production and HIF-1α protein levels in these cells. Similar results were obtained in mice exposed to high altitude (18000 ft ≈ 5500 m above sea level) for 24 hours. The animals showed hypoxia-induced pulmonary vascular leakage and responded with increased HIF-1α and VEGF protein levels in pulmonary vessels, which could be reverted upon administration of antioxidants (Irwin et al., 2009). In human volunteers exposed to an altitude of 4300 m above sea level, corresponding to roughly 12% inspiratory oxygen concentration, HIF-1α protein levels and HIF-1 DNA binding were enhanced in circulating leukocytes and total glutathione levels in the plasma were strikingly decreased by 35% (Tissot van Patot et al., 2009). Such data might suggest that under hypoxic conditions the glutathione pool, serving as the major physiological antioxidant in humans, gets exhausted, which in turn could potentiate hypoxic HIF-1α activation.

The role of antioxidants in erythropoiesis has been studied in cell culture models *in vitro* as well as *in vivo*. EPO secretion from isolated rat kidneys perfused with an arterial pO_2 of 35 mm Hg was increased upon treatment with vitamins A, E and C (Jelkmann et al., 1997). Yet, vitamins E and C failed to increase Epo secretion from the human hepatoma cell lines Hep3B and HepG2 (Jelkmann et al., 1997). Oxidative stress has also been observed in haematopoietic disorders. Patients suffering from inherited forms of anemia such as sickle cell anemia, thalassemia and glucose-6-phosphate-dehydrogenase deficiency, levels of certain antioxidants (predominantly vitamins E and C) are often decreased (Chan et al., 1999).

Physiological wound healing requires oxygen for an optimal healing process (Schreml et al., 2010). ROS produced during wound healing have been discussed to serve as signalling molecules in regulating cytokine release and cell proliferation, while they also contribute to killing harmful bacteria in the wound environment (Schreml et al., 2010). On the other hand, oxygen deprivation is supportive in wound healing as it stimulates VEGF expression and neovascularization (Hopf and Rollins, 2007; Scheid et al., 2000). Importantly, levels of ascorbate, vitamin E and glutathione are decreased in healing skin wounds and a reduced level of these antioxidants correlates with a delay in the healing process (Schafer and Werner, 2008). Consequently, detoxifying enzymes, such SODs, catalase and glutathione peroxidase and others, are involved in wound healing and responsible for maintaining a cellular redox balance (Schafer and Werner, 2008). Very likely, hypoxia, ROS and antioxidative pathways interact with each other to contribute to successive wound healing, though experimental proof of such a hypothesis is required.

Antioxidants also play an important role in aging and aging is associated with increased oxidative stress (Rockenfeller and Madeo, 2010). Mice lacking senescence marker protein 30, which functions as gluconolactonase and participates in ascorbate synthesis, displayed symptoms of scurvy and shortage in lifespan (Kondo et al., 2006). Moreover, ascorbate was shown to prevent premature aging in mice displaying the phenotype of Werner syndrome due to a lack of helicase of WRN homolog involved in DNA repair (Massip et al., 2009). Whether there is a direct link between HIF and antioxidants in the context of aging remains to be investigated.

Antioxidants in HIF-mediated tumourigenesis

In the 1970s, Linus Pauling reported that ascorbate can prolong the survival time of terminally ill cancer patients (Cameron and Pauling, 1976; Cameron and Pauling, 1978). Moreover, he claimed that ascorbate is applicable in the prevention of common cold and schizophrenia (Pauling, 1971; Pauling, 1977). However, his hypotheses did not find general approval by the scientific community and other studies failed to confirm these results (Creagan et al., 1979; Moertel et al., 1985). An impressive number of studies on ascorbate and cancer have been performed since that time and the general idea of using ascorbate in cancer treatment has experienced a renaissace in recent years: growing a collection of tumour cell lines as subcutaneous tumours in mice revealed that ascorbate administered at "pharmacological doses" could decrease the growth of aggressive tumour xenografts (Chen et al., 2008). In these studies, and somehow paradoxically, ascorbate has been proposed to function as a pro-drug which facilitates the generation of hydrogen peroxide in a Fenton-like reaction and selectively kills cancer cells (Chen et al., 2005; Chen et al., 2007). Of note, millimolar doses of ascorbate can be achieved only by intravenous application and the findings have not been perceived without controversy (Borst, 2008; Frei and Lawson, 2008). Moreover, such studies do not consider the role of HIF-1/2α in cancer progression. It is known that high expression of HIF-1/2α correlates with high mortality of cancer patients, especially in the case of solid tumours (Semenza, 2010). Little is known, however, about the correlation between ascorbate levels in patients and cancer progression in the context of HIF-1/2α expression and stability. It has been shown for endometrial cancers only that low ascorbate levels in cancer tissue is associated with increased HIF-1α activity and elevated expression of HIF-target genes (VEGF, GLUT-1 and BNIP3) (Kuiper et al., 2010). Endometrial cancers are associated with high expression of HIF-1/2α and increased angiogenesis, which is linked to poor prognosis of patients (Sivridis et al., 2002). Therefore, finding a way to overcome HIF-driven effects in these tumours by antioxidants could be a potential therapy target. Ascorbate can suppress HIF-1α protein levels and secretion of VEGF in pancreatic tumour in athymic mice, but ascorbate could reduce tumour size only at early and middle stages of cancer progression (Chen et al., 2009). In cancer cells *in vitro*, ascorbate supplementation could reduce HIF-1α protein levels in normoxic prostate cancer cells, which have high basal levels of this protein (Knowles et al., 2003). Moreover, ascorbate decreased HIF-1α protein levels stimulated by insulin and insulin growth factor I (IGF-1) in human breast cancer cells (Knowles et al., 2003). Interestingly, ascorbate had no effect on hypoxia-induced HIF-1α protein levels. Since iron(II) is a crucial co-factor for the activity of PHDs, its depletion from cells results in the stabilization of HIF-1α and activation of target genes. It has been shown that inhibition of transferrin receptor by monoclonal antibodies and thus decrease in iron uptake leads to the stabilization of HIF-1α and upregulation of its targets in cancer cells (Jones et al., 2006). These effects were suppressed by physiological concentration of ascorbate (25 µM). At this point, it is important to mention that DHA, the oxidized form of ascorbate, can be transported to cells by glucose transporters (GLUT 1, 3 and 4) (Corti et al., 2010). Interestingly, GLUT1 and GLUT3 are also HIF-target genes, therefore DHA uptake could be increased in hypoxia providing an additional feedback loop mechanism to balance HIF homeostasis, especially in cancer cells.

HIF-1α can mediate the inhibitory effects of antioxidants on tumour growth also *in vivo*. Benign prostatic hyperplasia (BPH) as well as prostate cancer are associated with hypoxia and angiogenesis. Moreover, testosterone induces HIF-1α levels in prostate cells (Mabjeesh et al., 2003). Ascorbate could reduce HIF-1α protein levels induced by testosterone treatment and decreased VEGF expression in prostate cells (Li et al., 2009). Moroever, ascorbate delayed prostate growth induced by testosterone in rats (Li et al., 2009).

Ascorbate deficiency had no effect on proline hydroxylation and colla-gen production in mammary tumour cells (4TI) grown in Gulo$^{-/-}$ mice (Par-sons et al., 2006). In contrast, ascorbic acid deficiency delayed growth of Lewis lung carcinoma in Gulo$^{-/-}$ (Telang et al., 2007). However, HIF-1α protein levels were not altered between ascorbate-free and ascorbate-supplemented tumours (Telang et al., 2007). These opposing effects could be explained by the different genetic background of Gulo$^{-/-}$ mice used in these experiments (Parsons et al., 2006; Telang et al., 2007). P493 human B cell xenografts grown in mice treated with N-acetyl cysteine (NAC, 40 mM) were significantly smaller than those in non-treated animals (Gao et al., 2007). Since P493 cells ectopically expressing non-degradable HIF-1α protein were more resistant to NAC treatment, HIF-1α might be involved in these effects (Gao et al., 2007). Moreover, NAC did not affect chromosomal stability, therefore excluding ROS-induced genomic instability as the reason for tumour growth. Similar effects were observed in P493 tumour xenografts when mice obtained a high concentration of ascorbate with drinking water (5 g/l) (Gao et al., 2007). NAC is an antioxidant itself but can also increase the intracellular pool of glutathione, since it is a precursor in the synthesis of this compound. Until recently, antioxidant effects on tumour growth were attributed to its ability to reduce oxidative stress and therefore genomic instability (Sablina et al., 2005). For the first time this data suggested that antioxidants could also prevent or delay tumour growth via mechanism mediated by PHDs/ HIF. Another protein linking HIF- and ROS-dependent pathways in can-cer cells is REDD1, a transcriptional target of HIF. REDD1 is also known as RT801 and is involved in the regulation of cell survival as well as ROS production (Ellisen et al., 2002; Shoshani et al., 2002). Increased ROS production and tumourigenesis has been shown for REDD1$^{-/-}$ cells, both mediated by HIF-1α, which can be blocked by treating the cells/animals with ascorbate and N-acetyl cysteine (Horak et al., 2010). JunD is a member of the AP-1 fam-ily of transcription factors and its lack in cells causes increased hydrogen peroxide generation and reduced antioxidative defense. As a result, these cells have increased HIF-1α levels which promotes angiogenesis and sur-vival of tumour cells (Gerald et al., 2004). These effects have been shown to be dependent on PHD2 activity, but reduced in JunD$^{-/-}$ cells by oxidation of iron (II) in the catalytic center of the enzyme. Interestingly, hydrogen peroxide concentrations and levels of HIF-1α proteins in JunD$^{-/-}$ cells were reduced by treatment with ascorbate, cysteine and reduced glutathione. These observations once again emphasise the role of these antioxidants in maintaining PHD activity and HIF-1α protein levels, especially under oxidative stress conditions.

Besides ascorbate and glutathione (or N-acetyl-cysteine) vitamin E has also been shown to exert antitumourigenic effects. Tocotrienol (unsaturated vitamin E) reduced hypoxia induced VEGF secretion from human colorectal adenocarcinoma cells (DLD-1) (Shibata et al., 2008). Considering that HIF-1α mediated angiogenesis is one of the major steps in cancer progression, this observation suggests vitamin E as a putative antitumourigenic agent.

As mentioned above, copper, nickel and other transition metals can deplete ascorbate (and other co-factors) required for PHD activity, stabilize HIF-1α and hence act as carcinogenic factors. These effects play an important role especially in cancers of the respiratory tract, since exposure to nickel(II), chromium(VI) and cobalt(II) via inhalation or ingestion causes primarily lung injury (Salnikow and Kasprzak, 2005). Moreover, advanced stages of lung cancer display decreased levels of ascorbate, reduced glutathione and other antioxidants (Esme et al., 2008).

Future perspectives

Whether antioxidants will serve as anti-cancer drugs in the context of the PHD/HIF oxygen sensing pathway remains speculative. The complexity of HIF responses together with the fact that in some tumours HIF down- and up-regulation exerts differential effects must be considered in such therapies. There is no doubt that HIF prolyl-4-hydroxylases require antioxidants for full activity. Whether this antioxidant is exclusively ascorbate, or if it can be replaced by other reducing compounds, needs to be elucidated. One has also to consider that there are three different PHD isoforms with partial redundancy but also distinct cellular and organ expression levels, inducibility and probably function. Furthermore, the specificity of antioxidant action on cells is very low with many enzymes/pathways being regulated and therefore difficult to control. Another point to be considered is a concentration-dependent dual function of ascorbate, either serving as an ROS scavenger or as a pro-oxidant (Levine et al., 2009). The border between these two states is very tightly regulated and depends on many factors that are difficult to control in vivo. Moreover, the half-life of most antioxidants is very short with intermediate states which exert differential effects. Thus, antioxidants can undergo rapid modifications/degradation while administered to organisms. The route of administration of antioxidants must also be considered. In Linus Pauling's studies, patients received ascorbate both orally and intravenously and in the follow-up studies, which failed to confirm Pauling's hypotheses, ascorbate was only orally applied to cancer patients, potentially explaining the opposing effects. Intravenous administration of ascorbate can result in 70 to 100-fold higher plasma concentrations of this compound (Levine et al., 2009). Overall, antioxidants have been proven to play an important role in the oxygen sensing pathway on almost all levels of HIF regulation: expression, stability and activity. However, further studies are required to elucidate their application in diseases mediated by PHDs/HIF oxygen sensing pathway.

References

Appelhoff RJ, Tian YM, Raval RR, Turley H, Harris AL, Pugh CW, Ratcliffe PJ, Gleadle JM (2004). Differential function of the prolyl hydroxylases PHD1, PHD2, and PHD3 in the regulation of hypoxia-inducible factor. J Biol Chem. 279(37): 38458-65.

Baron JH (2009). Sailors' scurvy before and after James Lind–a reassessment. Nutr Rev. 67(6): 315-32.

Belaiba RS, Bonello S, Zahringer C, Schmidt S, Hess J, Kietzmann T, Gorlach A (2007). Hypoxia up-regulates hypoxia-inducible factor-1alpha transcription by involving phosphatidylinositol 3-kinase and nuclear factor kappaB in pulmonary artery smooth muscle cells. Mol Biol Cell. 18(12): 4691-7.

Berchner-Pfannschmidt U, Yamac H, Trinidad B, Fandrey J (2007). Nitric oxide modulates oxygen sensing by hypoxia-inducible factor 1-dependent induction of prolyl hydroxylase 2. J Biol Chem. 282(3): 1788-96.

Bonello S, Zahringer C, BelAiba RS, Djordjevic T, Hess J, Michiels C, Kietzmann T, Gorlach A (2007). Reactive oxygen species activate the HIF-1alpha promoter via a functional NFkappaB site. Arterioscler Thromb Vasc Biol. 27(4): 755-61.

Borst P (2008). Mega-dose vitamin C as therapy for human cancer? Proc Natl Acad Sci U S A. 105(48): E95; author reply E96.

Cameron E, Pauling L (1976). Supplemental ascorbate in the supportive treatment of cancer: Prolongation of survival times in terminal human cancer. Proc Natl Acad Sci U S A. 73(10): 3685-9.

Cameron E, Pauling L (1978). Supplemental ascorbate in the supportive treatment of cancer: reevaluation of prolongation of survival times in terminal human cancer. Proc Natl Acad Sci U S A. 75(9): 4538-42.

Chan AC, Chow CK, Chiu D (1999). Interaction of antioxidants and their implication in genetic anemia. Proc Soc Exp Biol Med. 222(3): 274-82.

Chan DA, Sutphin PD, Yen SE, Giaccia AJ (2005). Coordinate regulation of the oxygen-dependent degradation domains of hypoxia-inducible factor 1 alpha. Mol Cell Biol. 25(15): 6415-26.

Chen C, Sun J, Liu G, Chen J (2009). Effect of small interference RNA targeting HIF-1alpha mediated by rAAV combined L: -ascorbate on pancreatic tumours in athymic mice. Pathol Oncol Res. 15(1): 109-14.

Chen Q, Espey MG, Krishna MC, Mitchell JB, Corpe CP, Buettner GR, Shacter E, Levine M (2005). Pharmacologic ascorbic acid concentrations selectively kill cancer cells: action as a pro-drug to deliver hydrogen peroxide to tissues. Proc Natl Acad Sci USA 102(38): 13604-9.

Chen Q, Espey MG, Sun AY, Lee JH, Krishna MC, Shacter E, Choyke PL, Pooput C, Kirk KL, Buettner GR, Levine M (2007). Ascorbate in pharmacologic concentrations selectively generates ascorbate radical and hydrogen peroxide in extracellular fluid in vivo. Proc Natl Acad Sci U S A. 104(21): 8749-54.

Chen Q, Espey MG, Sun AY, Pooput C, Kirk KL, Krishna MC, Khosh DB, Drisko J, Levine M (2008). Pharmacologic doses of ascorbate act as a prooxidant and decrease growth of aggressive tumour xenografts in mice. Proc Natl Acad Sci USA 105(32): 11105-9.

Cho H, Lee HY, Ahn DR, Kim SY, Kim S, Lee KB, Lee YM, Park H, Yang EG (2008). Baicalein induces functional hypoxia-inducible factor-1alpha and angiogenesis. Mol Pharmacol. 74(1): 70-81.

Ciafre SA, Niola F, Giorda E, Farace MG, Caporossi D (2007). CoCl(2)-simulated hypoxia in skeletal muscle cell lines: Role of free radicals in gene up-regulation and induction of apoptosis. Free Radic Res. 41(4): 391-401.

Corti A, Casini AF, Pompella A (2010). Cellular pathways for transport and efflux of ascorbate and dehydroascorbate. Arch 500(2): 107-15.

Coulet F, Nadaud S, Agrapart M, Soubrier F (2003). Identification of hypoxia-response element in the human endothelial nitric-oxide synthase gene promoter. J Biol Chem. 278(47): 46230-40.

Creagan ET, Moertel CG, O'Fallon JR, Schutt AJ, O'Connell MJ, Rubin J, Frytak S (1979). Failure of high-dose vitamin C (ascorbic acid) therapy to benefit patients with advanced cancer. A controlled trial. N Engl J Med. 301(13): 687-90.

Dao JH, Kurzeja RJ, Morachis JM, Veith H, Lewis J, Yu V, Tegley CM, Tagari P (2009). Kinetic characterization and identification of a novel inhibitor of hypoxia-inducible factor prolyl hydroxylase 2 using a time-resolved fluorescence resonance energy transfer-based assay technology. Anal Biochem. 384(2): 213-23.

Davidson TL, Chen H, Di Toro DM, D'Angelo G, Costa M (2006). Soluble nickel inhibits HIF-prolyl-hydroxylases creating persistent hypoxic signalling in A549 cells. Mol Carcinog. 45(7): 479-89.

de Jong L, Albracht SP, Kemp A (1982). Prolyl 4-hydroxylase activity in relation to the oxidation state of enzyme-bound iron. The role of ascorbate in peptidyl proline hydroxylation. Biochim Biophys Acta. 704(2): 326-32.

Dioum EM, Chen R, Alexander MS, Zhang Q, Hogg RT, Gerard RD, Garcia JA (2009). Regulation of hypoxia-inducible factor 2alpha signalling by the stress-responsive deacetylase sirtuin 1. Science. 324(5932): 1289-93.

Ellisen LW, Ramsayer KD, Johannessen CM, Yang A, Beppu H, Minda K, Oliner JD, McKeon F, Haber DA (2002). REDD1, a developmentally regulated transcriptional target of p63 and p53, links p63 to regulation of reactive oxygen species. Mol Cell. 10(5): 995-1005.

Epstein AC, Gleadle JM, McNeill LA, Hewitson KS, O'Rourke J, Mole DR, Mukherji M, Metzen E, Wilson MI, Dhanda A, Tian YM, Masson N, Hamilton DL, Jaakkola P, Barstead R, Hodgkin J, Maxwell PH, Pugh CW, Schofield CJ, Ratcliffe PJ (2001). C. elegans EGL-9 and mammalian homologs define a family of dioxygenases that regulate HIF by prolyl hydroxylation. Cell. 107(1): 43-54.

Esme H, Cemek M, Sezer M, Saglam H, Demir A, Melek H, Unlu M (2008). High levels of oxidative stress in patients with advanced lung cancer. Respirology. 13(1): 112-6.

Fedulova N, Hanrieder J, Bergquist J, Emren LO (2007). Expression and purification of catalytically active human PHD3 in Escherichia coli. Protein Expr Purif. 54(1): 1-10.

Flashman E, Davies SL, Yeoh KK, Schofield CJ (2010). Investigating the dependence of the hypoxia-inducible factor hydroxylases (factor inhibiting HIF and prolyl hydroxylase domain 2) on ascorbate and other reducing agents. Biochem 427(1): 135-42.

Frede S, Stockmann C, Freitag P, Fandrey J (2006). Bacterial lipopolysaccharide induces HIF-1 activation in human monocytes via p44/42 MAPK and NF-kappaB. Biochem J. 396(3): 517-27.

Frei B, Lawson S (2008). Vitamin C and cancer revisited. Proc Natl Acad Sci U S A. 105(32): 11037-8.

Furusawa H, Sato Y, Tanaka Y, Inai Y, Amano A, Iwama M, Kondo Y, Handa S, Murata A, Nishikimi M, Goto S, Maruyama N, Takahashi R, Ishigami A (2008). Vitamin C is not essential for carnitine biosynthesis in vivo: verification in vitamin C-depleted senescence marker protein-30/gluconolactonase knockout mice. Biol Pharm Bull. 31(9): 1673-9.

Gao P, Zhang H, Dinavahi R, Li F, Xiang Y, Raman V, Bhujwalla ZM, Felsher DW, Cheng L, Pevsner J, Lee LA, Semenza GL, Dang CV (2007). HIF-dependent antitumourigenic effect of antioxidants in vivo. Cancer Cell 12(3): 230-8.

Gerald D, Berra E, Frapart YM, Chan DA, Giaccia AJ, Mansuy D, Pouyssegur J, Yaniv M, Mechta-Grigoriou F (2004). JunD reduces tumour angiogenesis by protecting cells from oxidative stress. Cell. 118(6): 781-94.

Goldberg MA, Dunning SP, Bunn HF (1988). Regulation of the erythropoietin gene: evidence that the oxygen sensor is a heme protein. Science. 242(4884): 1412-5.

Halliwell B, Gutteridge JM (2007). Free radicals in biology and medicine. Oxford University Press, Oxford, p.184.

Hewitson KS, McNeill LA, Riordan MV, Tian YM, Bullock AN, Welford RW, Elkins JM, Oldham NJ, Bhattacharya S, Gleadle JM, Ratcliffe PJ, Pugh CW, Schofield CJ (2002). Hypoxia-inducible factor (HIF) asparagine hydroxylase is identical to factor inhibiting HIF (FIH) and is related to the cupin structural family. J Biol Chem. 277(29): 26351-5.

Hirsilä M, Koivunen P, Günzler V, Kivirikko KI, Myllyharju J (2003). Characterization of the human prolyl 4-hydroxylases that modify the hypoxia-inducible factor. J Biol Chem 278(33): 30772-80.

Hopf HW, Rollins MD (2007). Wounds: an overview of the role of oxygen. Antioxid Redox Signal. 9(8): 1183-92.

Hopfer U, Hopfer H, Jablonski K, Stahl RA, Wolf G (2006). The novel WD-repeat protein Morg1 acts as a molecular scaffold for hypoxia-inducible factor prolyl hydroxylase 3 (PHD3). J Biol Chem. 281(13): 8645-55.

Horak P, Crawford AR, Vadysirisack DD, Nash ZM, DeYoung MP, Sgroi D, Ellisen LW (2010). Negative feedback control of HIF-1 through REDD1-regulated ROS suppresses tumourigenesis. Proc 107(10): 4675-80.

Howitz KT, Bitterman KJ, Cohen HY, Lamming DW, Lavu S, Wood JG, Zipkin RE, Chung P, Kisielewski A, Zhang LL, Scherer B, Sinclair DA (2003). Small molecule activators of sirtuins extend Saccharomyces cerevisiae lifespan. Nature. 425(6954): 191-6.

Huang LE, Arany Z, Livingston DM, Bunn HF (1996). Activation of hypoxia-inducible transcription factor depends primarily upon redox-sensitive stabilization of its alpha subunit. J Biol Chem. 271(50): 32253-9.

Huang LE, Willmore WG, Gu J, Goldberg MA, Bunn HF (1999). Inhibition of hypoxia-inducible factor 1 activation by carbon monoxide and nitric oxide. Implications for oxygen sensing and signalling. J Biol Chem. 274(13): 9038-44.

Hutton JJ, Jr., Kaplan A, Udenfriend S (1967). Conversion of the amino acid sequence gly-pro-pro in protein to gly-pro-hyp by collagen proline hydroxylase. Arch Biochem Biophys. 121(2): 384-91.

Irwin DC, McCord JM, Nozik-Grayck E, Beckly G, Foreman B, Sullivan T, White M, T. Crossno J J, Bailey D, Flores SC, Majka S, Klemm D, van Patot MC (2009). A potential role for reactive oxygen species and the HIF-1alpha-VEGF pathway in hypoxia-induced pulmonary vascular leak. Free Radic Biol Med. 47(1): 55-61.

Ivan M, Kondo K, Yang H, Kim W, Valiando J, Ohh M, Salic A, Asara JM, Lane WS, Kaelin WG, Jr. (2001). HIFa targeted for VHL-mediated destruction by proline hydroxylation: implications for O2 sensing. Science 292(5516): 464-8.

Jaakkola P, Mole DR, Tian YM, Wilson MI, Gielbert J, Gaskell SJ, Kriegsheim A, Hebestreit HF, Mukherji M, Schofield CJ, Maxwell PH, Pugh CW, Ratcliffe PJ (2001). Targeting of HIF-a to the von Hippel-Lindau ubiquitylation complex by O2-regulated prolyl hydroxylation. Science 292(5516): 468-72.

Jelkmann W, Pagel H, Hellwig T, Fandrey J (1997). Effects of antioxidant vitamins on renal and hepatic erythropoietin production. Kidney Int. 51(2): 497-501.

Jeon H, Kim H, Choi D, Kim D, Park SY, Kim YJ, Kim YM, Jung Y (2007). Quercetin activates an angiogenic pathway, hypoxia inducible factor (HIF)-1-vascular endothelial growth factor, by inhibiting HIF-prolyl hydroxylase: a structural analysis of quercetin for inhibiting HIF-prolyl hydroxylase. Mol Pharmacol. 71(6): 1676-84.

Jones DT, Trowbridge IS, Harris AL (2006). Effects of transferrin receptor blockade on cancer cell proliferation and hypoxia-inducible factor function and their differential regulation by ascorbate. Cancer Res. 66(5): 2749-56.

Kaczmarek M, Timofeeva OA, Karaczyn A, Malyguine A, Kasprzak KS, Salnikow K (2007). The role of ascorbate in the modulation of HIF-1alpha protein and HIF-dependent transcription by chromium(VI) and nickel(II). Free Radic Biol Med. 42(8): 1246-57.

Kaelin WG, Jr., Ratcliffe PJ (2008). Oxygen sensing by metazoans: the central role of the HIF hydroxylase pathway. Mol Cell. 30(4): 393-402.

Kasuno K, Takabuchi S, Fukuda K, Kizaka-Kondoh S, Yodoi J, Adachi T, Semenza GL, Hirota K (2004). Nitric oxide induces hypoxia-inducible factor 1 activation that is dependent on MAPK and phosphatidylinositol 3-kinase signalling. J Biol Chem. 279(4): 2550-8.

Kimura H, Weisz A, Ogura T, Hitomi Y, Kurashima Y, Hashimoto K, D'Acquisto F, Makuuchi M, Esumi H (2001). Identification of hypoxia-inducible factor 1 ancillary sequence and its function in vascular endothelial growth factor gene induction by hypoxia and nitric oxide. J Biol Chem. 276(3): 2292-8.

Kivirikko KI, Myllyharju J (1998). Prolyl 4-hydroxylases and their protein disulfide isomerase subunit. Matrix Biol. 16(7): 357-68.

Knowles HJ, Raval RR, Harris AL, Ratcliffe PJ (2003). Effect of ascorbate on the activity of hypoxia-inducible factor in cancer cells. Cancer Res 63(8): 1764-8.

Koivunen P, Tiainen P, Hyvarinen J, Williams KE, Sormunen R, Klaus SJ, Kivirikko KI, Myllyharju J (2007). An endoplasmic reticulum transmembrane prolyl 4-hydroxylase is induced by hypoxia and acts on hypoxia-inducible factor alpha. J Biol Chem. 282(42): 30544-52.

Kondo Y, Inai Y, Sato Y, Handa S, Kubo S, Shimokado K, Goto S, Nishikimi M, Maruyama N, Ishigami A (2006). Senescence marker protein 30 functions as gluconolactonase in L-ascorbic acid biosynthesis, and its knockout mice are prone to scurvy. Proc Natl Acad Sci U S A. 103(15): 5723-8.

Kuiper C, Molenaar IG, Dachs GU, Currie MJ, Sykes PH, Vissers MC (2010). Low Ascorbate Levels Are Associated with Increased Hypoxia-Inducible Factor-1 Activity and an Aggressive Tumour Phenotype in Endometrial Cancer. Cancer Res. 70(14): 5749-58.

Laughner E, Taghavi P, Chiles K, Mahon PC, Semenza GL (2001). HER2 (neu) signalling increases the rate of hypoxia-inducible factor 1alpha (HIF-1alpha) synthesis: novel mechanism for HIF-1-mediated vascular endothelial growth factor expression. Mol Cell Biol. 21(12): 3995-4004.

Levine M, Espey MG, Chen Q (2009). Losing and finding a way at C: new promise for pharmacologic ascorbate in cancer treatment. Free Radic Biol Med. 47(1): 27-9.

Li SH, Ryu JH, Park SE, Cho YS, Park JW, Lee WJ, Chun YS (2009). Vitamin C supplementation prevents testosterone-induced hyperplasia of rat prostate by downregulating HIF-1alpha. J Nutr Biochem 21(9): 801-8.

Li Y, Schellhorn HE (2007). New developments and novel therapeutic perspectives for vitamin C. J Nutr. 137(10): 2171-84.

Lim JH, Lee YM, Chun YS, Chen J, Kim JE, Park JW (2010). Sirtuin 1 modulates cellular responses to hypoxia by deacetylating hypoxia-inducible factor 1alpha. Mol 38(6): 864-78.

Lind J (1753). A Treatise of the Scurvy in Three Parts. Containing an Inquiry into the Nature, Causes and Cure of that Disease, together with a Critical and Chronological View of what has been published on the subject.

Linster CL, Van Schaftingen E (2007). Vitamin C. Biosynthesis, recycling and degradation in mammals. Febs J. 274(1): 1-22.

Mabjeesh NJ, Willard MT, Frederickson CE, Zhong H, Simons JW (2003). Androgens stimulate hypoxia-inducible factor 1 activation via autocrine loop of tyrosine kinase receptor/phosphatidylinositol 3'-kinase/protein kinase B in prostate cancer cells. Clin Cancer Res. 9(7): 2416-25.

Maeda N, Hagihara H, Nakata Y, Hiller S, Wilder J, Reddick R (2000). Aortic wall damage in mice unable to synthesize ascorbic acid. Proc Natl Acad Sci USA 97(2): 841-6.

Mandl J, Szarka A, Banhegyi G (2009). Vitamin C: update on physiology and pharmacology. Br J Pharmacol. 157(7): 1097-110.

Martensson J, Han J, Griffith OW, Meister A (1993). Glutathione ester delays the onset of scurvy in ascorbate-deficient guinea pigs. Proc Natl Acad Sci USA 90(1): 317-21.

Martin F, Linden T, Katschinski DM, Oehme F, Flamme I, Mukhopadhyay CK, Eckhardt K, Troger J, Barth S, Camenisch G, Wenger RH (2005). Copper-dependent activation of hypoxia-inducible factor (HIF)-1: implications for ceruloplasmin regulation. Blood. 105(12): 4613-9.

Martini E (2002). Jacques Cartier witnesses a treatment for scurvy. Vesalius. 8(1): 2-6.

Massip L, Garand C, Paquet ER, Cogger VC, O'Reilly JN, Tworek L, Hatherell A, Taylor CG, Thorin E, Zahradka P, Le Couteur DG, Lebel M (2009). Vitamin C restores healthy aging in a mouse model for Werner syndrome. Faseb J 24(1): 158-72.

Masson N, Appelhoff RJ, Tuckerman JR, Tian YM, Demol H, Puype M, Vandekerckhove J, Ratcliffe PJ, Pugh CW (2004). The HIF prolyl hydroxylase PHD3 is a potential substrate of the TRiC chaperonin. FEBS Lett. 570(1-3): 166-70.

McDonough MA, Li V, Flashman E, Chowdhury R, Mohr C, Lienard BM, Zondlo J, Oldham NJ, Clifton IJ, Lewis J, McNeill LA, Kurzeja RJ, Hewitson KS, Yang E, Jordan S, Syed RS, Schofield CJ (2006). Cellular oxygen sensing: Crystal structure of hypoxia-inducible factor prolyl hydroxylase (PHD2). Proc Natl Acad Sci U S A. 103(26): 9814-9.

Melillo G, Taylor LS, Brooks A, Musso T, Cox GW, Varesio L (1997). Functional requirement of the hypoxia-responsive element in the activation of the inducible nitric oxide synthase promoter by the iron chelator desferrioxamine. J Biol Chem. 272(18): 12236-43.

Metzen E, Berchner-Pfannschmidt U, Stengel P, Marxsen JH, Stolze I, Klinger M, Huang WQ, Wotzlaw C, Hellwig-Burgel T, Jelkmann W, Acker H, Fandrey J (2003). Intracellular localisation of human HIF-1 alpha hydroxylases: implications for oxygen sensing. J Cell Sci. 116(Pt 7): 1319-26.

Moertel CG, Fleming TR, Creagan ET, Rubin J, O'Connell MJ, Ames MM (1985). High-dose vitamin C versus placebo in the treatment of patients with advanced cancer who have had no prior chemotherapy. A randomized double-blind comparison. N Engl J Med. 312(3): 137-41.

Muellner MK, Schreier SM, Schmidbauer B, Moser M, Quehenberger P, Kapiotis S, Goldenberg H, Laggner H (2010). Vitamin C inhibits NO-induced stabilization of HIF-1alpha in HUVECs. Free 44(7): 783-91.

Myllyharju J (2008). Prolyl 4-hydroxylases, key enzymes in the synthesis of collagens and regulation of the response to hypoxia, and their roles as treatment targets. Ann Med 23: 1-16.

Nagel S, Talbot NP, Mecinovic J, Smith TG, Buchan AM, Schofield CJ (2010). Therapeutic manipulation of the HIF hydroxylases. Antioxid 12(4): 481-501.

Nakayama K, Gazdoiu S, Abraham R, Pan ZQ, Ronai Z (2007). Hypoxia-induced assembly of prolyl hydroxylase PHD3 into complexes: implications for its activity and susceptibility for degradation by the E3 ligase Siah2. Biochem J. 401(1): 217-26.

Nishikimi M, Koshizaka T, Ozawa T, Yagi K (1988). Occurrence in humans and guinea pigs of the gene related to their missing enzyme L-gulono-gamma-lactone oxidase. Arch Biochem Biophys. 267(2): 842-6.

Nytko KJ, Spielmann P, Camenisch G, Wenger RH, Stiehl DP (2007). Regulated function of the prolyl-4-hydroxylase domain (PHD) oxygen sensor proteins. Antioxid Redox Signal 9(9): 1329-38.

Nytko KJ, Maeda N, Schläfli P, Spielmann P, Wenger RH, Stiehl DP (2011) Vitamin C is dispensable for oxygen sensing in vivo. Blood. 117(20): 5485-93.

Oehme F, Ellinghaus P, Kolkhof P, Smith TJ, Ramakrishnan S, Hutter J, Schramm M, Flamme I (2002). Overexpression of PH-4, a novel putative proline 4-hydroxylase, modulates activity of hypoxia-inducible transcription factors. Biochem Biophys Res Commun. 296(2): 343-9.

Page EL, Chan DA, Giaccia AJ, Levine M, Richard DE (2008). Hypoxia-inducible factor-1alpha stabilization in nonhypoxic conditions: role of oxidation and intracellular ascorbate depletion. Mol Biol Cell. 19(1): 86-94.

Palmer LA, Semenza GL, Stoler MH, Johns RA (1998). Hypoxia induces type II NOS gene expression in pulmonary artery endothelial cells via HIF-1. Am J Physiol. 274(2 Pt 1): L212-9.

Park YK, Ahn DR, Oh M, Lee T, Yang EG, Son M, Park H (2008). Nitric oxide donor, (+/-)-S-nitroso-N-acetylpenicillamine, stabilizes transactive hypoxia-inducible factor-1alpha by inhibiting von Hippel-Lindau recruitment and asparagine hydroxylation. Mol Pharmacol. 74(1): 236-45.

Parsons KK, Maeda N, Yamauchi M, Banes AJ, Koller BH (2006). Ascorbic acid-independent synthesis of collagen in mice. Am J Physiol Endocrinol Metab 290(6): E1131-9.

Pauling L (1971). The significance of the evidence about ascorbic acid and the common cold. Proc Natl Acad Sci U S A. 68(11): 2678-81.

Pauling L (1977). Vitamin homeostasis in the brain and megavitamin therapy. N Engl J Med. 297(14): 790-1.

Qiao H, Li L, Qu ZC, May JM (2009). Cobalt-induced oxidant stress in cultured endothelial cells: prevention by ascorbate in relation to HIF-1alpha. Biofactors. 35(3): 306-13.

Richard DE, Berra E, Gothie E, Roux D, Pouyssegur J (1999). p42/p44 mitogen-activated protein kinases phosphorylate hypoxia-inducible factor 1alpha (HIF-1alpha) and enhance the transcriptional activity of HIF-1. J Biol Chem. 274(46): 32631-7.

Rius J, Guma M, Schachtrup C, Akassoglou K, Zinkernagel AS, Nizet V, Johnson RS, Haddad GG, Karin M (2008). NF-kappaB links innate immunity to the hypoxic response through transcriptional regulation of HIF-1alpha. Nature. 453(7196): 807-11.

Rockenfeller P, Madeo F (2010). Ageing and eating. Biochim Biophys Acta 1803(4): 499-506.

Sablina AA, Budanov AV, Ilyinskaya GV, Agapova LS, Kravchenko JE, Chumakov PM (2005). The antioxidant function of the p53 tumour suppressor. Nat Med. 11(12): 1306-13.

Salnikow K, Donald SP, Bruick RK, Zhitkovich A, Phang JM, Kasprzak KS (2004). Depletion of intracellular ascorbate by the carcinogenic metals nickel and cobalt results in the induction of hypoxic stress. J Biol Chem 279(39): 40337-44.

Salnikow K, Kasprzak KS (2005). Ascorbate depletion: a critical step in nickel carcinogenesis? Environ Health Perspect 113(5): 577-84.

Sang N, Stiehl DP, Bohensky J, Leshchinsky I, Srinivas V, Caro J (2003). MAPK signalling up-regulates the activity of hypoxia-inducible factors by its effects on p300. J Biol Chem. 278(16): 14013-9.

Sasabe E, Yang Z, Ohno S, Yamamoto T (2010). Reactive oxygen species produced by the knockdown of manganese-superoxide dismutase up-regulate hypoxia-inducible factor-1alpha expression in oral squamous cell carcinoma cells. Free Radic Biol Med 48(10): 1321-9.

Schafer M, Werner S (2008). Oxidative stress in normal and impaired wound repair. Pharmacol Res. 58(2): 165-71.

Scheid A, Wenger RH, Christina H, Camenisch I, Ferenc A, Stauffer UG, Gassmann M, Meuli M (2000). Hypoxia-regulated gene expression in fetal wound regeneration and adult wound repair. Pediatr Surg Int. 16(4): 232-6.

Schreml S, Szeimies RM, Prantl L, Karrer S, Landthaler M, Babilas P (2010). Oxygen in acute and chronic wound healing. Br J Dermatol. 163(2): 257-68.

Semenza G (2002). Signal transduction to hypoxia-inducible factor 1. Biochem Pharmacol. 64(5-6): 993-8.

Semenza GL (2010). Defining the role of hypoxia-inducible factor 1 in cancer biology and therapeutics. Oncogene 29(5): 625-34.

Shibata A, Nakagawa K, Sookwong P, Tsuduki T, Tomita S, Shirakawa H, Komai M, Miyazawa T (2008). Tocotrienol inhibits secretion of angiogenic factors from human colorectal adenocarcinoma cells by suppressing hypoxia-inducible factor-1alpha. J Nutr. 138(11): 2136-42.

Shoshani T, Faerman A, Mett I, Zelin E, Tenne T, Gorodin S, Moshel Y, Elbaz S, Budanov A, Chajut A, Kalinski H, Kamer I, Rozen A, Mor O, Keshet E, Leshkowitz D, Einat P, Skaliter R, Feinstein E (2002). Identification of a novel hypoxia-inducible factor 1-responsive gene, RTP801, involved in apoptosis. Mol Cell Biol. 22(7): 2283-93.

Sivridis E, Giatromanolaki A, Gatter KC, Harris AL, Koukourakis MI (2002). Association of hypoxia-inducible factors 1alpha and 2alpha with activated angiogenic pathways and prognosis in patients with endometrial carcinoma. Cancer. 95(5): 1055-63.

Stiehl DP, Jelkmann W, Wenger RH, Hellwig-Burgel T (2002). Normoxic induction of the hypoxia-inducible factor 1alpha by insulin and interleukin-1beta involves the phosphatidylinositol 3-kinase pathway. FEBS Lett 512(1-3): 157-62.

Stiehl DP, Wirthner R, Köditz J, Spielmann P, Camenisch G, Wenger RH (2006).

Increased prolyl 4-hydroxylase domain proteins compensate for decreased oxygen levels. Evidence for an autoregulatory oxygen-sensing system. J Biol Chem 281(33): 23482-91.

Telang S, Clem AL, Eaton JW, Chesney J (2007). Depletion of ascorbic acid restricts angiogenesis and retards tumour growth in a mouse model. Neoplasia 9(1): 47-56.

Tissot van Patot MC, Serkova NJ, Haschke M, Kominsky DJ, Roach RC, Christians U, Henthorn TK, Honigman B (2009). Enhanced leukocyte HIF-1alpha and HIF-1 DNA binding in humans after rapid ascent to 4300 m. Free Radic Biol Med. 46(11): 1551-7.

Triantafyllou A, Mylonis I, Simos G, Bonanou S, Tsakalof A (2008). Flavonoids induce HIF-1alpha but impair its nuclear accumulation and activity. Free Radic Biol Med. 44(4): 657-70.

Tsukiyama F, Nakai Y, Yoshida M, Tokuhara T, Hirota K, Sakai A, Hayashi H, Katsumata T (2006). Gallate, the component of HIF-inducing catechins, inhibits HIF prolyl hydroxylase. Biochem Biophys Res Commun. 351(1): 234-9.

Vissers MC, Gunningham SP, Morrison MJ, Dachs GU, Currie MJ (2007). Modulation of hypoxia-inducible factor-1 alpha in cultured primary cells by intracellular ascorbate. Free Radic Biol Med. 42(6): 765-72.

Vissers MC, Wilkie RP (2007). Ascorbate deficiency results in impaired neutrophil apoptosis and clearance and is associated with up-regulation of hypoxia-inducible factor 1a. J Leukoc Biol 81(5): 1236-44.

Welsh SJ, Bellamy WT, Briehl MM, Powis G (2002). The redox protein thioredoxin-1 (Trx-1) increases hypoxia-inducible factor 1alpha protein expression: Trx-1 overexpression results in increased vascular endothelial growth factor production and enhanced tumour angiogenesis. Cancer Res. 62(17): 5089-95.

Wenger RH, Camenisch G, Stiehl DP, Katschinski DM (2009). HIF prolyl-4-hydroxylase interacting proteins: consequences for drug targeting. Curr Pharm Des. 15(33): 3886-94.

Wingrove JA, O'Farrell PH (1999). Nitric oxide contributes to behavioral, cellular, and developmental responses to low oxygen in Drosophila. Cell. 98(1): 105-14.

Wirthner R, Balamurugan K, Stiehl DP, Barth S, Spielmann P, Oehme F, Flamme I, Katschinski DM, Wenger RH, Camenisch G (2007). Determination and modulation of prolyl-4-hydroxylase domain oxygen sensor activity. Methods Enzymol 435: 43-60.

Wolf J, Levy IJ (1954). Treatment of sickle cell anemia with cobalt chloride. AMA Arch Intern Med. 93(3): 387-96.

Yee Koh M, Spivak-Kroizman TR, Powis G (2008). HIF-1 regulation: not so easy come, easy go. Trends Biochem Sci. 33(11): 526-34.

Yuan Y, Hilliard G, Ferguson T, Millhorn DE (2003). Cobalt inhibits the interaction between hypoxia-inducible factor-alpha and von Hippel-Lindau protein by direct binding to hypoxia-inducible factor-alpha. J Biol Chem. 278(18): 15911-6.

Zhong H, Chiles K, Feldser D, Laughner E, Hanrahan C, Georgescu MM, Simons JW, Semenza GL (2000). Modulation of hypoxia-inducible factor 1alpha expression by the epidermal growth factor/phosphatidylinositol 3-kinase/PTEN/AKT/FRAP pathway in human prostate cancer cells: implications for tumour angiogenesis and therapeutics. Cancer Res. 60(6): 1541-5.

Zhong L, D'Urso A, Toiber D, Sebastian C, Henry RE, Vadysirisack DD, Guimaraes A, Marinelli B, Wikstrom JD, Nir T, Clish CB, Vaitheesvaran B, Iliopoulos O, Kurland I, Dor Y, Weissleder R, Shirihai OS, Ellisen LW, Espinosa JM, Mostoslavsky R (2010). The histone deacetylase Sirt6 regulates glucose homeostasis via Hif1alpha. Cell. 140(2): 280-93.

Zhou J, Damdimopoulos AE, Spyrou G, Brune B (2007). Thioredoxin 1 and thioredoxin 2 have opposed regulatory functions on hypoxia-inducible factor-1alpha. J Biol Chem. 282(10): 7482-90.

Part II

Hypoxia-induced phenomena

Hypoxia-driven angiogenesis and other means of blood vessel formation in tumours – implication for anti-tumour therapy

Agnieszka Loboda[*], Halina Was, Urszula Florczyk, Alicja Jozkowicz, and Jozef Dulak[*]

[*]Authors for correspondence:
Department of Medical Biotechnology, Faculty of Biochemistry, Biophysics and Biotechnology, Jagiellonian University; Gronostajowa 7, 30-387 Krakow, Poland; phone: +48-12-664-63-75; fax: +48-12-664-69-18; email: jozef.dulak@.uj.edu.pl & agnieszka.loboda@uj.edu.pl

Contents

Key points

— Tumour growth is dependent on the formation of blood vessels; hypoxia arising inside tumours effectively stimulates vessel growth.

— Mechanisms of neovascularization in tumours include sprouting and intussusceptive angiogenesis, vessel co-option, vasculogenic mimicry and lymphangiogenesis.

— The recruitment of endothelial progenitor cells (EPCs) in response to local tumour hypoxia is also considered a means of blood vessel formation.

— Tumour blood vessels are structurally/functionally abnormal and are characterized by increased permeability, lack of pericytes and impaired flow.

— Hypoxia causes tumour resistance to radiation therapy; anti-angiogenic therapies increase radiation-induced tumour vasculature destruction.

Summary

Although tumours are not generally controlled by normal regulatory mechanisms, their growth is highly dependent on oxygen and nutrient supply. It is well established that pre-neoplastic proliferating cells cannot give origin to a tumour without an appropriate blood supply. In fact, angiogenesis could be considered the rate-limiting step of tumour growth. The formation of a tumour blood network is triggered by hypoxia and many studies demonstrate the importance of the critical mediators of the hypoxic response, hypoxia inducible factors (HIFs) for tumour survival. Such results suggested HIFs as the attractive targets for anti-cancer therapy and recent anti-angiogenic therapies are focused on HIFs inhibitors. However, a growing body of evidence also indicates that tumours may evade such treatment via induction of compensatory pathways to maintain angiogenic response. The understanding of molecular mechanisms of such processes may help to establish a powerful anti-tumour therapy.

Introduction

In 1971 Judah Folkman proposed that a "tumour growth is angiogenesis-dependent" (Folkman, 1971). The idea of association between cancer and blood vessels was even older; in the late 40's, Algire and Chalkley concluded that the development of an intrinsic vascular network is connected to the growth of solid tumours (Algire et al., 1950). However, until Folkman's theory, it was believed that excessive vascularity of tumours is a side effect of growing tumours or dying tumour cells.

Since 1971 a new era in angiogenesis research has started. Folkman predicted that most tumours would be unable to grow beyond 1-2 mm in diameter without blood supply and he stressed the importance of blood vessels for the tumour growth as well as metastatis. He also postulated that if new blood vessels were indeed essential for tumour development, then inhibiting angiogenesis should stop tumour expansion.

In fact, anti-angiogenic therapy has been shown to prevent tumour growth and to even cause tumour regression in various experimental models. Moreover, certain anti-angiogenic agents can transiently "normalize" the abnormal structure and function of tumour vasculature to make it more efficient for oxygen and drug delivery. Importantly, normalizing agents decrease hypoxia in tumours, improve blood flow and increase the efficacy of cytotoxic drug delivery to tumours. Nowadays, the idea of anti-angiogenic therapy is rapidly expanding with numerous of ongoing clinical trials.

Angiogenesis in tumours

Angiogenesis, (also called sprouting angiogenesis), the formation of blood vessels from pre-existing capillaries, is an essential process for normal physiological functions including development, reproduction, wound heal-ing, tissue repair or hair growth and its normal functioning is the result of the balance of many positive and negative regulators. However, in malig-nant angiogenesis, due to improper controlling of angiogenic homeostasis, a signalling cascade contributing to tumour neovascularization is induced thereby forming a complex, multi-step process that enables tumours to receive a new blood supply.

Angiogenesis starts when specific growth factors, after binding to their receptors, activate endothelial cells which form the inner part of the large blood vessels. Under the influence of locally activated/released matrix metal-loproteinases (MMPs), the degradation of the basement membrane and the extracellular matrix occurs, followed by migration of endothelial cells into the extracellular space and their proliferation in the later stage of formation of capillary structures. An important role in the maturation of blood vessels is played by pericytes and smooth muscle cells that stabilize the capillaries providing the scaffold for a delicate layer of endothelial cells (Risau, 1997).

Angiogenesis is controlled by positive and negative regulators. In tumours, the level of pro-angiogenic factors overcomes the effect of angio-static factors and the tumours acquire an angiogenic phenotype that leads to blood vessel formation (Bergers and Benjamin, 2003). In the early phase, called the avascular phase, tumours lack their own vascular network. The necessary oxygen and nutrients are supplied by surrounding normal tis-sues, but at this time cellular proliferation is equivalent to apoptosis. In the next step, avascular tumours become vascularized in a mechanism called an "angiogenic switch", which helps the tumour to overcome growth limi-tations imposed by an insufficient blood supply (Hanahan and Folkman, 1996), (Figure 5.1).

The angiogenic switch: a balance between pro- and anti-angiogenic factors

Hanahan and Folkman suggested that the equilibrium between positive and negative regulators of angiogenesis governs the angiogenic switch (Hanahan and Folkman, 1996). Both tumour and host cells secrete a variety of molecules to stimulate blood vessel formation. Cancer cells can produce several angiogenic mediators, mostly vascular endothelial growth factor (VEGF, also named VEGF-A), but also epidermal growth factor (EGF), basic fibroblast growth factor (bFGF), angiopoietin-1 (Ang1), transforming growth factor β (TGFβ) and others. On the other hand, angiogenic factors may be released by tumour endothelial cells, stroma cells and circulating host cells such as endothelial progenitor cells, macrophages and platelets (Ferrara and Kerbel, 2005). Blood platelets for instance carry a large pool of mediators including VEGF, bFGF, EGF, platelet-derived growth factor (PDGF) or hepatocyte growth factor (HGF), and such factors in turn can stimulate the growth of endothelial cells (Eichhorn et al., 2007).

The angiogenic switch is correlated with the hypoxic conditions within the tumour. It is known that rapid cell division and aberrant blood vessel formation in tumours are responsible for severe oxygen deprivation. Over the past decade, work from many laboratories has indicated that hypoxic microenvironments contribute to cancer progression by activating adaptive transcriptional programs that promote cell survival, motility, and tumour angiogenesis. In this program the hypoxia-inducible factors (HIFs), main transcription factors induced by hypoxia play a critical role. Among three isoforms of HIFs, HIF-1 and HIF-2 are closely related and mediate transcriptional responses to localized hypoxia in normal tissues and in cancers. HIFs may promote tumour progression by altering cellular metabolism and stimulating angiogenesis (Keith and Simon, 2007). In fact, evidence that HIFs play a fundamental role in angiogenesis arose from a study performed on HIF-1 subunits knockout mice, both HIF-1α and HIF-1β, which are lethal to the embryo and are characterized by defects in blood vessel development (Pugh and Ratcliffe, 2003).

Apart from „real" microenvironmental hypoxia, HIF expression or activity may be increased in response to genetic alterations causing inactivation of tumour suppressor genes or activation of oncogenes. About 100 years ago von Hippel and Lindau described the so-called von Hippel-Lindau (VHL) disease, which is caused by germline inactivating mutations of the *VHL* tumour suppressor gene. VHL inactivation is frequently

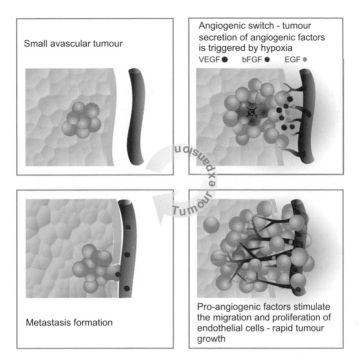

Figure 5.1 _ Sprouting angiogenesis drives the angiogenic switch and tumour progression.

detected in sporadic hemangioblastomas (retinal, cerebellar, spinal cord hemangioblastoma), clear cell renal carcinoma, pheochromocytoma, pancreatic islet cell tumour and others (Kaelin, 2007). Clinical features of VHL-associated tumours led to the recognition that the VHL gene product, pVHL, is a critical negative regulator of hypoxia–induced response. VHL loss of function creates an angiogenic phenotype with increased expression of VEGF. Moreover, overexpression of the other HIF-induced gene, erythropoietin, is also connected with VHL syndrome.

Nowadays it is well known, that VHL protein plays a special role in the ubiquitination of HIF-1α and its degradation. In normal oxygen conditions HIF-1α is hydroxylated by prolyl hydroxylase enzymes (PHDs) on specific proline residues (Pro 402, Pro 564) and then recognized by pVHL. Such direct interaction between pVHL and HIF-1α is a signal for forming a multimeric complex with additional proteins, namely elongin B, elongin C, Cul2, Rbx1 and triggering HIF-1α for proteasomal degradation (reviewed in Zagorska and Dulak, 2004).

The key angiogenic factor, VEGF, is HIF-regulated

The most crucial pro-angiogenic factor, VEGF, discovered as a vascular permeability factor (VPF) (Senger et al., 1983), is regulated in a HIF-dependent manner. Regulation of VEGF expression in hypoxic conditions is mediated on the transcriptional level and is dependent on HIF-1 binding to the hypoxia response element (HRE) present in the promoter of the VEGF gene (Levy et al., 1995). Low oxygen concentration also increases the stability of VEGF mRNA (Shima et al., 1995), which in normal concentrations of oxygen is unstable (half-life is 15 to 40 minutes in vitro). This is mediated by binding of proteins, like HuR, to specific sequences in the 3' UTR VEGF mRNA (Levy, 1998). In addition, effective VEGF translation under hypoxia is possible due to the existence of an internal ribosomal entry site (IRES) in the 5'UTR sequence (Stein et al., 1998).

Hypoxia-induced up-regulation of VEGF in tumour cells has been subsequently demonstrated in various experimental models (Levy et al., 1995). A number of studies have also demonstrated the correlation between HIF expression and intratumoural microvascular density as a measure of tumour angiogenesis (Brahimi-Horn and Pouyssegur, 2005).

Interestingly, hypoxia, which was thought to only induce expression of pro-angiogenic mediators, may exert a more complex effect on the production of factors, which stimulate blood vessel formation. We have recently focused our attention on the effect of hypoxia on the interleukin-8 (IL-8) expression, known as not only chemoattractant for neutrophiles and T lymphocytes but also a potent mediator of angiogenesis, cancer growth and metastasis (Xie, 2001). In contrast to increased level of VEGF, low oxygen tension diminishes the expression of IL-8 in endothelial cells and was associated with lowered activity of Nrf2 transcription factor (Loboda et al., 2009). Moreover, the expression of placental-growth factor (PlGF), the other factor with pro-angiogenic properties, was also diminished in hypoxic endothelial cells (Loboda et al., 2006). In contrast, inhibition of HIF-1α by RNA interference caused increase in the levels of several angiogenic factors such as IL-6, IL-8, and MCP-1 with concomitant down-regulation of VEGF production (Forooghian and Das, 2007; Loboda et al., 2009).

Such data presenting a diminished level of pro-angiogenic factors by HIF-1 induction may have strong significance in clinics. Accordingly, using the therapies based on HIF-1 inhibition it should be noted that down-regulation of one angiogenic factor may not be enough to inhibit angiogenesis in tumours and more importantly, some compensatory pathways may be activated to preserve angiogenic response. In fact, Mizukami et al. (2005)

noticed that after injection of either wild type or HIF-1α knockdown colon cancer cells to nude mice, the vascularization of tumours was high and comparable. The authors suggested that some compensatory pathways have to be activated to maintain angiogenic response in the absence of HIF-1. They showed that IL-8 was induced by hypoxia in colon cancer deprived of HIF-1 and this occurred in a NF-κB dependent manner. These results suggest that anti-HIF therapy may not be sufficient for inhibition of tumour angiogenesis. The targeting of both HIF-1 and IL-8 may be more efficient for treatment of tumours.

Additionally, it was observed in many clinical trials, that although efficient in the early phase of treatment, anti-VEGF therapy ultimately leads to disease progression and tumour regrowth. The mechanism of this phenomenon was nicely presented by Casanovas et al. (2005). In the initial phase, blockage of VEGF receptor, VEGFR2 leads to vascular and tumoural regression, and as a consequence it also causes regions of hypoxia. This may lead to the increased production of other pro-angiogenic factors, including bFGF and such induction may be sufficient for the reestablishment of tumour vasculature.

In summary, this indicates that inhibition of one pro-angiogenic factor may lead to increased expression of other pro-angiogenic factors what can circumvent the blockade, to promote a new wave of angiogenesis and tumour growth. Inhibition of e.g. VEGF may lead to an increase in IL-8, IL-6, MCP-1, bFGF, which may in fact, stimulate angiogenesis, even in the absence/reduction of VEGF.

The mechanisms of tumour vascularization

When diffusion from surrounding blood vessels is no longer sufficient to sustain tumour growth, there are several ways by which tumours may expand their own vasculature. Although for 30 years the sprouting angiogenesis was considered an exclusive mean of tumour vascularization, studies published in recent years revealed several additional mechanisms of neovascularization in tumours including vessel co-option, intussusceptive angiogenesis, vasculogenic mimicry, recruitment of endothelial progenitor cells and lymphangiogenesis (Hillen and Griffioen, 2007), (Figure 5.2). Thus, it could be concluded that anti-cancer targeting therapies based on anti-angiogenic strategies should be more complex than initially thought. It is

believed that such treatment might be more beneficial when based on mul-
timodal anti-angiogenic, anti-vasculogenic mimicry and anti-lymphangiogenic approaches.

Co-option

As mentioned above, it is generally established that tumours initiate as an
avascular mass and cannot grow beyond a few millimeters in size without
the development of new vessels (Folkman, 1971). Though it has been observed
that tumours can enlarge mainly when localized in well-vascularized tissues such as brain or lungs (Wesseling et al., 1994; Holmgren et al., 1995; Pezzella et
al., 1997). This process has been defined as vessel co-option (Holash et al., 1999a).
Although initially co-option seemed to be restricted to the initial phases of
tumourigenesis, further studies discovered that this process might persist
during the entire period of tumour growth. Cutaneous melanoma has been
shown to grow by co-opting the massive vascular plexus present in the peri-
tumoural connective tissue (Dome et al., 2002). Furthermore, non-small cell
lung carcinoma can grow without evidence of neoangiogenesis (Pezzella et
al., 1997). Vessel co-option has also been demonstrated in human colorectal
carcinomas (Vermeulen et al., 2001), murine ovarian cancer (Zhang et al., 2003)
and human neuroblastoma (Kim et al., 2002).

Interestingly, Holash and colleagues observed that two weeks after
tumour cells implantation, co-opted blood vessels underwent a dramatic
regression in the center of the tumour, whereas in the tumour periphery, a
strong angiogenic response was detected (Holash et al., 1999a). Therefore, it has
been hypothesized that cross talk between angiogenic antagonist angiopoi-
etin-2 (Ang-2) and pro-angiogenic VEGF could be responsible for regression of originally co-opted tumour vessels and following neovascularization
(Holash et al., 1999b). Indeed, in co-opted blood vessels, the up-regulation of
Ang-2 disrupted the interaction between angiogenic agonist Ang-1 and its
receptor Tie-2, which in turn caused the detachment of pericytes from the
vessel wall and massive death of endothelial cells. The regression of the
initial co-opted vessels might be considered as a host defense mechanism.
On the other hand, necrosis in the centre of the tumour leads to hypoxia
and subsequently evokes angiogenic response. As a result robust VEGF-
induced sprouting angiogenesis in the periphery of the tumour takes place
and remaining tumour cells can re-grow at a later stage (Holash et al., 1999b).

The important role of VEGF in vessel co-option may suggest that anti-
VEGF therapies can be considered not only for blocking angiogenesis but

also to inhibit vessel co-option. As the systemic injection of a glioblastoma with anti-VEGFR2 antibodies was able to diminish tumour angiogenesis but led to an augmented co-option of host vessels in the brain (Kunkel et al., 2001), targeting of VEGF together with Ang-2, could overcome the growth of tumours along existing vessels.

Intussusception

Intussusceptive angiogenesis was described for the first time in postnatal lungs as a splitting of a pre-existing vessel into two new capillaries by the formation of transvascular tissue pillar into the lumen of the vessel (Caduff et al., 1986). This is a fast process, requiring little energy, because it occurs

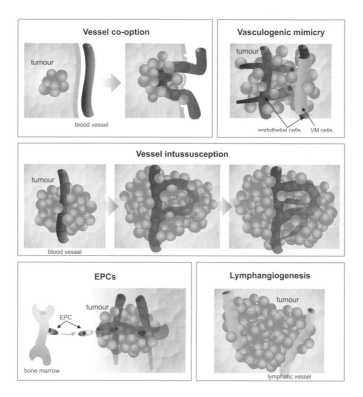

Figure 5.2 _ Alternative means of blood vessel formation in tumours: vasculogenic mimicry, intussusception, vessel co-option, EPCs involvement and lymphangiogenesis. Furthermore, non-small cell lung carcinoma can grow without evidence of neoangiogenesis.

without proliferation of endothelial cells, but only with their remodeling (Burri et al., 2004). Intussusception plays a role both in physiological situations, e.g. during tissue repair processes, but is also characteristic for tumour development. As intussusception involves migration of endothelial cells and vascular remodeling but not cell proliferation, anti-proliferative agents commonly used in anti-angiogenic therapies nowadays may not be able to prevent intussusception and inhibit tumour growth. Thus, to develop effective anti-vascular strategies, novel compounds should also block vessel intussusception.

Tissue pillars were detected for the first time in a colon carcinoma xenograft model (Patan et al., 1996), where intussusception occurred together with sprouting angiogenesis dependently on the tumour region: at the growing edge of the tumour both mechanisms of blood formation were detected, whereas in the more stabilised regions mainly intussusception took place. Although many different cell types are considered to play a role in intussusceptive angiogenesis, it seems to be primarily mediated by endothelial cell-endothelial cell and endothelial cell-pericyte interactions. Molecularly, VEGF and Ang-1 and its Tie receptors are likely to synergistically regulate intussusceptive vascular expansion (Makanya et al., 2009).

Recently, a connection between hypoxia and intussusception has been established not only in tumours, where it is a known hypoxia-adaptation mechanism (Dome et al., 2007). This method of blood formation accompanied the healing of the hypoxic tissue in a murine model of ovarian pedicle repair (Patan et al., 2001). Additionally, Taylor et al. showed that chronic systemic hypoxia results in the enlargement of vessel diameters along the arteriolar tree and induces intussesceptive angiogenesis in the adult mouse retina (Taylor et al., 2010). Interestingly, a comparison of sprouting and intussesceptive angiogenesis in a computational model of oxygen transport in skeletal muscle, indicated that intussusception growth provided better oxygen delivery to the tissue than sprouting or control networks and resulted in the lowest volume of hypoxic tissue (Ji et al., 2006).

Vasculogenic mimicry

In 1999, the term "vasculogenic mimicry" (VM) was introduced by Maniotis and coworkers (Maniotis et al., 1999) to describe the process in which tumour cells dedifferentiate to an endothelial phenotype and form tube-like structures. Interestingly, such tumour cells overexpressed endothelium-associated genes, which promote cell migration, invasion and matrix remodeling.

Importantly, vascular channels formation via VM may be regulated by hypoxia.

This unique property of tumour cells to mimic endothelial cells was firstly observed in highly aggressive human melanoma cells (Maniotis et al., 1999), but it has since presented in other malignant tumours, including breast, prostatic, ovarian and clear renal cell carcinomas (references in: Hillen and Griffioen, 2007). Importantly, presence of such networks was coupled with a worse patient outcome (Folberg et al., 1993).

Yao et al. suggested that in epithelial ovarian carcinoma the VM is induced by hypoxia. The increased formation of tumour channels was observed under decreased oxygen concentration and interestingly, sirolimus (rapamycin, used as an anti-angiogenic agent) was able to decrease hypoxia-induced VM by blocking HIF-1α at transcription level (Yao et al., 2005). In contrast, it has been shown that anti-angiogenic targeting strategies do not block the VM in Ewing sarcoma (van der Schaft et al., 2005). Moreover, there is no correlation between VM and the expression of several pro-angiogenic factors such as bFGF, VEGF, TGF-β, and PDGF (Maniotis et al., 1999), which may suggest different signalling pathways for angiogenesis and VM. Additionally, HIF-1α and VEGF expression was significantly increased in retinoblastoma with VM (Niu et al., 2009). However, the study performed by Li et al. (2010) on paraffin-embedded human samples from gastric adenocarcinoma did not show any differences between HIF-1α and pro-angiogenic VEGF, MMP-2 and MMP-9 in the VM and non-VM group. On the contrary, the correlation between identical factors and VM was present in hepatocellular carcinoma (Liu et al., 2010).

The involvement of additional factors, like VE-cadherin, ephrin-A1 and its receptor EPHA2 as well as matrix related components, e.g. laminin 5γ-2 chain fibronectin, collagen IV α2, collagen I (Hendrix et al., 2003) in the VM was underlined. The inhibition of VE-cadherin in melanoma cells resulted in a reduction of their ability to create vasculogenic-like structures (Hendrix et al., 2001), whereas MT1-MMP/MMP-2-induced breakdown of laminin 5γ-2 chain into pro-migratory fragments has been shown to play an important role in formation of vasculogenic-like networks (Seftor et al., 2001; Hendrix et al., 2003). In turn, the significance of the extracellular matrix in the VM was shown elegantly by studies demonstrating that matrix preconditioned with aggressive melanoma cells reprograms normal melanocytes to express genes associated with a multipotent, plastic phenotype similar to aggressive melanoma cells (Seftor et al., 2005).

Furthermore, VM-positive melanoma cells seemed to dedifferentiate to embryonic-like phenotype as genes responsible for melanocytic phenotype, such as Melan-A, microphthalmia-associated transcription factor (MTIF) and tyrosinase, were strongly reduced in melanoma (Hendrix et al., 2003), whereas pluripotency marker Notch-4 has been reported to be elevated in aggressive melanoma cells in the context of VM (Hendrix et al., 2003; Demou and Hendrix, 2008).

The above results suggest that VM-positive cells, stimulated by hypoxia, are characterized by an undifferentiated molecular signature together with embryonic-like differentiation plasticity, thereby implying a link between cancer stem cells and aggressive tumour cells capable of VM (Schatton and Frank, 2008).

The role of endothelial progenitor cells in tumour angiogenesis

The discovery of CD34-enriched subpopulation of mononuclear blood cells in 1997 (Asahara et al., 1999) changed the appearance of growth of new blood vessels in adults. CD34-positive cells, named endothelial progenitor cells (EPCs), circulate in the blood and can be recruited to newly formed blood vessels. EPCs apart from CD34, exhibit expression of several endothelial specific markers such as CD31, VEGFR2, Tie-2 (Asahara et al., 1997) and CD14 (Kalka et al., 2000).

Growth factors, cytokines and chemokines, which are generated during tissue ischaemia, physical exercise or tumour growth can promote mobilization and recruitment of EPCs. Factors such as PLGF and VEGF (Asahara et al., 1999; Hattori et al., 2002), stromal cell-derived factor (SDF-1), Ang-1 (Moore et al., 2001), nitric oxide (Aicher et al., 2003), granulocyte colony-stimulating factor and granulocyte-macrophage colony-stimulating factor (Takahashi et al., 1999) have been identified as bone marrow stem cell mobilizing factors. Moreover, expression of P-selectin, E-selectin and integrins seems to be crucial in the adhesion of EPCs to the vessel wall and in transendothelial migration (Vajkoczy et al., 2003; Deb et al., 2004; Chavakis et al., 2007). Additionally, CD31 and CD99 can facilitate diapedesis of EPCs (Liao et al., 1995; Schenkel et al., 2002). Finally, VEGF is a key player in the differentiation of EPCs to mature endothelial cells (Asahara et al., 1997; Gehling et al., 2000).

Recently, it has been proposed that postnatal vasculogenesis is driven primarily by local tissue ischaemia related to the release of soluble factors that promote EPCs recruitment (Takahashi et al., 1999). SDF-1 in particular has been shown to be involved in hypoxia-mediated recruitment of EPCs in mouse models of tissue ischaemia (Ceradini et al., 2004; De Falco et al., 2004), whereas another hypoxia-upregulated factor – VEGF (Ferrara, 2001) has been demonstrated to promote mobilization of immature hematopoietic progenitors into peripheral circulation as well as the numbers of EPCs/ml of peripheral blood in mice (Asahara et al., 1999; Hattori et al., 2001).

Importantly, EPCs can also home in at the site of neovascularization in tumours. It has been reported that EPCs facilitate the initial establishment of tumour endothelium (Nolan et al., 2007), control tumour growth (Lyden et al., 2001) and metastasis transition (Gao et al., 2008), and can also affect the sensitivity of a tumour to chemotherapy (Shaked et al., 2008). Similarly, hypoxia-induced VEGF and PlGF have been shown to promote tumour vasculogenesis by enhancing EPCs recruitment and vessel formation (Li et al., 2006), whereas locally generated insulin-like growth factor 2 (IGF2) at either ischemic or tumour sites may contribute to postnatal vasculogenesis by augmenting the recruitment of EPCs through IGF2/IGF2R/PLCβ2 axis (Maeng et al., 2009).

Although, most clinical applications of EPCs are in the field of ischaemic tissue recovery, inhibition of EPCs actions might have remarkable potential in anti-cancer strategies. For example, simultaneous inhibition of VEGFR-2 and VEGFR-1 reduced mobilization and incorporation of EPCs in tumour vasculature (Lyden et al., 2001). EPCs can be also used as a marker for the validation of effectiveness of anti-angiogenic therapy. A strong correlation between bFGF- of VEGF-induced angiogenesis and the level of EPCs has been shown in 8 different mouse strains (Shaked et al., 2005). Alternatively, EPCs might be used as a vehicle in targeted anti-cancer treatment. CD34+ cells harboring suicide gene of thymidine kinase showed a co-localization with tumour vasculature and led to inhibited tumour growth (Arafat et al., 2000).

Nevertheless, there is contradictory data regarding the contribution of EPCs to vessel development in tumours (Lyden et al., 2001; Machein et al., 2003; Ruzinova et al., 2003; Gothert et al., 2004; Peters et al., 2005). Notably, in studies with cancer patients similar mixed results were found (Kim et al., 2003; Sussman et al., 2003). This could be due to variance in methodology, as there is still controversy on specific markers of EPCs as well as possible contamination of the EPCs population with other cell types resulting from: cell fusion, cell engulfment or transfer of microparticles. Additional possible explanations of such differences include: the tumour type, size at time of analysis, mouse genetic background, site of implantation, or time-point of analysis (Patenaude et al., 2010).

These results show that the influence of EPCs in tumour vascularization cannot be ignored and the development of targeting strategies to prevent EPCs from incorporating in regions of neovascularization in the tumour could be beneficial in anti-cancer therapy. Nevertheless, better characterisation of EPCs, improvement of purification of these progenitor cells and study of their long-term actions are needed.

Lymphangiogenesis

The entry of tumour cells into lymphatic vessels in the early phase of tumour progression has been known for years, however only recently has it been discovered that this is not a passive process, but that tumours can actively promote the growth of lymphatic vessels (Stacker et al., 2002). Tumour lymphangiogenesis and its possible role in promoting lymph node metastasis in human malignancy were originally recognized in cutaneous malignant melanomas (Dadras et al., 2003). Moreover, in certain cancer types, such as breast cancer, lymphatic metastasis is one of the major routes of cancer spread in the organism (Perou et al., 2000). The mechanism of tumour-associated lymphangiogenesis has not yet been fully discovered. Apart from lymphatic endothelial cells, bone marrow-derived endothelial precursors (such as bone marrow derived podoplanin(+) cells, (Lee et al., 2010)) and, through vascular mimicry or transdifferentiation, CD11b positive macrophages (Maruyama et al., 2005) can both contribute to the lymphatic vasculature in tumours.

Increasing evidence, principally concerning lymphatic vessel specific markers and lymphangiogenic growth factors, resulted in the identification of tumour-associated lymphangiogenesis (Karpanen et al., 2001; Skobe et al., 2001; Stacker et al., 2001). Several lymphatics markers including Fms-related tyrosine kinase 4 (FLT4)/vascular endothelial growth factor receptor-3 (VEGFR-3) (Kaipainen et al., 1995) to which VEGF-C and VEGF-D are bound, lymphatic vascular endothelial hyaluronan receptor-1 (LYVE-1) (Banerji et al., 1999), mutin-type glycoprotein T1α/podoplanin (Breiteneder-Geleff et al., 1999) and homeobox transcription factor Prox-1 (Wigle et al., 2002) have been identified. In turn, the best-known signalling pathway implicated in tumour lymphangiogenesis involves two members of the VEGF family, VEGF-C and VEGF-D. VEGF-C has been shown to stimulate proliferation, migration and survival of lymphatic endothelial cells (Makinen et al., 2001). Concomitantly, VEGF-C null mouse embryos completely lack a lymphatic vasculature and die prenatally (Karkkainen et al., 2004), whereas VEGF-D does not play a major role in lymphatic development (Baldwin et al., 2005). In the case of tumour tissue, both VEGF-C and -D increased intratumoural lymphangiogenesis and metastasis (Skobe et al., 2001; Stacker et al., 2001). Interestingly, VEGF-D, possessing hypoxia-regulated promoter activity (Teng et al., 2002), has been recently shown to be associated with HIF-1α in breast cancer (Currie et al., 2004). In turn, VEGF-C mRNA levels have been demonstrated to be elevated by hypoxia in some endothelial cells (Nilsson et al., 2004), whereas in human esophageal cancer cells levels of HIF-1α correlate with VEGF-C expression and lymphatic metastasis (Katsuta et al., 2005; Liang et al., 2008). Finally, it has been shown that overexpression of cold shock domain protein A (CSDA) that binds directly to hypoxia response element (HRE) and serum response element (SRE) led to diminished VEGF-A and VEGF-C production, resulting in blocked tumour growth, inhibited regional lymph-node metastasis, and reduced the density of blood vessels and lymphatic vessels in primary squamous carcinoma tumours in vivo (Matsumoto et al., 2010).

Accordingly, many results show that inhibition of lymphatic development could be considered as an anti-cancer treatment. Indeed, blocking VEGF-D with a monoclonal antibody had been demonstrated to diminish lymphatic spread (Stacker et al., 2001), whereas injection of a VEGFR-3 fusion protein inhibited the growth of tumour-associated lymphatic vessels and led to reduced tumour metastasis (Karpanen et al., 2001). Thus, cancer patients could benefit from anti-lymphangiogenic therapy, although better understanding of the process and additional information on specific tumour lymphatic markers are needed.

Interestingly, a growing body of evidence highlights the existence of cross talk between VEGF-C/VEGF-D/VEGF-R3 and VEGF/VEGFR-2 signalling, suggesting that some growth factors previously known to stimulate angiogenesis can also induce lymphangiogenesis. The VEGF/VEGFR-2 signalling pathway stimulates the growth of lymphatics (Nagy et al., 2002). Cultured lymphatic endothelial cells quickly proliferate in the presence of VEGF under physiological conditions (Hirakawa et al., 2003), whereas chemically-induced squamous cell carcinomas in VEGF transgenic mice potently induce tumour angiogenesis and lymphangiogenesis (Hirakawa et al., 2005). However, VEGF was not pro-lymphangiogenic in a mouse model of pancreatic cancer (Gannon et al., 2002) or in a tumour xenograft model using human embryonic kidney HEK293 cells (Stacker et al., 2001). This may indicate that specific conditions promote lymphangiogenic properties of VEGF. However, such cross talk must be taken into consideration for the design of therapeutic agents to block tumour associated angiogenesis and lymphangiogenesis.

Tumour blood vessels

Independently of the process in which blood vessels are formed, the new tumour vasculature is structurally and functionally abnormal. Compared to regular blood vessels, tumour vessels are characterized by increased permeability, lack of supporting cells such as pericytes and impaired blood flow (Table 5.1).

Morphological abnormalities in tumour blood vessels were found using three-dimensional plaster casting and scanning electron microscopy (Konerding et al., 1999; Baluk et al., 2005; McDonald and Baluk, 2005). Unlike normal blood vessels, those supplying tumours are formed by a chaotic mixture of disorganized serpentines, which branch irregularly, and on average, are larger than their normal counterparts but their walls are thin (Eberhard et al., 2000; Hashizume et al., 2000). This results in an altered surface area to volume ratio that impairs tissue nutrition and causes poor clearance of carbon dioxide and other metabolites. Additionally, high rate of aerobic glycolysis instead of oxidative phosphorylation in tumour cell causes special, acidic tumour microenvironment, as compared with normal tissues (pH ~ 7.2 versus pH ~ 7.4) (Stubbs et al., 2000). Together these create the special zones of metabolic insufficiency, ischaemia, and necrosis leading to activation of HIF-1 factor which promotes the formation of new blood vessels (Semenza, 2001).

The morphological changes are found in different cells/structures from which blood vessels are composed such as endothelial cells, pericytes and the basement membrane. The endothelial cells in tumours are characterized by large nucleus, and are very often aneuploid. Molecularly they

Table 5.1 _ Morphological and functional characteristics of normal and tumour vasculature.

Properties	Vessel type	
	Normal blood vessels	Tumour blood vessels
GLOBAL ORGANIZATION	normal	disturbed
PERICYTES	present	absent or detached
BASEMENT MEMBRANE	present	absent
BLOOD FLOW	normal	impaired
PERMEABILITY	non-permeable	leaky
OXYGEN STATUS	normoxic	hypoxic

are characterized by high activity of the MAPK signalling cascade, protein kinase C and activation of protein Akt, which promote their survival (Furuya et al., 205). Furthermore, by the use of serial analysis of gene expression (SAGE) method, St Croix and coworkers (St Croix et al., 2000) have identified almost 50 genes that were specifically up-regulated in the colon cancer endothelium compared to normal endothelial cells. Such experiments led to discovery of a set of specific tumour endothelial markers – (TEMs), such as TEM5 and TEM8, which show strong tumour endothelial expression but are essentially absent from normal tissue (Carson-Walter et al., 2001). Nowadays, TEMs are considered specific targets for anti-cancer therapies.

Moreover, fragmentation of basement membrane, openings and wide inter-endothelial junctions are the main differences between normal and tumour vessel walls. This results in hyperpermeability of tumour blood vessels to plasma and plasma proteins which leads to local oedema and extravascular clotting of plasma. Because of the deposition of fibrin gel which may serve as a matrix for cell migration, angiogenic signalling is induced in endothelial cells (Dvorak, 2003). The leakiness of blood vessels is also the result of diminished adherence of pericytes. Leaky vasculature causes easier entry of tumour cells to circulation, migration to distant sites and even implantation to other organs. In fact, the degree of permeability varies between tumour type and this is taken into consideration for new approaches for cancer treatment.

Another characteristic of tumour blood vessels, caused by their chaotic structure and disproportion in vessels shunts and branching, is impaired flow. In individual cases, the flow of blood through the tumour capillaries may be sluggish and may be stationary or the direction of blood flow may be reversed (Tozer et al., 1990; Tozer et al., 2005).

All characteristics of blood vessels described above cause functional abnormalities of blood flow, and stress the importance of tumour vessel normalization approach to improve access to standard chemotherapy (*see next paragraph*).

microRNAs and tumour angiogenesis

Recent studies have established a link between a specific group of microRNAs (miRNAs), hypoxia and tumour microenvironment miRNAs were described for the first time in 1993 as small, non-coding RNA molecules which bind to the 3' untranslated regions (UTRs) of target mRNAs to negatively regulate gene expression (Lee et al., 1993). However, miRNAs can also influence a positive regulation of gene expression. miRNAs control numerous cellular processes, including proliferation, differentiation, metabolism and motility (Miska, 2005). Importantly, all those processes may also be influenced by HIFs (Carmeliet et al., 1998), implying possible connection between the main hypoxia-activated transcription factors and miRNAs.

A significant number of hypoxia-regulated miRNAs are overexpressed in human cancers, suggesting that they play a crucial role in tumourigenesis. They have recently been named "hypoxamirs" (Chan and Loscalzo, 2010) and divided to three main groups, with different effects on HIFs and being dependent or independent of hypoxia induction (Figure 5.3).

The first group of miRNAs, represented by miR-210 and miR-373, is induced by HIFs under hypoxic conditions but do not affect HIFs reciprocally. To the second group belong miRNAs, such as miR-20b and miR-424, which are induced by hypoxia and they in turn affect expression of HIFs. The third group is comprised of miRNAs, such as miR-17-92 cluster, miR-107 or miR-519c, which affect HIF expression but are not hypoxia-dependent (Loscalzo, 2010).

miR-210 is probably the most consistently and predominantly up-regulated miRNA in hypoxic conditions (Huang et al., 2010). It was shown to be regulated by both HIF-1α (Camps et al., 2008; Zhang et al., 2009) and HIF-2α (Zhang

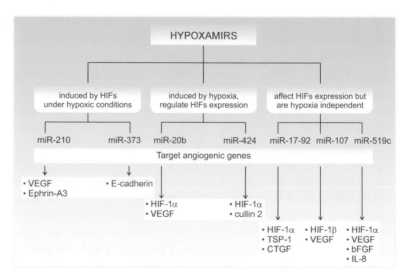

Figure 5.3 _ Three groups of hypoxamirs and their molecular targets.

et al., 2009). miR-210 apart from many other functions, may contribute to tumour growth and progression by influencing angiogenesis, as it mostly targets VEGF (Hua et al., 2006) as well as the receptor tyrosine kinase ligand Ephrin-A3 (Fasanaro et al., 2008). Importantly, miR-210 has been suggested to be a novel prognostic biomarker in cancer patients, drawing particular attention to the fact that it can be used as a biomarker for the noninvasive detection of tumour hypoxia. This is based on the observation that miR-210 expression is increased in plasma in highly hypoxic pancreatic cancer patients (Ho et al., 2010) or was shown to correlate with VEGF expression, hypoxia and angiogenesis in breast cancer patients (Foekens et al., 2008).

The second group of miRNAs (induced by hypoxia and regulating HIF expression) is represented by miR-20b (Lei et al., 2009) and miR-424 (Ghosh et al., 2010). miR-20b seems to play an important role in fine-tuning the adaptation of tumour cells to oxygen concentration: in normoxic tumours the inhibition of miR-20b increased the protein level of HIF-1α and VEGF, whereas in hypoxic tumours the up-regulation of miR-20b decreased HIF-1α and VEGF levels (Lei et al., 2009). Interestingly, and in contrast to miR-210, widely overexpressed in response to hypoxia (Huang et al., 2010), the increase of miR-424 level in hypoxia is restricted to endothelial cells. miR-424 targets cullin 2, a protein involved in the multimeric complex regulating HIFs destruction in normoxic conditions, and it turn it increases HIF-1α (Ghosh et al., 2010).

Finally, there are miRNAs, which influence HIFs expression in a hypoxia-independent manner. miR-107 is induced by p53 tumour suppressor gene and in turn decreases hypoxia signalling by inhibition of HIF-1β expression in human colon cancer cells (Yamakuchi et al., 2010). Both *in vitro* (HCT116 colorectal carcinoma cell lines) and *in vivo* (human colon cancer specimens) studies showed the inverse association between miR-107 and VEGF – expression of VEGF was the highest in the group with low miR-107 level and was the lowest in the high miR-107 group. As p53 is very often mutated in human cancers and it might regulate hypoxic signalling, the mechanism of miR-107 mediated inhibition of HIF signalling has to be taken into consideration when new anti-angiogenic strategies are developed.

The other two miRNAs, the miR-17-92 cluster induced by c-Myc oncogene (Taguchi et al., 2008) and miR-519c suppressed by hepatocyte growth factor (HGF) (Cha et al., 2010), also down-regulate expression of HIF-1α and angiogenesis. miR-519c has been suggested to be a tumour suppressor as its overexpression was observed in early-stage lung cancer patients compared with late-stage patients (Cha et al., 2010). All of this and other data indicate that the modulation of miRNAs expression and/or activity may be a promising therapeutic strategy to control tumour angiogenesis.

Inhibition of blood vessel growth in tumours – anti-angiogenic therapy

The idea of targeting the blood supply by inhibiting blood vessel formation in order to arrest the tumour growth or even to induce tumour shrinkage was, as previously mentioned, first published by Folkman (Folkman, 1971) and is now more than 40 years old. Inhibition of angiogenesis is a promising strategy for treatment of cancer and major progress towards this has been achieved over the past few years, with the first anti-angiogenic agents having recently been approved for use in several countries (Ferrara and Kerbel, 2005). Specific inhibitors of blood vessel formation have been identified, on the basis of preclinical *in vitro* and *in vivo* studies, to block tumour growth and metastases. Thus, several strategies for angiogenesis intervention, which trigger of different steps of blood vessel formation might be applied (Mauriz and Gonzalez-Gallego, 2008).

Inhibition of endothelial cell proliferation was the first experimental strategy for the screening of new anti-angiogenic drugs and has been investigated as a candidate for anticancer cytostatic treatments. Nowadays, several drugs exist such as endogenously produced angiostatin and endostatin, fumagilin and its less toxic semisynthetic analogue TNP-470 (AGM-1470) and rapamycin (Sirolimus). The mechanism of their action is related to down-regulation of cyclin-dependent kinase 5 (CDK5), methionine aminopeptidases (MetAP) or mammalian target of rapamycin (mTOR) inhibition repectively. Noteworthy, the anti-angiogenic effect of rapamycin is associated with a decrease of VEGF production and inhibited response of endothelial cells to VEGF stimulation (Mauriz and Gonzalez-Gallego, 2008).

Because of the important function of MMPs in blood vessel formation, the inhibitors of their activity have been used to develop another anti-cancer strategy. Both, endogenous (tissue inhibitors of matrix metalloproteinases, TIMPs) or synthetic MMP inhibitors such as batimastat, marimastat, or neovastat have been shown to possess anti-angiogenic activity. TIMP-1, for example, inhibits basal and VEGF-induced migration of endothelial cells (Oh et al., 2004). Synthetic MMP inhibitors have been tested in several clinical trials, however with limited response clinical trials, principally to treat tumour angiogenesis (reviewed in Overall and Kleifeld, 2006; Mauriz and Gonzalez-Gallego, 2008; Dorman et al. 2010).

Furthermore, since endothelial cell migration depends on adhesion to extracellular matrix proteins through receptors called integrins, cell adhesion peptides were being investigated to target anti-tumour drugs for cells with enhanced expression of specific integrin (reviewed in Price and Thompson, 2002; Mauriz and Gonzalez-Gallego, 2008).

From a variety of the growth factors involved in tumour angiogenesis, VEGF seems to play the most relevant role, and different drugs and experimental strategies have been developed to counteract its production and function (Mauriz and Gonzalez-Gallego, 2008). Leading anti-angiogenic inhibitors block VEGF-mediated endothelial cell functions during blood vessel formation, influencing endothelial proliferation, migration and survival. Bevacizumab (Avastin), a monoclonal antibody against VEGF received Food and Drug Administration (FDA) approval for use in combination with fluorouracil based chemotherapy for metastatic colorectal cancer treatment in 2004 (Hurwitz et al., 2004). In October 2006, the FDA granted approval for bevacizumab administered in combination with carboplatin and paclitaxel for the first-line treatment of patients with unresectable, locally advanced, recurrent or metastatic nonsquamous, non-small cell lung cancer (Cohen et al., 2007). On the other hand, a soluble decoy receptor, which incorporates both VEGFR-1 and VEGFR-2 domains (VEGF-Trap) and binds VEGF with significantly high affinity (Holash et al., 2002) has shown a robust antitumour effect in numerous models of cancer and was tested in phase I and II clinical trials (Teng et al., 2010).

Apart from antibody-based drugs, the second leading class of anti-angiogenic agents are small molecule receptor tyrosine kinase inhibitors, which have been investigated in several preclinical and clinical trials (reviewed in Eichhorn et al., 2007 ; Longo et al., 2002; Mauriz and Gonzalez-Gallego, 2008). For instance, sorafenib, a small molecular inhibitor of Raf kinase, PDGF and VEGFR-2 kinase, was approved by FDA in 2005 for treatment of advanced renal cell cancer.

As already underlined, many key aspects of tumour progression are promoted by adaptation to hypoxia. Because a major mechanism mediating adaptive response to reduced oxygen availability is regulation of HIF-1, a growing number of its inhibitors have been investigated. A large body of clinical data shows the association between HIF protein level with increased patient mortality in many human cancers, with early stage breast, cervical and endometrial cancers being particularly striking (Semenza, 2009). Thus, anticancer agents with anti-angiogenic effects, due to inhibition of HIF-1, have been recently identified and validated (Table 5.2). Among them one can find inhibitors of HIF-1 DNA binding – anthracyclines (doxorubicin); inhibitors of HIF-1α synthesis – epidermal growth factor receptor inhibitors (gefitinib/Iressa, erlotinib/Tarceva, Cetuximab/C225), inhibitors of mTOR-dependent translation of HIF-1α mRNA (rapamycin, temsirolimus/CCI-779, everolimus/RAD-001), topoisomerase I inhibitors (topotecan); drugs increasing HIF-1α degradation – histone deacetylases inhibitors (trichostatin A, TSA); factors decreasing HIF-1α transactivation – proteasome inhibitors (Bortezomib) (reviewed in Semenza, 2009). Besides those, many other chemical compounds have been reported to possess anti-HIF-1 activity and are in preclinical development (Melillo, 2007).

Importantly, hypoxia may cause tumour resistance to radiation therapy, due to reduced generation of oxygen radicals (Moeller et al., 2007). Moreover, radiation was shown to activate HIF-1 and subsequently increase pro-angiogenic growth factor production, which protects endothelial cells of tumour blood vessels from radiation-induced death (Moeller et al., 2004). It had long been assumed that an angiogenesis inhibitors would impair the effect of ionizing radiation by inducing tumour hypoxia. Paradoxically, many studies with HIF-1 inhibitors demonstrated increased radiation-induced tumour vasculature destruction (Moeller et al., 2004; Schwartz et al., 2009; Semenza, 2009) and thus the important role of HIF-1 in mediating radiation resistance. Although HIF-1 blockade seems to be a viable strategy for tumour radiosensitisation, the mechanisms of this phenomenon have not yet been fully described. One explanation is that anti-angiogenic therapies temporarily normalized tumour blood vessels (Jain, 2005), resulting in improved tumour oxygenation and enhanced response to radiation therapy. However, clinical strategies combining HIF-1 inhibitors and radiation therapy may need to be optimized on a cancer and patient-specific basis.

Anti-angiogenic drugs seem to be very attractive for treatment of malignant tumours, however, only sorafenib and sunitinib, tyrosine kinase inhibitors are effective as a monotherapy, and have been approved for treatment

Table 5.2 _ Selected classes of anticancer drugs inhibiting HIF-1.

Mechanism	Drug class	Example
Inhibition of HIF-1α synthesis	EGF inhibitors mTOR inhibitors topoisomerase I inhibitors	erlotinib, gefitinib, cetuximab, rapamycin, temsirolimus, everolimus topotecan
Increase in HIF-1α degradation	histone deacetylases inhibitor	trichostatin A
Inhibition of HIF-1 DNA binding	anthracyclines	doxorubicin
Inhibition of HIF-1α transactivation	proteasome inhibitors	bortezomib

EGF – epidermal growth factor, mTOR – mammalian target of rapamycin kinase.

of gastrointestinal tumours. It has already been suggested (Jain, 2005) that certain anti-angiogenic agents can transiently "normalize" the abnormal structure and function of tumour vasculature to make it more efficient for oxygen and drug delivery. Jain postulated the use of combined therapy of both anti-angiogenic factor and (2005) chemotherapeutic agent, which is now a widely used approach for tumour treatment (e.g. described above for Avastin). This approach appears to be a very attractive: normalizing agent decreases hypoxia in abnormal blood vessels, improves blood flow and increases the efficacy of cytotoxic drug delivery to tumours. Accordingly, on the basis of such results, it has been recently suggested that anti-angiogenic drugs represent universal chemosensitizing agents for cancer treatment (Kerbel, 2006) and are most effective in increasing survival of patients when combined with traditional therapies, particularly chemotherapy.

Conclusions

The association between cancer and blood vessel formation has been observed for more than a century. It is now well established, that besides sprouting angiogenesis, tumour tissue can acquire its vasculature by a number of additional mechanisms, such as vessel co-option, intussusceptive angiogenesis, vasculogenic mimicry or EPCs recruitment. A fundamental condition, which drives all those processes, is hypoxia. However, these different types of vascularization are also characterized by some unique properties, which have to be taken into consideration, when anti-angiogenic strategies are being developed.

Acknowledgments _ Supported by the grants No DWM/N148/INCA/08, 311/N-COST/2008, N N301 144336 and statutory funds from the Polish Ministry of Science and Higher Education. Department of Medical Biotechnology participates in the COST CM0602 (ANGIOKEM) and TD0901 (HypoxiaNet) Actions, both supported by European Commission. The Faculty of Biochemistry, Biophysics and Biotechnology of the Jagiellonian University is a beneficiary of the structural funds from the European Union and the Polish Ministry of Science and Higher Education (grants No: POIG.02.01.00-12 064/08, POIG 01.01.02-00-109/09, POIG.02.02.00-014/08 and 01.01.02-00-069/09). AJ is a recipient of the Wellcome Trust Senior Research Fellowship in Basic Biomedical Science. AL is supported by the Foundation for Polish Science – Parent-Bridge Programme co-financed by the European Union within European Regional Development Fund. UF is the recipient of the Foundation for Polish Science START Programme.

References

Aicher A, Heeschen C, Mildner-Rihm C, Urbich C, Ihling C, Technau-Ihling K, Zeiher AM, Dimmeler S (2003). Essential role of endothelial nitric oxide synthase for mobilization of stem and progenitor cells. Nat Med 9(11): 1370-6.

Algire GH, Chalkley HW, Earle WE, Legallais FY, Park HD, Shelton E, Schilling EL (1950). Vascular reactions of normal and malignant tissues in vivo. III. Vascular reactions' of mice to fibroblasts treated in vitro with methylcholanthrene. J Natl Cancer Inst 11(3): 555-80.

Arafat WO, Casado E, Wang M, Alvarez RD, Siegal GP, Glorioso JC, Curiel DT, Gomez-Navarro J (2000). Genetically modified CD34+ cells exert a cytotoxic bystander effect on human endothelial and cancer cells. Clin Cancer Res 6(11): 4442-8.

Asahara T, Murohara T, Sullivan A, Silver M, van der Zee R, Li T, Witzenbichler B, Schatteman G, Isner JM (1997). Isolation of putative progenitor endothelial cells for angiogenesis. Science 275(5302): 964-7.

Asahara T, Takahashi T, Masuda H, Kalka C, Chen D, Iwaguro H, Inai Y, Silver M, Isner JM (1999). VEGF contributes to postnatal neovascularization by mobilizing bone marrow-derived endothelial progenitor cells. EMBO J 18(14): 3964-72.

Baldwin ME, Halford MM, Roufail S, Williams RA, Hibbs ML, Grail D, Kubo H, Stacker SA, Achen MG (2005). Vascular endothelial growth factor D is dispensable for development of the lymphatic system. Mol Cell Biol 25(6): 2441-9.

Banerji S, Ni J, Wang SX, Clasper S, Su J, Tammi R, Jones M, Jackson DG (1999). LYVE-1, a new homologue of the CD44 glycoprotein, is a lymph-specific receptor for hyaluronan. J Cell Biol 144(4): 789-801.

Bergers G, Benjamin LE (2003). Tumourigenesis and the angiogenic switch. Nat Rev Cancer 3(6): 401-10.

Brahimi-Horn MC, Pouyssegur J (2005). The hypoxia-inducible factor and tumour progression along the angiogenic pathway. Int Rev Cytol 242: 157-213.

Breiteneder-Geleff S, Soleiman A, Kowalski H, Horvat R, Amann G, Kriehuber E, Diem K, Weninger W, Tschachler E, Alitalo K, Kerjaschki D (1999). Angiosarcomas express mixed endothelial phenotypes of blood and lymphatic capillaries: podoplanin as a specific marker for lymphatic endothelium. Am J Pathol 154(2): 385-94.

Burri PH, Hlushchuk R, Djonov V (2004). Intussusceptive angiogenesis: its emergence, its characteristics, and its significance. Dev Dyn 231(3): 474-88.

Caduff JH, Fischer L.C, Burri PH (1986). Scanning electron microscope study of the developing microvasculature in the postnatal rat lung. Anat Rec 216(2): 154-64.

Carson-Walter EB, Watkins DN, Nanda A, Vogelstein B, Kinzler KW, St Croix B (2001). Cell surface tumour endothelial markers are conserved in mice and humans. Cancer Res 61(18): 6649-55.

Casanovas O, Hicklin DJ, Bergers G, Hanahan D (2005). Drug resistance by evasion of antiangiogenic targeting of VEGF signalling in late-stage pancreatic islet tumours. Cancer Cell 8(4): 299-309.

Ceradini DJ, Kulkarni, AR, Callaghan MJ, Tepper OM, Bastidas N, Kleinman ME, Capla JM, Galiano RD, Levine, JP, Gurtner GC (2004). Progenitor cell trafficking is regulated by hypoxic gradients through HIF-1 induction of SDF-1. Nat Med 10:(8) 858-64.

Chan SY, Loscalzo J (2010). MicroRNA-210: A unique and pleiotropic hypoxamir. Cell Cycle 9(6): 1072 – 83.

Chavakis E, Hain A, Vinci M, Carmona G, Bianchi ME, Vajkoczy P, Zeiher AM, Chavakis T, Dimmeler S (2007). High-mobility group box 1 activates integrin-dependent homing of endothelial progenitor cells. Circ Res 100(2): 204-12.

Cohen MH, Gootenberg J, Keegan P, Pazdur R (2007). FDA drug approval summary: bevacizumab (Avastin) plus Carboplatin and Paclitaxel as first-line treatment of advanced/metastatic recurrent nonsquamous non-small cell lung cancer. Oncologist 12(6): 713-8.

Currie MJ, Hanrahan V, Gunningham SP, Morrin HR, Frampton C, Han C, Robinson BA, Fox SB (2004). Expression of vascular endothelial growth factor D is associated with hypoxia inducible factor (HIF-1alpha) and the HIF-1alpha target gene DEC1, but not lymph node metastasis in primary human breast carcinomas. J Clin Pathol 57(8): 829-34.

Dadras SS, Paul T, Bertoncini J, Brown LF, Muzikansky A, Jackson DG, Ellwanger U, Garbe C, Mihm MC, Detmar M (2003). Tumour lymphangiogenesis: a novel prognostic indicator for cutaneous melanoma metastasis and survival. Am J Pathol 162(6): 1951-60.

De Falco E, Porcelli D, Torella AR, Straino S, Iachininoto MG, Orlandi A, Truffa S, Biglioli P, Napolitano M, Capogrossi MC, Pesce M (2004). SDF-1 involvement in endothelial phenotype and ischaemia-induced recruitment of bone marrow progenitor cells. Blood 104(12): 3472-82.

Deb A, Skelding KA, Wang S, Reeder M, Simper D, Caplice NM (2004). Integrin profile and in vivo homing of human smooth muscle progenitor cells. Circulation 110(17): 2673-7.

Demou ZN, Hendrix MJ (2008). Microgenomics profile the endogenous angiogenic phenotype in subpopulations of aggressive melanoma. J Cell Biochem 105(2): 562-73.

Dome B, Hendrix MJ, Paku S, Tovari J, Timar J (2007). Alternative vascularization mechanisms in cancer: Pathology and therapeutic implications. Am J Pathol 170(1): 1-15.

Dome B, Paku S, Somlai B, Timar J (2002). Vascularization of cutaneous melanoma involves vessel co-option and has clinical significance. J Pathol 197(3): 355-62.

Dorman G, Cseh S, Hajdu I, Barna L, Konya D, Kupai K, Kovacs L, Ferdinandy P (2010). Matrix metalloproteinase inhibitors: a critical appraisal of design principles and proposed therapeutic utility. Drugs 70(8): 949-64.

Dvorak HF (2003). Rous-Whipple Award Lecture. How tumours make bad blood vessels and stroma. Am J Pathol 162(6): 1747-57.

Eberhard A, Kahlert S, Goede V, Hemmerlein B, Plate KH, Augustin HG (2000). Heterogeneity of angiogenesis and blood vessel maturation in human tumours: implications for antiangiogenic tumour therapies. Cancer Res 60(4): 1388-93.

Eichhorn ME, Kleespies A, Angele MK, Jauch KW, Bruns CJ (2007). Angiogenesis in cancer: molecular mechanisms, clinical impact. Langenbecks Arch Surg 392(3): 371-9.

Fasanaro P, D'Alessandra Y, Di Stefano V, Melchionna R, Romani S, Pompilio G, Capogrossi MC, Martelli F (2008). MicroRNA-210 modulates endothelial cell response to hypoxia and inhibits the receptor tyrosine kinase ligand Ephrin-A3. J Biol Chem 283(23): 15878-83.

Ferrara N (2001). Role of vascular endothelial growth factor in regulation of physiological angiogenesis. Am J Physiol Cell Physiol 280(6): C1358-66.

Ferrara N, Kerbel RS (2005). Angiogenesis as a therapeutic target. Nature 438(7070): 967-74.

Foekens JA, Sieuwerts AM, Smid M, Look MP, de Weerd V, Boersma AW, Klijn JG, Wiemer EA, Martens JW (2008). Four miRNAs associated with aggressiveness of lymph node-negative, estrogen receptor-positive human breast cancer. Proc Natl Acad Sci U S A 105(35): 13021-6.

Folberg R, Rummelt V, Parys-Van Ginderdeuren R, Hwang T, Woolson RF, Pe'er J, Gruman LM (1993). The prognostic value of tumour blood vessel morphology in primary uveal melanoma. Ophthalmology 100(9): 1389-98.

Folkman J (1971). Tumour angiogenesis: therapeutic implications. N Engl J Med 285(21): 1182-6.

Forooghian F, Das B (2007). Anti-angiogenic effects of ribonucleic acid interference targeting vascular endothelial growth factor and hypoxia-inducible factor-1alpha. Am J Ophthalmol 144(5): 761-8.

Furuya M, Nishiyama M, Kasuya Y, Kimura S, Ishikura H (2005). Pathophysiology of tumour neovascularization. Vasc Health Risk Manag 1(4): 277-90.

Gannon G, Mandriota SJ, Cui L, Baetens D, Pepper MS, Christofori G (2002). Overexpression of vascular endothelial growth factor-A165 enhances tumour angiogenesis but not metastasis during beta-cell carcinogenesis. Cancer Res 62(2): 603-8.

Gao D, Nolan DJ, Mellick AS, Bambino K, McDonnell K, Mittal V (2008). Endothelial progenitor cells control the angiogenic switch in mouse lung metastasis. Science 319(5860): 195-8.

Gehling UM, Ergun S, Schumacher U, Wagener C, Pantel K, Otte M, Schuch G, Schafhausen P, Mende, T, Kilic, N, Kluge K, Schafer B, Hossfeld DK, Fiedler W (2000). In vitro differentiation of endothelial cells from AC133-positive progenitor cells. Blood 95(10): 3106-12.

Ghosh G, Subramanian IV, Adhikari N, Zhang X, Joshi, HP, Basi D, Chandrashekhar YS, Hall JL, Roy S, Zeng Y, Ramakrishnan S (2010). Hypoxia-induced microRNA-424 expression in human endothelial cells regulates HIF-alpha isoforms and promotes angiogenesis. J Clin Invest 120(11): 4141-54.

Gothert JR, Gustin SE, van Eekelen JA, Schmidt U, Hall MA, Jane SM, Green AR, Gottgens B, Izon DJ, Begley CG (2004). Genetically tagging endothelial cells in vivo: bone marrow-derived cells do not contribute to tumour endothelium. Blood 104(6): 1769-77.

Hanahan D, Folkman J (1996). Patterns and emerging mechanisms of the angiogenic switch during tumourigenesis. Cell 86(3): 353-64.

Hashizume H, Baluk P, Morikawa S, McLean JW, Thurston G, Roberge S, Jain RK, McDonald DM (2000). Openings between defective endothelial cells explain tumour vessel leakiness. Am J Pathol 156(4): 1363-80.

Hattori K, Heissig B, Wu Y, Dias S, Tejada R, Ferris B, Hicklin DJ, Zhu Z, Bohlen P, Witte L, Hendrikx J, Hackett NR, Crystal RG, Moore MA, Werb Z, Lyden D, Rafii S (2002). Placental growth factor reconstitutes hematopoiesis by recruiting VEGFR1(+) stem cells from bone-marrow microenvironment. Nat Med 8(8): 841-9.

Hendrix MJ, Seftor EA, Hess AR, Seftor RE (2003). Vasculogenic mimicry and tumour-cell plasticity: lessons from melanoma. Nat Rev Cancer 3(6): 411-21.

Hendrix MJ, Seftor, EA, Meltzer PS, Gardner LM, Hess AR, Kirschmann DA, Schatteman GC, Seftor RE (2001). Expression and functional significance of VE-cadherin in aggressive human melanoma cells: role in vasculogenic mimicry. Proc Natl Acad Sci U S A 98(14): 8018-23.

Hillen F, Griffioen AW (2007). Tumour vascularization: sprouting angiogenesis and beyond. Cancer Metastasis Rev 26(3-4): 489-502.

Hirakawa S, Hong YK, Harvey N, Schacht V, Matsuda K, Libermann T, Detmar M (2003). Identification of vascular lineage-specific genes by transcriptional profiling of isolated blood vascular and lymphatic endothelial cells. Am J Path 162(2): 575-86.

Hirakawa S, Kodama S, Kunstfeld R, Kajiya K, Brown LF, Detmar M (2005). VEGF-A induces tumour and sentinel lymph node lymphangiogenesis and promotes lymphatic metastasis. J Exp Med 201(7): 1089-99.

Ho AS, Huang X, Cao H, Christman-Skieller C, Bennewith K, Le QT, Koong AC (2010). Circulating miR-210 as a Novel Hypoxia Marker in Pancreatic Cancer. Transl Oncol 3(2): 109-13.

Holash J, Davis S, Papadopoulos N, Croll SD, Ho L, Russell M, Boland P, Leidich R, Hylton D, Burova E, Ioffe E, Huang T, Radziejewski C, Bailey K, Fandl JP, Daly T, Wiegand SJ, Yancopoulos GD, Rudge JS (2002). VEGF-Trap: a VEGF blocker with potent antitumour effects. Proc Natl Acad Sci U S A 99(17): 11393-8.

Holash J, Maisonpierre PC, Compton D, Boland P, Alexander CR, Zagzag D, Yancopoulos GD, Wiegand SJ (1999a). Vessel cooption, regression, and growth in tumours mediated by angiopoietins and VEGF. Science 284(5422): 1994-8.

Holash J, Wiegand SJ, Yancopoulos GD (1999b). New model of tumour angiogenesis: dynamic balance between vessel regression and growth mediated by angiopoietins and VEGF. Oncogene 18(38): 5356-62.

Holmgren L, O'Reilly MS, Folkman J (1995). Dormancy of micrometastases: balanced proliferation and apoptosis in the presence of angiogenesis suppression. Nat Med 1(2): 149-53.

Hua Z, Lv Q, Ye W, Wong CK, Cai G, Gu D, Ji Y, Zhao C, Wang J, Yang BB, Zhang Y (2006). MiRNA-directed regulation of VEGF and other angiogenic factors under hypoxia. PLoS One 1: e116.

Huang X, Le, QT, Giaccia AJ (2010). MiR-210-micromanager of the hypoxia pathway. Trends Mol Med 16(5): 230-7.

Hurwitz H, Fehrenbacher L, Novotny W, Cartwright T, Hainsworth J, Heim W, Berlin J, Baron A, Griffing S, Holmgren E, Ferrara N, Fyfe G, Rogers B, Ross, R, Kabbinavar F (2004). Bevacizumab plus irinotecan, fluorouracil, and leucovorin for metastatic colorectal cancer. N Engl J Med 350(23): 2335-42.

Jain RK (2005). Normalization of tumour vasculature: an emerging concept in antiangiogenic therapy. Science 307(5706): 58-62.

Ji JW, Tsoukias NM, Goldman D, Popel AS (2006). A computational model of oxygen transport in skeletal muscle for sprouting and splitting modes of angiogenesis. J Theor Biol 241(1): 94-108.

Kaelin WG (2007). Von Hippel-Lindau disease. Annu Rev Pathol 2: 145-73.

Kaipainen A, Korhonen J, Mustonen T, van Hinsbergh VW, Fang GH, Dumont D, Breitman M, Alitalo K (1995). Expression of the fms-like tyrosine kinase 4 gene becomes restricted to lymphatic endothelium during development. Proc Natl Acad Sci U S A 92(8): 3566-70.

Kalka C, Masuda H, Takahashi T, Kalka-Moll WM, Silver M, Kearney M, Li T, Isner JM, Asahara T (2000). Transplantation of ex vivo expanded endothelial progenitor cells for therapeutic neovascularization. Proc Natl Acad Sci U S A 97(7): 3422-7.

Karkkainen MJ, Haiko P, Sainio K, Partanen J, Taipale J, Petrova TV, Jeltsch M, Jackson DG, Talikka M, Rauvala H, Betsholtz C, Alitalo K (2004). Vascular endothelial growth factor C is required for sprouting of the first lymphatic vessels from embryonic veins. Nat Immunol 5(1): 74-80.

Karpanen T, Egeblad M, Karkkainen MJ, Kubo H, Yla-Herttuala S, Jaattela M, Alitalo K (2001). Vascular endothelial growth factor C promotes tumour lymphangiogenesis and intralymphatic tumour growth. Cancer Res 61(5): 1786-90.

Katsuta M, Miyashita M, Makino H, Nomura T, Shinji S, Yamashita K, Tajiri T, Kudo M, Ishiwata T, Naito Z (2005). Correlation of hypoxia inducible factor-1alpha with lymphatic metastasis via vascular endothelial growth factor-C in human esophageal cancer. Exp Mol Pathol 78(2): 123-30.

Keith B, Simon MC (2007). Hypoxia-inducible factors, stem cells, and cancer. Cell 129(3): 465-72.

Kerbel RS (2006). Antiangiogenic therapy: a universal chemosensitization strategy for cancer? Science 312(5777): 1171-5.

Kim ES, Serur A, Huang J, Manley CA, McCrudden KW, Frischer JS, Soffer SZ, Ring L, New T, Zabski S, Rudge JS, Holash J, Yancopoulos GD, Kandel JJ, Yamashiro DJ (2002). Potent VEGF blockade causes regression of coopted vessels in a model of neuroblastoma. Proc Natl Acad Sci U S A 99(17): 11399-404.

Kim HK, Song KS, Kim HO, Chung JH, Lee KR, Lee YJ, Lee DH, Lee ES, Kim HK, Ryu KW, Bae JM (2003). Circulating numbers of endothelial progenitor cells in patients with gastric and breast cancer. Cancer Lett 198(1): 83-8.

Kunkel P, Ulbricht U, Bohlen P, Brockmann MA, Fillbrandt R, Stavrou D, Westphal M, Lamszus K (2001). Inhibition of glioma angiogenesis and growth in vivo by systemic treatment with a monoclonal antibody against vascular endothelial growth factor receptor-2. Cancer Res 61(18): 6624-8.

Lee JY, Park C, Cho YP, Lee E, Kim H, Kim P, Yun SH, Yoon YS (2010). Podoplanin-expressing cells derived from bone marrow play a crucial role in postnatal lymphatic neovascularization. Circulation 122(14): 1413-25.

Lee RC, Feinbaum RL, Ambros V (1993). The C. elegans heterochronic gene lin-4 encodes small RNAs with antisense complementarity to lin-14. Cell 75(5): 843-54.

Lei Z, Li B, Yang Z, Fang H, Zhang GM, Feng ZH, Huang B (2009). Regulation of HIF-1alpha and VEGF by miR-20b tunes tumour cells to adapt to the alteration of oxygen concentration. PLoS One 4(10): e7629.

Levy AP (1998). Hypoxic regulation of VEGF mRNA stability by RNA-binding proteins. Trends Cardiovasc Med 8(6): 246-50.

Levy AP, Levy NS, Wegner S, Goldberg MA (1995). Transcriptional regulation of the rat vascular endothelial growth factor gene by hypoxia. J Biol Chem 270(22): 13333-40.

Li B, Sharpe EE, Maupin AB, Teleron AA, Pyle AL, Carmeliet P, Young PP (2006). VEGF and PlGF promote adult vasculogenesis by enhancing EPC recruitment and vessel formation at the site of tumour neovascularization. FASEB J 20(9): 1495-7.

Li M, Gu Y, Zhang Z, Zhang S, Zhang D, Saleem AF, Zhao X, Sun B (2010). Vasculogenic mimicry: a new prognostic sign of gastric adenocarcinoma. Pathol Oncol Res 16(2): 259-66.

Liang X, Yang D, Hu J, Hao X, Gao J, Mao Z (2008). Hypoxia inducible factor-alpha expression correlates with vascular endothelial growth factor-C expression and lymphangiogenesis /angiogenesis in oral squamous cell carcinoma. Anticancer Res 28(3A): 1659-66.

Liao F, Huynh HK, Eiroa A, Greene T, Polizzi E, Muller WA (1995). Migration of monocytes across endothelium and passage through extracellular matrix involve separate molecular domains of PECAM-1. J Exp Med 182(5): 1337-43.

Liu WB, Xu GL, Jia WD, Li JS, Ma JL, Chen K, Wang ZH, Ge YS, Ren WH, Yu JH, Wang W, Wang XJ (2011). Prognostic significance and mechanisms of patterned matrix vasculogenic mimicry in hepatocellular carcinoma. Med Oncol. 28, S1: 5228-38.

Loboda A, Jazwa A, Jozkowicz A, Molema G, Dulak J (2006). Angiogenic transcriptome of human microvascular endothelial cells: Effect of hypoxia, modulation by atorvastatin. Vascul Pharmacol 44(4): 206-14.

Loboda A, Stachurska A, Florczyk U, Rudnicka D, Jazwa A, Wegrzyn J, Kozakowska M, Stalinska K, Poellinger L, Levonen AL, Yla-Herttuala S, Jozkowicz A, Dulak J (2009). HIF-1 induction attenuates Nrf2-dependent IL-8 expression in human endothelial cells. Antioxid Redox Signal 11(7): 1501-17.

Longo R, Sarmiento R, Fanelli M, Capaccetti B, Gattuso D, Gasparini G (2002). Anti-angiogenic therapy: rationale, challenges and clinical studies. Angiogenesis 5(4): 237-56.

Loscalzo J (2010). The cellular response to hypoxia: tuning the system with microRNAs. J Clin Invest 120(11): 3815-7.

Lyden D, Hattori K, Dias S, Costa C, Blaikie P, Butros L, Chadburn A, Heissig B, Marks, W, Witte L, Wu Y, Hicklin D, Zhu Z, Hackett NR, Crystal RG, Moore MA, Hajjar KA, Manova K, Benezra R, Rafii S (2001). Impaired recruitment of bone-marrow-derived endothelial and hematopoietic precursor cells blocks tumour angiogenesis and growth. Nat Med 7(11): 1194-1201.

Machein MR, Renninger S, de Lima-Hahn E, Plate KH (2003). Minor contribution of bone marrow-derived endothelial progenitors to the vascularization of murine gliomas. Brain Pathol 13(4): 582-97.

Maeng YS, Choi HJ, Kwon JY, Park YW, Choi KS, Min JK, Kim YH, Suh PG, Kang KS, Won MH, Kim YM, Kwon YG (2009). Endothelial progenitor cell homing: prominent role of the IGF2-IGF2R-PLCbeta2 axis. Blood 113(1): 233-43.

Makanya AN, Hlushchuk R, Djonov VG (2009). Intussusceptive angiogenesis and its role in vascular morphogenesis, patterning, and remodeling. Angiogenesis 12(2): 113-23.

Makinen T, Veikkola T, Mustjoki S, Karpanen T, Catimel B, Nice EC, Wise L, Mercer A, Kowalski H, Kerjaschki D, Stacker SA, Achen MG, Alitalo K (2001). Isolated lymphatic endothelial cells transduce growth, survival and migratory signals via the VEGF-C/D receptor VEGFR-3. EMBO J 20(17): 4762-73.

Maniotis AJ, Folberg R, Hess A, Seftor EA, Gardner LM, Pe'er J, Trent JM, Meltzer PS, Hendrix MJ, (1999). Vascular channel formation by human melanoma cells in vivo and in vitro: vasculogenic mimicry. Am J Pathol 155(3): 739-52.

Maruyama K, Ii M, Cursiefen C, Jackson DG, Keino H, Tomita M, Van Rooijen N, Takenaka H, D'Amore PA, Stein-Streilein J, Losordo DW, Streilein JW (2005). Inflammation-induced lymphangiogenesis in the cornea arises from CD11b-positive macrophages. J Clin Invest 115(9): 2363-72.

Matsumoto G, Yajima N, Saito H, Nakagami H, Omi Y, Lee U, Kaneda Y (2010). Cold shock domain protein A (CSDA) overexpression inhibits tumour growth and lymph node metastasis in a mouse model of squamous cell carcinoma. Clin Exp Metastasis 27(7): 539-47.

Mauriz JL, Gonzalez-Gallego J (2008). Antiangiogenic drugs: current knowledge and new approaches to cancer therapy. J Pharm Sci 97(10): 4129-54.

Melillo G (2007). Targeting hypoxia cell signalling for cancer therapy. Cancer Metastasis Rev 26(2): 341-52.

Miska EA (2005). How microRNAs control cell division, differentiation and death. Curr Opin Genet Dev 15(5): 563-8.

Mizukami Y, Jo WS, Duerr EM, Gala M, Li J, Zhang X, Zimmer MA, Iliopoulos O, Zukerberg LR, Kohgo Y, Lynch MP, Rueda BR, Chung DC (2005). Induction of interleukin-8 preserves the angiogenic response in HIF-1alpha-deficient colon cancer cells. Nat Med 11(9): 992-7.

Moeller BJ, Cao Y, Li CY, Dewhirst MW (2004). Radiation activates HIF-1 to regulate vascular radiosensitivity in tumours: role of reoxygenation, free radicals, and stress granules. Cancer Cell 5(5): 429-41.

Moeller BJ, Richardson RA, Dewhirst MW (2007). Hypoxia and radiotherapy: opportunities for improved outcomes in cancer treatment. Cancer Metastasis Rev 26(2): 241-8.

Moore MA, Hattori K, Heissig B, Shieh JH, Dias S, Crystal RG, Rafii S (2001). Mobilization of endothelial and hematopoietic stem and progenitor cells by adenovector-mediated elevation of serum levels of SDF-1, VEGF, and angiopoietin-1. Ann N Y Acad Sci 938: 36-45.

Nagy JA, Vasile E, Feng D, Sundberg C, Brown LF, Detmar MJ, Lawitts JA, Benjamin L, Tan X, Manseau EJ, Dvorak AM, Dvorak HF (2002). Vascular permeability factor/

vascular endothelial growth factor induces lymphangiogenesis as well as angiogenesis. J Exp Med 196(11): 1497-1506.

Nilsson I, Shibuya M, Wennstrom S (2004). Differential activation of vascular genes by hypoxia in primary endothelial cells. Exp Cell Res 299(2): 476-85.

Niu YJ, Liu FL, Yang Y, Yuan CY (2009). Relationship between vasculogenic mimicry and clinical pathological characters in retinoblastoma. Zhonghua Yan Ke Za Zhi 45(4): 318-22.

Nolan DJ, Ciarrocchi A, Mellick AS, Jaggi JS, Bambino K, Gupta S, Heikamp E, McDevitt MR, Scheinberg DA, Benezra R, Mittal V (2007). Bone marrow-derived endothelial progenitor cells are a major determinant of nascent tumour neovascularization. Genes Dev 21(12): 1546-58.

Oh J, Seo DW, Diaz T, Wei B, Ward Y, Ray JM, Morioka Y, Shi S, Kitayama H, Takahashi C, Noda M, Stetler-Stevenson WG (2004). Tissue inhibitors of metalloproteinase 2 inhibits endothelial cell migration through increased expression of RECK. Cancer Res 64(24): 9062-9.

Overall CM, Kleifeld O (2006). Towards third generation matrix metalloproteinase inhibitors for cancer therapy. Br J Cancer 94(7): 941-6.

Patan S, Munn LL, Jain RK (1996). Intussusceptive microvascular growth in a human colon adenocarcinoma xenograft: a novel mechanism of tumour angiogenesis. Microvasc Res 51(2): 260-72.

Patan S, Munn LL, Tanda S, Roberge S, Jain, RK, Jones RC (2001). Vascular morphogenesis and remodeling in a model of tissue repair: blood vessel formation and growth in the ovarian pedicle after ovariectomy. Circ Res 89(8): 723-31.

Patenaude A, Parker J, Karsan A (2010). Involvement of endothelial progenitor cells in tumour vascularization. Microvasc Res 79(3): 217-23.

Perou CM, Sorlie T, Eisen MB, van de Rijn M, Jeffrey SS, Rees CA, Pollack JR, Ross DT, Johnsen H, Akslen LA, Fluge O, Pergamenschikov A, Williams C, Zhu SX, Lonning PE, Borresen-Dale AL, Brown PO, Botstein D (2000). Molecular portraits of human breast tumours. Nature 406(6797): 747-52.

Peters BA, Diaz LA, Polyak K, Meszler L, Romans K, Guinan EC, Antin JH, Myerson D, Hamilton SR, Vogelstein B, Kinzler KW, Lengauer C (2005). Contribution of bone marrow-derived endothelial cells to human tumour vasculature. Nat Med 11(3): 261-2.

Pezzella F, Pastorino U, Tagliabue E, Andreola S, Sozzi G, Gasparini G, Menard S, Gatter KC, Harris AL, Fox S, Buyse M, Pilotti S, Pierotti M, Rilke F (1997). Non-small-cell lung carcinoma tumour growth without morphological evidence of neo-angiogenesis. Am J Pathol 151(5): 1417-23.

Price JT, Thompson EW (2002). Mechanisms of tumour invasion and metastasis: emerging targets for therapy. Expert Opin Ther Targets 6(2): 217-33.

Pugh CW, Ratcliffe PJ (2003). Regulation of angiogenesis by hypoxia: role of the HIF system. Nat Med 9(6): 677-84.

Risau W (1997). Mechanisms of angiogenesis. Nature 386(6626): 671-4.

Ruzinova MB, Schoer RA, Gerald W, Egan JE, Pandolfi PP, Rafii S, Manova K, Mittal V, Benezra R (2003). Effect of angiogenesis inhibition by Id loss and the contribution of bone-marrow-derived endothelial cells in spontaneous murine tumours. Cancer Cell 4(4): 277-89.

Schatton T, Frank MH (2008). Cancer stem cells and human malignant melanoma. Pigment Cell Melanoma Res 21(1): 39-55.

Schenkel AR, Mamdouh Z, Chen X, Liebman RM, Muller WA (2002). CD99 plays a major role in the migration of monocytes through endothelial junctions. Nat Immunol 3(2): 143-50.

Schwartz DL, Powis G, Thitai-Kumar A, He Y, Bankson J, Williams R, Lemos R, Oh J, Volgin A, Soghomonyan S, Nishii R, Alauddin M, Mukhopadhay U, Peng Z, Bornmann W, Gelovani J (2009). The selective hypoxia inducible factor-1 inhibitor PX-478 provides in vivo radiosensitization through tumour stromal effects. Mol Cancer Ther 8(4): 947-58.

Seftor EA, Brown KM, Chin L, Kirschmann DA, Wheaton WW, Protopopov A, Feng B, Balagurunathan Y, Trent JM, Nickoloff BJ, Seftor RE, Hendrix MJ (2005). Epigenetic transdifferentiation of normal melanocytes by a metastatic melanoma microenvironment. Cancer Res 65(22): 10164-9.

Seftor RE, Seftor EA, Koshikawa N, Meltzer PS, Gardner LM, Bilban M, Stetler-Stevenson WG, Quaranta V, Hendrix MJ (2001). Cooperative interactions of laminin 5 gamma2 chain, matrix metalloproteinase-2, and membrane type-1-matrix/metalloproteinase are required for mimicry of embryonic vasculogenesis by aggressive melanoma. Cancer Res 61(17): 6322-7.

Semenza GL (2009). Defining the role of hypoxia-inducible factor 1 in cancer biology and therapeutics. Oncogene 29(5): 625-34.

Semenza GL (2001). Hypoxia-inducible factor 1: oxygen homeostasis and disease pathophysiology. Trends Mol Med 7(8): 345-50.

Senger DR, Galli SJ, Dvorak AM, Perruzzi CA, Harvey VS, Dvorak HF (1983). Tumour cells secrete a vascular permeability factor that promotes accumulation of ascites fluid. Science 219(4587): 983-5.

Shaked Y, Bertolini F, Man S, Rogers M.S, Cervi D, Foutz T, Rawn K, Voskas D, Dumont DJ, Ben-David Y, Lawler J, Henkin J, Huber J, Hicklin DJ, D'Amato RJ, Kerbel RS (2005). Genetic heterogeneity of the vasculogenic phenotype parallels angiogenesis; Implications for cellular surrogate marker analysis of antiangiogenesis. Cancer Cell 7(1): 101-11.

Shaked, Y, Henke E, Roodhart JM, Mancuso P, Langenberg MH, Colleoni M, Daenen LG, Man S, Xu P, Emmenegger U, Tang T, Zhu Z, Witte L, Strieter RM, Bertolini F, Voest EE, Benezra R, Kerbel RS (2008). Rapid chemotherapy-induced acute endothelial progenitor cell mobilization: implications for antiangiogenic drugs as chemosensitizing agents. Cancer cell 14(3): 263-73.

Shima DT, Deutsch U, D'Amore PA (1995). Hypoxic induction of vascular endothelial growth factor (VEGF) in human epithelial cells is mediated by increases in mRNA stability. FEBS Lett 370(3): 203-8.

Skobe M, Hawighorst T, Jackson DG, Prevo R, Janes L, Velasco P, Riccardi L, Alitalo K, Claffey K, Detmar M (2001). Induction of tumour lymphangiogenesis by VEGF-C promotes breast cancer metastasis. Nat Med 7(2): 192-8.

St Croix B, Rago C, Velculescu V, Traverso G, Romans KE, Montgomery E, Lal A, Riggins GJ, Lengauer C, Vogelstein B, Kinzler KW (2000). Genes expressed in human tumour endothelium. Science 289(5482): 1197-202.

Stacker SA, Achen MG, Jussila L, Baldwin ME, Alitalo K (2002). Lymphangiogenesis and cancer metastasis. Nat Rev Cancer 2(8): 573-83.

Stacker SA, Caesar C, Baldwin ME, Thornton GE, Williams RA, Prevo R, Jackson DG, Nishikawa S, Kubo H, Achen MG (2001). VEGF-D promotes the metastatic spread of tumour cells via the lymphatics. Nat Med 7(2): 186-91.

Stein I, Itin A, Einat P, Skaliter R, Grossman Z, Keshet E (1998). Translation of vascular endothelial growth factor mRNA by internal ribosome entry: implications for translation under hypoxia. Mol Cell Biol 18(6): 3112-9.

Stubbs M, McSheehy PM, Griffiths JR, Bashford CL (2000). Causes and consequences of tumour acidity and implications for treatment. Mol Med Today 6(1): 15-9.

Sussman LK, Upalakalin JN, Roberts MJ, Kocher O, Benjamin LE (2003). Blood markers for vasculogenesis increase with tumour progression in patients with breast carcinoma. Cancer Biol Ther 2(3): 255-6.

Takahashi T, Kalka C, Masuda H, Chen D, Silver M, Kearney M, Magner M, Isner JM, Asahara T (1999). Ischaemia- and cytokine-induced mobilization of bone marrow-derived endothelial progenitor cells for neovascularization. Nat Med 5(4): 434-8.

Taylor AC, Seltz LM, Yates PA, Peirce SM (2010). Chronic whole-body hypoxia induces intussusceptive angiogenesis and microvascular remodeling in the mouse retina. Microvasc Res 79(2): 93-101.

Teng LS, Jin KT, He KF, Zhang J, Wang HH, Cao J (2010). Clinical applications of VEGF-trap (aflibercept) in cancer treatment. J Chin Med Assoc 73(9): 449-56.

Teng X, Li D, Johns RA (2002). Hypoxia up-regulates mouse vascular endothelial growth factor D promoter activity in rat pulmonary microvascular smooth-muscle cells. Chest 121(3 Suppl): 82S-83S.

Tozer GM, Ameer-Beg SM, Baker J, Barber PR, Hill SA, Hodgkiss RJ, Locke R, Prise VE, Wilson I, Vojnovic B (2005). Intravital imaging of tumour vascular networks using multi-photon fluorescence microscopy. Adv Drug Deliv Rev 57(1): 135-52.

Tozer GM, Lewis S, Michalowski A, Aber V (1990). The relationship between regional variations in blood flow and histology in a transplanted rat fibrosarcoma. Br J Cancer 61(2): 250-7.

Vajkoczy P, Blum S, Lamparter M, Mailhammer R, Erber R, Engelhardt B, Vestweber D, Hatzopoulo AK (2003). Multistep nature of microvascular recruitment of ex vivo-expanded embryonic endothelial progenitor cells during tumour angiogenesis. J Exp Med 197(12): 1755-65.

van der Schaft DW, Hillen F, Pauwels P, Kirschmann DA, Castermans K, Egbrink MG, Tran MG, Sciot R, Hauben E, Hogendoorn PC, Delattre O, Maxwell PH, Hendrix MJ, Griffioen AW (2005). Tumour cell plasticity in Ewing sarcoma, an alternative circulatory system stimulated by hypoxia. Cancer Res 65(24): 11520-8.

Vermeulen PB, Colpaert C, Salgado R, Royers R, Hellemans H, Van Den Heuvel E, Goovaerts G, Dirix LY, Van Marck E (2001). Liver metastases from colorectal adenocarcinomas grow in three patterns with different angiogenesis and desmoplasia. J Pathol 195(3): 336-42.

Wesseling P, van der Laak JA, de Leeuw H, Ruiter DJ, Burger PC (1994). Quantitative immunohistological analysis of the microvasculature in untreated human glioblastoma multiforme. Computer-assisted image analysis of whole-tumour sections. J Neurosurg 81(6): 902-9.

Wigle JT, Harvey N, Detmar M, Lagutina I, Grosveld G, Gunn MD, Jackson DG, Oliver G (2002). An essential role for Prox1 in the induction of the lymphatic endothelial cell phenotype. EMBO J 21(7): 1505-13.

Xie K (2001). Interleukin-8 and human cancer biology. Cytokine Growth Factor Rev 12(4): 375-91.

Zagorska A, Dulak J (2004). HIF-1: the knowns and unknowns of hypoxia sensing. Acta Biochim Pol 51(3): 563-85.

Zhang L, Yang N, Park JW, Katsaros D, Fracchioli S, Cao G, O'Brien-Jenkins A, Randall TC, Rubin SC, Coukos G (2003). Tumour-derived vascular endothelial growth factor up-regulates angiopoietin-2 in host endothelium and destabilizes host vasculature, supporting angiogenesis in ovarian cancer. Cancer Res 63(12): 3403-12.

Chapter 6

Cell cycle alterations by hypoxic microenvironment

Erik Olai Pettersen[*]

[*]Address for correspondence:
Department of Physics, The University of Oslo, P.O.Box 1048 Blindern, 0316 Oslo, Norway
Tel. +47 228 556 44, Fax. +47 228 556 71, E-mail: e.o.pettersen@fys.uio.no

Contents

Key points

— Hypoxia affects cell cycle regulation and thereby contributes to poor response to radiotherapy.

— Extreme hypoxia (below 0.1%) induces G1 arrest via mechanism involving hypophosphorylation of pRb and induction of p27.

— Moderate hypoxia regulates cell cycle in a HIF-dependent manner.

— Hypoxia also blocks DNA synthesis through deactivation of DNA precursors-producing enzymes and activates ATM-related DNA machinery.

— Hypoxia inhibits protein synthesis and thus slows down progression through various stages of cell cycle.

Historical development of the field of cell cycle regulation in eukaryotic cells

Modern studies of the cell cycle started in the 1950s. Howard and Pelc (1953) demonstrated, using incorporation of [^{32}P] into DNA of vicia faba roots and visualizing the incorporation by autoradiography, that DNA synthesis takes place only in a limited part of interphase and that this phase can be divided into 3: Apart from the synthesis (S) phase there is one period before and one after the S phase without any synthetic activity. Later, several groups developed methods with DNA-incorporation of [^{3}H]-labeled thymidine during DNA-synthesis. With the ultra-short range of the β-particles from [^{3}H] one could determine the exact location within the cell where the precursor was incorporated. Possibly even the effect of hypoxia may have been seen during the early experiments: As early as 1958 Firket and Verly reported autoradiography data on chicken fibroblasts after [^{3}H]-thymidine incorporation demonstrating the time it takes between the end of S-phase and the start of mitosis. Their curve illustrates use of the PLM-method (per cent labelled mitosis), which was fully developed by Quastler and Sherman (1959). Together with the continuous labelling method, the PLM method was later used to determine the relative role of all kinetic parameters, such as duration of all cell-cycle phases, growth fraction and cell loss fraction in tumour tissue growth (see Steel *et al.* 1966 and Steel 1967). Firket and Verly grew their cells in a hanging drop culture and found that at least 30 % of the cells *"mainly in the inner part of the growth zone"* did not cycle. With the knowledge we have today concerning the role of respiration to determine the pericellular oxygen concentration in cell cultures (Pettersen *et al.* 2005) some of the resting cells may well have been brought out of the cell cycle due to strict hypoxia.

In the 1960s observations on cells in tumours as well as in normal tissues indicated that G1 was the cell-cycle phase with the largest variation both in transplanted tumours (Steel et al 1966) and (even more so) in human solid tumours in man (Gavosto and Pileri 1971). The complex question of how cells can regulate cell cycling and protein accumulation to ascertain a true doubling of all components before mitosis gave rise to different interpretations over a period of about 15 years. From studies primarily on yeast cells (Nash *et al.* 1988) the molecular machinery for the regulation of the normal eukaryotic cell cycle was finally clarified and shown to have similar regulatory mechanisms both for the G1/S and G2/M transitions through the kinase function of Cdk/cyclin complexes (Murray and Kirschner 1989). Thus, around 1990 the main machinery of cell-cycle regulation was largely clarified, although many pathways of regulation from the huge number of different external growth- or growth-inhibiting signals and to this machinery was still obscure.

The problem of tumour hypoxia and treatment

Tumour hypoxia has been considered a problem in radiotherapy since the 1930s at least (Mottram 1936). The problem was that cells irradiated under low oxygen could survive larger radiation doses than cells irradiated under normal oxygenation, and low oxygen was associated with solid tumours and not with normal tissues. Even in these early studies observations indicated to pathologists that cell cycling as reflected by the mitotic activity was of importance for cellular responses to radiation and hypoxia. The problem was brought into focus for the whole radiotherapy and radiobiology fields in the early to mid 50s (Gray *et al.* 1953, Thomlinson and Gray 1955) when the effect was quantified: Hypoxic cells were shown to tolerate 3 times more radiation than aerobic cells. Tumour hypoxia has since been an important aspect of radiotherapy and radiobiology.

More recent studies have shown that there is a strong correlation between tumour hypoxia and poor prognosis for the patient, and even that the prognosis gets worse as the degree of hypoxia increases (Nordsmark *et al.* 1996, 2005, Hockel *et al.* 1996). This is a very serious observation from a patient point of view reaching far above the traditional problem defined in radiotherapy. Prognosis is not delimited to a certain treatment, but represents an over-all factor describing the chances of the patient group including all types of treatment in use.

It has been shown that hypoxia in solid tumours is even more complex than first anticipated and that there is both a permanent limitation in oxygen diffusion and transient limitations in blood perfusion (Hockel and Vaupel 2001, Brown and Giaccia 1998). Of particular importance is perhaps the variation in oxygenation experienced by individual cells involving rapid changes between severe hypoxia and reoxygenation. This process has been shown to correlate with increased propensity to metastasize (Rofstad 2000, Subarsky and Hill 2003).

Cell cycle regulation under severe hypoxia: The oxygen region below 0.1%

The influence of hypoxia on cell cycle regulation has been studied by radiobiologists interested in the radiobiological oxygen effect since the late 1960s. It was not fully recognized at the time that different cell types in culture might respond differently due to genetic differences between cells. Still the findings showed some common effects, which gave Kruuv and Sinclair (1968) reason to address the possibility that hypoxia arrested cells in G1. Soon Harris *et al.* (1970) showed that there was an accumulation of Ehrlich ascites tumour cells in G1 in animals breathing a mixture of 6 or 9% O_2 in nitrogen. Other types of growth inhibition, such as contact inhibition or starvation had shown various other types of cell cycle phase accumulation, but Harris *et al.*'s findings in their *in vivo* model were soon confirmed for Chinese hamster V-79 cells *in vitro* by Koch *et al.* (1973a, b). Furthermore, Koch *et al.* (1973b), using cells which under normal growth conditions had been shown to have a very short G1, could demonstrate that these cells accumulated almost completely in G1 after 4 days of extreme hypoxia (<25ppm O_2 in the medium). In this case the cell cycle distribution was determined by photometric cytometry measuring DNA content in individual cells and therefore represented all cells visible after hypoxia, and not just those that were able to cycle after hypoxia (which would result by use of the PLM technique). Koch *et al.* also found that the cells, which accumulated in G1 by hypoxia had a sensitivity for radiation which was different from cells synchronized (by mitotic selection) in an undisturbed G1. Thus, the arrested cells did not behave as undisturbed G1-cells.

This was to some extent a break-through, indicating that an oxygen-sensitive restriction point must exist in the G1-phase. It is important to note that the pericellular oxygen concentration used was in this case so low that the rate of cell respiration due to diffusion limitation was inhibited down to almost zero (Froese 1962, Boag 1970). A general criticism of many studies in the field of hypoxia is that it is difficult to evaluate the pericellular oxygenation in the experimental systems used. The diffusion rate of oxygen in an unstirred aqueous solution is so slow compared to cell respiration rate that the oxygen concentration at the bottom of an ordinary cell culture flask, where cells are routinely covered by almost 2 mm medium has to be measured in order to know what the pericellular oxygen concentration is (Chapman *et al.* 1970, Pettersen *et al.* 2005). In order to secure that the atmospheric O_2 concentration expresses the pericellular concentration without stirring, the cells have to be covered by little more than moisture of medium. There-fore, some care must be taken when results from different laboratories are compared. As long as extreme hypoxia was used, however, the few groups in the world who used set-ups, which could guarantee reproducible oxy-genation control at that level could reproduce each other's data well. The G1-arrest induced by extreme hypoxia was confirmed by different labora-tories using cells of different origin (Bedford and Mitchell, 1974, Born et al. 1976, Löffler et al. 1978), and found to be functional in all. Bedford and Mitchell (1974) and later Pettersen and Lindmo (1983) showed that the G1-arrest was only induced at oxygen concentrations below about 1000 ppm (0.1%) and that it was complete only if the concentration dropped below 100 ppm. The data of Bedford and Mitchell (1974) and later by Born et al. (1976), Löffler (1987) and Pettersen and Åmellem (1993) all showed that mammalian cells of different origin were not able to complete S-phase, but did proceed from G2 through mitosis and into G1 under extremely hypoxic conditions before they were arrested in G1.

The observation by Koch et al. (1973) that cells, which arrested in G1 during extreme hypoxia had a different radiosensitivity compared to cells in a normal cell cycle was followed up by later studies, which showed that chronic hypoxia tends to increase radiosensitivity of the cells (Shrieve and Harris 1985, Pettersen and Wang 1996), and that this lasts for several hours after reoxygenation (Koritzinsky et al. 2001).

Although the pericellular oxygen concentrations inducing the specific G1 arrest can be seen as extreme in relation to solid tumours this mecha-nism may well have some practical importance for cell survival in hypoxic microenvironments. Respiration is uninhibited down to about 0.1% oxygen (~1000 ppm or ~1.4 μM or ~1 mm Hg) (Froese 1962). Therefore there is no reason to rule out the possibility that extremely hypoxic regions, i.e. far below 100 ppm O_2 may exist in tumours, particularly for acutely hypoxic cells. In any case the early data of Harris et al. (1970) indicates that such low concentrations were obtained in the abdomen of Ehrlich ascites-bearing mice breathing low oxygen.

Cells have been shown to be particularly sensitive to damaging effects by extreme hypoxia in S phase (Pettersen and Lindmo 1983, Åmellem and Pettersen 1991) and recent reports (see Olcina et al. 2010 for a review) have indicated that this is related to activation of ATM/ATR (see below) and disassembly of the replisome after 8 to 12 hours under severely hypoxic ($<0.1\%$ O_2) conditions. Thus, the oxygen sensitive restriction point in G1 under respiration-limiting hypoxia may well function as a protection for cancer cells against the start of DNA-synthesis, which would otherwise be lethal after just a few hours under such extreme conditions. In this respect it is possible that abolition of the oxygen-sensitive restriction point in G1 could be one way of specifically killing acutely hypoxic cancer cells.

The mechanism for the onset of the G1-arrest under extreme hypoxia was later found to be independent of the cell cycle regulatory tumour suppressor proteins p53 and pRB which both otherwise actively regulate G1-transition (Graeber *et al.* 1994; Åmellem *et al.* 1996). Still data has indicated that both may play important roles in the maintenance of cellular homeo-stasis under as well as after hypoxia (Graeber et al. 1996, Åmellem et al 1996, 1997).

The accumulation of cells in G1 was reported to be a result of 3 pro-cesses: Firstly, the retinoblastoma protein (pRB) is dephosphorylated and rebound in the cell nucleus under both extreme and more moderate (1300ppm O_2) hypoxia and thereby mediates cell cycle arrest in mid-G1. Secondly, there is activation of an oxygen-sensitive restriction point in late G1 close to the G1/S-border. And thirdly, DNA replication is inhibited prob-ably by several mechanisms including lack of DNA precursors (see below) (Åmellem *et al.* 1991, Åmellem *et al.* 1996, Åmellem *et al.* 1998). Thus, this data indicated that cells in G2, mitosis or early G1 by the onset of hypoxia progress to the pRB checkpoint in mid G1 during hypoxia, while RB-incompetent cells or cells that have already passed this checkpoint in G1 progress until they become arrested in a restriction point close to the G1/S-border. Krtolica *et al.* (1998) showed that the pRB-activation entailed decreased activity in Cdk4, Cdk2 and cyclin D and E protein levels, but also showed that there was an increase in the level of CKI p27 associated with cyclin E/Cdk2.

This final observation is of particular importance since earlier data had indicated that the G1-arrest seen under extreme hypoxia is general for mammalian cells, observed in all cell types studied, independent of func-tionality of the G1 regulatory proteins p53 and pRB. The dependency of p27 and p21 was reported by Green *et al.* (2001) to be on the re-entry of the cell cycle after reoxygenation. Parallel however, Gardner *et al.* (2001) showed that the G1/S transition is dependent on the presence of p27 that the induc-tion of p27 by hypoxia is transcriptional and is Hif-1 independent. This last conclusion was opposed by data reported by Goda *et al.* (2003) indicating that the enhanced expression of p27 was Hif-1α dependent. Data published by Wang *et al.* (2003) showed, however that the enhanced p27 expression was ARNT (Hif-1β) dependent and indicated that ARNT could have a func-tion independent of Hif-1α. The view of Green *et al.* (2003) that p27 is neces-sary for re-entry of the cell cycle after reoxygenation was supported by Graff *et al.* (2005), but their data also indicated that p27 was important for the induction of the cell cycle arrest in late G1 upon exposure to hypoxia.

Gardner *et al.* (2003) showed that the G1 checkpoint can be bypassed by over-expression of E2F under moderate hypoxia, but under extreme hypoxia this was not enough. However the viral protein E1a which disassembles the binding between pRB and E2F thus inactivating the regulatory function of pRB (Gardner *et al.* 2003) was found to drive the cells into apoptosis under extreme hypoxia or, if the antiapoptotic protein Bcl-2 was simultaneously overexpressed, to start DNA-synthesis. Thus, even the oxygen sensitive restriction point in G1 can be bypassed during hypoxia, possibly leading to proliferation of genomically instable cells.

As was elegantly formulated by Green and Giaccia (1998) it is difficult to know from these data what the cause and effect among these various gene products affecting the cell cycle is since the regulatory pathways are so interlaced. For example, as pointed out by Green and Giaccia, the observation that cyclin A is down-regulated under hypoxia (Ludlow et al 1993, Seim et al. 2003) could be a result of the hypophosphorylation of pRB which inhibits E2F activity and which in turn leads to a decrease in cyclin A. If cell cycle progression is stopped by quite another mechanism all these changes in gene expression could just follow as a natural consequence. Therefore, other mechanisms like the hypoxia-induced decrease in deoxyribonucleotides for DNA synthesis (see below) are important to follow up.

Oxygen sensing at moderate hypoxia and cell cycle regulation influenced by HIF

Although extreme hypoxia stopped protein accumulation, early observations showed an up-regulation of specific gene-products (Heacock *et al.* 1986, Shi *et al.* 1993, Kraggerud *et al.* 1995) even under such conditions. This regulation of specific genes, although first seen for extreme hypoxia and involving proteins which not necessarily represented prime hypoxia-regulated genes or post-transcriptional hypoxia-regulated cascades, is perhaps a harbinger of one of the fundamental regulatory principles in cellular biology. The cloning and characterisation of the oxygen-regulated transcription factor HIF (Hypoxia-inducible factor) (Wang *et al.* 1995) and the subsequent characterisation of hypoxia-regulated cascades in cells (see for example the recent review by Lendahl *et al.* 2009) brought hypoxia into the focus of cellular and molecular biology on a far broader scale than before.

In the present paper it is cell cycle regulatory effects of HIF which are of interest, but it is important to notice that the HIF transcription factor is the pivotal regulator of oxygen homeostasis in cells and therefore influences cell survival, growth and cell cycle regulation in complex and often indirect ways. It consists of HIFα (of which there are 3 paralogues denoted HIF-1α, HIF-2α and HIF-3α) which form complexes with another subunit, ARNT (Arylhydrocarbon Receptor Nuclear Translocator). Normally HIFα is degraded under aerobic conditions by ubiquitylation after binding to the VHL (von Hippel Lindau) protein, but under hypoxic conditions activation is done by post-translational O_2-dependent hydroxylation, which stabilizes the protein. Thus, seemingly the first-line O_2-sensing process activated by moderate reductions in oxygenation is done by the prolyl-4-hydroxylases which are denoted PHD1, PHD2 and PHD3 (Prolyl Hydroxylase Domain containing enzymes).

HIF is involved in various regulatory cascades, some of which have the consequence of deactivation or suppression of genes (Mole et al. 2009), but the direct function is activation by transcription. Generally HIF activates processes which increase the ability for the tissues to function during low oxygenation, such as inhibition of apoptosis, oxygen-independent metabolism and pH-control (see Brahimi-Horn et al. 2010 for an overview). It also induces cell growth and cell cycling through different mechanisms. HIF induces angiogenesis through its target gene VEGF (Vascular Endothelial Growth Factor) which is a secreted protein attracted to endothelial cells, stimulating them to growth and to form new blood vessels (Forsythe et al. 1996).

The role of the PHD proteins on cell proliferation has recently been shown to be more complex than earlier anticipated (see review by Jokilehto and Jaakkola 2010) indicating both that these may act independently of HIF and that they may have dualistic effects on cell proliferation under hypoxic conditions. Their tumour suppressive effect may for example partly be due to inhibition of hypoxia-induced endothelial cell proliferation (Takeda and Fong 2007, Chan et al 2009).

Hypoxia was also shown to induce angiogenesis through c-Myc (Baudino et al. 2002, Knies-Bamforth et al. 2004). This is a cell-cycle-driving mechanism of potentially carcinogenic importance since c-Myc is involved in the driving of cells into the cell cycle from G0 (see for example Blanchard et al. 1985), and is one of the factors through which pRB via E2F exerts its growth- and cell-cycle regulation (Salcedo et al. 1995). Later studies have shown that both Hif-1α and Hif-2α inhibit c-Myc activity under physiologic conditions but that the role of Hif-2α seems to be dualistic and can promote cell growth by enhancing oncogenic Myc transcriptional activity (Gordan et al. 2007). Recently high constitutive HIF-1α has also been shown to be associated with oncogenic c-Myc in multiple myeloma (Zhang et al. 2009). The mechanism through which c-Myc induces its regulation of the cell cycle as well as other processes is well described in recent reviews (Dang *et al.* 2008, Podar and Anderson 2010).

Oxygen sensing by DNA-precursor production and a subsequent stop of DNA synthesis

Apart from the accumulation of cells in G1 there is also a halt of DNA-synthesis during severe hypoxia and this effect is also seen to some extent under more moderate hypoxia, i. e. at least up to about 1300 ppm (0.13%) O_2 (Åmellem et al 1998). The mechanism for this effect is probably to some extent related to deactivation of two enzymes, which depend on molecular oxygen in a tyrosyl radical for activation. These enzymes are important in the biosynthesis of nucleosides: Firstly, dihydroorotate dehydrogenase is a respiratory chain-dependent protein synthesizing uridine monophosphate. This protein is located in the mitochondrial membrane, has its activity coupled with the respiratory chain and the radical has a half-life of just 10 min under hypoxic conditions (Thelander et al. 1983). Secondly, ribonucleotid reductase (RNR) is producing the deoxyribonucleotides as precursors for DNA synthesis (Löffler 1992, Löffler et al. 1997). The deactivation of these two DNA-precursor-producing proteins during severe hypoxia has been considered to be a candidate for a hypoxia-sensing mechanism. This sensing may have a protective function for the tissue since cells are rapidly accumulating lethal damage by severe hypoxia while in S-phase (Pettersen and Lindmo 1981) and a halt in DNA synthesis would inhibit further proliferation of damaged cells. In particular focus has been on the effect, which the deactivation of ribonucleotide reductase has on reduction of the dCTP pool (Brischwein *et al.* 1997). The protein was found to reversibly lose its free tyrosyl radical in the oxygen concentration range from 2 down to 0.02 % oxygen (200 ppm). At the low level of this range dCTP was severely reduced while the other dNTP pools were less affected. This observation, done in both Ehrlich ascites cells and in HeLa cells (Probst *et al.* 1999) indicates that the down-regulation of the dCTP-pool due to deactivation of ribonucleotid reductase is a sensing signal which regulates DNA synthesis under relatively severe hypoxia (200 ppm O_2).

The testing of this possibility by addition of nucleosides and/or deoxy-nucleosides to the hypoxic cells and observing re-stimulation of DNA synthesis have indicated that this mechanism is of importance (Löffler 1987, 1992,

Brischwein *et al.* 1997). It is, however, obvious that some other cell-cycle regulatory factors are involved as well (Green *et al.* 2001). For example, in cervical cancer cells of type NHIK 3025, which express HPV18 E7 protein (Åmellem et al. 1998) and therefore are pRB non-functional, it was found that addition of dCTP during 100 ppm O_2 hypoxia could restore DNA synthesis. Similarly, in human osteosarcoma cells SAOS-2 which also lack functional pRB (Ewen *et al.* 1993) the same result was seen at 1300 ppm O_2 (Åmellem *et al.* 1998). But in human breast cancer T-47D cells, which are pRB-functional, it turned out that pRB was activated in cells arrested by hypoxia in S-phase and rebound in the nucleus. In these cells re-phosphrylation of pRB was found to be the rate-limiting step for re-entry into the cell cycle following reoxygenation (Åmellem *et al.* 1996). In these cells it turned out that addition of dCTP during moderat hypoxia (1300 ppm O_2) did not reverse the DNA synthesis arrest (Åmellem *et al.* 1998). In fact, further studies indicated that cells having pRB rebound in the nucleus during hypoxia were irreversibly arrested (Seim *et al.* 2003) and could not re-enter the cell cycle following reoxygenation.

In a further study of the role of ribonucleotide reductase the T-47D cells were grown continuously over half a year with steadily increasing concentrations of hydroxyurea in the medium, ending with cells that could grow well in contact with 0.5 mM. These cells (denoted T-47DHU-res) were shown by EPR analysis to contain about 8 times more ribonucleotid reductase radical than wild-type T-47D cells (Graff *et al.* 2002) and the level was high in all cell cycle phases. In opposition to the wild type cells it turned out that the pRB rebinding in the nucleus during hypoxia had lost its rate-limiting effect in the subline with elevated ribonucleotid reductase (Graff *et al.* 2004). An elevated level of ribonucleotid reductase could therefore function to drive cell cycle progression after reoxygenation for cells that were otherwise arrested in S-phase following a prolonged period of hypoxia. It was also shown that cervical cancer NHIK 3025 cells (which are non-functional for both pRB and p53), like the T-47DHU-res cells were able to start proliferation from S-phase after reoxygenation. Perhaps the most thought-provoking observation was that in both cases where cells were able to restart DNA-synthesis from a hypoxia-induced arrest in S-phase, a significant subpopulation of cells continued into the next cell cycle without completing mitosis and performed a complete endoreduplication of their DNA (Graff *et al.* 2004). The suggestion was that increased ribonucleotid reductase through such doubling of DNA could represent genomic instability and thus be a driver towards increased malignancy. In recent studies based on time-lapse cytometry it has been shown that polyploidy cells, although senescent and not able to undergo mitosis by themselves, may still produce proliferating descendant cells through the process of neosis (Rajaraman *et al.* 2007, Singh *et al.* 2010) where chromosomes are distributed to daughter cells by budding with an intact nuclear envelope and subsequent asymmetric cytokinesis. Thus, a combination of elevated ribonucleotid reductase and hypoxia could be a driver to start this process.

Fast effect of hypoxia: Influence of over-all growth regulation on cell cycling

For cancer research in general, tumour hypoxia is highly interesting from the metabolic point of view: The question is how cancer cells adjust their metabolism in a low-oxygen micro-environment to enable the cells to regulate energy homeostasis and survive? This aspect is of utmost importance (Semenza *et al.* 2001, Brahimi-Horn *et al.* 2010) and may have great potential in the further development of new ways to treat cancers (see for example Sonveax *et al.* 2008), but cannot be given much space in the present paper. One aspect, however, is so closely related to cell-cycle control that it needs to be commented on:

Early observations indicated that inhibition of general protein accumulation by itself reduces cell-cycle progression (Terasima and Yakusawa 1966, Brooks 1977). Later, detailed analysis of progression in the various cell-cycle stages indicated that severe inhibition of protein synthesis may in fact slow down progression in the various stages of the cell cycle (Rønning *et al.* 1981). Parallel to these observations, chemical synchronization techniques based on inhibition of DNA synthesis by use of excess thymidine or hydroxyurea had shown that such arrest did not stop cell growth: Neither synthesis of RNA nor synthesis of protein were halted during the arrest (Young and Hodas 1964, Studzinski and Lambert 1969) and cell populations synchronized by these techniques had been characterized as being in unbalanced growth (Nias and Fox 1971). Thus, there may be a general relation between cell-cycle- and growth control: While inhibition of DNA synthesis has no influence on cell growth, stopping cell growth by protein synthesis inhibition stops the cell cycle in all phases.

When protein synthesis and –degradation was measured under extreme hypoxia it was found that the rate of protein synthesis was abruptly reduced to a level below protein degradation (the degradation rate was slightly increased) (Pettersen *et al.* 1986). This creates a slightly negative balance much similar to the one seen by use of cycloheximide (Rønning *et al.* 1981). Thus, extreme hypoxia induces a primary effect on protein synthesis/-accumulation, which is almost immediate (Kraggerud *et al.* 1995).

Even under prolonged extremely hypoxic conditions cells were shown to complete G2 and mitosis to be halted in their cell cycle before the next S-phase (Koritzinsky *et al.* 2001). Thus, protein accumulation is not necessary for the cells to complete the cell cycle, a finding well in line with the observation that the cell cycle can be shorter than the protein doubling time in an environment of low serum *in vitro* (Rønning and Pettersen 1984) and therefore the coupling is less stringent than early observations indicated.

Still, growth reduction is probably the fastest response to severe hypoxia and the mechanisms have been studied intensely for the last two decades. The fast reduction in protein synthesis is related to a reduction in mRNA translation and can be seen as a way of increasing cellular tolerance to hypoxia by promoting energy homeostasis since protein synthesis is the major energy-consuming process (Hochachka *et al.* 1996). The mechanisms are known to a large extent (for a review, see Koritzinsky and Wouters 2007).

HIF also stimulates expression of some membrane-associated Carbonic Anhydrase proteins (CA IX and CA XII), which seem to increase cellular ability to grow through stimulation of the PI-3 kinase (Dorai *et al.* 2005).

Another process related to protein metabolism and energy homeostasis is regulation of protein folding in the ER (Endoplasmic Reticulum) by the UPR (Unfolded Protein Response). Protein folding is also an energy-requiring process and UPR protects cells against accumulation of misfolded protein (for a review see Koumenis *et al.* 2007).

Induction of DNA-repair machinery, ATM and the DNA damage response

Cells from ataxia telangiectasia patients are extremely radiosensitive. This has to do with a lack of radiation-induced cell-cycle delay which gives cells from healthy individuals time to repair double strand DNA breaks before entering S-phase or mitosis (Painter and Young, 1980, Zampetti-Bosseler and Scott 1981, Beamish and Lavin 1994). The lack of this checkpoint control has turned out to depend on a mutation in a gene denoted ATM (Ataxia Telangiectasia Mutated) which normally codes for a kinase belonging to the phosphatidyl-3-kinase-like kinase (PIKK) family (as does ATR, DNA-PK and mTOR) (Bencokova *et al.* 2009). The ATM protein has been shown to be recruited to sites of DNA strand breaks and halt cell-cycle progression, induce apoptosis or DNA-repair through activation of genes like p53, Chk2 and BRCA. This protein was for example suspected to be pivotal in the explanation of the low dose hyper-radiosensitivity, seen for small radiation doses, i.e. below about 0.5 Gy (Lambin *et al.* 1993) when it was shown that higher doses were needed to activate ATM and induce G2-arrest in cells irradiated in G2 (Xu *et al.* 2002). Thus, cells irradiated with very small radiation doses while in G2, proceed uninhibited into mitosis without time to repair double strand breaks in their DNA. At slightly higher doses (>0.5Gy) ATM was found to be activated (Marples *et al.* 2003), cells were delayed in a restriction point in G2 and thereby gained time to repair DNA strand breaks before mitosis. The consequence is that for some cell types, cell survival increases rather than falls with increasing radiation dosage in the dose range 0.3 to 0.5 Gy (for a review see Marples *et al.* 2004). Several of the regulatory cascades induced by ATM are now known and have been described (Wykes *et al.* 2006, Marples and Collis 2008). Recent findings indicate that these mechanisms are also of importance with respect to cell damaging effects induced in microenvironments characterized by chronic as well as cycling hypoxia (Olcina *et al.* 2010).

Hypoxia itself has not been shown to induce DNA damage and therefore does not activate the ATM or ATR genes through the DNA damage response. However, hypoxia has been shown to activate ATM even in the absence of DNA damage (Bakkenist *et al.* 2003). Furthermore, with fluctuating hypoxia, as is found in solid tumours, reoxygenation or cycling hypoxia creates reactive oxygen species (ROS) which has been shown to induce such DNA damage (Hammond *et al.* 2002, 2003). Thus, under such conditions the ATM-Chk2-mediated arrest in G2 is activated allowing pre-mitotic DNA repair (Bencocova *et al.* 2009) and it has been shown that replication fork integrity during severe hypoxia is dependent on this DNA damage response (Hammond *et al.* 2003).

Summing up

As discussed above, molecular oxygen influences aspects of both cell metabolism and of macromolecular functionality. In addition hypoxia is a complex notion characterized by variations in the level of oxygenation, the duration of hypoxia and also the influence of reoxygenation; all aspects,

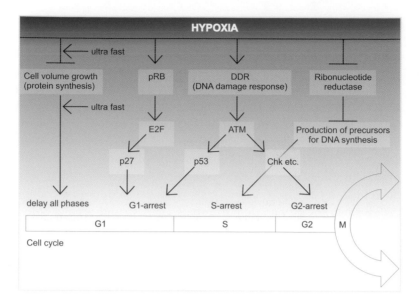

Figure 6.1 _ In this drawing 4 different pathways are indicated which all are induced at relatively severe hypoxia (< 1000 ppm O_2). Reduced protein synthesis induces inhibition in all cell-cycle phases while the molecular deactivation of enzymes producing dexyribonucleotides for DNA-synthesis halts DNA-synthesis only. The G1-arrest induced by p27 in G1 is related to pRB, but has been shown to be induced even in pRB-incompetent cells. Activation of ATM can be induced by hypoxia even without the induction of DNA double-strand breaks while reoxygenation can give rise to DNA damage; ATM can induce inhibition in both G1 and in G2.

which are challenging to control and even reproduce in experimental models. The influence of hypoxic microenvironments on the cell-cycle progression of mammalian cells is therefore a subject of many aspects. In Figure 6.1 only some major pathways of cell-cycle regulatory effects of hypoxia are summed up.

A c k n o w l e d g e m e n t s _ The author is supported by the METOXIA project no. 222741 under the 7th Research Framework Programme of the European Union

References

Åmellem, Ø. and Pettersen, E.O.: Cell inactivation and cell cycle inhibition as induced by extreme hypoxia: the possible role of cell cycle arrest as a protection against hypoxia-induced lethal damage. Cell Prolif. 24; (1991) 127-141.

Åmellem, Ø., Stokke, T., Sandvik, J.A. and Pettersen, E.O.: The retinoblastoma gene product is reversibly dephosphorylated and bound in the nucleus in S and G2 phase during hypoxic stress. Exp. Cell Res. 227; (1996) 106-115.

Åmellem, Ø., Stokke, T., Sandvik, J.A., Smedshammer, L. and Pettersen, E.O.: Hypoxia-induced apoptosis in human cells with normal p53 status and function, without any alteration in the nuclear protein level. Exp. Cell Res. 232; (1997) 361-370.

Åmellem, Ø., Sandvik, J.A., Stokke, T. and Pettersen, E.O.: The retinoblastoma protein-associated cell cycle arrest in S-phase under moderate hypoxia is dirupted in cells expressing HPV18 E7 oncoprotein. Br. J. Cancer 77; (1998) 862-872.

Bakkenist, C.J. and Kastan, M.B.: DNA damage activates ATM through intermolecular autophosphrylation and dimer dissociation. Nature 421; (2003) 499-506.

Baudino, T.A., McKay, C., Pendeville-Samain, H., Nilsson, J.A., Maclean, K.H., White, E.L., Davis, A.C., Ihle, J.N. and Cleveland, J.L.: c-Myc is essential for vasculogenesis and angiogenesisduring development and tumour progression. Genes Dev 16; (2002) 2530–2543.

Beamish, H., and M. F. Lavin. 1994. Radiosensitivity in ataxia-telangiectasia: Anomalies in radiation-induced cell cycle delay. Int. J. Radiat. Biol. 65; (1994) 175 184

Bedford, J.S. and Mitchell, J.B.: The effect of hypoxia on the growth and radiation response ofmammalian cells in culture. Br. J. Radiol. 47; (1974) 687-696.

Bencokova, Z., Kaufmann, M.R., Pires, I.M., Lecane, P.S., Giaccia, A.J. and Hammond, E.M.: ATM activation and signalling under hypoxic conditions. Mol. Cell. Biol. 29; (2009) 526-537.

Blanchard, J.M., Piechaczyk, M., Dani, C., Chambard, J.C., Franchi, A., Pouyssegur, J. and Jeanteur, P.: c-myc gene is transcribed at high rate in G0-arrested fibroblasts and is post-transcriptionally regulated in response to growth factors. Nature 317; (1985) 443-445.

Boag, J.W.: Cell respiration as a function of oxygen tension. Int J. Radiat. Biol. 18; (1970) 475-478.

Born, R., Hug, O. and Trott, K.R.: The effect of prolonged hypoxia on growth and viability of Chinese hamster cells. Int. J. Radiat. Oncol. Biol. Phys. 12 (1976) 687-697.

Brahimi-Horn, M.C., Bellotand, G. and Pouyssegur, J.: Hypoxia and energetic tumour metabolism. Curr. Opin. Gen. Dev. 21; (2010) 1–6.

Brischwein, K., Engelcke, M., Riedinger, H.J. and Probst, H.: Role of ribonucleotide reductase and deoxynucleotide pools in the oxygen-dependent control of DNA replication in Ehrlich ascites cells. Eur. J. Biochem. 244; (1997) 286-293.

Brooks, R.F.: Continuous protein synthesis is required to maintain the probability of entry into S phase. Cell 12; (1977) 311-317.

Brown, J.M. and Giaccia, A.J.: The unique physiology of solid tumours: opportunities (and problems) for cancer therapy. Cancer Res. 58; (1998) 1408-1416.

Chan, D.A., Kawahara, T.L.A., Sutphin, P.D., Chang, H.Y., Chi, J.T. and Giaccia, A.J.: Tumour vasculature is regulated by PHD2-mediated angiogenesis and bone marrow-derived cell recruitment. Cancer Cell. 15; (2009) 527-538.

Chapman, J.D., Sturrock, J., Boag, J.W. and Crookall, J.O.: Factors affecting the oxygen tension around cells growing in plastic Petri dishes. Int. J. Radiat. Biol. Relat. Stud. Phys. Chem. Med. 17; (1970) 305-328.

Dang, C.V., Kim, J.W., Gao, P. and Yustein, J.: The interplay between MYC and HIF in cancer. Nat. Rev. Cancer 8; (2008) 51-56.

Dorai, T., Sawczuk, I.S., Pastorek, J., Wiernik, P.H. and Dutcher, J,P.: The role of carbonic anhydrase IX overexpression in kidney cancer. Eur. J. Cancer. 41; (2005) 2935-2947.

Ewen, M.E., Sluss, H.K., Sherr, C.J., Matsushime, H., Kato, J. and Livingston, D.M.: Functional interactions of the retinoblastoma protein with mammalian D-type cyclins. Celol 73; (1993) 487-497.

Firket, H. and Verly, W.G.: Autoradiographic visualization of synthesis of deoxyribonucleic acid in tissue culture with tritium-labelled thymidine. Nature 181 (1958) 274-275.

Forsythe, J.A., Jiang, B.H., Iyer, N.V., Agani, F., Leung, S.W., Koos, R.D. and Semenza, G.L.: Activation of vascular endothelial growth factor gene transcription by hypoxia-inducible factor 1. Mol. Cell. Biol. 16; (1996) 4604-4613.

Froese, G.: The respiration of ascites tumour cells at low oxygen concentrations. Biochim. Biophys. Acta 57; (1962) 509-519.

Gardner, L.B., Li, F., Yang, X. and Dang, C.V.: Anoxic fibroblasts activate a replication checkpoint that is bypassed by E1a. Mol. Cell Biol. 23; (2003) 9032-45.

Gavosto, F. and Pileri A.: Cell cycle of cancer cells in man. In: Renato Baserga (Ed.) *The cell cycle and cancer*. Marcel Dekker Inc., New York 1971, pp 99-125.

Goda, N., Ryan, H.E., Khadivi, B., McNulty, W., Rickert, R.C. and Johnson, R.S.: Hypoxia-inducible factor 1alpha is essential for cell cycle arrest during hypoxia. Mol. Cell Biol. 23; (2003) 359-369.

Gordan, J.D., Bertout, J.A., Hu, J.A., Diehl, C.J. and Simon, M.C.: HIF-2α promotes hypoxic cell proliferation by enhancing c-myc transcriptional activity. Cancer Cell 11; (2007) 335-347.

Graeber, T. G., J. F. Peterson, M. Tsai, K. Monica, A. J. Fornace and A. J. Giaccia.: Hypoxia induces accumulation of p53 protein, but activation of a G1 phase checkpoint by low oxygen conditions is independent of p53 status. Mol. Cell. Biol. 14; (1994) 6264-6277.

Graeber, T.G., Osmanian, C., Jacks, T., Housman, D.E., Koch, C.J., Lowe, S.W. and Giaccia, A.J.: Hypoxia-mediated selection of cells with diminished apoptotic potential in solid tumours. Nature 379; (1996) 6264-6277.

Graff, P., Åmellem, Ø., Andersson, K. K. & Pettersen, E. O.: Role of ribonucleotide reductase in regulation of cell cycle progression during and after exposure to moderate hypoxia. Anticancer Res. 22; (2002) 59-68.

Graff, P., Seim, J., Åmellem, Ø., Arakawa, H., Nakumura, Y., Andersson, K. K., Stokke, T. and Pettersen, E. O.: Counteraction of pRB-dependent protection after extreme hypoxia by elevated ribonucleotide reductase. Cell Prolif. 37; (2004) 367-383.

Graff, P,. Åmellem, Ø., Seim, J., Stokke, T. and Pettersen, E.O.: The role of p27 in controlling the oxygen-sensitive checkpoint of mammalian cells in late G_1. Anticancer Res. 25; (2005) 2259-2268.

Green, S.L. and Giaccia, A.J.: Tumour hypoxia and the cell cycle: Implications for malignant progression and response to therapy. Cancer J. Sci. Am. 4; (1998)218-223.

Green, S.L., Freiberg, R.A. and Giaccia, A.J.: p21^{Cip} and p27^{Kip} regulate cell cycle reentry after hypoxic stress but are not necessary for hypoxia-induced arrest. Mol. Cell. Biol. 21; (2001) 1196-1206.

Hammond, E.M., Denko, N.C., Dorie, M.J., Abraham, R.T. and Giaccia, A.J.: Hypoxia links ATR and p53 through replication arrest. Mol. Cell. Biol. 22; (2002) 1834-43.

Hammond, E.M., Dorie, M.J. and Giaccia, A.J.: ATR/ATM targets are phosphorylated by ATR in response to hypoxia and ATM in response to reoxygenation. J. Biol. Chem. 278; (2003) 12207-12213.

Harris, J.W., Meyskens, F. and Patt, H.M: Biochemical Studies of Cytokinetic Changes during Tumour Growth. Cancer Res. (1970) 1937-1946.

Heacock, C.S. and Sutherland, R.M.: Induction characteristics of oxygen regulated proteins. International Journal of Radiation Oncology Biology and Physics, 12; (1986) 1287-1290.

Hochachka, P.W., Buck, L.T., Doll, C.J. and Land, S.C.: Unifying theory of hypoxia tolerance: Molecular/metabolic defence and rescue mechanisms for surviving oxygen lack. Proc. Natl. Acad. Sci. USA 93; (1996) 9493-9498.

Hockel, M., Schlenger, K., Aral, B., Mitze, M., Schaffer, U. and Vaupel P: Association between tumour hypoxia and malignant progression in advanced cancer of the uterine cervix. Cancer Res. 56; (1996) 4509-4515.

Hockel, M., and Vaupel P: Tumour hypoxia: definitions and current clinical, biologic, and molecular aspects. J. Natl. Cancer Inst. 93; (2001) 266-276.

Howard, A. and Pelc, S.R.: Synthesis of desoxyribobucleic acid in normal and irradiated cells and its relationship to chromosome breakage. Heredity (Suppl.), 6; (1953) 261-273.

Jokilehto, T., and Jaakkola, P.M.: The role of HIF prolyl hydroxylases in tumour growth. J. Cell. Mol. Med. 14; (2010) 758-770.

Knies-Bamforth, U.E., Fox, S.B., Poulsom, R., Evan, G.I. and Harris AL.: c-Myc interacts with hypoxia to induce angiogenesis in vivo by a vascular endothelial growth factor-dependent mechanism. Cancer Res. 64; (2004) 6563–6570.

Koch, C.J., Kruuv, J. and Frey, H.E.: The effect of hypoxia on the generation time of mammalian cells. Radiat. Res. 53; (1973a) 43-48.

Koch, C.J., Kruuv, J., Frey, H.E. and Snyder, R.A.: Plateau phase in growth induced by hypoxia. Int. J. Radiat. Biol. 23; (1973b) 67-74.

Koritzinsky, M. and Wouters, B.G.: Hypoxia and regulation of messenger RNA translation. Meth. Enzymol. 435; (2007) 247-273.

Koritzinsky, M., Wouters, B.G., Åmellem, Ø., Pettersen, E.O.: Cell cycle progression and radiation survival following prolonged hypoxia and re-oxygenation. Int. J. Radiat. Biol. 77; (2001) 319-328.

Koumenis, C., Bi, M., Ye, J., Feldman, D. and Koong, A.C.: Hypoxia and the unfolded protein response. Meth. Enzymol. 435; (2007) 275-291.

Kraggerud, S.M., Sandvik, J.A. and Pettersen, E.O.: Regulation of protein synthesis in human cells exposed to extreme hypoxia. Anticancer Res. 15; (1995) 683-686.

Krek W, Xu, G. and Livingston, D.M.: Cyclin A-kinase regulation of E2F-1 DNA binding function underlies suppression of an S phase checkpoint. Cell. 83; (1995) 1149-1158.

Kruuv, J. and Sinclair, W.K.: X-ray sensitivity of synchronized Chinese hamster cells irradiated during hypoxia. Radiat. Res. 36; (1968) 45-54.

Ludlow, J.W., Howell, R.L., Smith, H.C.: Hypoxic stress induces reversible hypophosphorylation of pRB and reduction in cyclin A abundance independent of cell cycle progression. Oncogene 8; (1993) 331-339.

Lambin, P., Marples,B., Fertil, B., Malaise, E.P. and Joiner, M.C.: Hypersensitivity of a human tumour cell line to very low radiation doses. Int. J. Radiat. Biol. 63; (1993) 639-650.

Lendahl, U., Lee, K.L., Yang, H. and Poellinger, L.: Generating specificity and diversity in the transcriptional response to hypoxia. Nat. Rev. Genet. 10; (2009) 821-32.

Löffler, M.: restimulation of cell cycle progression by hypoxic tumour cells with deoxynucleosides requires ppm oxygen tension. Exp. Cell Res. 169; (1987) 255-261.

Löffler, M.: A cytokinetic approach to determine the range of O_2-dependence of pyrimidine(deoxy)nucleotide biosynthesis relevant for cell proliferation. Cell Prolif. 25; (1992) 169–179.

Löffler, M., Jockel, J., Schuster, G. and Becker, C.: Dihydroorotat-ubiquinone oxidoreductase links mitochondria in the biosynthesis of pyrimidine nucleotides. Mol. Cell Biochem. 174; (1997) 125–129.

Marples, B., Wouters, B.G. and Joiner, M.C.: An association between the radiation-induced arrest of G2-phase cells and low-dose hyper-radiosensitivity: a plausible underlying mechanism? Radiat. Res. 160; (2003) 38-45.

Marples, B., Wouters, B.G., Collis, S.J., Chalmers, A.J. and Joiner, M.C.: Low-dose hyper-radiosensitivity: A consequence of ineffective cell cycle arrest of radiation-damaged G2-phase cells. Radiation Res. 161; (2004) 247–255.

Marples, B. and Collis, S.J.: Low-dose hyper-radiosensitivity: Past, present and future. Int. J. Radiation Oncology Biol. Phys. 70; (2008) 1310–1318.

Mole, D.R., Blancher, C., Copley, R.R., Pollard, P.J., Gleadle, J.M., Ragoussis,. J. and Ratcliffe, P.J.: Genome-wide association of hypoxia-inducible factor (HIF)-1alpha and HIF-2alpha DNA binding with expression profiling of hypoxia-inducible transcripts. J. Biol. Chem. 284; (2009) 16767-16775.

Mottram J.C.: A factor of importance in the radio sensitivity of tumours. Br. J. Radiol. 9; (1936) 606-614.

Murray W. and Kirschner, M.W.: Dominoes and clocks: The union of two views of the cell cycle. Science 246; (1989) 614-621.

Nash, R., Tokiwa, G., Anand, S., Erikson, K. and Futcher, A.B.: The WHI1⁺ gene of

S. cerevisiae tethers cell division to cell size and is a cycling homolog. EMBO J. 7; (1988) 4335-4346.

Nias, A.H.W. and Fox, M.: Synchronization of mammalian cells with respect to the mitotic cycle. Cell Tissue Kinet. 4; (1971) 375-398.

Nordsmark, M., Overgaard. M. and Overgaard, J.: Pretreatment oxygenation predicts radiation response in advanced squamous cell carcinoma of the head and neck. Radiother. Oncol. 41; (1996) 31-39.

Nordsmark, M., Bentzen, S.M., Rudat, V., Brizel, D., Lartigau, E., Stadler, P., Becker, A., Adam, M., Molls, M. and Dunst, J., Terris, D.J. and Overgaard, J.: Prognostic value of tumour oxygenation in 397 head and neck tumours after primary radiation therapy. An international multi-center study. Radiothe.r Oncol. 77; (2005) 18-24.

Olcina, M., Lecane, P.S. and Hammond, E.: Targeting hypoxic cells through the DNA damage response. Clin. Cancer Res. 16; (2010) 5624-5629.

Painter, R.B. and Young, B.R.: Radiosensitivity in ataxia telangiectasia: A new explanation. Proc. Natl. Acad. Sci., USA 77; (1980) 7315-7317.

Pettersen, E.O. and Lindmo T.: Inhibition of cell-cycle progression by acute treatment with various degrees of hypoxia. Modifications induced by low concentrations of misonidazole present during hypoxia. Br. J. Cancer 48; (1983) 809-817.

Pettersen, E.O., Juul, N.O. & Rønning, Ø.W.: Regulation of protein metabolism of human cells during and after acute hypoxia. Cancer Res. 46; (1986) 4346-4351.

Pettersen, E.O., Larsen. L.H., Ramsing, N.B., Ebbesen, P.: Pericellular oxygen depletion during ordinary tissue culturing, measured with oxygen microsensors. Cell Proliferation 38; (2005) 257-267.

Pettersen, E.O., Bjørhovde, I., Søvik, Å , Edin, N.F.J., Zachar, V., Hole, E.O., Sandvik, J.A. and Ebbesen, P.: Response of chronic hypoxic cells to low dose-rate irradiation. Int. J. Radiat. Biol. 83; (2007) 331-345.

Podar, K. and Anderson, K.C.: A therapeutic role for targeting c-Myc/Hif-1-dependent signalling pathways. Cell Cycle 9; (2010) 1722-1728.

Quastler, H , and Sherman, F.G.: Cell population kinetics in the intestinal epithelium of the mouse. Exptl. Cell Res. 17; (1959) 420-438.

Rajaraman, R., Guernsey, D.L., Rajaraman, M.M. and Rajaraman, S.R.: Neosis – a parasexual somatic reduction division in cancer. Int. J. Human Genet. 7; (2007) 29-48.

Rofstad, E.K.: Microenvironment-induced cancer metastasis. Int. J. Radiat. Biol. 76; (2000) 589-605.

Rønning, Ø.W., Lindmo, T., Pettersen, E.O. and Seglen, P.O.: The role of protein accumulation in the cell cycle control of human NHIK 3025 cells. J. Cell. Physiol. 109; (1981) 411-418.

Salcedo, M., Garrido, E., Taja, L. and Gariglio, P.: The retinoblastoma gene product negatively regulates cellular or viral oncogene promoters in vivo. Arch. Med. Res.: 26; (1995) S157-162.

Semenza, G.L., Artemov, D., Bedi, A., Bhujwalla, Z., Chiles, K., Feldser, D., Laughner, E., Ravi, R., Simons, J., Taghavi, P. and Zhong, H.: "The metabolism of tumours": 70 years later. Novartis Found. Symp. 240; (2001) 251-60; Discussion 260-264.

Shi, Y., Åmellem, Ø. and Pettersen, E.O.: Hypoxia-associated proteins in human cells cultivated in vitro: lack of association with hypoxia-induced cell cycle regulation. Apmis 101; (1993) 75-82.

Singh, R., George, J. And Shukla, Y.: Role of senescence and mitotic catastrophe in cancer therapy. Cell Division 5; (2010) doi: 10.1186/1747-1028-5-4.

Sonveaux, P., Végran, F., Schroeder, T., Wergin, M.C., Verrax, J., Rabbani, Z.N., De Saedeleer, C.J., Kennedy, K.M., Diepart, C., Jordan, B.F., Kelley, M.J., Gallez, B., Wahl, M.L., Feron, O. and Dewhirst, M.W.: Targeting lactate-fueled respiration selectively kills hypoxic tumour cells in mice. J. Clin. Invest. 118; (2008) 3930-3942.

Steel, G.G., Adams, K. and Barrett, J.C.; Analysis of the cell population kinetics of transplanted tumours of widely-differing growth rate. Br. J. Cancer 20; (1966) 784-800.

Steel, G.G: Cell loss as a factor in the growth rate of human tumours, Eur. J. Cancer 3; (1967) 381-387.

Studzinski, G.P. and Lambert, W.C.: Thymidine as a synchronizing agent. I. Nucleic acid and protein formation in synchronous HeLa cultures treated with excess thymidine. J. Cell. Physiol. 73; (1969) 109-118.

Subarsky, P. and Hill, R.P.: The hypoxic tumour microenvironment and metastatic progression. Clin. Exp. Metastasis 20; (2003) 237-250.

Takeda, K. and Fong, G.H.: Prolyl hydroxylase domain 2 protein suppresses hypoxia-induced endothelial cell proliferation. Hypertension 49; (2007) 178-184.

Terasima, T. and Yakusawa, M.: Synthesis of G1 protein preceding DNA synthesis in cultured mammalian cells. Exp. Cell Res. 44; (1966) 669-672.

Thelander, L., Graslund, A., Thelander, M.: Continual Presence Of Oxygen And Iron Required For Mammalian Ribonucleotide Reduction – Possible Regulation Mechanism. Biochem. Bioph. Res. Co. 110; (1983) 859-865.

Wang, G.L. Jiang, B.H., Rue, E.A. and Semenza, G.L.: Hypoxia-inducible factor 1 is a basic-helix-loop-helix-PAS heterodimer regulated by cellular O_2 tension. Proc. Natl. Acad. Sci. U S A. 92; (1995) 5510-5514.

Wang, G., Reisdorph, R., Clark, R.E.Jr., Miskimins, R., Lindahl, R. and Miskimins, W.K.: Cyclin dependent kinase inhibitor p27(Kip1) is upregulated by hypoxia via an ARNT dependent pathway. J Cell Biochem. 90; (2003) 548-60.

Wykes, S.M. Piasentin, E., Joiner, M.C., Wilson, G.D. and Marples, B.: Low-dose hyper-radiosensitivity is not caused by a failure to recognize DNA double-strand breaks. Radiat. Res. 165; (2006) 516-524.

Young, C.W. and Hodas, S.: Hydroxyurea: Inhibitory effect on DNA metabolism. Science 146; (1964) 1172-1174.

Zampetti-Bosseler, F. and Scott, D.: Cell death, chromosome damage and mitotic delay in normal human, ataxia telangiectasia and retinoblastoma fibroblasts after X-irradiation. Int. J. Radiat. Biol. 39; (1981) 547-558.

Zhang, J., Sattler, M., Tonon, G., Grabher, C., Lababidi, S., Zimmerhackl, A., Raab, M.S., Vallet, S., Zhou, Y., Cartron, M.A., Hideshima, T., Tai, Y.T., Chauhan, D., Anderson, K.C. and Podar, K.: Targeting angiogenesis via a c-MYC/hypoxia-inducible factor-1α-dependent pathway in multiple myeloma. Cancer Res. 69; (2009) 5082-5090.

Chapter 7

The role of NF-κB in hypoxia-induced gene expression

Eoin P. Cummins[1], Susan F. Fitzpatrick[1,2] and Cormac T. Taylor[1,2*]

[1]UCD Conway Institute and [2]Systems Biology Ireland, University College Dublin, Belfield, Dublin 4, Ireland.

*Author for correspondence:
UCD Conway Institute, School of Medicine and Medical Science, College of Life Sciences, University College Dublin, Belfield, Dublin 4, Ireland. Tel: (353)-1-716-6732, FAX: (353)-1-716-6701, E-mail: cormac.taylor@ucd.ie

Contents

Key points

—   NF-κB is a family of transcription factors, which regulate the expression
      of genes involved in innate immunity, inflammation and apoptosis.

—   Hypoxia regulates NF-κB through multiple mechanisms including
      inhibition of HIF-hydroxylase activity.

—   NF-κB regulates gene expression in hypoxia directly through regulation
      of target genes and indirectly through regulation of HIF-1α.

—   Hypoxia-dependent NF-κB activation has important implications in
      diseases including chronic inflammation and cancer.

Introduction

Hypoxia and inflammation occur coincidentally in tissues in a range of pathophysiologic conditions including chronic inflammation, ischaemic vascular disease and cancer (Taylor and Colgan, 2010; Imtiyaz et al., 2010; Semenza, 2010). It is highly likely that the crosstalk, which exists between inflammatory and hypoxic signalling pathways, has significant implications for disease development. Hypoxia-inducible factor (HIF) and nuclear factor-kappaB (NF-κB) are two key hypoxia-sensitive transcriptional regulators, which govern the transcriptional response to hypoxia. While HIF is a key regulator of the adaptive transcriptional response, NF-κB plays a governing role in controlling the expression of genes regulating innate immunity, inflammation and apoptosis. NF-κB regulates gene expression in response to hypoxia directly by activating the expression of pro-inflammatory target genes including cyclooxygenase-2 (COX-2; Fitzpatrick et al. 2010). Furthermore, NF-κB plays a role in the regulation of HIF-1-dependent gene expression through controlling the basal rate of HIF-1α mRNA expression (Frede et al., 2006; reviewed by Taylor, 2008). Thus, NF-κB is a key transcriptional regulator of the cellular response to hypoxia, which regulates the expression of genes, which promote inflammation, innate immunity and the prevention of apoptosis. In this chapter, we will review our current knowledge of mechanisms leading to NF-κB activity in hypoxia and describe the consequence of this for cells, tissues, organs and organisms.

The NF-κB pathway

NF-κB is the generic name for a family of transcriptional regulators which regulate the expression of a wide range of genes including those involved in the promotion of innate immunity, inflammation and cell survival (Chen and Greene, 2004; Gilmore, 2006). There are five members of the NF-κB family (RelA/p65, RelB, c-Rel, p50 and p52), which share a conserved Rel homology domain and can form either homo- or hetero-dimers. The p50-p65 heterodimer is the most commonly encountered NF-κB complex during inflammation. There are two primary pathways by which NF-κB can be activated termed the canonical and the non-canonical pathways respectively (Moynagh, 2005).

A general schematic of the canonical and non-canonical NF-κB pathways is provided in Figure 7.1. In the resting state, NF-κB is sequestered in the cytosol through association with co-repressor IκB molecules via multiple ankyrin repeat domains. Upon activation, IκB is phosphorylated by components of the IκB kinase (IKK) complex and proteolytically processed resulting in the liberation of NF-κB allowing its translocation to the nucleus. The presence of specific κB-binding sites within the promoters of target genes facilitates NF-κB binding with subsequently enhanced mRNA transcription. Target genes for NF-κB include adhesion molecules, cytokines, inflammatory enzymes and inhibitors of apoptosis (Chen and Greene, 2004; Gilmore, 2006; Moynagh 2005; Oliver et al., 2009).

The NF-κB pathway can be activated in response to a number of ligand stimuli including cytokines, bacterial and viral components, cell surface molecules and antigens. These ligands act via receptor-specific signal transduction cascades to activate either the canonical or the non-canonical NF-κB pathways (summarized in Figure 7.1). Recently, it has become appreciated that NF-κB can also be modulated in response to non-ligand stimuli including ultraviolet light, hypercapnia, acidosis and hypoxia (Cooper and Bowden, 2007; Tsuchiya et al 2010; O'Toole et al, 2009; Cummins et al, 2010; Oliver et al., 2009). In this chapter, we will focus our attention on the mechanisms and consequences of the activation of NF-κB by hypoxia.

Stimulation of NF-κB may be via the canonical pathway, which is activated in response to ligands such as LPS, TNF, IL-1. These ligands bind to receptors including the Toll-like receptors (TLRs), TNFα receptors (TNFR) or the interleukin-1 receptor (IL-1R) leading to the activation of the IKK complex resulting in the phosphorylation and subsequent proteosomal degradation of IκB. The liberated NF-κB dimer (most commonly p50/p65) is then free to translocate to the nucleus to regulate gene expression.

Alternatively, the non-canonical pathway can be activated by ligands such as lymphotoxin or CD40. Binding of these stimuli to their cognate receptors leads to activation of IKKα dimers leading to the processing of p100 and the liberation and nuclear translocation of RelB/p52 dimers (Bakkar and Guttridge, 2010). Activation of the non-canonical pathway leads to the expression of genes important in B-cell maturation and lymphangiogenesis.

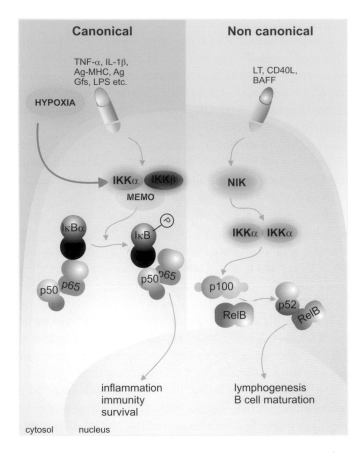

Figure 7.1 _ Hypoxia activates NF-κB signalling through the canonical pathway. Multiple stimuli including tumour necrosis factor (TNF), Interleukin-1 (IL-1), MHC-Antigen complexes (Ag-MHC), Antigen (Ag), Growth factors (Gfs) and lipopolysaccharide (LPS) and hypoxia activate NF-κB signalling through the canonical signalling pathway. The non-canonical pathway can be activated by Lymphotoxin (LT), CD40 ligand (CD40L) and B-cell activating factor (BAFF) but is not activated by hypoxia.

Evidence that hypoxia activates NF-κB

The first demonstration that the NF-κB pathway is responsive to hypoxia was published in 1994 (Koong et al, 1994). This was followed by a series of in vitro studies confirming that upon exposure to hypoxia, a range of cell types including endothelial cells, macrophages, epithelial cells and neurons demonstrated hypoxic sensitivity with respect to NF-κB activation (Karakurum et al, 1994; Muraokaet al., Leeper-Woodford and Detmer, 1999; Taylor et al 1999; Shi et al, 1999; Chandel et al, 2000; Rius et al, 2008). While these studies identified robust hypoxic sensitivity in the NF-κB pathway in multiple cell types, they predominantly demonstrated hypoxia to be a relatively mild activator of NF-κB activity when compared to classical inflammatory stimuli such as LPS or TNFα. Evidence that NF-κB is a bona fide hypoxia responsive transcription factor is strengthened by in vivo studies which have demonstrated that hypoxia activates NF-κB in a range of tissues including the brain, heart and lungs (Simakajornboon et al., 2001; Qui et al., 2001; Fitzpatrick et al 2011).

Mechanism of hypoxia-activated NF-κB

As outlined above, a significant amount of evidence now exists that NF-κB is a hypoxia-responsive transcription factor with consequences for the regulation of genes involved in innate immunity, inflammation and apoptosis. Thus, developing our understanding of how hypoxia leads to the activation of NF-κB is important in understanding the role of this pathway in regulating the nature of the hypoxic transcriptome in cells. Of note, it appears that it is the canonical arm rather than the non-canonical arm of the NF-κB pathway, which is responsive to hypoxia (Oliver et al, 2009). In support of this, several studies in this area identify the phosphorylation of IKKβ as being associated with hypoxia-induced NF-κB (Winning et al, 2010; Cummins et al, 2006; Rius et al, 2008). A number of studies have proposed distinct mechanisms by which changes in oxygen tension may be transduced to activate the canonical NF-κB pathway. These pathways are summarized in Figure 7.2 and are described in detail below:

Tyrosine phosphorylation of IκBα

Initial studies into the mechanism by which hypoxia activates NF-κB proposed that this was via signalling through Ras and Raf-1 kinase-dependent signalling pathways. These studies demonstrated that pharmacologic tyrosine kinase inhibition or transfection with dominant negative alleles of Ras or Raf-1 inhibited IκBα degradation, NF-κB-DNA binding and transac-

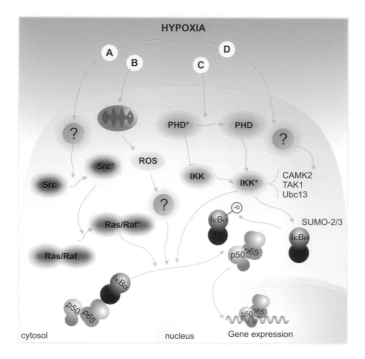

Figure 7.2 _ Proposed mechanisms for hypoxic activation of NF-κB. (A) Hypoxia leads to activation of Src through via a unknown oxygen sensor resulting in Raf/Ras activation which promotes tyrosine phosphorylation of IκBα leading to its degradation with the subsequent liberation and transcriptional activation of IκBα. (B) Hypoxia induces mitochondrial reactive oxygen species (ROS) production leading through an unknown mechanism to IκBα phosphorylation and subsequent NF-κB activation. (C) Hypoxia decreases activity of prolyl hydroxylases, which suppress IKK activity leading to IKK activation, phosphorylation of IκBα and activation of NF-κB. (D) Hypoxia, through an undefined oxygen sensing mechanism leads to activation of the IKK complex via CaMK2, TAK1 and Ubc13 which promotes the modification of IκBα by SUMO-2/3 leading to its disassociation from p50/p65 and subsequent activation of NF-κB.

tivation of an NF-κB reporter gene in response to hypoxia (Koong et al 1994a). Furthermore, tyrosine phosphorylation status of IκBα was increased with hypoxia. This response was independent of Erk1/Erk2 kinase activity and instead was dependent upon the early activation of Src kinase. This led to the phosphorylation of IκBα on tyrosine residues with a subsequent dissociation from the active p50/p65 NF-κB and the induction of inflammatory gene expression (Koong et al, 1994b).

Reactive Oxygen Species

Hypoxia-induced generation of mitochondrial reactive oxygen species (ROS) in cells and the role of these ROS in signalling the activation of transcription factors were first proposed for HIF in 1998 (Chandel et al 1998). While the role of ROS in mediating signalling during hypoxia has remained controversial, these and subsequent studies identified a clear role for the mitochondrial electron transport chain in the regulation of the cellular response to hypoxia (reviewed by Taylor, 2008). The potential role of ROS in activation of the NF-κB pathway is also controversial (Reuter et al., 2010; Bowie and O'Neill, 2000). However, studies into the role of hypoxia-induced ROS in NF-κB signalling implicated the generation of reactive oxygen species by mitochondria during hypoxic stress as being key signalling molecules (Chandel et al, 2000). In these studies, it was demonstrated that hypoxia increased mitochondrial ROS production as well as NF-κB activity and downstream gene expression in a manner which was abolished by pretreatment with antioxidants. Furthermore, antioxidants did not impact upon LPS-stimulated NF-κB indicating that while hypoxia-dependent NF-κB is ROS-dependent, LPS-dependent NF-κB activation is ROS-independent (Chandel et al, 2000). Further studies demonstrate that ROS-mediated response to hypoxia results in increased expression of pro-inflammatory cytokines including IL-6 and was reversible through treatment with anti-oxidants (Pearlstein et al, 2002).

Hydroxylase inhibition

A series of studies investigating parallels between oxygen sensing mechanisms in the HIF and NF-κB pathways revealed that the same hydroxylase enzymes responsible for conferring oxygen sensitivity to HIF also regulate NF-κB. Four such HIF hydroxylases have been described which are termed Prolyl Hydroxylase (PHD)-1, PHD-2, PHD-3 and factor inhibiting HIF (FIH) (reviewed by Kaelin and Ratcliffe, 2008). Initially, global proteomic analysis revealed that components of NF-κB pathway including IκBα and p105 were subject to hydroxylation by FIH (Cockman et al, 2006). This observation was later shown to occur on many proteins containing ankyrin repeat domains (Cockman et al., 2009). While hydroxylation of IκBα by FIH appears to be largely inconsequential for basal NF-κB activity (Cockman et al, 2006; Devries et al., 2010), further studies into the possible modulatory role of FIH in the regulation of stimulated NF-κB activity are required to fully describe its potential role in NF-κB signalling.

In contrast to FIH, in vitro and in vivo studies examining the effects of PHD 1, 2 & 3 have revealed a significant contribution to NF-κB signalling but without empirical verification of post-translational hydroxylation of NF-κB family members. Indeed, the contribution of the catalytic activity of the hydroxylases to NF-κB signalling has been equivocal. We previously demonstrated that hypoxia, hydroxylase inhibition and isoform specific siRNAs to PHD-1 and PHD-2 activated NF-κB signalling. This resulted in increased activity of the IKK complex, increased nuclear p65 localization and enhanced p65 DNA binding (Cummins et al, 2006). We made similar observations in vivo using the pharmacologic pan-hydroxylase inhibitor, DMOG (Cummins et al., 2008). Recently, Chan and colleagues identified a PHD-2-dependent angiogenic phenotype through the use of shRNA against PHD-2. This phenotype was HIF-independent and NF-κB dependent. Interestingly, while the authors observed hypoxia induced NF-κB activity, the effects of PHD-2 on angiogenesis were found to be independent of the enzyme's catalytic hydroxylase activity. Similarly, a role for PHD-3 as a negative regulator of NF-κB signalling has been described recently. Again the authors report a hypoxia-dependent increase in NF-κB signalling but demonstrate a suppressive role for PHD-3, independent of its catalytic activity. The mechanism for this inhibition involves PHD-3 mediated repression of the IKK complex through competition for IKKβ's chaperone HSP-90 (Xue et al., 2010). However, Fu and colleagues implicate hypoxia, hydroxylase inhibition and PHD-3 in myoblast differentiation in a manner that is dependent on the canonical NF-κB pathway, independent of HIF and is dependent on the catalytic hydroxylase activity of PHD-3 (Fu and Taubman., 2010). Finally, PHD-1s role in NF-κB signalling has been further supported by in vivo and in vitro studies implicating this hydroxylase isoform in NF-κB-dependent myocardial protection in ischaemia/reperfusion injury (Adluri et al., 2010) and hypoxia-induced monocyte adherence respectively (Winning et al. 2010). Taken together there is strong evidence for the PHDs negatively regulating the NF-κB pathway through suppression of canonical NF-κB signalling. The catalytic activity of the PHDs is suppressed in hypoxia and with pharmacological inhibition, which consistently results in enhanced NF-κB signalling. However, an emerging role for non-enzymatic functions of the PHDs with respect to NF-κB signalling should be considered.

SUMO-modification of IκB

A further mechanism by which hypoxia regulates NF-κB activity has been recently proposed. This study confirmed previous studies indicating a role for activation of the canonical NF-κB pathway in response to hypoxia. In this model however, increased post-translational modification of IκBα by the small ubiquitin related modifier (SUMO)-2/3 through increased SUMO modification of IκBα on key lysine residues is implicated (Culver et al., 2010). How specific oxygen/hypoxia sensing fits into this model remains unclear.

Impact of hypoxic NF-κB on gene expression

Direct regulation of gene expression

Hypoxia-dependent canonical NF-κB activation can result in direct regulation of inflammatory gene expression through binding of p50/p65 heterodimers to promoter elements within specific target genes. A number of direct NF-κB targets, which are activated in response to hypoxia, have been reported including the key pro-inflammatory enzyme cyclooxygenase-2 (COX-2). While it is clear that COX-2 expression is increased in hypoxia, this has been variously attributed to being mediated by HIF (Csiki et al, 2006, Lukiw et al., 2003; Cook Johnson et al., 2006; Kaidi et al., 2006;) or NF-κB (Lukiw et al., 2003; Schmedtje et al., 1997). However, more recent evidence demonstrates direct binding of the p65 subunit of NF-κB to the COX-2 promoter leading to increased gene transcription (Fitzpatrick et al., 2010).

Indirect regulation of gene expression (via HIF)

It has recently become clear that in addition to its direct role in the regulation of gene expression, NF-κB can also play an important indirect role through the regulation of HIF-dependent gene expression (reviewed by Taylor, 2008). As well as being responsive to hypoxia through decreased hydroxylase activity, HIF can be regulated by a range of non-hypoxic stimuli through NF-κB including TNFα, hepatocyte growth factor, lipopolysaccharide, microtubule disrupting agents, reactive oxygen species and IL-18 (Figuora et al, 2002; Jung et al, 2003a,b; Zhou et al., 2003; Tacchini et al 2004; Frede et al, 2006; Bonello et al 2007; Sun et al, 2007; Belaiba et al, 2007; Kim et al, 2008; van Uden et al.,

2008). Of interest, hypoxia has also been reported to regulate HIF-1α mRNA levels through NF-κB (Frede et al., 2006; Belaiba et al, 2007). As well as mediating stimulated increases in HIF-1α mRNA in response to the stimuli outlined above, NF-κB has been recently reported to be important in the regulation of basal HIF-1α mRNA expression both *in vitro* and *in vivo* (Rius et al, 2008, van Uden et al., 2008). The HIF-1α promoter has been reported to contain a functional NF-κB-response element −197/−188 base pairs upstream of the transcriptional start site (van Uden et al 2008).

NF-κB can also regulate HIF signalling via a direct interaction between the IKKγ subunit of the IKK complex (also known as NEMO) and the HIF-2α isoform which increases the transcriptional activity of HIF-2α through promoting it's interaction with CREB binding protein (CBP; Bracken et al, 2005).

Consequences of NF-κB activation in hypoxia

NF-κB is a key regulator of apoptotic pathways in a number of cell types including both normal and malignant cells (Karin and Lin, 2002; Luo et al., 2005). NF-κB inhibits apoptosis through promoting the expression of genes, which suppress the cellular apoptotic response including members of the Bcl-2 family (e.g. Bcl-X$_L$) and cellular inhibitors of apoptosis (c-IAPs; Luo et al., 2005). NF-κB plays a role in the regulation of apoptotic response to hypoxia in a range of cell types including endothelial cells, hippocampal tissues and neutrophils (Mutsushita et al., 2000; Qiu et al., 2001; Walmsley et al, 2005). Thus a primary consequence of the activation of NF-κB by hypoxia is the inhibition of apoptotic responses. This pro-survival response may function to complement the adaptive response activated through the HIF pathway and promote cell survival during periods of hypoxic stress.

A second consequence of NF-κB activation during hypoxia is the promotion of inflammation. Hypoxia and inflammation are co-incidental features of a number of chronic inflammatory disease states (Colgan and Taylor 2010). NF-κB activates the expression of a wide range of inflammatory mediators including cytokines, adhesion molecules and pro-inflammatory enzymes. Hypoxia promotes NF-κB-dependent inflammatory activity through a number of pathways including directly regulating the expression of inflammatory genes such as cytokines and promoting monocyte adhesion (Winning et al., 2010; Cummins et al, 2006) and indirectly through the promotion of immune cell survival via HIF (Nitzet and Johnson 2009). Thus, a second consequence of hypoxia-induced NF-κB activity may be the promotion of innate immune and inflammatory responses.

Conclusions and Perspectives

Hypoxia is a prominent feature of the microenvironment in a range of pathophysiologic conditions where inflammation also occurs. HIF and NF-κB are key hypoxia-responsive transcription factors, which determine the transcriptional response to hypoxia and thus play a role in tissue adaptation, survival and inflammation. Developing our understanding of the mechanisms by which hypoxia regulates these pathways will help us to understand the role of the microenvironment in regulating the expression of genes which contribute to disease development. NF-κB is regulated by hypoxia through a mechanism, which is at least in part dependent upon the same oxygen sensing hydroxylases which confer oxygen sensitivity to HIF. Furthermore, hypoxia-induced NF-κB activity results in direct transcriptional regulation of some genes such as COX-2 as well as indirect regulation of genes via the HIF pathway, the latter role being through the upregulation of HIF-1α mRNA expression. Thus NF-κB is a bona fide hypoxia responsive transcription factor, which likely plays an important role in the ultimate shaping of the transcriptional response to hypoxia.

Acknowledgements _ Work from the author's lab is funded by a grant from Science Foundation Ireland.

References

Bakkar N, Guttridge DC (2010). NF-kappaB signalling: a tale of two pathways in skeletal myogenesis. Physiol Rev. 90(2):495-511.

Belaiba RS, Bonello S, Zähringer C, Schmidt S, Hess J, Kietzmann T, Görlach A (2007). Hypoxia up-regulates hypoxia-inducible factor-1alpha transcription by involving phosphatidylinositol 3-kinase and nuclear factor kappaB in pulmonary artery smooth muscle cells. Mol Biol Cell. 18(12):4691-7.

Bonello S, Zähringer C, BelAiba RS, Djordjevic T, Hess J, Michiels C, Kietzmann T,

Görlach A (2007). Reactive oxygen species activate the HIF-1alpha promoter via a functional NFkappaB site. Arterioscler Thromb Vasc Biol. 27(4):755-61

Bowie A, O'Neill LA (2000). Oxidative stress and nuclear factor-kappaB activation: a reassessment of the evidence in the light of recent discoveries. Biochem Pharmacol. 59(1):13-23.

Bracken CP, Whitelaw ML, Peet DJ (2005). Activity of hypoxia-inducible factor 2alpha is regulated by association with the NF-kappaB essential modulator. J Biol Chem. 280(14):14240-51.

Chan DA, Kawahara TL, Sutphin PD, Chang HY, Chi JT, Giaccia AJ (2009). Tumour vasculature is regulated by PHD2-mediated angiogenesis and bone marrow-derived cell recruitment. Cancer Cell. 15(6):527-38.

Chandel NS, Maltepe E, Goldwasser E, Mathieu CE, Simon MC, Schumacker PT (1998). Mitochondrial reactive oxygen species trigger hypoxia-induced transcription. Proc Natl Acad Sci U S A. 95(20):11715-20.

Chandel NS, Trzyna WC, McClintock DS, Schumacker PT (2000). Role of oxidants in NF-kappa B activation and TNF-alpha gene transcription induced by hypoxia and endotoxin. J Immunol. 165(2):1013-21.

Chen LF, Greene WC (2004). Shaping the nuclear action of NF-kappaB. Nat Rev Mol Cell Biol. 5(5):392-401.

Cockman ME, Lancaster DE, Stolze IP, Hewitson KS, McDonough MA, Coleman ML, Coles CH, Yu X, Hay RT, Ley SC, Pugh CW, Oldham NJ, Masson N, Schofield CJ, Ratcliffe PJ (2006). Posttranslational hydroxylation of ankyrin repeats in IkappaB proteins by the hypoxia-inducible factor (HIF) asparaginyl hydroxylase, factor inhibiting HIF (FIH). Proc Natl Acad Sci U S A. 103(40):14767-72.

Cockman ME, Webb JD, Ratcliffe PJ (2009). FIH-dependent asparaginyl hydroxylation of ankyrin repeat domain-containing proteins. Ann N Y Acad Sci. 1177:9-18.

Colgan SP, Taylor CT (2010). Hypoxia: an alarm signal during intestinal inflammation. Nat Rev Gastroenterol Hepatol. 7(5):281-7

Cook-Johnson RJ, Demasi M, Cleland LG, Gamble JR, Saint DA, James MJ (2006). Endothelial cell COX-2 expression and activity in hypoxia. Biochem. Biophys. Acta 1761, 1443-1449.

Cooper SJ, Bowden GT (2007). Ultraviolet B regulation of transcription factor families: roles of nuclear factor-kappa B (NF-kappaB) and activator protein-1 (AP-1) in UVB-induced skin carcinogenesis. Curr Cancer Drug Targets. 7(4):325-34.

Csiki I, Yanagisawa K, Haruki N, Nadaf S, Morrow JD, Johnson DH, Carbone, DP (2006). Thioredoxin-1 modulates transcription of Cyclooxygenase-2 via hypoxia-inducible factor-1alpha in non-small cell lung carcinoma. Cancer Res. 66(1); 143-150.

Culver C, Sundqvist A, Mudie S, Melvin A, Xirodimas D, Rocha S (2010). Mechanism of hypoxia-induced NF-kappaB. Mol Cell Biol. 30(20):4901-21.

Cummins EP, Berra E, Comerford KM, Ginouves A, Fitzgerald KT, Seeballuck F, Godson C, Nielsen JE, Moynagh P, Pouyssegur J, Taylor CT (2006). Prolyl hydroxylase-1 negatively regulates IkappaB kinase-beta, giving insight into hypoxia-induced NFkappaB activity. Proc Natl Acad Sci U S A. 103(48):18154-9.

Cummins EP, Seeballuck F, Keely SJ, Mangan NE, Callanan JJ, Fallon PG, Taylor CT

(2008). The hydroxylase inhibitor dimethyloxalylglycine is protective in a murine model of colitis. Gastroenterology. 134(1):156-65.

Cummins EP, Oliver KM, Lenihan CR, Fitzpatrick SF, Bruning U, Scholz CC, Slattery C, Leonard MO, McLoughlin P, Taylor CT (2010). NF-kB links CO2 sensing to innate immunity and inflammation in mammalian cells. J Immunol. 185(7):4439-45.

Devries IL, Hampton-Smith RJ, Mulvihill MM, Alverdi V, Peet DJ, Komives EA (2010). Consequences of IkappaB alpha hydroxylation by the factor inhibiting HIF (FIH). FEBS Lett. 2010 Dec 1;584(23):4725-30. Epub 2010 Nov 5.

Figueroa YG, Chan AK, Ibrahim R, Tang Y, Burow ME, Alam J, Scandurro AB, Beckman BS (2002). NF-kappaB plays a key role in hypoxia-inducible factor-1-regulated erythropoietin gene expression. Exp Hematol. 30(12):1419-27.

Fitzpatrick SF, Tambuwala MM, Bruning U, Schaible B, Scholz CC, Byrne A, O'Connor A, Gallagher WM, Lenihan CR, Garvey JF, Howell K, Fallon PG, Cummins EP, Taylor CT (2011). An intact canonical NF-κB pathway is required for inflammatory gene expression in response to hypoxia. J Immunol. 2011 Jan 15;186(2):1091-6. Epub 2010 Dec 13.

Frede S, Stockmann C, Freitag P, Fandrey J (2006) Bacterial lipopolysaccharide induces HIF-1 activation in human monocytes via p44/42 MAPK and NF-kappaB. Biochem J. 396(3):517-27.

Fu J, Taubman MB (2010). Prolyl hydroxylase EGLN3 regulates skeletal myoblast differentiation through an NF-kappaB-dependent pathway. J Biol Chem. 285(12):8927-35.

Gilmore TD (2006). Introduction to NF-kappaB: players, pathways, perspectives. Oncogene. 25(51):6680-84.

Imtiyaz HZ, Simon MC (2010). Hypoxia-inducible factors as essential regulators of inflammation. Curr Top Microbiol Immunol. 345:105-20.

Jung Y, Isaacs JS, Lee S, Trepel J, Liu ZG, Neckers L (2003). Hypoxia-inducible factor induction by tumour necrosis factor in normoxic cells requires receptor-interacting protein-dependent nuclear factor kappa B activation. Biochem J. 370(Pt 3):1011-7.

Jung YJ, Isaacs JS, Lee S, Trepel J, Neckers L (2003). Microtubule disruption utilizes an NFkappa B-dependent pathway to stabilize HIF-1alpha protein. J Biol Chem. 278(9):7445-52.

Kaelin WG Jr, Ratcliffe PJ (2008). Oxygen sensing by metazoans: the central role of the HIF hydroxylase pathway. Mol Cell. 30(4):393-402.

Kaidi A, Qualtrough D, Williams AC, Paraskeve C (2006). Direct transcriptional upregulation of cyclooxgenase-2 by hypoxia inducible factor (HIF)-1 promotes colorectal tumour cell survival and enhances HIF-1 transcriptional activity during hypoxia. Cancer Res. 60(13); 6683-6691.

Kim J, Shao Y, Kim SY, Kim S, Song HK, Jeon JH, Suh HW, Chung JW, Yoon SR, Kim YS, Choi I (2008). Hypoxia-induced IL-18 increases hypoxia-inducible factor-1alpha expression through a Rac1-dependent NF-kappaB pathway. Mol Biol Cell. 19(2):433-44.

Koong AC, Chen EY, Giaccia AJ (1994). Hypoxia causes the activation of nuclear factor kappa B through the phosphorylation of I kappa B alpha on tyrosine residues. Cancer Res. 54(6):1425-30.

Koong AC, Chen EY, Mivechi NF, Denko NC, Stambrook P, Giaccia AJ (1994). Hypoxic activation of nuclear factor-kappa B is mediated by a Ras and Raf signalling pathway and does not involve MAP kinase (ERK1 or ERK2). Cancer Res. 54(20):5273-9.

Leeper-Woodford SK, Detmer K (1999). Acute hypoxia increases alveolar macrophage tumour necrosis factor activity and alters NF-kappaB expression. Am J Physiol. 276(6 Pt 1):L909-16

Lukiw WJ, Ottlecz A, Lambrou G, Grueninger M, Finley J, Thompson HW, Bazan NG (2003). Coordinate activation of HIF-1 and NF- B DNA binding and COX-2 and VEGF expression in retinal cells by hypoxia. Invest. Opthamol Vis. Sci. 44, 4163-4170.

Matsushita H, Morishita R, Nata T, Aoki M, Nakagami H, Taniyama Y, Yamamoto K, Higaki J, Yasufumi K, Ogihara T (2000). Hypoxia-induced endothelial apoptosis through nuclear factor-kappaB (NF-kappaB)-mediated bcl-2 suppression: in vivo evidence of the importance of NF-kappaB in endothelial cell regulation. Circ Res. 86(9):974-81.

Moynagh PN (2005). The NF-kappaB pathway. J Cell Sci. 118(Pt 20):4589-92.

Muraoka K, Shimizu K, Sun X, Zhang YK, Tani T, Hashimoto T, Yagi M, Miyazaki I, Yamamoto K (1997). Hypoxia, but not reoxygenation, induces interleukin 6 gene expression through NF-kappa B activation. Transplantation. 63(3):466-70.

Nizet V, Johnson RS (2009). Interdependence of hypoxic and innate immune responses. Nat Rev Immunol. 9(9):609-17.

Oliver KM, Garvey JF, Ng CT, Veale DJ, Fearon U, Cummins EP, Taylor CT (2009). Hypoxia activates NF-kappaB-dependent gene expression through the canonical signalling pathway. Antioxid Redox Signal. 11(9):2057-64.

O'Toole D, Hassett P, Contreras M, Higgins BD, McKeown ST, McAuley DF, O'Brien T, Laffey JG (2009). Hypercapnic acidosis attenuates pulmonary epithelial wound repair by an NF-kappaB dependent mechanism. Thorax. 64(11):976-82.

Qiu J, Grafe MR, Schmura SM, Glasgow JN, Kent TA, Rassin DK, Perez-Polo JR (2001). Differential NF-kappa B regulation of bcl-x gene expression in hippocampus and basal forebrain in response to hypoxia. J Neurosci Res. 64(3):223-34.

Reuter S, Gupta SC, Chaturvedi MM, Aggarwal BB (2010). Oxidative stress, inflammation, and cancer: how are they linked? Free Radic Biol Med. 49(11):1603-16.

Rius J, Guma M, Schachtrup C, Akassoglou K, Zinkernagel AS, Nizet V, Johnson RS, Haddad GG, Karin M (2008). NF-kappaB links innate immunity to the hypoxic response through transcriptional regulation of HIF-1alpha. Nature. 453(7196):807-11.

Semenza GL (2010). Vascular responses to hypoxia and ischaemia. Arterioscler Thromb Vasc Biol. 30(4):648-52

Schmedtje JF Jr, Ji YS, Liu WL, DuBois RN, Runge MS (1997). Hypoxia induces cyclooxygenase-2 via the NF-kappaB p65 transcription factor in human vascular endothelial cells. J Biol Chem. 272(1):601-8.

Shen RR, Hahn WC (2010). Emerging roles for the non-canonical IKKs in cancer. Oncogene. 2011 Feb 10;30(6):631-41. Epub 2010 Nov 1. Review.

Shi Q, Le X, Abbruzzese JL, Wang B, Mujaida N, Matsushima K, Huang S, Xiong Q, Xie K (1999). Cooperation between transcription factor AP-1 and NF-kappaB in the induction of interleukin-8 in human pancreatic adenocarcinoma cells by hypoxia. J Interferon Cytokine Res. 19(12):1363-71.

Simakajornboon N, Gozal E, Gozal D (2001). Developmental patterns of NF-kappaB activation during acute hypoxia in the caudal brainstem of the rat. Brain Res Dev Brain Res. 127(2):175-83.

Sun HL, Liu YN, Huang YT, Pan SL, Huang DY, Guh JH, Lee FY, Kuo SC, Teng CM (2007). YC-1 inhibits HIF-1 expression in prostate cancer cells: contribution of Akt/NF-kappaB signalling to HIF-1alpha accumulation during hypoxia. Oncogene 26(27):3941-51.

Tacchini L, De Ponti C, Matteucci E, Follis R, Desiderio MA (2004). Hepatocyte growth factor-activated NF-kappaB regulates HIF-1 activity and ODC expression, implicated in survival, differently in different carcinoma cell lines. Carcinogenesis. 25(11):2089-100.

Taylor CT (2008). Interdependent roles for hypoxia inducible factor and nuclear factor-kappaB in hypoxic inflammation. J Physiol. 586(Pt 17):4055-9.

Taylor CT (2008). Mitochondria and cellular oxygen sensing in the HIF pathway. Biochem J. 409(1):19-26.

Taylor CT, Fueki N, Agah A, Hershberg RM, Colgan SP (1999). Critical role of cAMP response element binding protein expression in hypoxia-elicited induction of epithelial tumour necrosis factor-alpha. J Biol Chem. 274(27):19447-54

Tsuchiya Y, Asano T, Nakayama K, Kato T Jr, Karin M, Kamata H (2010). Nuclear IKKbeta is an adaptor protein for IkappaBalpha ubiquitination and degradation in UV-induced NF-kappaB activation. Mol Cell. 39(4):570-82.

van Uden P, Kenneth NS, Rocha S (2008). Regulation of hypoxia-inducible factor-1alpha by NF-kappaB. Biochem J. 412(3):477-84.

Walmsley SR, Print C, Farahi N, Peyssonnaux C, Johnson RS, Cramer T, Sobolewski A, Condliffe AM, Cowburn AS, Johnson N, Chilvers ER (2005). Hypoxia-induced neutrophil survival is mediated by HIF-1alpha-dependent NF-kappaB activity. J Exp Med. 201(1):105-15.

Winning S, Splettstoesser F, Fandrey J, Frede S (2010). Acute hypoxia induces HIF-independent monocyte adhesion to endothelial cells through increased intercellular adhesion molecule-1 expression: the role of hypoxic inhibition of prolyl hydroxylase activity for the induction of NF-kappa B. J Immunol. 185(3):1786-93.

Zhou J, Schmid T, Brüne B (2003). Tumour necrosis factor-alpha causes accumulation of a ubiquitinated form of hypoxia inducible factor-1alpha through a nuclear factor-kappaB-dependent pathway. Mol Biol Cell. 14(6):2216-25.

Chapter 8

Hypoxia and p53

Roman Hrstka, Petr Müller, Philip J. Coates, Borivoj Vojtesek[*]

[1] Regional Centre for Applied Molecular Oncology, Masaryk Memorial Cancer Institute, Zluty kopec 7, 656 53 Brno, Czech Republic, [2]Tayside Tissue Bank, Medical Research Institute, Ninewells Hospital and Medical School, University of Dundee, Dundee DD1 9SY, UK

[*]Author for correspondence:
Tel: +420543133300, E-mail: vojtesek@mou.cz

Contents

Key points

— The *TP53* gene has a major role as an integrator of cellular stresses and is commonly mutated or inactivated in human cancers.

— As well as inducing growth arrest and cell death by transcriptional activation of target genes after genotoxic stress, p53 also responds to hypoxia.

— Under hypoxic conditions, p53 acts largely as a transcriptional repressor but also enhances HIF-1-mediated activation of apoptosis.

— Mutation to *TP53* in tumours allows increased survival in hypoxia, suggesting that these pathways could be therapeutically useful.

— The two other members of the p53-family, p63 and p73, also influence hypoxic responses in poorly defined ways.

Introduction to p53

The p53 protein was first discovered in 1979 (Lane & Crawford, 1979; Linzer & Levine, 1979) and was considered to be an oncogene until 1989, when its anti-oncogenic functions were first described (Baker et al., 1989; Nigro et al., 1989). Functional inactivation of this protein is the most frequent feature of human cancers. p53 is a transcription factor that maintains genomic integrity by regulating the expression of a large number of genes involved in cell cycle arrest, DNA repair and programmed cell death, in response to various stress stimuli such as DNA damage and hypoxia (Oren, 1997; Asker et al., 1999). The level and activity of p53 in the cell is the result of a constant balance between synthesis, stabilisation and degradation. Stabilisation of p53 under stress conditions is linked either to inhibition of degradation, a similar mechanism known for some other transcription factors such as hypoxia-inducible factor (HIF) (Nikinmaa & Rees, 2005), or to an increase of p53 translation directly linked to protein synthesis (Takagi et al., 2005). Its functions as a transcription factor and efficient accumulation under stress conditions are crucial for suppression of tumour growth (Pietenpol et al., 1994; Miled et al., 2005) as this protein suppresses tumour progress mainly by inducing cell cycle arrest and apoptosis (Avivi et al., 2005).

Human p53 has 393 residues and is composed of at least four functional domains that regulate its function as a stress-activated sequence-specific DNA-binding protein and transcription factor. The N-terminus of p53 contains the transactivation domain through which p53 interacts with components of the transcriptional machinery (Pietenpol et al., 1994) and a smaller N-terminal highly conserved Box 1 domain (BOX-I), which directs the binding of p53 to Mdm2 (mouse double minute 2) protein. p53 has a short half-life in proliferating cells due to the binding of Mdm2 protein to p53 followed by degradation of p53 through the ubiquitin-dependent degradation machinery (Oren, 1997). The central core domain of p53 contains the sequence-specific DNA-binding domain, which is highly conserved in vertebrates and in two recently identified human homologues: p73 and p63 (Bargonetti et al., 1993; Kaghad et al., 1997; Yang et al., 1998). A C-terminal tetramerization domain is required to assemble p53 into a fully competent tetrameric transcription factor (Hupp et al., 1993; Cho et al., 1994). Although most research has focused on identifying the downstream signalling pathways regulated by p53, leading to identification of hundreds of p53-target genes, other approaches have concentrated on the identification of upstream factors that control p53 activity by post-translational modifications.

In the normal cellular environment, p53 is expressed at very low levels with a short half-life. When cells are exposed to stress stimuli, p53 is stabilised and activated via N-terminal and C-terminal modifications that include multiple phosphorylation, acetylation and other events (reviewed in (Appella & Anderson, 2001; Lavin & Gueven, 2006; Carter & Vousden, 2009)). In particular, the N-terminal residues of p53 are phosphorylated by ataxia telangiectasia-mutated (Atm) and DNA-dependent protein kinase (DNA-PK), proteins activated during DNA damage, leading to p53 phosphorylation at Ser15. This phosphorylation is responsible for a reduction in the ability of p53 to bind to Mdm2, resulting in stabilisation and increased activity of p53 (Banin et al., 1998; Canman et al., 1998; Woo et al., 1998). The dephosphorylation of Ser376 at the C-terminus of p53 induces binding to a 14-3-3 protein, leading to higher DNA binding activity of p53 (Waterman et al., 1998). Phosphorylation of at least three sites, at Ser366, Ser378 and Thr387, is induced by DNA damage, and the induction at Ser366 and Thr387 is inhibited by small interfering RNA targeting Chk1 and Chk2. This data supports an interplay between p53 C-terminal phosphorylation and acetylation and provides an additional mechanism for the control of the activity of p53 by Chk1 and Chk2 (Ou et al., 2005).

Cellular properties are influenced by complex factors inherent to their microenvironments and one major factor in this environment is oxygen deprivation (hypoxia). Cells respond to hypoxia by stabilising hypoxia-inducible factors (HIFs), which are known to function by altering cellular metabolism and blood vessel architecture. In tumours, hypoxia occurs due to rapid cell proliferation and aberrant blood vessel formation. Direct molecular links have been found between HIFs and critical cell signalling pathways such as c-Myc and p53. These novel links suggest a new role for HIFs in tumour regulation.

The above-described regulation of p53 implies that both 53 and HIF share several common characteristics in terms of their regulation. Both HIF and p53 serve as transcription factors that integrate upstream cellular signalling events resulting in their activation and the triggering of transcription of their target genes. The regulation of p53 and HIF lies in the control of protein ubiquitination and degradation, while mRNA expression does not change. The levels of both p53 and HIF proteins are maintained low in unstressed normal cells due to negative feedback loops, which are realized by specific E3 ubiquitin ligases. From this perspective, Mdm2 and VHL play analogous roles in the regulation of p53 and HIF, respectively. Although the mechanism of regulation of both transcription factors is similar, the consequences of their alteration in cancers are very different. While VHL and p53 act as tumour suppressors, Mdm2 and HIF function as oncogenes.

Hypoxia as a p53 activating signal to induce apoptosis

The wild-type p53 protein is well known as a "guardian of the genome" responsible for monitoring cellular state and responding to stress by inducing cell cycle arrest, senescence, or apoptosis. When p53 function is lost, the cell loses an efficient gatekeeper, allowing cells to survive and proliferate unchecked. Thus, it could be expected that selection pressures exist to lose or inactivate p53, resulting in clonal expansion of cells. Human cancers are characterized by intra-tumoural hypoxia and physiological responses triggered by hypoxia impact on all critical aspects of cancer progression, including immortalization, transformation, differentiation, genetic instability, angiogenesis, metabolic adaptation, autocrine growth factor signalling, invasion, metastasis and resistance to therapy.

Interestingly, one of the first links between tumour hypoxia and a specific cancer genetic programme was demonstrated by Giaccia and colleagues, showing that loss of the functional p53 tumour suppressor protein reduced hypoxia-induced cell death (Graeber et al., 1996). The authors proposed that O_2 deprivation provides a selective pressure within tumours for the clonal expansion of rare cells that bear p53 mutations. Although it is now generally accepted that hypoxia triggers accumulation of p53, there are still many unanswered questions. The molecular mechanism responsible for delivery of the hypoxic signal to p53 was proposed by An et al., who showed that p53 is stabilised by direct interaction with HIF-1α (An et al., 1998). However there is still considerable confusion within the field as to the exact nature of the relationship between HIF-1α and p53 (Pan et al., 2004). The complexity of this relationship is confounded by the finding that HIF-1α and p53 are differentially expressed and stabilised in response to differing oxygen concentrations (reviewed in Hammond & Giaccia, 2005).

Following DNA damage, p53 assembles as a homo-tetramer that binds to specific target sequences on DNA and can thereby activate or repress expression of a relatively large number of genes that ultimately influence cell cycle arrest or apoptosis, genome stability, cellular senescence and angiogenesis. In response to a wide range of stress stimuli, wild type (wt) p53 becomes active as a transcription factor and promotes transcription of cell cycle regulating genes such as *CDKN1A* (p21[waf1/cip1]) as well as genes involved in apoptotic events such as *BAX* or *FAS*, that are involved in the intrinsic and extrinsic apoptotic pathways, respectively. Importantly, p53 is also sensitive to hypoxia, although the manner of p53 expression, activation and transactivation capacity is different under hypoxia from other stresses, showing increase in protein level, reduction of transcriptional activity, enhancement of transrepression and promoting apoptosis.

Both *in vitro* and *in vivo* experiments showed that these effects are not cell-type specific and that the increase in p53 levels after hypoxia is through a post-transcriptional mechanism (Koumenis et al., 2001). In contrast to genotoxic stress, hypoxia-induced p53 induces apoptosis through a trans-activation-independent mechanism (Ashcroft et al., 2000). Accordingly, p53 induced by hypoxic conditions fails to associate with the coactivator p300 but is instead in complex with the co-repressor molecule mSin3A (Koumenis et al., 2001). Hammond and co-workers identified a set of genes repressed by hypoxia in a p53-dependent manner. They also investigated p53 regions involved in this response and identified residues 25-26 and 53-54, which are present in p53 transactivation domains, as essential for repression of gene transcription, since mutation of all four of these residues is sufficient to abolish both p53-dependent repression and the ability to induce apoptosis under hypoxia in oncogenically transformed cells (Hammond et al., 2006b).

Thus, the decrease in p53 transactivation and increase in p53 transrepression under hypoxia is a strategy for the cell to adapt to hypoxia. Inducing a series of genes to synthesize new mRNA costs much energy and thus consumes more oxygen. In cells under hypoxia, it is much easier for p53 to inhibit expression of a series of genes than to transactivate them. This is partly attributed to the transactivation of HIF-1, which requires the presence of the transcriptional coactivator CBP/p300. HIF-1 may attract CBP/p300 away from p53, inhibiting p53 transactivation under hypoxia.

Different mechanisms of p53 regulated apoptosis in response to hypoxia

The important role of p53 in mediating apoptosis in the hypoxic regions of tumours has been demonstrated in many publications. During the initial phases, hypoxia induces inner mitochondrial membrane permeabilization resulting in cytochrome c release from mitochondria and the formation of the apoptosome, which includes Apaf-1 and caspase-9. The loss of either caspase-9 or Apaf-1 leads to an increase in tumourigenicity, which was attributed to the loss of p53-dependent apoptosis within hypoxic regions of tumours (Soengas et al., 1999). It is well appreciated that p53 activation can lead to the induction of numerous proteins with pro-apoptotic activity. In particular, *PUMA*, *NOXA* and *BAX* are p53-regulated genes that play a role in mitochondrial apoptosis. Puma and Noxa belong to the BH-3 only proteins, which antagonize the effect of the anti-apoptotic protein Bcl-2, whereas Bax leads to the formation of pores in the inner mitochondrial membrane, causing release of cytochrome c into the cytoplasm and activation of Apaf.

HIF-1 is also able to induce several pro-apoptotic BH3-only genes, including *BNIP3*, *NIX* and *NOXA*. *BNIP3* is up-regulated under hypoxic conditions through an HRE-element located in its promoter region (Bruick, 2000). Its death promoting activities are characterized by mitochondrial localization, loss of mitochondrial membrane potential and ROS formation (Van de Velde et al., 2000). Using cDNA arrays and serial analysis of gene expression, a homologue of BNIP3, NIX, was identified as hypoxia-inducible and reported to be expressed at higher rates in breast carcinoma compared with normal tissue (Sowter et al., 2001). Another BH3-only protein regulated by HIF-1 is Noxa, which, like the two above-mentioned BH3-only proteins, increases the permeability of mitochondria and leads to the release of cytochromec into the cytoplasm.

The fact that both HIF-1 and p53 induce pro-apoptotic gene expression suggests that HIF-1 potentiates the effect of p53 to induce apoptosis. However, the situation in hypoxic tumour cells is more complex. Thus, the effect of anti-apoptotic pro-survival genes e.g. *IGF2* and *TGF-α* that are also induced by HIF-1 can outweigh the effect of proteins that lead to the induction of apoptosis. Moreover, the effect of pro-apoptotic gene induction by HIF-1 can be reduced by promoter methylation; hypermethylation of CpG islands in the *BNIP3* promoter may account for down-regulation of the protein in pancreatic adenocarcinomas compared with normal pancreas (Okami et al., 2004). Thus, silencing of pro-apoptotic genes may contribute to the survival and progression of cancers in a hypoxic environment. In addition to these complexities in regulation of apoptotic genes in hypoxic cancer cells, several investigators have shown that hypoxia and activation of HSF-1 are responsible for restricting the ability of p53 to trigger apoptosis, suggesting that simultaneous activation of HIF-1 and p53 may contribute to resistance of tumours to chemotherapy (Achison & Hupp, 2003; Li et al., 2004).

At least some of the apparent discrepancies in the roles of p53 and HIF-1 in regulating apoptosis during hypoxia are accounted for by the unusual properties of hypoxia-activated p53. Yu et al showed that p53-dependent, hypoxia-induced apoptosis is mediated via Puma and its effect on Bax (Yu et al., 2003). On the other hand, some studies have also determined that Puma is induced by hypoxia and leads to Bax-mediated apoptosis by a p53-independent mechanism (Nelson et al., 2004). Similarly, hypoxia-induced endoplasmic reticulum stress has been shown to increase Puma levels in a p53-independent manner (Reimertz et al., 2003; Romero-Ramirez et al., 2004). Although Noxa is a p53 target in response to many stresses, in response to hypoxia it is not p53 but HIF-1α that drives Noxa expression (Kim et al., 2004). Taken together, recent investigations suggest that the BH3 proapoptotic downstream targets of p53 do not appear to be direct p53 targets under hypoxic conditions. In fact, as mentioned above, hypoxia-induced p53 was dubbed transcriptionally incompetent due to an apparent failure to trans-activate many of the previously identified p53 target genes (Ashcroft et al., 2000). These observations suggest that in response to hypoxia, p53 plays a less important role as a transcriptional activator, but rather functions as a transrepressor and it is HIF-1α that takes over the role of p53 in inducing pro-apoptotic genes.

The mechanism for hypoxia-induced transrepression by p53 is related to interactions of p53 with co-repressors. Following hypoxia, p53 was shown to interact with the mSin3a co-repressor molecule and with histone dea-cetylases (HDACs) to form a repression complex specifically recogniz-ing promoters of target genes such as *survivin*, a well known inhibitor of apoptosis (Hassig et al., 1998; Mirza et al., 2002). The N-terminus of p53 includes a proline-rich domain (amino acids 61–75), which has been identified as the mSin3a binding site. Importantly, the interaction of p53 with mSin3a was demonstrated to protect p53 from proteasome-mediated degradation through an MDM2-independent mechanism (Zilfou et al., 2001). One likely explanation for induction of transrepression is that at the low oxygen con-centrations required to induce p53 accumulation and DNA-synthesis stops, followed by a rapid decrease in both transcription and translation levels (Koumenis et al., 2002; Denko et al., 2003). Thus, it could be speculated that in this stressful environment it is more efficient to act negatively than to induce synthesis of mRNA and proteins. On the other hand, it should be added that HIF-1 transactivates genes important for adaptation to low oxygen levels. Alternatively, hypoxia could also down-regulate or inhibit the inter-action of p53 with an accessory factor required for p53-transactivation, or hypoxia-induced p53 may not be modified appropriately to be transactiva-tion competent (Figure 8.1). None of these hypotheses are mutually exclusive and are supported to different degrees by data in the literature.

Finally, in relation to the mechanisms of p53-mediated apoptosis, it is worth noting that several reports indicate a role for p53 in the cytoplasm and specifically at the mitochondria, implying that stabilised p53 acts directly at the mitochondria to affect the release of cytochrome c to trigger

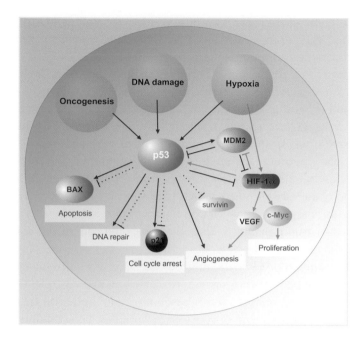

Figure 8.1 _ Schematic representation of p53 regulation under hypoxia and other stress stimuli. In response to stress (e.g. DNA damage; oncogene activation), p53 protein levels are elevated and trigger cellular response (red lines/ arrows) such as apoptosis, cell cycle arrest and DNA repair. Under hypoxia, p53 transcriptional activity is at least partially reduced, or p53 acts as transrepressor (dashed black lines/arrows). Activation of HIF-1α (blue lines/arrows) in response to hypoxia involves *inter alia* the accumulation of p53, which can destabilize HIF-1α by activating MDM2 expression. The combination of these effects results in the growth arrest or cell death observed in normal cells exposed to hypoxia.

apoptosis (Sansome et al., 2001; Chipuk et al., 2004). Although most data indicates that hypoxia-induced p53 is entirely nuclear, it is certainly conceivable that a portion of hypoxia-stabilised p53 translocates from the nucleus to the cytoplasm.

P53, cell cycle arrest and genome maintenance in hypoxia and acidic pH

A major role of wild-type p53 is in the activation of cell cycle checkpoints after genotoxic damage, to allow efficient repair and ensure genomic stability. The most important p53-induced proteins are p21[waf1/cip1] (the product of the *CDKN1A* gene), stopping the cell cycle at G_1 phase, and 14-3-3-σ leading to cell cycle arrest at G_2. Experimental evidence to date suggests that many human tumours contain hypoxic sub-populations and that hypoxia can induce G_1 or intra-S phase growth arrest. It was also shown that activation of HIF-1 interferes with p53-dependent cell cycle arrest. Thus, HIF-1 induces expression of proteins that stimulate proliferation, such as Insulin-like growth factor-2 (IGF2) and Transforming growth factor-α (TGF-α).

However, activated HIF-1 may also participate directly in cell cycle arrest at G_1/S. The crucial effector in this checkpoint is again p21[waf1/cip1], which is regulated by several transcription factors including p53, SMAD and Myc. The tumour suppressor proteins, p53, SMAD3 and SMAD4, enhance the expression of p21[waf1/cip1], whereas the oncogenic Myc protein functions as a repressor. HIF-1 induces cell cycle arrest by functionally counteracting Myc by displacing Myc from the *CDKN1A* promoter (Koshiji et al., 2004). It would seem logical to expect that the induction of p21[waf1/cip1] is beneficial to suppress the tumour phenotype. However, the cell cycle arrest induced by p21[waf1/cip1] may promote cancer cell survival by allowing DNA repair and preventing the initiation of apoptosis, and this pro-survival property may counteract its tumour-suppressive functions as a growth inhibitor.

Hypoxia may or may not always cause DNA damage during S-phase, but it has been suggested that re-oxygenation produces reactive oxygen species (ROS) that generate DNA damage, including DNA single-strand breaks (SSBs) and possibly DNA double-strand breaks (DSBs), that elicits a Chk2-dependent G_2 checkpoint. Indeed, *CHK2*-deficient cells do not undergo G_2 arrest following hypoxia and instead undergo apoptosis (Gibson et al., 2005; Freiberg et al., 2006). In these conditions, hypoxia-induced cell cycle checkpoints are controlled by the p21[waf1/cip1]–Cyclin E–Cdk2 (cyclin-dependent kinase 2); Atm–p53–Chk2; and Atr–Chk1 pathways, and by the regulation of Brca1 (Bindra et al., 2005; Hammond et al., 2006a).

In addition to hypoxia, low pH and nutrient deprivation are common features of the tumour microenvironment and pH is another potentially important stress signal involved in regulation of p53 signalling under hypoxic conditions. Indeed, recent research has focused on the effects of hypoxia and acidity on the apoptotic and DNA repair pathways in human cells. Several studies suggest that genetic instability due to low pH and hypoxia is the additive result of increased DNA damage, defective DNA repair and enhanced mutagenesis (Yuan et al., 2000; Mihaylova et al., 2003). Dregoesc et al. examined the effect of hypoxia alone and hypoxia combined with decreased pH on p53 expression, nucleotide excision repair, cellular sensitivity to UV-damage and viability in human primary fibroblasts and tumour-derived cell lines. Interestingly, they found early up-regulation of p53 and increased repair of UV-damaged DNA under hypoxia coupled with low pH compared to hypoxia alone, indicating different cellular response relating to the specific cellular conditions (Dregoesc & Rainbow, 2009). These results suggest that an early transient p53-dependent increase in nucleotide excision repair is due to the low pH conditions, rather than hypoxia. The data highlights the role of tumour microenviroment in modifying the response of tumours to radiation and/or chemotherapy, as DNA repair is a crucial factor for differential tumour radiosensitivity and chemosensitivity.

The role of p53 in hypoxia induced angiogenesis

The formation of new blood vessels is a crucial step in tumour growth and progression to alleviate hypoxia. HIF-1 is the principal transcription factor involved in the hypoxic response and is responsible for, among other things, inducing angiogenesis and glycolytic metabolism. The expression of HIF-1 correlates with hypoxia-induced angiogenesis mainly as a result of the induction of the major HIF-1 target gene, vascular endothelial cell growth factor (*VEGF*). Moeller *et al* found that ionizing radiation significantly up-regulates HIF-1 activity in tumours (Moeller et al., 2004). Radiation causes tumour oxygenation to increase both the accumulation of tumour-reactive oxygen/nitrogen species and the depolymerization of stress granules. These two events lead to increased expression and activity of HIF-1. As a result, expression of HIF-1-regulated cytokines delivers survival signals to tumour endothelium, resulting in radioresistance through vascular radioprotection. However, HIF-1 may also serve to radiosensitize tumours through mechanisms that include increasing apoptotic potential, proliferation rates, and ATP metabolism (Moeller et al., 2005). *Inter alia*, HIF-1 is also a requisite for enhancement of radiation-induced p53 activation by hypoxia and ultimately may be needed for HIF-1-mediated potentiation of radiation-induced apoptosis by hypoxia.

   Oncogenic regulation of angiogenesis has also been suggested, either alone or working in combination with hypoxia. For example, up-regulation of H-Ras and Epidermal Growth Factor Receptor (EGFR) and inactivation of p53 can increase rates of synthesis of HIF-1α to a level that overwhelms the capacity of the degradation pathway to eliminate it (Feldkamp et al., 1999). The increase in HIF-1α synthesis appears to be regulated by the PI3K–AKT pathway (Jiang & Liu, 2008). Thus, tumours may stimulate angiogenesis even before hypoxia arises.

HIF-1 – p53 protein interactions

As discussed elsewhere, the hypoxia inducible transcription factor (HIF) is a key regulator of the cellular response to hypoxia. HIF is composed of 2 subunits, an α-subunit that is oxygen labile but which is rapidly stabilised in response to low oxygen conditions and a β-subunit that is constitutively expressed. Together the α and β subunits form a potent transcription factor, which recognizes specific promoter elements known as hypoxia response elements (HREs). HIF-1 also mediates the accumulation of p53 in response to hypoxia (An et al., 1998), as well as there being a role for p53 in inhibiting HIF-1α stabilisation (Ravi et al., 2000). More recently, the Fersht laboratory showed that HIF-1α exists as an unfolded protein and, because of this feature, resembles DNA. They speculate that the DNA binding or core domain of p53 therefore recognizes HIF-1α and binds to the oxygen-dependent degradation domain region (Sanchez-Puig et al., 2005), which fits with the findings that hypoxia-induced p53 does not transactivate its usual target genes, but rather acts as a transcriptional repressor.

HIF and p53 interaction with molecular chaperones

Molecular chaperones are known to maintain protein homeostasis by folding polypeptide chains, protecting proteins from denaturation and removing unfolded or aggregated proteins. The molecular chaperones are particularly important for the survival of cancer cells due to their exposure to different kinds of stress including genetic instability and hypoxia. The molecular chaperone Hsp90 is often termed a "cancer chaperone" due to exclusive roles in the activation of several oncogenic proteins. Hsp90 is unique in its ability to stabilise certain mutated proteins, which enables them to express the oncogenic phenotype. Hsp90 activity is highly increased in advanced tumours compared to normal tissues and tumour cells become dependent on Hsp90 function. Hsp90 is a major regulator of transcription factors that play important roles in cancer. Both p53 and HIF-1 interact with Hsp90, which is involved in their stabilisation and folding. The pro-oncogenic properties of Hsp90 are particularly expressed in stabilisation of p53 mutants and HIF-1 under hypoxia. The inhibition of Hsp90 results in ubiquitination and proteasomal degradation of its client proteins. The unfolded client proteins bind the chaperone Hsp70, which leads to ubiquitination by Chaperone Interacting Protein (CHIP) which functions as an E3 ubiquitin ligase. Several recent studies show that CHIP may act as a tumour suppressor that counterbalances the hyperactivity of Hsp90 in tumours, because CHIP was shown to ubiquitinate not only chaperone clients but also Hsp70 and Hsp90 themselves. The tumour-suppressor function of CHIP is further supported by observations of its down-regulation during malignant transformation, where the CHIP levels negatively correlate with tumour progression. Naito et al. has also shown that the level of CHIP is decreased under hypoxic conditions in myocardium. This observation suggests that HIF may be involved in the activation of the Hsp90 chaperone system by silencing the expression of CHIP (Naito et al., 2010).

p53 and HIF in the regulation of glucose metabolism

Otto Warburg discovered that cancer cells have consistently higher rates of glycolysis than normal cells, known as the Warburg effect, and this phenomenon is characteristic of virtually all cancers (Gatenby & Gillies, 2004). Although for many years considered to be a by-product of the oncogenic process, recent evidence suggests that this shift to high rates of glycolysis (which persists even under conditions of normal oxygen, and is therefore known as aerobic glycolysis) is required for malignant progression (Bui & Thompson, 2006). The underlying mechanisms leading to the Warburg effect include mitochondrial changes, up-regulation of rate-limiting glycolytic enzymes, intracellular pH regulation, hypoxia-induced switch to anaerobic metabolism and metabolic reprogramming after loss of p53 function.

p53 is well described as a sensor of genotoxic stress but also serves as a sensor of many other stresses including glucose starvation and hypoxia. Glucose or oxygen starvation in proliferating cells is reflected by an increase of adenosine mono-phosphate AMP, which leads to the activation of AMPK (AMP kinase) (Jones et al., 2005). p53 is a direct target of AMPK which is phosphorylated and activated in response of increased AMP. This activation of p53 is followed by gene expression changes resulting in reversible G1/S cell cycle arrest. This glucose-dependent cell cycle check-point demonstrates the importance of p53 for protection of proliferating cells against metabolic stress.

The role of p53 in regulating glucose metabolism is analogous to HIF in the sense that they both participate in the regulation of genes that are directly involved in glucose metabolism (Figure 8.2). Activation of HIF under hypoxic conditions switches glucose metabolism to anaerobic glycolysis by enhancing the expression of key enzymes of this metabolic pathway. Thus, HIF enhances expression of Adenylate kinase-3, Aldolase-A,C (*ALDA,C*), Enolase-1 (*ENO1*). Glucose transporter-1,3 (*GLU1,3*), Glyceraldehyde phosphate dehydrogenase (*GAPDH*), Hexokinase 1,2 (*HK1,2*), Lactate dehydrogenase-A (*LDHA*), Pyruvate kinase M (*PKM*), Phosphofructokinase L (*PFKL*), Phosphoglycerate kinase 1 (PGK1) and 6-phosphofructo-2-kinase/gructose-2,6-bisphosphate-3 (*PFKFB3*). In general terms, it seems that p53 activation leads to the expression of genes that facilitate the utilization of pyruvate in mitochondrial respiration. Therefore, p53 activation prevents the metabolic switch towards glycolysis. Recently, p53 was shown to regulate the expression of *SCO2* (Synthesis of cytochrome c oxidase 2). This enzyme plays the key role in cytochrome c synthesis, an essential cofactor for enzymes involved in mitochondrial respiration. Levels of p53 in normal tissue appear to be sufficient to induce *SCO2* expression, which ensures the maintenance of the cytochrome c oxidase complex. Cells that lack functional p53 show lower oxygen consumption by mitochondrial respiration and a shift to glycolysis for the production of energy, thereby contributing to the Warburg effect.

The transrepression of genes participating in glycolysis is another mechanism through which p53 can reduce the rate of glycolysis in cancer cells. Kondoh et al. demonstrated that p53 is involved in repression of phosphoglycerate mutase (*PGM*) which is responsible for conversion of 3-phosphoglycerate to 2-phosphoglycerate during glycolytic process (Kondoh et al., 2005).

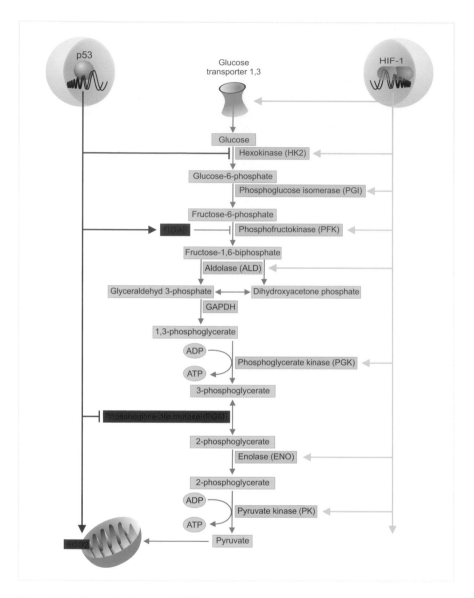

Figure 8.2 _ The role of p53 and HIF in glycolysis and respiration. The tumour suppressor p53 decelerates anaerobic glycolysis by induction of TIGAR and suppression of phosphoglycerate mutase (PGM). The utilization of pyruvate for oxidative phosphorylation is enhanced by p53 mediated induction of SCO2. In contrast to p53, HIF enhances the expression of enzymes that accelerate the glycolytic process in the absence of oxygen.

The role of p53-family members, p63 and p73, in hypoxia

Although p53 was thought to be unique for many years due to failure to identify similar proteins, 13 years ago two homologues were identified by chance (Kaghad et al., 1997; Schmale & Bamberger, 1997). These proteins are similar to p53 in sequence and structure, containing similar N-terminal transactivation (TA) domains, highly homologous DNA binding domains, and related tetramerization domains. It was quickly realized that these two genes, now known as *TP63* and *TP73* to reflect their similarity with *TP53*, each give rise to a variety of different protein isoforms through the use of alternative promoters and alternative splicing of 3' exons (Moll & Slade, 2004). In particular, both p63 and p73 can be produced as N-terminally shortened proteins that lack the transactivation (TA) domain, and these ΔN isoforms are therefore able to act as antagonists for the TA isoforms. Although highly similar in sequence to p53, the main functions of p63 and p73 seem to lie in the regulation of development, as evidenced by the developmental abnormalities and lack of tumours seen in p63-null and p73-null mice (Yang et al., 1999; Yang et al., 2000). On the other hand, p63 and p73 are able to transactivate a wide range of genes that are also subject to regulation by p53.

When considering the functions of p63 and p73, it is vital to recognize the tissue- and cell specific expression of the different isoforms, and their relative capacities for transactivation and repression. For example, ΔNp63 isoforms are highly expressed in epithelial tissues, particularly in basal epithelia and in squamous cancers (Nylander et al., 2002; Thurfjell et al., 2004), whereas TAp63 isoforms are expressed in some lymphocytes and lymphomas (Nylander et al., 2002). In most cases, p63α isoforms are the most prevalent, although other C-terminal isoforms can also be found (Thurfjell et al., 2004). Notably, there is good evidence that the p63β isoforms have more transactivation ability than p63α or p63γ, with the latter showing a higher repression capacity (Boldrup et al., 2009). In the same way, p73 isoforms show a highly restricted expression pattern (Nenutil et al., 2003) and different isoforms show different DNA-binding and transcriptional activities (Blint et al., 2002; Holcakova et al., 2008), making it difficult to identify the overall effects of p63 or p73 expression in any individual circumstance.

In relation to the role of p63 in response to hypoxia, TAp63γ, like p53, can repress the expression of VEGF, whilst ΔNp63α induces VEGF expression. In both cases, p63 regulation of VEGF operates through a HIF-1 binding site in the VEGF promoter (Senoo et al., 2002). The mechanism for reciprocal regulation of VEGF was proposed to relate to the ability of TAp63γ to target HIF-1 for degradation and of ΔNp63α to stabilise HIF-1. Two-hybrid assays provided evidence that HIF-1-dependent transcription is repressed by TAp63 and p53, but is enhanced by DNp63 through cooperation with the p300 co-activator (Senoo et al., 2002). Similarly, p73 was shown to repress VEGF expression, similar to p53 (Salimath et al., 2000), although p73 has also been shown to induce VEGF (Vikhanskaya et al., 2001). In these studies, the effect of p73 was related to p53 status, with p73 repressing VEGF in cells that lack p53 or express a mutant p53, suggesting that p73 acts as a competitor of wild-type p53 (Vikhanskaya et al., 2001). However, it is not clear, which p73 isoform was expressed in these experiments. Further evidence for a role of p73 in reducing hypoxia in tumour growth comes from clinical studies that have shown that p73 expression correlates with both VEGF expression and with tumour vascularity, although again it is unclear which p73 isoforms are responsible (Guan et al., 2003). More recently, the levels of VEGF were found to correlate with both TAp73 and ΔNp73 isoforms in human cancers and it was suggested that this may be a property of the ΔNp73 isoforms dominantly inhibiting TAp73 isoforms (Diaz et al., 2008). These studies highlight the complexity of p73 expression patterns and the difficulty of surmising function from protein or mRNA levels of isoforms that may have opposing functions.

In addition to the ability to regulate HIF-1 and angiogenesis, there is also data to indicate that hypoxia can itself regulate the expression of p63 and p73. In an ischaemia model in the brain, the levels of ΔNp63 and ΔNp73 were found to increase, with a particular rise in the levels of p63β isoforms. The levels of TAp63 and TAp73 decrease in association with increases in the ZEB1 transcriptional repressor that is responsible for silencing TAp73 expression, and ΔNp63β was shown to promote ZEB1 expression (Bui et al., 2009). This data indicates a complex interplay of p63 and p73 in regulating cell survival under reduced oxygen conditions and indicates that distinct isoforms of both p63 and p73 have different functions. The role of this ΔNp63β -ZEB1-TAp73 axis in neuronal hypoxia requires further investigation in other hypoxic conditions, including cancer.

Concluding remarks

The p53 protein has multiple interactions with hypoxia, including effects on HIF-1 activity. In particular, wild-type p53 acts as a repressor of adaptation to hypoxia, such that loss of p53 activity in human tumour cells allows them to survive more easily under hypoxic growth conditions. Indeed, hypoxia may itself serve as a selective pressure for the emergence of tumour cell clones that have acquired p53 mutation or inactivation. The effects of p53 on HIF-1 and hypoxia can be modified by the actions of the p63 and p73 family members, particularly the ΔN isoforms of these proteins that can antagonize p53 function. The complexity of expression of each of these proteins and the production of distinct isoforms with distinct properties implies that our understanding of the role(s) of p53 in influencing the effects of hypoxia is far from complete.

A c k n o w l e d g e m e n t s _ RH, PM and BV are funded by MZ0MOU2005, IGA MZCR NT/13794-4/2012 and the European Regional Development Fund (RECAMO; CZ 1.05/2.1.00/03.0101). All authors declare that there are no conflicts of interest.

References

Achison M, Hupp TR (2003). Hypoxia attenuates the p53 response to cellular damage. Oncogene 22(22): 3431-40.

An WG, Kanekal M, Simon MC, Maltepe E, Blagosklonny MV, Neckers LM (1998). Stabilisation of wild-type p53 by hypoxia-inducible factor 1alpha. Nature 392(6674): 405-8.

Appella E, Anderson CW (2001). Post-translational modifications and activation of p53 by genotoxic stresses. Eur J Biochem 268(10): 2764-72.

Ashcroft M, Taya Y, Vousden KH (2000). Stress signals utilize multiple pathways to stabilize p53. Mol Cell Biol 20(9): 3224-33.

Asker C, Wiman KG, Selivanova G (1999). p53-induced apoptosis as a safeguard against cancer. Biochem Biophys Res Commun 265(1): 1-6.

Avivi A, Ashur-Fabian O, Amariglio N, Nevo E, Rechavi G (2005). p53–a key player in tumoural and evolutionary adaptation: a lesson from the Israeli blind subterranean mole rat. Cell Cycle 4(3): 368-72.

Baker SJ, Fearon ER, Nigro JM, Hamilton SR, Preisinger AC, Jessup JM, vanTuinen P, Ledbetter DH, Barker DF, Nakamura Y, White R, Vogelstein B (1989). Chromosome 17 deletions and p53 gene mutations in colorectal carcinomas. Science 244(4901): 217-21.

Banin S, Moyal L, Shieh S, Taya Y, Anderson CW, Chessa L, Smorodinsky NI, Prives C, Reiss Y, Shiloh Y, Ziv Y (1998). Enhanced phosphorylation of p53 by ATM in response to DNA damage. Science 281(5383): 1674-7.

Bargonetti J, Manfredi JJ, Chen X, Marshak DR, Prives C (1993). A proteolytic fragment from the central region of p53 has marked sequence-specific DNA-binding activity when generated from wild-type but not from oncogenic mutant p53 protein. Genes Dev 7(12B): 2565-74.

Bindra RS, Gibson SL, Meng A, Westermark U, Jasin M, Pierce AJ, Bristow RG, Classon MK, Glazer PM (2005). Hypoxia-induced down-regulation of BRCA1 expression by E2Fs. Cancer Res 65(24): 11597-604.

Blint E, Phillips AC, Kozlov S, Stewart CL, Vousden KH (2002). Induction of p57(KIP2) expression by p73beta. Proc Natl Acad Sci U S A 99(6): 3529-34.

Boldrup L, Coates PJ, Gu X, Nylander K (2009). DeltaNp63 isoforms differentially regulate gene expression in squamous cell carcinoma: identification of Cox-2 as a novel p63 target. J Pathol 218(4): 428-36.

Bruick RK (2000). Expression of the gene encoding the proapoptotic Nip3 protein is induced by hypoxia. Proc Natl Acad Sci U S A 97(16): 9082-7.

Bui T, Thompson CB (2006). Cancer's sweet tooth. Cancer Cell 9(6): 419-20.

Bui T, Sequeira J, Wen TC, Sola A, Higashi Y, Kondoh H, Genetta T (2009). ZEB1 links p63 and p73 in a novel neuronal survival pathway rapidly induced in response to cortical ischaemia. PLoS One 4(2): e4373.

Canman CE, Lim DS, Cimprich KA, Taya Y, Tamai K, Sakaguchi K, Appella E, Kastan MB, Siliciano JD (1998). Activation of the ATM kinase by ionizing radiation and phosphorylation of p53. Science 281(5383): 1677-9.

Carter S, Vousden KH (2009). Modifications of p53: competing for the lysines. Curr Opin Genet Dev 19(1): 18-24.

Chipuk JE, Kuwana T, Bouchier-Hayes L, Droin NM, Newmeyer DD, Schuler M, Green DR (2004). Direct activation of Bax by p53 mediates mitochondrial membrane permeabilization and apoptosis. Science 303(5660): 1010-4.

Cho Y, Gorina S, Jeffrey PD, Pavletich NP (1994). Crystal structure of a p53 tumour suppressor-DNA complex: understanding tumourigenic mutations. Science 265(5170): 346-55.

Denko N, Wernke-Dollries K, Johnson AB, Hammond E, Chiang CM, Barton MC (2003). Hypoxia actively represses transcription by inducing negative cofactor 2 (Dr1/DrAP1) and blocking preinitiation complex assembly. J Biol Chem 278(8): 5744-9.

Diaz R, Pena C, Silva J, Lorenzo Y, Garcia V, Garcia JM, Sanchez A, Espinosa P, Yuste R, Bonilla F, Dominguez G (2008). p73 Isoforms affect VEGF, VEGF165b and PEDF expression in human colorectal tumours: VEGF165b downregulation as a marker of poor prognosis. Int J Cancer 123(5): 1060-7.

Dregoesc D, Rainbow AJ (2009). Differential effects of hypoxia and acidosis on p53 expression, repair of UVC-damaged DNA and viability after UVC in normal and tumour-derived human cells. DNA Repair (Amst) 8(3): 370-82.

Feldkamp MM, Lau N, Rak J, Kerbel RS, Guha A (1999). Normoxic and hypoxic regulation of vascular endothelial growth factor (VEGF) by astrocytoma cells is mediated by Ras. Int J Cancer 81(1): 118-24.

Freiberg RA, Hammond EM, Dorie MJ, Welford SM, Giaccia AJ (2006). DNA damage during reoxygenation elicits a Chk2-dependent checkpoint response. Mol Cell Biol 26(5): 1598-609.

Gatenby RA, Gillies RJ (2004). Why do cancers have high aerobic glycolysis? Nat Rev Cancer 4(11): 891-9.

Gibson SL, Bindra RS, Glazer PM (2005). Hypoxia-induced phosphorylation of Chk2 in an ataxia telangiectasia mutated-dependent manner. Cancer Res 65(23): 10734-41.

Graeber TG, Osmanian C, Jacks T, Housman DE, Koch CJ, Lowe SW, Giaccia AJ (1996). Hypoxia-mediated selection of cells with diminished apoptotic potential in solid tumours. Nature 379(6560): 88-91.

Guan M, Peng HX, Yu B, Lu Y (2003). p73 Overexpression and angiogenesis in human colorectal carcinoma. Jpn J Clin Oncol 33(5): 215-20.

Hammond EM, Giaccia AJ (2005). The role of p53 in hypoxia-induced apoptosis. Biochem Biophys Res Commun 331(3): 718-25.

Hammond EM, Freiberg RA, Giaccia AJ (2006a). The roles of Chk 1 and Chk 2 in hypoxia and reoxygenation. Cancer Lett 238(2): 161-7.

Hammond EM, Mandell DJ, Salim A, Krieg AJ, Johnson TM, Shirazi HA, Attardi LD, Giaccia AJ (2006b). Genome-wide analysis of p53 under hypoxic conditions. Mol Cell Biol 26(9): 3492-504.

Hassig CA, Tong JK, Fleischer TC, Owa T, Grable PG, Ayer DE, Schreiber SL (1998). A role for histone deacetylase activity in HDAC1-mediated transcriptional repression. Proc Natl Acad Sci U S A 95(7): 3519-24.

Holcakova J, Ceskova P, Hrstka R, Muller P, Dubska L, Coates PJ, Palecek E, Vojtesek B (2008). The cell type-specific effect of TAp73 isoforms on the cell cycle and apoptosis. Cell Mol Biol Lett 13(3): 404-20.

Hupp TR, Meek DW, Midgley CA, Lane DP (1993). Activation of the cryptic DNA binding function of mutant forms of p53. Nucleic Acids Res 21(14): 3167-74.

Jiang BH, Liu LZ (2008). AKT signalling in regulating angiogenesis. Curr Cancer Drug Targets 8(1): 19-26.

Jones RG, Plas DR, Kubek S, Buzzai M, Mu J, Xu Y, Birnbaum MJ, Thompson CB (2005). AMP-activated protein kinase induces a p53-dependent metabolic checkpoint. Mol Cell 18(3): 283-93.

Kaghad M, Bonnet H, Yang A, Creancier L, Biscan JC, Valent A, Minty A, Chalon P, Lelias JM, Dumont X, Ferrara P, McKeon F, Caput D (1997). Monoallelically expressed gene related to p53 at 1p36, a region frequently deleted in neuroblastoma and other human cancers. Cell 90(4): 809-19.

Kim JY, Ahn HJ, Ryu JH, Suk K, Park JH (2004). BH3-only protein Noxa is a mediator of hypoxic cell death induced by hypoxia-inducible factor 1alpha. J Exp Med 199(1): 113-24.

Kondoh H, Lleonart ME, Gil J, Wang J, Degan P, Peters G, Martinez D, Carnero A, Beach D (2005). Glycolytic enzymes can modulate cellular life span. Cancer Res 65(1): 177-85.

Koshiji M, Kageyama Y, Pete EA, Horikawa I, Barrett JC, Huang LE (2004). HIF-1alpha induces cell cycle arrest by functionally counteracting Myc. Embo J 23(9): 1949-56.

Koumenis C, Alarcon R, Hammond E, Sutphin P, Hoffman W, Murphy M, Derr J, Taya Y, Lowe SW, Kastan M, Giaccia A (2001). Regulation of p53 by hypoxia: dissociation of transcriptional repression and apoptosis from p53-dependent transactivation. Mol Cell Biol 21(4): 1297-310.

Koumenis C, Naczki C, Koritzinsky M, Rastani S, Diehl A, Sonenberg N, Koromilas

A, Wouters BG (2002). Regulation of protein synthesis by hypoxia via activation of the endoplasmic reticulum kinase PERK and phosphorylation of the translation initiation factor eIF2alpha. Mol Cell Biol 22(21): 7405-16.

Lane DP, Crawford LV (1979). T antigen is bound to a host protein in SV40-transformed cells. Nature 278(5701): 261-3.

Lavin MF, Gueven N (2006). The complexity of p53 stabilisation and activation. Cell Death Differ 13(6): 941-50.

Li J, Zhang X, Sejas DP, Bagby GC, Pang Q (2004). Hypoxia-induced nucleophosmin protects cell death through inhibition of p53. J Biol Chem 279(40): 41275-9.

Linzer DI, Levine AJ (1979). Characterisation of a 54K dalton cellular SV40 tumour antigen present in SV40-transformed cells and uninfected embryonal carcinoma cells. Cell 17(1): 43-52.

Mihaylova VT, Bindra RS, Yuan J, Campisi D, Narayanan L, Jensen R, Giordano F, Johnson RS, Rockwell S, Glazer PM (2003). Decreased expression of the DNA mismatch repair gene Mlh1 under hypoxic stress in mammalian cells. Mol Cell Biol 23(9): 3265-73.

Miled C, Pontoglio M, Garbay S, Yaniv M, Weitzman JB (2005). A genomic map of p53 binding sites identifies novel p53 targets involved in an apoptotic network. Cancer Res 65(12): 5096-104.

Mirza A, McGuirk M, Hockenberry TN, Wu Q, Ashar H, Black S, Wen SF, Wang L, Kirschmeier P, Bishop WR, Nielsen LL, Pickett CB, Liu S (2002). Human survivin is negatively regulated by wild-type p53 and participates in p53-dependent apoptotic pathway. Oncogene 21(17): 2613-22.

Moeller BJ, Cao Y, Li CY, Dewhirst MW (2004). Radiation activates HIF-1 to regulate vascular radiosensitivity in tumours: role of reoxygenation, free radicals, and stress granules. Cancer Cell 5(5): 429-41.

Moeller BJ, Dreher MR, Rabbani ZN, Schroeder T, Cao Y, Li CY, Dewhirst MW (2005). Pleiotropic effects of HIF-1 blockade on tumour radiosensitivity. Cancer Cell 8(2): 99-110.

Moll UM, Slade N (2004). p63 and p73: roles in development and tumour formation. Mol Cancer Res 2(7): 371-86.

Naito AT, Okada S, Minamino T, Iwanaga K, Liu ML, Sumida T, Nomura S, Sahara N, Mizoroki T, Takashima A, Akazawa H, Nagai T, Shiojima I, Komuro I (2010). Promotion of CHIP-mediated p53 degradation protects the heart from ischemic injury. Circ Res 106(11): 1692-702.

Nelson DA, Tan TT, Rabson AB, Anderson D, Degenhardt K, White E (2004). Hypoxia and defective apoptosis drive genomic instability and tumourigenesis. Genes Dev 18(17): 2095-107.

Nenutil R, Ceskova P, Coates PJ, Nylander K, Vojtesek B (2003). Differential expression of p73alpha in normal ectocervical epithelium, cervical intraepithelial neoplasia, and invasive squamous cell carcinoma. Int J Gynecol Pathol 22(4): 386-92.

Nigro JM, Baker SJ, Preisinger AC, Jessup JM, Hostetter R, Cleary K, Bigner SH, Davidson N, Baylin S, Devilee P, et al. (1989). Mutations in the p53 gene occur in diverse human tumour types. Nature 342(6250): 705-8.

Nikinmaa M, Rees BB (2005). Oxygen-dependent gene expression in fishes. Am J Physiol Regul Integr Comp Physiol 288(5): R1079-90.

Nylander K, Vojtesek B, Nenutil R, Lindgren B, Roos G, Zhanxiang W, Sjostrom B, Dahlqvist A, Coates PJ (2002). Differential expression of p63 isoforms in normal tissues and neoplastic cells. J Pathol 198(4): 417-27.

Okami J, Simeone DM, Logsdon CD (2004). Silencing of the hypoxia-inducible cell death protein BNIP3 in pancreatic cancer. Cancer Res 64(15): 5338-46.

Oren M (1997). Lonely no more: p53 finds its kin in a tumour suppressor haven. Cell 90(5): 829-32.

Ou YH, Chung PH, Sun TP, Shieh SY (2005). p53 C-terminal phosphorylation by CHK1 and CHK2 participates in the regulation of DNA-damage-induced C-terminal acetylation. Mol Biol Cell 16(4): 1684-95.

Pan Y, Oprysko PR, Asham AM, Koch CJ, Simon MC (2004). p53 cannot be induced by hypoxia alone but responds to the hypoxic microenvironment. Oncogene 23(29): 4975-83.

Pietenpol JA, Tokino T, Thiagalingam S, el-Deiry WS, Kinzler KW, Vogelstein B (1994). Sequence-specific transcriptional activation is essential for growth suppression by p53. Proc Natl Acad Sci U S A 91(6): 1998-2002.

Ravi R, Mookerjee B, Bhujwalla ZM, Sutter CH, Artemov D, Zeng Q, Dillehay LE, Madan A, Semenza GL, Bedi A (2000). Regulation of tumour angiogenesis by p53-induced degradation of hypoxia-inducible factor 1alpha. Genes Dev 14(1): 34-44.

Reimertz C, Kogel D, Rami A, Chittenden T, Prehn JH (2003). Gene expression during ER stress-induced apoptosis in neurons: induction of the BH3-only protein Bbc3/PUMA and activation of the mitochondrial apoptosis pathway. J Cell Biol 162(4): 587-97.

Romero-Ramirez L, Cao H, Nelson D, Hammond E, Lee AH, Yoshida H, Mori K, Glimcher LH, Denko NC, Giaccia AJ, Le QT, Koong AC (2004). XBP1 is essential for survival under hypoxic conditions and is required for tumour growth. Cancer Res 64(17): 5943-7.

Salimath B, Marme D, Finkenzeller G (2000). Expression of the vascular endothelial growth factor gene is inhibited by p73. Oncogene 19(31): 3470-6.

Sanchez-Puig N, Veprintsev DB, Fersht AR (2005). Binding of natively unfolded HIF-1alpha ODD domain to p53. Mol Cell 17(1): 11-21.

Sansome C, Zaika A, Marchenko ND, Moll UM (2001). Hypoxia death stimulus induces translocation of p53 protein to mitochondria. Detection by immunofluorescence on whole cells. FEBS Lett 488(3): 110-5.

Schmale H, Bamberger C (1997). A novel protein with strong homology to the tumour suppressor p53. Oncogene 15(11): 1363-7.

Senoo M, Matsumura Y, Habu S (2002). TAp63gamma (p51A) and dNp63alpha (p73L), two major isoforms of the p63 gene, exert opposite effects on the vascular endothelial growth factor (VEGF) gene expression. Oncogene 21(16): 2455-65.

Soengas MS, Alarcon RM, Yoshida H, Giaccia AJ, Hakem R, Mak TW, Lowe SW (1999). Apaf-1 and caspase-9 in p53-dependent apoptosis and tumour inhibition. Science 284(5411): 156-9.

Sowter HM, Ratcliffe PJ, Watson P, Greenberg AH, Harris AL (2001). HIF-1-dependent regulation of hypoxic induction of the cell death factors BNIP3 and NIX in human tumours. Cancer Res 61(18): 6669-73.

Takagi M, Absalon MJ, McLure KG, Kastan MB (2005). Regulation of p53 translation and induction after DNA damage by ribosomal protein L26 and nucleolin. Cell 123(1): 49-63.

Thurfjell N, Coates PJ, Uusitalo T, Mahani D, Dabelsteen E, Dahlqvist A, Sjostrom B, Roos G, Nylander K (2004). Complex p63 mRNA isoform expression patterns in squamous cell carcinoma of the head and neck. Int J Oncol 25(1): 27-35.

Van de Velde C, Cizeau J, Dubik D, Alimonti J, Brown T, Israels S, Hakem R, Greenberg AH (2000). BNIP3 and genetic control of necrosis-like cell death through the mitochondrial permeability transition pore. Mol Cell Biol 20(15): 5454-68.

Vikhanskaya F, Bani MR, Borsotti P, Ghilardi C, Ceruti R, Ghisleni G, Marabese M, Giavazzi R, Broggini M, Taraboletti G (2001). p73 Overexpression increases VEGF and reduces thrombospondin-1 production: implications for tumour angiogenesis. Oncogene 20(50): 7293-300.

Waterman MJ, Stavridi ES, Waterman JL, Halazonetis TD (1998). ATM-dependent activation of p53 involves dephosphorylation and association with 14-3-3 proteins. Nat Genet 19(2): 175-8.

Woo RA, McLure KG, Lees-Miller SP, Rancourt DE, Lee PW (1998). DNA-dependent protein kinase acts upstream of p53 in response to DNA damage. Nature 394(6694): 700-4.

Yang A, Kaghad M, Wang Y, Gillett E, Fleming MD, Dotsch V, Andrews NC, Caput D, McKeon F (1998). p63, a p53 homolog at 3q27-29, encodes multiple products with transactivating, death-inducing, and dominant-negative activities. Mol Cell 2(3): 305-16.

Yang A, Schweitzer R, Sun D, Kaghad M, Walker N, Bronson RT, Tabin C, Sharpe A, Caput D, Crum C, McKeon F (1999). p63 is essential for regenerative proliferation in limb, craniofacial and epithelial development. Nature 398(6729): 714-8.

Yang A, Walker N, Bronson R, Kaghad M, Oosterwegel M, Bonnin J, Vagner C, Bonnet H, Dikkes P, Sharpe A, McKeon F, Caput D (2000). p73-deficient mice have neurological, pheromonal and inflammatory defects but lack spontaneous tumours. Nature 404(6773): 99-103.

Yu J, Wang Z, Kinzler KW, Vogelstein B, Zhang L (2003). PUMA mediates the apoptotic response to p53 in colorectal cancer cells. Proc Natl Acad Sci U S A 100(4): 1931-6.

Yuan J, Narayanan L, Rockwell S, Glazer PM (2000). Diminished DNA repair and elevated mutagenesis in mammalian cells exposed to hypoxia and low pH. Cancer Res 60(16): 4372-6.

Zilfou JT, Hoffman WH, Sank M, George DL, Murphy M (2001). The corepressor mSin3a interacts with the proline-rich domain of p53 and protects p53 from proteasome-mediated degradation. Mol Cell Biol 21(12): 3974-85.

Chapter 9

Hypoxia: A powerful signal to induce metabolic changes

Thomas Kietzmann[*]

[*]Author for correspondence:

Oulun yliopisto, Biokemian laitos, PL 3000, 90014 Oulun Yliopisto, Oulu, Finland

Tel: +358-85537713, Fax: +358-8-5531141, Thomas.Kietzmann@oulu.fi

Contents

Key points

— Most if not all cells of the human body possess the ability to activate an adaptive metabolic program responding to hypoxia.

— Hypoxia is ultimately linked to increased expression and activity of the hypoxia-inducible transcription factors (HIFs). Of the three HIFs known to date, HIF-1α is the best characterized.

— Many of the HIF-1α regulated genes encode enzymes of metabolic pathways. In addition, appearance of HIF-1α is associated with poor prognosis in cancer.

— Therefore, studying links and feedbacks between HIF-1α and metabolism is of major importance to find new therapeutic strategies for hypoxia-associated diseases.

Introduction

Aerobic living cells need a reliable system allowing adequate metabolic adaptation under limited oxygen concentrations, i.e. hypoxia. These adaptations aimed at supplying sufficient ATP necessary to maintain the vital cellular functions are achieved by changes in the redox and phosphorylation status of enzymes as well as by changes in the gene expression pattern. Hypoxia thereby increases expression and activity of hypoxia-inducible transcription factors, especially HIF-1α. In addition to the central role in the adaptive cellular program responding to hypoxia in normal tissues, enhanced levels of HIF-1α are also associated with intratumoural hypoxia and a poor prognosis in cancer patients. This has increased the interest in HIF-1α as a cancer drug target and understanding the links and feedback mechanisms between hypoxia and metabolism will help to find new and more specific therapeutic options.

Oxygen and metabolism

The regulation of oxygen delivery into cells and the control of cellular functions in response to oxygen are essential for all mammals. Under physiological conditions, the average oxygen tension in human arterial blood is between 74 and 104 mm Hg (104-146 µmol/l) and in venous blood between 34 and 46 mm Hg (48-64 µmol/l) (Piiper 1996; Greger and Bleich 1996). Under these normal physiological conditions, mammalian cells produce energy in the form of adenosine triphosphate (ATP), predominantly by aerobic conversion of glucose, fatty acids and amino acids to CO_2, H_2O and urea, respectively. In addition, small amounts of energy can be produced from the aerobic oxidative metabolism of lactate, glycerol or ethanol and by formation and utilisation of ketone bodies.

Once the major nutrient glucose has entered the cells via glucose transporters, it is converted to acetyl-CoA in the glycolytic pathway. Acetyl-CoA, which can also be gained from proteins and fatty acids is then transported to the mitochondria where it enters the citric acid (Krebs) cycle and becomes dehydrogenated to CO_2 and reducing equivalents in the form of three NADH and one $FADH_2$. The reducing equivalents are then required for the formation of a trans-membrane proton-motive force enabling ATP generation in mitochondria. The generated electrons thereby react with O_2, which is subsequently reduced to H_2O. Thus, under aerobic conditions, energy production might also be referred to as a redox process that occurs during combustion of food-derived energy substrates serving as electron donors, and molecular oxygen serving as an electron acceptor.

By contrast, under anaerobic conditions, energy can only be gained by conversion of carbohydrates which are only partially dehydrogenated to pyruvate under formation of NADH. The electrons from NADH are then transferred to pyruvate, which is converted to lactate thereby regenerating NAD+. The net amount of 2 ATP is then formed by conversion of one molecule of glucose via substrate level phosphorylation. Thus, molecular oxygen is an essential component of energy metabolism and its availability can limit the energy balance of the cell.

In line with this, it was shown that in primary rat hepatocytes, net glucose uptake started under hypoxia (2% O_2) whereas CO_2 formation increased in direct proportion to oxygen concentration. Concomitantly, the gluconeogenic-dependent net glucose output and net lactate uptake increased under higher pO_2 values. By contrast, the net glucose output initiated by glycogen breakdown and the net lactate output started to increase under hypoxia. Thus, the net flow between glucose 6-phosphate and pyruvate in the gluconeogenic direction was enhanced with increasing pO_2 and, conversely, it was increased in the glycolytic direction with decreasing pO_2 (Nauck et al., 1981; Wolfle et al., 1983; Wolfle and Jungermann 1985; Jungermann and Kietzmann 1996, Kietzmann and Jungermann 1997).

To operate efficiently under varying O_2 tensions, cells need a reliable O_2 sensing system allowing adequate adaptation of cellular functions to the O_2 available. The first threshold of cellular hypoxia occurs when a decrease in ATP production is measurable; however, sufficient ATP necessary to maintain the vital cellular functions is still produced by metabolic adaptations involving changes in the redox and phosphorylation status of enzymes and increased glycolysis (Connett et al., 1990; Duke 1999). The second threshold occurs when the ATP demand can be met only by anaerobic glycolysis; and the third threshold is reached when glycolysis is not sufficient to produce enough ATP for cell survival (Connett and others 1990; Duke 1999). Adaptation may be achieved by short-term enzymatic reactions or by long-term regulations via modulating gene expression patterns. Within the latter, hypoxia-inducible factor-1 (HIF-1) appears to be a master regulator for the expression of genes which are activated under low oxygen levels, i.e. hypoxia (Semenza 2001).

Hypoxia-inducible transcription factors (HIFs)

Hypoxia-inducible factors are heterodimers composed of α- and β-subunits (also termed ARNT) both belonging to the basic-helix-loop-helix (bHLH) Per/Arnt/Sim (PAS) transcription factor family (Kewley et al., 2004). The heterodimers bind to hypoxia-responsive elements (HRE) localised in regulatory regions of the target genes. Of the three HIFs described so far, HIF-1 is the best characterized and the sensitivity towards oxygen is brought about by the HIF-α subunits. While HIF-1α appears to be ubiquitously expressed, HIF-2α also known as EPAS1 (endothelial PAS protein), HLF (HIF-like factor) or HRF (HIF-related factor), is predominantly expressed in highly vascularized tissues suggesting that HIF-2α may represent an important regulator of vascularisation, and may modulate the regulation of endothelial cell gene expression in response to hypoxia (Flamme et al., 1997; Tian et al., 1997; Ema et al., 1997). Although HIF-1α and HIF-2α have some overlapping targets, they appear to be needed independently of each other, since knock out of HIF-1α and HIF-2α are lethal in utero due to major vascularisation defects (Tian et al., 1998; Ryan et al., 1998; Yu et al., 1999). Both, HIF-1α and HIF-2α contain two nuclear localisation sequences, one is N-terminal and the other is C-terminal (Kallio et al., 1998). Transactivation activity is brought about by two transactivation domains (TAD), the N-terminal and the C-terminal (TAD) (Pugh et al., 1997; Jiang et al., 1997; Ema et al. 1997)

In contrast to the other proteins from that family, HIF-3α does not contain the C-terminal TAD (Gu et al., 1998; Kietzmann et al., 2001). Interestingly, several HIF-3α splice variants have been described from which the inhibitory PAS protein (IPAS) additionally lacks the TADN and exerts inhibitory effects possibly by binding to HIF-1α (Makino et al., 2001; Makino et al., 2002).

HIF-α subunit regulation

While the levels of ARNT remain constant under different oxygen tensions, HIF-1α and HIF-2α protein levels rise dramatically in response to hypoxia. This is primarily caused by mechanisms affecting HIF-α subunit protein stability (Kaelin, Jr. and Ratcliffe 2008) and to a lesser extent by transcriptional regulation (Gorlach 2009). Hypoxia-dependent stabilization of HIF-α subunits is governed by the oxygen-dependent degradation domain termed ODD.

Under normoxia this domain becomes hydroxylated at critical proline residues. The hydroxylation is carried out by O_2-dependent prolyl hydroxylases (PHDs) which also require iron, α-ketoglutarate and ascorbate as cofactors (Schofield and Ratcliffe 2005; Chowdhury et al., 2008; Kaelin, Jr. and Ratcliffe 2008).

Four different HIF prolyl hydroxylases have been identified so far: PHD1 (prolyl hydroxylase domain 1; EglN2), PHD2 (EglN1), PHD3 (EglN3) and PHD4 (C-P4H-I) (Ivan et al., 2001; Epstein et al., 2001; Bruick and McKnight 2002; Oehme et al., 2002; Hirsila et al., 2003). However, the impact of the latter on HIF-1α appears not to be as strong as that of the other types (Koivunen et al., 2007b). The extent to which these enzymes are redundant is not fully elucidated although PHD2 appears to be the primary regulator of HIF-1α, since a decrease in PHD2 activity by RNA interference (knockdown) was sufficient to activate HIF-1α in most cells under standard conditions whereas depletion of PHD1 was less effective (Berra et al., 2003; Appelhoff et al., 2004). However, all PHDs contribute to HIF-1α destabilization since maximal HIF-1α stabilization can only be observed when all PHDs are knocked-down (Berra et al., 2003; Appelhoff et al., 2004). Once the prolines within the ODD of HIF-1α are hydroxylated they become recognized by the von Hippel-Lindau tumour suppressor protein (pVHL) that is part of a multiprotein ubiquitin ligase which initiates the ubiquitinylation and degradation by the 26S proteasome system (Salceda and Caro 1997; Kallio et al., 1999). Interaction between HIF-1α and pVHL, and therefore HIF-1α proteasomal degradation seems to be further enhanced by HIF-1α acetylation by arrest-defective-1 (ARD1) at K532 (Jeong et al., 2002). Interestingly, recent data showed that histone deacetylase-1 is activated under hypoxia thus decreasing acetylated HIF-1α levels which would allow its activation (Arnesen et al., 2005; Bilton et al., 2005). Moreover, it appears to be of interest that the NAD+-dependent deacetylase sirtuin 1 (SIRT1) could interact and deacetylate HIF-2α but not HIF-1α thereby inducing HIF-2α transactivity (Dioum et al., 2009) In line with this it was found that the NAD+-dependent poly(ADP-ribose) polymerase 1 (PARP1) bound to HIF-1α and promoted transactivation through a PARP1-dependent mechanism (Elser et al., 2008).

Recently, the protein small ubiquitin like modifier-1 (SUMO-1) was associated with modification of HIF-1α at K391 and K477 and, in contrast to ubiquitination which promotes proteasomal degradation, sumoylation acts antagonistically, thus promoting HIF-1α stability and activation (Bae et al., 2004).

The factor inhibiting HIF-1 (FIH) was identified in a yeast-two-hybrid system (Mahon et al., 2001) and shown to be an asparagine hydroxylase (Lando et al., 2002) which controls the recruitment of coactivators such as CREB binding protein (CBP)/p300 to the c-terminal TAD. Like with PHDs hypoxic conditions decrease hydroxylation, which allows CBP/p300 to contact and to activate HIF a-subunits. In addition to CBP/p300, other coactivators have been shown to bind HIF-1α and a complete list of those can be found in another excellent review (Wenger et al., 2005).

HIF-1α is also regulated at the translational level. Hypoxia impairs translation in order to limit energy consumption but HIF-1α escapes this rule because of an internal ribosome entry site (IRES) in the 5' UTR (Gorlach et al., 2000; Lang et al., 2002).

In addition, the redox state of HIF-1α seems to be important for its activity (Kietzmann and Gorlach 2005). Ref-1 (redox factor-1) and its regulator thioredoxin (Trx) have been found to interact with both TADN and TADC and to increase its transactivation (Huang et al., 1996; Welsh et al., 2002). In the TADC, Ref-1 reduces C800 thereby potentiating coactivator binding. Moreover, reactive oxygen species (ROS) appear to mediate the induction of HIF-1α in response to many stimuli including thrombin, growth factors, insulin and angiotensin II under normoxic conditions (Richard et al., 2000; Gorlach et al., 2001; BelAiba et al., 2004; Kietzmann and Gorlach 2005) suggesting that the redox balance of the cell is a major regulator of HIF-1α (Kietzmann and Gorlach 2005).

Furthermore, HIF-1α levels can also be regulated by different signalling cascades. The PI3K (phosphatidyl 3-inositol kinase) and the PI3K target protein kinase B, PKB, thereby appear to have a dual role since downstream components of PKB are said to either activate or inactivate HIF-1α. The PKB target GSK3 (glycogen synthase kinase-3) therefore directly phosphorylates HIF-1α and destabilizes it (Flugel et al., 2007) while PTEN (phosphatase and tensin homologue) overexpression decreases HIF-1α (Zundel et al., 2000). The PKB target HDM2 (mouse double minute homologue) directly interacts with HIF-1α preventing destabilization of HIF-1α independently of pVHL (Bardos et al., 2004). In addition, mTOR (mammalian target of rapamycin) was shown to positively regulate HIF-1α under hypoxia whereas rapamycin decreased hypoxia-induced HIF-1α levels independently of PTEN, involving the ODD domain of HIF-1α (Hudson et al., 2002). In addition, the mTOR pathway undergoes an interplay with the AMP-activated protein kinase (AMPK) signalling pathway which can be activated allosterically under hypoxia due to an increased AMP:ATP ratio.

The MAPK (mitogen-activated protein kinase) pathways have also been shown to contribute to the regulation of HIF-1α. Indeed, inhibitors of these pathways, such as the MEK1 inhibitor PD98059 or the p38MAPK inhibitor SB203580, decreased hypoxia-induced HIF-1α expression (Kaluz et al., 2002; Kietzmann et al., 2003; Dimova et al., 2009). ERK-1 (Extracellular-regulated kinase) was shown to phoshorylate both the TADN and TADC. These events enhanced not only the stability of HIF-1α but also its transactivation in response to hypoxia (Minet et al., 2000; Lee et al., 2002; Mylonis et al., 2006). Moreover, overexpression of MKK3 or MKK6 (mitogen-activated kinase kinase), two upstream kinases of p38MAPK, elevated HIF-1α protein levels and activity by hypoxia (for review see (Dimova et al., 2009).

Role of HIF-1 in cellular metabolism

So far, more than 100 targets of HIF-1 have been identified (refer to Wenger et al. 2005 and Rosenberger et al. 2005). HIF-1-regulated genes are coding for proteins involved in several processes (Dimova et al., 2004; Eckardt et al., 2005). However, one of the most important roles that HIF-1 is playing in the adaptive response to hypoxia is the regulation and the control of energy metabolism (Table 9.1).

HIF-1 seems to regulate the expression of almost every single gene whose protein product is involved in glucose uptake and glycolysis (reviewed by Stoeltzing et al., 2004; Wenger and others 2005). However, this appeared to occur in an isoenzyme-specific manner (Ebert et al., 1996). This isoenzyme-specific regulation by hypoxia was also found in embryonic stem cells from mice containing intact hif-1α alleles (HIF-1α ⁺/⁺). By contrast, cells deficient for HIF-1α (HIF-1α⁻/⁻) did not display hypoxia-dependent induction of mRNAs encoding glycolytic enzymes such as hexokinase-1, -2, glucosephosphate isomerase, phosphofructokinase L, aldolase A and C, triosephosphate isomerase, glyceraldehyde-3-phosphate dehydrogenase, phosphoglycerate kinase 1, enolase 1, pyruvate kinase M and lactate dehydrogenase A (Wood et al., 1998; Iyer et al., 1998). In addition, these cells showed reduced expression of mRNA for GLUT1, GLUT3, hexokinase-1, -2, phosphofructokinase L, aldolase A and C, triosephosphate isomerase, glyceraldehyde-3-phosphate dehydrogenase, phosphoglycerate kinase 1 and lactate dehydrogenase A indicating significant alterations in energy metabolism (Wood et al., 1998; Iyer et al., 1998; Ryan et al., 1998).

Aside from hexokinase 1 and 2, the key enzyme of glucose utilisation in liver, glucokinase or hexokinase IV, has also been shown to be induced in a HIF-1-dependent manner (Roth et al., 2004). Further, liver-type pyruvate kinase L (PK_L) gene expression was hypoxia-inducible, whereas under normoxia the predominant mode of activation was glucose-dependent; moreo-

Table 9.1 _ Hypoxia and HIF-1 regulated genes of major metabolic pathways.

Carbohydrate metabolism		Hypoxia inducible	HIF-1 inducible
Glucose transport	Glucose transporter-1	+	+
Glycolysis	Insulin receptor	+	+
	Glucokinase	+	+
	Phosphofructokinase L	+	+
	PFKFB3 and PFKFB4	+	+
	Aldolase A and C	+	+
	GAPDH	+	+
	Phosphoglycerate kinase 1	+	+
	Phosphoglycerate mutase B	+	+
	Enolase 1	+	+
	Pyruvate kinase M	+	+
	Lactate dehydrogenase A	+	+
Amino acid metabolism	L-Arginine transporter	+	-
	Arginase-1	+	-
Lipid metabolism	Leptin	+	+
	Leptin receptor	+	+
Xenobiotic metabolism	CYP4B1	+	+
	CYP3A6	+	+
	CYP2C11	+	+
	CYP2C11	+	+
Polyamine metabolism	Ornithine decarboxylase	+	-
	Ornithine aminotransferase	+	-
	Spermidine acetyltransferase	+	-
Iron metabolism	Transferrin	+	+
	Transferrin receptor	+	+
	Heme oxygenase 1	+	+[*]
Energy phosphate metabolism	Adenylate kinase 3	+	+
	AMP-activated protein kinase family member 5	+	+
pH regulation	CA IX	+	+

For a further detailed list see (Wood et al.,1998; Gong et al., 2001; Manalo et al., 2005; Wenger et al., 2005) and the references therein.

ver, the glucose-responsive element within the PK_L promoter seems to be a low affinity HIF-1 binding site, suggesting a crosstalk between oxygen and glucose signalling pathways (Krones et al., 2001), for review see (Kietzmann et al., 2002).

The activation of phosphofructokinase 1 (PFK-1), which is also a rate-limiting enzyme in glycolysis, is dependent on fructose 2,6 phosphate and is allosterically modified by ADP and citrate. Therefore, maintenance of fructose 2,6 phosphate levels by a family of bi-functional 6-phosphofructo-2-kinase/fructose-2,6-bisphosphatase (PFKFB) enzymes is important not only for the glycolytic but also for the gluconeogenic pathway (Pilkis et al., 1995; Okar et al., 2001). Four different genes encode isoforms of the PFKFB (1-4) family (Okar and others 2001). Interestingly, all four can be activated by hypoxia in a more or less tissue-specific manner. PFKFB-1, highly expressed in liver, heart and skeletal muscle, showed the strongest response to hypoxia in testis. PFKFB-2, which is mainly expressed in lung, brain and heart, displayed the strongest response to hypoxia in liver and testis. PFKFB-3 is highly expressed in skeletal muscle although all other organs show a variable low basal level of expression; however, hypoxia strongly induced PFKFB-3 expression in lung, liver, kidney, brain, heart and testis. Furthermore, PFKFB-4 was only induced by hypoxia in testis (Minchenko et al., 2002; Bobarykina et al., 2006). Despite various implications that the whole family is regulated by HIF-1, this appeared to be the case only for PFKFB 3 and PFKFB-4 as revealed by assays detecting the binding of HIF-1 to their promoters (Fukasawa et al., 2000, Obach et al., 2004).

By contrast to the genes encoding glycolytic enzymes, the transcription of the gene encoding phosphoenolpyruvate carboxykinase 1 (PCK1), a rate-limiting enzyme in gluconeogenesis was induced to higher levels by glucagon under aerobic conditions (Bratke et al., 1999). Using transient transfections, a normoxia-responsive element was identified within its promoter, which is a binding target for a yet unknown transcription factor (Bratke et al., 1999).

Under hypoxic conditions, increased glycolysis is paralleled by down-regulation of the mitochondrial fatty acid-β-oxidation (Hochachka et al., 1996) and by decreased expression of genes encoding respiratory chain components e.g. mitochondrial DNA-encoded cytochrome oxidase subunit III, ATP synthase subunit 6, NADH dehydrogenase subunits 1 and 2, and 16S ribosomal RNA, nuclear encoded ATP synthase beta subunit and adenine nucleotide translocase (Webster et al., 1990). These adaptative effects might partially be explained by the HIF-1-mediated pyruvate dehydrogenase kinase gene expression. The pyruvate dehydrogenase kinase phosphorylates and inhibits pyruvate dehydrogenase (PDH), an enzyme converting pyruvate to acetyl-CoA. The hypoxia-induced inhibition of PDH would reduce formation of acetyl-CoA, its conversion within the citric acid cycle and the subsequent production of the reducing equivalents NADH and FADH. This in turn would lower the activity of the mitochondrial respiratory chain and may result in decreased mitochondrial oxygen consumption (Kim et al., 2006; Papandreou et al., 2006).

The importance of HIF-1 in cellular energy metabolism is also pointed out by the fact that HIF-1α stability can be influenced by changes in specific glycolytic and Krebs cycle metabolites. Glucose metabolites, such as pyruvate and oxalacetate, can activate HIF-1α via downregulation of PHDs reversal of this response by ascorbate, cysteine, histidine and Fe(II) (Dalgard et al., 2004; Koivunen et al., 2007a). Additionally, two enzymes of the citric acid cycle, succinate dehydrogenase (SDH) and fumarate hydratase (FH) appear to play a role in O_2-dependent energy metabolism. Loss-of-function mutations within those two genes cause accumulation of two intermediate products from the citric acid cycle, succinate and fumarate, respectively. Both can lead to stabilization of HIF-1α probably via an inhibition of the PHDs. This enhanced HIF-1α stability might be one of the reasons for the inherited cancer syndromes observed in clinical cases characterized with SDH and FH mutations (Tomlinson et al., 2002; Vanharanta et al., 2004; Selak et al., 2005; Esteban and Maxwell 2005; Pollard et al., 2007). Thus, the potential of the PHDs to be regulated by various metabolic intermediates coming from glycolysis and TCA need to be further elucidated.

The upregulation of anaerobic glycolysis under hypoxia also results in increased lactate production and accumulation and therefore alterations in lactate export and clearance lead to acidosis (review by (Duke 1999)). Acidosis is also among common metabolic tumour phenotype features and promotes tumour cell invasiveness (Griffiths et al., 2002). In addition, a potential link between metabolism and pH regulation appears to be the carbonic anhydrases (CA), enzymes that catalyze the interconversion of carbon dioxide and water into carbonic acid, protons, and bicarbonate ions. Carbon dioxide can freely diffuse in and out of the cell, while bicarbonate must be transported. Thus, the conversion of bicarbonate to carbon dioxide facilitates its transport into the cell, while the conversion of carbon dioxide to bicarbonate helps to trap the carbon dioxide inside the cell. Additionally, those enzymes have been implicated in ammonia transport, gastric acidity, muscle contraction, gluconeogenesis, renal acidification and normal brain development (Wykoff et al., 2000a; Pastorekova et al., 2004; Swietach et al., 2007; Pastorekova et al., 2008). Several isozymes have been involved in disease states and two isozymes, carbonic anhydrases 9 and 12, are strongly induced by hypoxia in many tumour cells and CA9 was shown to be a HIF-1-responsive gene (Wykoff et al., 2000a).

Leptin, an adipocytokine was first described as a hormone produced by adipose tissue (Ahima 2008). The main function of leptin in the human body is the regulation of energy homeostasis especially under conditions of restricted energy availability but it also plays a role in immune response, inflammation, hematopoiesis, angiogenesis and reproduction. Leptin stimulates growth, migration and invasion of cancer cells *in vitro* and potentiates angiogenesis thus having the capacity of promoting cancer *in vivo* (reviewed by (Ahima and Flier 2000; Ahima and Osei 2008; Fantuzzi 2009)). Additionally, diabetes, obesity, and sterility are associated with leptin administration in ob/ob mice, which have a mutation in the leptin gene. Hypoxia markedly increases human leptin gene expression in skin dermal fibroblasts and BeWo cells, a process mediated via a HIF-1-regulated pathway (Grosfeld et al., 2002; Koda et al., 2007). In addition, hypoxia has been shown to induce leptin expression in 3T3-F442A adipocyte cells, increasing the possibility that hypoxia, if occurring in adipose tissue, might be a modulator of the angiogenic process through the HIF-1 pathway (Lolmede et al., 2003). Additionally, HIF-1 appears to play a role in the regulation of the transglutaminase 2 gene (Wykoff et al., 2000b). The primary enzymatic activity of transglutaminase 2 (TG2) is the Ca^{2+}-dependent transamidation of polypeptide chains through their glutamine and lysine residues (or through polyamines). In addition, it may participate in cell adhesion processes and extra cellular matrix (ECM) stabilization (Verderio et al., 1999) and might thus have a role in cell proliferation (Birckbichler and Patterson, Jr. 1978; Birckbichler et al., 1981) or in receptor-mediated endocytosis (Levitzki et al., 1980).

Moreover, HIF-1 plays a role in iron metabolism by increasing transferrin (Rolfs et al., 1997), transferrin receptor (Tacchini et al., 1999) and ceruloplasmin (Mukhopadhyay et al., 2000) gene expression. Thus, regulation of the iron availability by HIF-1 represents an important feedback mechanism since the activity of PHDs strictly depends on iron (see above).

HIF-1 and cancer cell metabolism

An intriguing observation already made by Otto Warburg about 80 years ago is the ability of tumour cells to maintain high rates of glycolysis even under aerobic conditions (Bartrons and Caro 2007). This so called Warburg effect has been further confirmed by many publications and a correlation between aggressive tumour phenotype and elevated glycolysis has been established (Bartrons and Caro 2007; Zhivotovsky and Orrenius 2009), although the circumstances promoting the switch from oxidative metabolism to increased glycolysis are still poorly understood. However, this switch and the increase in glycolysis appear to be very important since they correlate with decreased tumour sensitivity to chemotherapy and increased tumour resistance to radiotherapy and therefore tumour aggressiveness (Brown 2002; Harris 2002; Koukourakis et al., 2002). The role of HIF-1 appears fundamental in such a switch since it acts as the major regulator of cell metabolism and at the same time changes in cellular metabolism influence HIF-1α stabilization and consequently HIF-1 target gene expression (Figure 9.1). Moreover, tumour cells with dysregulated HIF-1α show not only increased glycolysis even under normoxic conditions but also a tendency towards more aggres-

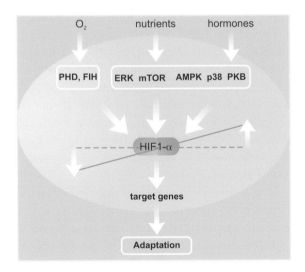

Figure 9.1 _ Hypoxia and HIF-1α are important for metabolic activation.

The role of HIF-1α appears fundamental in metabolic adaptation since it integrates signals from hypoxia, nutrient availability and hormonal signals. At the same time, up-or down-regulation of HIF-1α levels is crucial for the transcription of target genes, the products of which mediate the adaptive programme. The role within this scenario makes HIF-1α and its regulators attractive candidates for pharmaceutical intervention.

AMPK, AMP regulated kinase; ERK, extracellular regulated kinase; FIH, factor inhibiting HIF; PHD, proline hydroxylase domain containing HIF proline hydroxylase; PKB, protein kinase B/Akt

sive tumours. It seems then likely that increased levels and HIF-1α activity might represent a link between enzyme dysregulation and cancer. Furthermore, glycolysis generates intermediates which are used as precursors in different anabolic pathways such as in the synthesis of glycine, serine and purine/pyrimidine; therefore, the flux through glycolysis is critical to maintain carbon skeletons for those synthetic pathways; those pathways in turn are essential for cell growth and proliferation (Harris 2002). Thus, accelerated glycolysis might facilitate hypoxic tumour growth (Griffiths et al., 2002).

Thus, HIF-α subunits and HIF-1α in particular appear to be attractive targets for pharmacological interventions to block tumour progression (Table 9.2).

Potential therapeutic agents may act directly on the HIF-1α protein itself, or in a more indirect manner via the mechanisms degrading it. Thus, compounds may specifically activate the HIF-hydroxylases (PHDs and/or

Table 9.2 _ Reported agents with HIF-1 inhibitory potential.

Mode of action	Agent
Angiogenesis inhibitor	• endostatin
Ca^{2+} blocker	• carboxyamido-triazole
Cyclin-dependent kinase inhibitor	• flavopiridol
Cyclooxygenase-2 inhibitor	• celecoxib (Celebrex®)
	• ibuprofen
	• NS-398
HIF-1α inhibitor	• PX-478
HIF-1α / p300 interaction inhibitor	• chetomin
Histone deacetylase inhibitor	• FK228
	• NVP-LAQ824
Hsp-90 inhibitor	• geldanamycin
	• 17-allyl-amino-geldanamycin
	• radicol and analogue KF58333
Cytotoxin	• TX-402
MAPK pathway inhibitors	• PD98095
Microtubule cytoskeleton targeting agent	• 2-methoxyestradiol
	• taxol
	• vincristine
HER2/neu (erbB2) monoclonal antibody	• trastuzumab (Herceptin®)

Mode of action	Agent
Flavoprotein inhibitor	• diphenylene iodonium
PI3K / PKB / mTOR pathway inhibitor	• LY294002
	• wortmannin
	• rapamycin
	• RAD-001
	• CCI-779
PKC inhibitor	• 7-hydroxystaurosporine (UCN-01)
Raf kinase inhibitor	• BAY 43-9006 (Sorafenib)
RNA synthesis inhibitor	• echinomycin
Thioredoxin inhibitor	• 1-methylpropyl-2-imidazolyl-disulfide (PX-12)
	• pleurotin
Soluble guanyl cyclase activator	• YC-1
Topoisomerase inhibitor	
• Topo I	• topotecan
• Topo II	• GL331
Tyrosine kinase inhibitor	• genistein
	• imatinib mesylate (Glivec®, Gleevec®)
	• OSI-774 (erlotinib, Tarceva®)
	• ZD1839 (gefitinib, Iressa®)
Unknown	• resveratrol

HIF: hypoxia-inducible factor; Hsp: heat-shock protein, MAPK: mitogen-activated protein kinases; PI3K: phosphatidylinositol 3-kinase; PKB: protein kinase B; PKC: protein kinase C; mTOR: mammalian target of rapamycin; For detailed references see (Semenza 2003; Zhang et al., 2004; Yeo et al., 2004; Quintero et al., 2004; Brahimi-Horn and Pouyssegur 2005; Belozerov and Van Meir 2006; Semenza 2006; Koh et al., 2009; Schwartz et al., 2009; Koh et al., 2010) and references therein.

FIH) or promote HIF-1α/VHL interaction. In addition, degradation may be promoted by compounds which act as cofactors for the HIF-hydroxylases. The inhibition of HIF-1α could also be achieved in a more indirect manner by interfering with growth factor signalling pathways which enhance HIF-1α levels. Further, preventing association of HIF-1α with its interacting coactivator proteins and regulation of the activities of those metabolic enzymes whose products participate in HIF-1α regulation could contribute to inhibition of HIF-1α. This matter is complex due to the presence of feedback loops. Thus, large-scale screening attempts might lead to the identification of only a few specific inhibitors.

From a metabolic point of view, interference with the HIF-1 system might be most attractive by controlling HIF-hydroxylase activities directly or by regulating the production of cofactors such as 2-oxoglutarate, Fe^{2+} or factors modulating the activity of enzymes controlling the pyruvate dehydrogenase activity.

Together, the use of HIF-1α inhibitors in combination with classical chemotherapy and radiotherapy might represent a new strategy in anti-cancer therapy for those patients with tumours containing high HIF-1 levels, especially when side-effects of the new drugs can be minimized.

Acknowledgments _ We apologize to all researchers who excellently contributed to the field and whose work has not been cited due to space limitations. This work was supported by grants from the Suomen Akatemia and Sigrid Juselius Foundation to TK. There is no conflict of interest.

References

Ahima RS (2008) Revisiting leptin's role in obesity and weight loss. J Clin Invest 118(7):2380-3.

Ahima RS, Flier JS (2000). Leptin. Annu Rev Physiol 62:413-37.

Ahima RS, Osei SY (2008). Adipokines in obesity. Front Horm Res 36:182-97.

Appelhoff RJ, Tian YM, Raval RR, Turley H, Harris AL, Pugh CW, Ratcliffe PJ, Gleadle JM (2004). Differential function of the prolyl hydroxylases PHD1, PHD2, and PHD3 in the regulation of hypoxia-inducible factor. J Biol Chem 279(37):38458-65.

Arnesen T, Kong X, Evjenth R, Gromyko D, Varhaug JE, Lin Z, Sang N, Caro J, Lillehaug JR (2005). Interaction between HIF-1 alpha (ODD) and hARD1 does not induce acetylation and destabilization of HIF-1 alpha. FEBS Lett 579(28):6428-32.

Bae SH, Jeong JW, Park JA, Kim SH, Bae MK, Choi SJ, Kim KW (2004). Sumoylation increases HIF-1alpha stability and its transcriptional activity. Biochem Biophys Res Commun 324(1):394-400.

Bardos JI, Chau NM, Ashcroft M (2004). Growth factor-mediated induction of HDM2 positively regulates hypoxia-inducible factor 1alpha expression. Mol Cell Biol 24(7):2905-14.

Bartrons R, Caro J (2007). Hypoxia, glucose metabolism and the Warburg's effect. J Bioenerg Biomembr 39(3):223-9.

BelAiba RS, Djordjevic T, Bonello S, Flugel D, Hess J, Kietzmann T, Gorlach A (2004). Redox-sensitive regulation of the HIF pathway under non-hypoxic conditions in pulmonary artery smooth muscle cells. Biol Chem 385(3-4):249-57.

Belozerov VE, Van Meir EG (2006). Inhibitors of hypoxia-inducible factor-1 signalling. Curr Opin Investig Drugs 7(12):1067-76.

Berra E, Benizri E, Ginouves A, Volmat V, Roux D, Pouyssegur J (2003). HIF prolyl-hydroxylase 2 is the key oxygen sensor setting low steady-state levels of HIF-1alpha in normoxia. EMBO J 22(16):4082-90.

Bilton R, Mazure N, Trottier E, Hattab M, Dery MA, Richard DE, Pouyssegur J, Brahimi-Horn MC (2005). Arrest-defective-1 protein, an acetyltransferase, does not alter stability of hypoxia-inducible factor (HIF)-1alpha and is not induced by hypoxia or HIF. J Biol Chem 280(35):31132-40.

Birckbichler PJ, Orr GR, Patterson MK, Jr., Conway E, Carter HA (1981). Increase in proliferative markers after inhibition of transglutaminase. Proc Natl Acad Sci U S A 78(8):5005-8.

Birckbichler PJ, Patterson MK, Jr. (1978). Cellular transglutaminase, growth, and transformation. Ann N Y Acad Sci 312:354-65.

Bobarykina AY, Minchenko DO, Opentanova IL, Moenner M, Caro J, Esumi H, Minchenko OH (2006). Hypoxic regulation of PFKFB-3 and PFKFB-4 gene expression in gastric and pancreatic cancer cell lines and expression of PFKFB genes in gastric cancers. Acta Biochim Pol 53(4):789-99.

Brahimi-Horn C, Pouyssegur J (2005). When hypoxia signalling meets the ubiquitin-proteasomal pathway, new targets for cancer therapy. Crit Rev Oncol Hematol 53(2):115-23.

Bratke J, Kietzmann T, Jungermann K (1999). Identification of an oxygen-responsive element in the 5'-flanking sequence of the rat cytosolic phosphoenolpyruvate carboxykinase-1 gene, modulating its glucagon-dependent activation. Biochem J 339(Pt 3):563-9.

Brown JM (2002). Tumour microenvironment and the response to anticancer therapy. Cancer Biol Ther 1(5):453-8.

Bruick RK, McKnight SL (2002). Transcription. Oxygen sensing gets a second wind. Science 295(5556):807-8.

Chowdhury R, Hardy A, Schofield CJ (2008). The human oxygen sensing machinery and its manipulation. Chem Soc Rev 37(7):1308-19.

Connett RJ, Honig CR, Gayeski TE, Brooks GA (1990). Defining hypoxia: a systems view of VO2, glycolysis, energetics, and intracellular PO2. J Appl Physiol 68(3):833-42.

Dalgard CL, Lu H, Mohyeldin A, Verma A (2004). Endogenous 2-oxoacids differentially regulate expression of oxygen sensors. Biochem J 380(Pt 2):419-24.

Dimova EY, Michiels C, Kietzmann T (2009). Kinases as Upstream Regulators of the HIF System: Their Emerging Potential as Anti-Cancer Drug Targets. Curr Pharm Des.

Dimova EY, Samoylenko A, Kietzmann T (2004). Oxidative stress and hypoxia: implications for plasminogen activator inhibitor-1 expression. Antioxid Redox Signal 6(4):777-91.

Dioum EM, Chen R, Alexander MS, Zhang Q, Hogg RT, Gerard RD, Garcia JA (2009). Regulation of hypoxia-inducible factor 2alpha signalling by the stress-responsive deacetylase sirtuin 1. Science 324(5932):1289-93.

Duke T (1999). Dysoxia and lactate. Arch Dis Child 81(4):343-50.

Ebert BL, Gleadle JM, O'Rourke JF, Bartlett SM, Poulton J, Ratcliffe PJ (1996). Iso-enzyme-specific regulation of genes involved in energy metabolism by hypoxia: similarities with the regulation of erythropoietin. Biochem J 313(Pt 3):809-14.

Eckardt KU, Bernhardt WM, Weidemann A, Warnecke C, Rosenberger C, Wiesener MS, Willam C (2005). Role of hypoxia in the pathogenesis of renal disease. Kidney Int Suppl(99):S46-S51.

Elser M, Borsig L, Hassa PO, Erener S, Messner S, Valovka T, Keller S, Gassmann M, Hottiger MO (2008). Poly(ADP-ribose) polymerase 1 promotes tumour cell survival by coactivating hypoxia-inducible factor-1-dependent gene expression. Mol Cancer Res 6(2):282-90.

Ema M, Taya S, Yokotani N, Sogawa K, Matsuda Y, Fujii-Kuriyama Y (1997). A novel bHLH-PAS factor with close sequence similarity to hypoxia-inducible factor 1alpha regulates the VEGF expression and is potentially involved in lung and vascular development. Proc Natl Acad Sci U S A 94(9):4273-8.

Epstein AC, Gleadle JM, McNeill LA, Hewitson KS, O'Rourke J, Mole DR, Mukherji M, Metzen E, Wilson MI, Dhanda A, Tian YM, Masson N, Hamilton DL, Jaakkola P, Barstead R, Hodgkin J, Maxwell PH, Pugh CW, Schofield CJ, Ratcliffe PJ (2001). C. elegans EGL-9 and mammalian homologs define a family of dioxygenases that regulate HIF by prolyl hydroxylation. Cell 107(1):43-54.

Esteban MA, Maxwell PH (2005). HIF, a missing link between metabolism and cancer. Nat Med 11(10):1047-8.

Fantuzzi G (2009). Three questions about leptin and immunity. Brain Behav Immun 23(4):405-10.

Flamme I, Frohlich T, von RM, Kappel A, Damert A, Risau W (1997). HRF, a putative basic helix-loop-helix-PAS-domain transcription factor is closely related to hypoxia-inducible factor-1 alpha and developmentally expressed in blood vessels. Mech Dev 63(1):51-60.

Flugel D, Gorlach A, Michiels C, Kietzmann T (2007). Glycogen synthase kinase 3 phosphorylates hypoxia-inducible factor 1alpha and mediates its destabilization in a VHL-independent manner. Mol Cell Biol 27(9):3253-65.

Fukasawa M, Takayama E, Shinomiya N, Okumura A, Rokutanda M, Yamamoto N, Sakakibara R (2000). Identification of the promoter region of human placental 6-phosphofructo-2-kinase/fructose-2,6-bisphosphatase gene. Biochem Biophys Res Commun 267(3):703-8.

Gong PF, Hu B, Stewart D, Ellerbe M, Figueroa YG, Blank V, Beckman BS, Alam J (2001). Cobalt induces heme oxygenase-1 expression by a hypoxia-inducible factor-independent mechanism in Chinese hamster ovary cells – Regulation by Nrf2 and MafG transcription factors. Journal of Biological Chemistry 276(29):27018-25.

Gorlach A (2009). Regulation of HIF-1alpha at the transcriptional level. Curr Pharm Des 15(33):3844-52.

Gorlach A, Camenisch G, Kvietikova I, Vogt L, Wenger RH, Gassmann M (2000). Efficient translation of mouse hypoxia-inducible factor-1alpha under normoxic and hypoxic conditions. Biochim Biophys Acta 1493(1-2):125-34.

Gorlach A, Diebold I, Schini-Kerth VB, Berchner-Pfannschmidt U, Roth U, Brandes RP, Kietzmann T, Busse R (2001). Thrombin activates the hypoxia-inducible factor-1 signalling pathway in vascular smooth muscle cells: Role of the p22(phox)-containing NADPH oxidase. Circ Res 89(1):47-54.

Greger R, Bleich M. 1996. Normal values for physiological parameters. In: Greger R, Windhorst U, editors. Comprehensive human physiology. Berlin-Heidelberg: Springer Verlag; p 2427-47.

Griffiths JR, McSheehy PM, Robinson SP, Troy H, Chung YL, Leek RD, Williams KJ, Stratford IJ, Harris AL, Stubbs M (2002). Metabolic changes detected by in vivo magnetic resonance studies of HEPA-1 wild-type tumours and tumours deficient in hypoxia-inducible factor-1beta (HIF-1beta): evidence of an anabolic role for the HIF-1 pathway. Cancer Res 62(3):688-95.

Grosfeld A, Andre J, Hauguel-De Mouzon S, Berra E, Pouyssegur J, Guerre-Millo M (2002). Hypoxia-inducible factor 1 transactivates the human leptin gene promoter. J Biol Chem 277(45):42953-7.

Gu YZ, Moran SM, Hogenesch JB, Wartman L, Bradfield CA (1998). Molecular characterization and chromosomal localization of a third alpha-class hypoxia inducible factor subunit, HIF3alpha. Gene Expr 7(3):205-13.

Harris AL (2002). Hypoxia–a key regulatory factor in tumour growth. Nat Rev Cancer 2(1):38-47.

Hirsila M, Koivunen P, Gunzler V, Kivirikko KI, Myllyharju J (2003). Characterization of the human prolyl 4-hydroxylases that modify the hypoxia-inducible factor. J Biol Chem 278(33):30772-80.

Hochachka PW, Buck LT, Doll CJ, Land SC (1996). Unifying theory of hypoxia tolerance: molecular/metabolic defense and rescue mechanisms for surviving oxygen lack. Proc Natl Acad Sci U S A 93(18):9493-8.

Huang LE, Arany Z, Livingston DM, Bunn HF (1996). Activation of hypoxia-inducible transcription factor depends primarily upon redox-sensitive stabilization of its alpha subunit. J Biol Chem 271(50):32253-9.

Hudson CC, Liu M, Chiang GG, Otterness DM, Loomis DC, Kaper F, Giaccia AJ, Abraham RT (2002). Regulation of hypoxia-inducible factor 1alpha expression and function by the mammalian target of rapamycin. Mol Cell Biol 22(20):7004-14.

Ivan M, Kondo K, Yang H, Kim W, Valiando J, Ohh M, Salic A, Asara JM, Lane WS, Kaelin WGJ (2001). HIFalpha targeted for VHL-mediated destruction by proline hydroxylation: implications for O2 sensing. Science 292(5516):464-8.

Iyer NV, Kotch LE, Agani F, Leung SW, Laughner E, Wenger RH, Gassmann M, Gearhart JD, Lawler AM, Yu AY, Semenza GL (1998). Cellular and developmental control of O2 homeostasis by hypoxia-inducible factor 1 alpha. Genes Dev 12(2):149-62.

Jeong JW, Bae MK, Ahn MY, Kim SH, Sohn TK, Bae MH, Yoo MA, Song EJ, Lee KJ, Kim KW (2002). Regulation and Destabilization of HIF-1alpha by ARD1-Mediated Acetylation. Cell 111(5):709-20.

Jiang BH, Zheng JZ, Leung SW, Roe R, Semenza GL (1997). Transactivation and inhibitory domains of hypoxia-inducible factor 1alpha. Modulation of transcriptional activity by oxygen tension. J Biol Chem 272(31):19253-60.

Jungermann K, Kietzmann T (1996). Zonation of parenchymal and nonparenchymal metabolism in liver. Annu Rev Nutr 16:179-203.

Kaelin WG, Jr., Ratcliffe PJ (2008). Oxygen sensing by metazoans: the central role of the HIF hydroxylase pathway. Mol Cell 30(4):393-402.

Kallio PJ, Okamoto K, O'Brien S, Carrero P, Makino Y, Tanaka H, Poellinger L (1998). Signal transduction in hypoxic cells: inducible nuclear translocation and recruitment of the CBP/p300 coactivator by the hypoxia-inducible factor-1alpha. EMBO J 17(22):6573-86.

Kallio PJ, Wilson WJ, O'Brien S, Makino Y, Poellinger L (1999). Regulation of the hypoxia-inducible transcription factor 1alpha by the ubiquitin-proteasome pathway. J Biol Chem 274(10):6519-25.

Kaluz S, Kaluzova M, Chrastina A, Olive PL, Pastorekova S, Pastorek J, Lerman MI, Stanbridge EJ (2002). Lowered oxygen tension induces expression of the hypoxia marker MN/carbonic anhydrase IX in the absence of hypoxia-inducible factor 1 alpha stabilization: a role for phosphatidylinositol 3'-kinase. Cancer Res 62(15):4469-77.

Kewley RJ, Whitelaw ML, Chapman-Smith A (2004). The mammalian basic helix-loop-helix/PAS family of transcriptional regulators. Int J Biochem Cell Biol 36(2):189-204.

Kietzmann T, Cornesse Y, Brechtel K, Modaressi S, Jungermann K (2001). Perivenous expression of the mRNA of the three hypoxia-inducible factor alpha-subunits, HIF1alpha, HIF2alpha and HIF3alpha, in rat liver. Biochem J 354(Pt 3):531-7.

Kietzmann T, Gorlach A (2005). Reactive oxygen species in the control of hypoxia-inducible factor-mediated gene expression. Semin Cell Dev Biol 16(4-5):474-86.

Kietzmann T, Jungermann K (1997). Modulation by oxygen of zonal gene expression in liver studied in primary rat hepatocyte cultures. Cell Biol Toxicol 13(4-5):243-55.

Kietzmann T, Jungermann K, Gorlach A (2003). Regulation of the hypoxia-dependent plasminogen activator inhibitor 1 expression by MAP kinases in HepG2 cells. Thromb Haemost 89:666-74.

Kietzmann T, Krones-Herzig A, Jungermann K (2002). Signalling cross-talk between hypoxia and glucose via hypoxia-inducible factor 1 and glucose response elements. Biochem Pharmacol 64(5-6):903-11.

Kim JW, Tchernyshyov I, Semenza GL, Dang CV (2006). HIF-1-mediated expression of pyruvate dehydrogenase kinase: a metabolic switch required for cellular adaptation to hypoxia. Cell Metab 3(3):177-85.

Koda M, Sulkowska M, Wincewicz A, Kanczuga-Koda L, Musiatowicz B, Szymanska M, Sulkowski S (2007). Expression of leptin, leptin receptor, and hypoxia-inducible factor 1 alpha in human endometrial cancer. Ann N Y Acad Sci 1095:90-8.:90-8.

Koh MY, Spivak-Kroizman TR, Powis G (2009). Inhibiting the hypoxia response for cancer therapy: the new kid on the block. Clin Cancer Res 15(19):5945-6.

Koh MY, Spivak-Kroizman TR, Powis G (2010). HIF-1alpha and cancer therapy. Recent Results Cancer Res 180:15-34.

Koivunen P, Hirsila M, Remes AM, Hassinen IE, Kivirikko KI, Myllyharju J (2007a). Inhibition of hypoxia-inducible factor (HIF) hydroxylases by citric acid cycle intermediates: possible links between cell metabolism and stabilization of HIF. J Biol Chem 282(7):4524-32.

Koivunen P, Tiainen P, Hyvarinen J, Williams KE, Sormunen R, Klaus SJ, Kivirikko KI, Myllyharju J (2007b). An endoplasmic reticulum transmembrane prolyl 4-hydroxylase is induced by hypoxia and acts on hypoxia-inducible factor alpha. J Biol Chem 282(42):30544-52.

Koukourakis MI, Giatromanolaki A, Sivridis E, Simopoulos C, Turley H, Talks K, Gatter KC, Harris AL (2002). Hypoxia-inducible factor (HIF1A and HIF2A), angiogenesis, and chemoradiotherapy outcome of squamous cell head-and-neck cancer. Int J Radiat Oncol Biol Phys 53(5):1192-202.

Krones A, Jungermann K, Kietzmann T (2001). Cross-talk between the signals hypoxia and glucose at the glucose response element of the L-type pyruvate kinase gene. Endocrinology 142(6):2707-18.

Lando D, Peet DJ, Gorman JJ, Whelan DA, Whitelaw ML, Bruick RK (2002). FIH-1 is an asparaginyl hydroxylase enzyme that regulates the transcriptional activity of hypoxia-inducible factor. Genes Dev 16(12):1466-71.

Lang KJ, Kappel A, Goodall GJ (2002). Hypoxia-inducible factor-1alpha mRNA contains an internal ribosome entry site that allows efficient translation during normoxia and hypoxia. Mol Biol Cell 13(5):1792-801.

Lee E, Yim S, Lee SK, Park H (2002). Two transactivation domains of hypoxia-inducible factor-1alpha regulated by the MEK-1/p42/p44 MAPK pathway. Mol Cells 14(1):9-15.

Levitzki A, Willingham M, Pastan I (1980). Evidence for participation of transglutaminase in receptor-mediated endocytosis. Proc Natl Acad Sci U S A 77(5):2706-10.

Lolmede K, Durand dSF, V, Galitzky J, Lafontan M, Bouloumie A (2003). Effects of hypoxia on the expression of proangiogenic factors in differentiated 3T3-F442A adipocytes. Int J Obes Relat Metab Disord 27(10):1187-95.

Mahon PC, Hirota K, Semenza GL (2001). FIH-1: a novel protein that interacts with HIF-1alpha and VHL to mediate repression of HIF-1 transcriptional activity. Genes Dev 15(20):2675-86.

Makino Y, Cao R, Svensson K, Bertilsson G, Asman M, Tanaka H, Cao Y, Berkenstam A, Poellinger L (2001). Inhibitory PAS domain protein is a negative regulator of hypoxia-inducible gene expression. Nature 414(6863):550-4.

Makino Y, Kanopka A, Wilson WJ, Tanaka H, Poellinger L (2002). Inhibitory PAS domain protein (IPAS) is a hypoxia-inducible splicing variant of the hypoxia-inducible factor-3alpha locus. J Biol Chem 277(36):32405-8.

Manalo DJ, Rowan A, Lavoie T, Natarajan L, Kelly BD, Ye SQ, Garcia JG, Semenza GL (2005). Transcriptional regulation of vascular endothelial cell responses to hypoxia by HIF-1. Blood 105(2):659-69.

Minchenko A, Leshchinsky I, Opentanova I, Sang N, Srinivas V, Armstead V, Caro J (2002). Hypoxia-inducible factor-1-mediated expression of the 6-phosphofructo-2-kinase/fructose-2,6-bisphosphatase-3 (PFKFB3) gene. Its possible role in the Warburg effect. J Biol Chem 277(8):6183-7.

Minet E, Arnould T, Michel G, Roland I, Mottet D, Raes M, Remacle J, Michiels C

(2000). ERK activation upon hypoxia: involvement in HIF-1 activation. FEBS Lett 468(1):53-8.

Mukhopadhyay CK, Mazumder B, Fox PL (2000). Role of hypoxia-inducible factor-1 in transcriptional activation of ceruloplasmin by iron deficiency. J Biol Chem 275(28):21048-54.

Mylonis I, Chachami G, Samiotaki M, Panayotou G, Paraskeva E, Kalousi A, Georgatsou E, Bonanou S, Simos G (2006). Identification of MAPK phosphorylation sites and their role in the localization and activity of hypoxia-inducible factor-1alpha. J Biol Chem 281(44):33095-106.

Nauck M, Wolfle D, Katz N, Jungermann K (1981). Modulation of the glucagon-dependent induction of phosphoenolpyruvate carboxykinase and tyrosine aminotransferase by arterial and venous oxygen concentrations in hepatocyte cultures. Eur J Biochem 119(3):657-61.

Obach M, Navarro-Sabate A, Caro J, Kong X, Duran J, Gomez M, Perales JC, Ventura F, Rosa JL, Bartrons R (2004). 6-Phosphofructo-2-kinase (pfkfb3) gene promoter contains hypoxia-inducible factor-1 binding sites necessary for transactivation in response to hypoxia. J Biol Chem 279(51):53562-70.

Oehme F, Ellinghaus P, Kolkhof P, Smith TJ, Ramakrishnan S, Hutter J, Schramm M, Flamme I (2002). Overexpression of PH-4, a novel putative proline 4-hydroxylase, modulates activity of hypoxia-inducible transcription factors. Biochem Biophys Res Commun 296(2).343-9.

Okar DA, Manzano A, Navarro-Sabate A, Riera L, Bartrons R, Lange AJ (2001). PFK-2/FBPase-2: maker and breaker of the essential biofactor fructose-2,6-bisphosphate. Trends Biochem Sci 26(1):30-5.

Papandreou I, Cairns RA, Fontana L, Lim AL, Denko NC (2006). HIF-1 mediates adaptation to hypoxia by actively downregulating mitochondrial oxygen consumption. Cell Metab 3(3):187-97.

Pastorekova S, Parkkila S, Pastorek J, Supuran CT (2004). Carbonic anhydrases: current state of the art, therapeutic applications and future prospects. J Enzyme Inhib Med Chem 19(3):199-229.

Pastorekova S, Ratcliffe PJ, Pastorek J (2008). Molecular mechanisms of carbonic anhydrase IX-mediated pH regulation under hypoxia. BJU Int 101 Suppl 4:8-15.

Piiper J. 1996. Oxygen supply and energy metabolism. In: Greger R, Windhorst U, editors. Comprehensive human physiology. Berlin-Heidelberg: Springer Verlag; p 2063-9.

Pilkis SJ, Claus TH, Kurland IJ, Lange AJ (1995). 6-Phosphofructo-2-kinase/fructose-2,6-bisphosphatase: a metabolic signalling enzyme. Annu Rev Biochem 64:799-835.

Pollard PJ, Spencer-Dene B, Shukla D, Howarth K, Nye E, El Bahrawy M, Deheragoda M, Joannou M, McDonald S, Martin A, Igarashi P, Varsani-Brown S, Rosewell I, Poulsom R, Maxwell P, Stamp GW, Tomlinson IP (2007). Targeted inactivation of fh1 causes proliferative renal cyst development and activation of the hypoxia pathway. Cancer Cell 11(4):311-9.

Pugh CW, O'Rourke JF, Nagao M, Gleadle JM, Ratcliffe PJ (1997). Activation of hypoxia-inducible factor-1; definition of regulatory domains within the alpha subunit. J Biol Chem 272(17):11205-14.

Quintero M, Mackenzie N, Brennan PA (2004). Hypoxia-inducible factor 1 (HIF-1) in cancer. Eur J Surg Oncol 30(5):465-8.

Richard DE, Berra E, Pouyssegur J (2000). Nonhypoxic pathway mediates the induction of hypoxia-inducible factor 1alpha in vascular smooth muscle cells. J Biol Chem 275(35):26765-71.

Rolfs A, Kvietikova I, Gassmann M, Wenger RH (1997). Oxygen-regulated transferrin expression is mediated by hypoxia-inducible factor-1. J Biol Chem 272(32):20055-62.

Rosenberger C, Rosen S, Heyman SN (2005). Current understanding of HIF in renal disease. Kidney Blood Press Res 28(5-6):325-340

Roth U, Curth K, Unterman TG, Kietzmann T (2004). The transcription factors HIF-1 and HNF-4 and the coactivator p300 are involved in insulin-regulated glucokinase gene expression via the phosphatidylinositol 3-kinase/protein kinase B pathway. J Biol Chem 279(4):2623-31.

Ryan HE, Lo J, Johnson RS (1998). HIF-1 alpha is required for solid tumour formation and embryonic vascularization. EMBO J 17(11):3005-15.

Salceda S, Caro J (1997). Hypoxia-inducible factor 1alpha (HIF-1alpha) protein is rapidly degraded by the ubiquitin-proteasome system under normoxic conditions. Its stabilization by hypoxia depends on redox-induced changes. J Biol Chem 272(36):22642-7.

Schofield CJ, Ratcliffe PJ (2005). Signalling hypoxia by HIF hydroxylases. Biochem Biophys Res Commun 338(1):617-26.

Schwartz DL, Powis G, Thitai-Kumar A, He Y, Bankson J, Williams R, Lemos R, Oh J, Volgin A, Soghomonyan S, Nishii R, Alauddin M, Mukhopadhay U, Peng Z, Bornmann W, Gelovani J (2009). The selective hypoxia inducible factor-1 inhibitor PX-478 provides in vivo radiosensitization through tumour stromal effects. Mol Cancer Ther 8(4):947-58.

Selak MA, Armour SM, Mackenzie ED, Boulahbel H, Watson DG, Mansfield KD, Pan Y, Simon MC, Thompson CB, Gottlieb E (2005). Succinate links TCA cycle dysfunction to oncogenesis by inhibiting HIF-alpha prolyl hydroxylase. Cancer Cell 7(1):77-85.

Semenza GL (2001). HIF-1 and mechanisms of hypoxia sensing. Curr Opin Cell Biol 13(2):167-71.

Semenza GL (2003). Targeting HIF-1 for cancer therapy. Nat Rev Cancer 3(10):721-32.

Semenza GL (2006). Development of novel therapeutic strategies that target HIF-1. Expert Opin Ther Targets 10(2):267-80.

Stoeltzing O, McCarty MF, Wey JS, Fan F, Liu W, Belcheva A, Bucana CD, Semenza GL, Ellis LM (2004). Role of hypoxia-inducible factor 1alpha in gastric cancer cell growth, angiogenesis, and vessel maturation. J Natl Cancer Inst 96(12):946-56.

Swietach P, Vaughan-Jones RD, Harris AL (2007). Regulation of tumour pH and the role of carbonic anhydrase 9. Cancer Metastasis Rev 26(2):299-310.

Tacchini L, Bianchi L, Bernelli ZA, Cairo G (1999). Transferrin receptor induction by hypoxia. HIF-1-mediated transcriptional activation and cell-specific post-transcriptional regulation. J Biol Chem 274(34):24142-6.

Tian H, Hammer RE, Matsumoto AM, Russell DW, McKnight SL (1998). The hypoxia-responsive transcription factor EPAS1 is essential for catecholamine homeostasis and protection against heart failure during embryonic development. Genes Dev 12(21):3320-4.

Tian H, McKnight SL, Russell DW (1997). Endothelial PAS domain protein 1 (EPAS1), a transcription factor selectively expressed in endothelial cells. Genes Dev 11(1):72-82.

Tomlinson IP, Alam NA, Rowan AJ, Barclay E, Jaeger EE, Kelsell D, Leigh I, Gorman P, Lamlum H, Rahman S, Roylance RR, Olpin S, Bevan S, Barker K, Hearle N, Houlston RS, Kiuru M, Lehtonen R, Karhu A, Vilkki S, Laiho P, Eklund C, Vierimaa O, Aittomaki K, Hietala M, Sistonen P, Paetau A, Salovaara R, Herva R, Launonen V, Aaltonen LA (2002). Germline mutations in FH predispose to dominantly inherited uterine fibroids, skin leiomyomata and papillary renal cell cancer. Nat Genet 30(4):406-10.

Vanharanta S, Buchta M, McWhinney SR, Virta SK, Peczkowska M, Morrison CD, Lehtonen R, Januszewicz A, Jarvinen H, Juhola M, Mecklin JP, Pukkala E, Herva R, Kiuru M, Nupponen NN, Aaltonen LA, Neumann HP, Eng C (2004). Early-onset renal cell carcinoma as a novel extraparaganglial component of SDHB-associated heritable paraganglioma. Am J Hum Genet 74(1):153-9.

Verderio E, Gaudry C, Gross S, Smith C, Downes S, Griffin M (1999). Regulation of cell surface tissue transglutaminase: effects on matrix storage of latent transforming growth factor-beta binding protein-1. J Histochem Cytochem 47(11):1417-32.

Webster KA, Gunning P, Hardeman E, Wallace DC, Kedes L (1990). Coordinate reciprocal trends in glycolytic and mitochondrial transcript accumulations during the in vitro differentiation of human myoblasts. J Cell Physiol 142(3):566-73.

Welsh SJ, Bellamy WT, Briehl MM, Powis G (2002). The redox protein thioredoxin-1 (Trx-1) increases hypoxia-inducible factor 1alpha protein expression: Trx-1 overexpression results in increased vascular endothelial growth factor production and enhanced tumour angiogenesis. Cancer Res 62(17):5089-95.

Wenger RH, Stiehl DP, Camenisch G (2005). Integration of oxygen signalling at the consensus HRE. Sci STKE 306:re12.

Wolfle D, Jungermann K (1985). Long-term effects of physiological oxygen concentrations on glycolysis and gluconeogenesis in hepatocyte cultures. Eur J Biochem 151(2):299-303.

Wolfle D, Schmidt H, Jungermann K (1983). Short-term modulation of glycogen metabolism, glycolysis and gluconeogenesis by physiological oxygen concentrations in hepatocyte cultures. Eur J Biochem 135(3):405-12.

Wood SM, Wiesener MS, Yeates KM, Okada N, Pugh CW, Maxwell PH, Ratcliffe PJ (1998). Selection and analysis of a mutant cell line defective in the hypoxia-inducible factor-1 alpha-subunit (HIF-1alpha). Characterization of hif-1alpha-dependent and -independent hypoxia-inducible gene expression. J Biol Chem 273(14):8360-8.

Wykoff CC, Beasley NP, Watson PH, Turner KJ, Pastorek J, Sibtain A, Wilson GD, Turley H, Talks KL, Maxwell PH, Pugh CW, Ratcliffe PJ, Harris AL (2000a). Hypoxiainducible expression of tumour-associated carbonic anhydrases. CANCER RESEARCH 60(24):7075-83.

Wykoff CC, Pugh CW, Maxwell PH, Harris AL, Ratcliffe PJ (2000b). Identification of novel hypoxia dependent and independent target genes of the von Hippel-Lindau

(VHL) tumour suppressor by mRNA differential expression profiling. Oncogene 19(54):6297-305.

Yeo EJ, Chun YS, Park JW (2004). New anticancer strategies targeting HIF-1. Biochem Pharmacol 68(6):1061-9.

Yu AY, Shimoda LA, Iyer NV, Huso DL, Sun X, McWilliams R, Beaty T, Sham JS, Wiener CM, Sylvester JT, Semenza GL (1999). Impaired physiological responses to chronic hypoxia in mice partially deficient for hypoxia-inducible factor 1alpha. J Clin Invest 103(5):691-6.

Zhang X, Kon T, Wang H, Li F, Huang Q, Rabbani ZN, Kirkpatrick JP, Vujaskovic Z, Dewhirst MW, Li CY (2004). Enhancement of hypoxia-induced tumour cell death in vitro and radiation therapy in vivo by use of small interfering RNA targeted to hypoxia-inducible factor-1alpha. Cancer Res 64(22):8139-42.

Zhivotovsky B, Orrenius S (2009). The Warburg Effect returns to the cancer stage. Semin Cancer Biol 19(1):1-3.

Zundel W, Schindler C, Haas KD, Koong A, Kaper F, Chen E, Gottschalk AR, Ryan HE, Johnson RS, Jefferson AB, Stokoe D, Giaccia AJ (2000). Loss of PTEN facilitates HIF-1-mediated gene expression. Genes Dev 14(4):391-6.

Chapter 10

Hypoxia, regulation of pH and cell migration/invasion

Eliska Svastova and Silvia Pastorekova[*]

[*]Authors for correspondence:
Institute of Virology, Slovak Academy of Sciences, Dubravska cesta 9, 84505 Bratislava,
Slovak Republic, Tel: +421259302404, Fax: +421254774284, viruelis@savba.sk, virusipa@savba.sk

Contents

Key points

—   Solid tumours display acidic extracellular pH resulting from the metabolic shift caused by hypoxia or oncogenic activation.

—   Hypoxia and extracellular acidosis contribute to remodeling of the extracellular matrix.

—   Many hypoxia-regulated genes encode proteins that actively participate in cell migration and invasion.

—   pH regulators promote cell migration and invasion by generating proper pH gradients at the leading edge and rear end of the moving cells.

—   pH gradients and local volume changes affect focal adhesion assembly and disassembly, formation of lamellipodia and invadopodia.

—   Inhibition of the pH-regulating machinery represents a promising anticancer strategy leading to reduced tumour cell migration and survival.

Introduction

Besides hypoxic environment, the metastatic process is controlled by tumour-stroma interactions. Surrounding mesenchymal cells produce cytokines that coordinate this complex cascade. The prototype of migratory factors is the hepatocyte growth factor (HGF). HGF receptor on cancer cells c-Met is a HIF-1α target gene overexpressed in many invading tumours. It is believed that the combination of acidic extracellular pH (pHe) with hypoxia induces invasive switch, which enables cancer cells to escape this hostile environment (Pennacchietti et al., 2003).

Human solid tumours display acidic pHe in a range between 6.2-6.8 compared to neutral pHe in normal tissues 7.2-7.4. This is the consequence of neutralisation demand to buffer intracellular acidification resulting from the metabolic shift to glycolysis caused by hypoxia or oncogenic activation. On the other hand, low pHe appears to give selective advantage for tumour growth and is involved in tumour progression and malignancy. Hypoxia-induced tumour invasiveness is a very complex process, which leads to disruption of cell-cell contacts, increased motility of tumour cells, neo-vascularisation, and activity of proteases necessary for cleavage of the extracellular matrix.

Hypoxia and the epithelial-mesenchymal transition

An important component of cell adhesion maintaining tissue integrity is E-cadherin that forms homophilic adherens junctions. Its intracellular domain binds β-catenin and α-catenin and thus provides a link to the actin cytoskeleton. Loss of E-cadherin function promotes cell migration and invasion (Christiansen et al., 2006). Hypoxia was shown to increase the expression of transcription factors Snail and Slug, which repress expression of E-cadherin. However, identification of hypoxia response elements within the promoters of these transcriptional repressors has not yet been reported. Indeed, Snail and Slug are expressed in response to different stimuli inducing epithelial-mesenchymal transition (EMT) such as Wnt signalling, or TGF-β signalling (Micalizzi et al, 2010), and hypoxic conditions as well as acidic pH microdomains in the tumour convert latent TGF-β into bioactive form. This conversion can be realised in protease-dependent and protease-independent manners, both being supported by hypoxia. Acidic pHe activates proteases like plasmin, cathepsin, MMP-2, MMP-9, which all proteolytically activate latent TGF-β complex (Wever et al, 2003). Non-proteolytically induced activation of TGF-β is based on binding to thrombospondin 1, which is elevated via a HIF-1α-dependent mechanism (Crawford et al, 1998, Osada-Oka et al, 2008). Activated TGF-β then transdifferentiates normal stromal fibroblasts into myofibroblasts, which then release invasion-stimulatory signals like HGF, KGF, bFGF, proteinases or ECM proteins (Wever et al, 2003). Such transdifferentiation is an excellent example of adaptation to tumour microenvironmental acidification.

Hypoxia, tumour acidity and remodeling of the extracellular matrix

HIF-1α regulates expression of proteolytic enzymes such as cathepsin D, MMP2, uPAR to degrade basement membrane and enable cancer cells to invade. HIF-1α-directed remodeling of ECM also comprises production of fibronectin and their specific receptors integrins, expression of intermediate filaments typical for motile mesenchymal cells (vimentin, keratin 14, 18, 19) and alteration of the matrix stiffness (Krishnamachary et al., 2003, Erler et al, 2009).

Digestion of extracellular matrix is accomplished by hypoxia-induced and acidosis-activated proteases. Low pHe in tumour stroma is optimal for the activity of uPA, cathepsin D or MMP3 (stromelysin), (Iessi et al, 2008). Indeed, acidic pHe stimulates the release of some cathepsins and MMP-9 from cells, and constitutes a source for protonation of proteins. Protonation of MMP-3 increases the affinity of the enzyme for the peptide substrates because of the influence on the binding pocket (Holman et al., 1999). Furthermore, protonation of fibrinogen as a substrate for MMP-2 is important for its proteolytic cleavage (Monaco et al, 2007).

The interesting connection between ECM component hyaluronan and local pH gradient represents activation of sodium-hydrogen exchanger NHE1 on breast tumour cells. Binding of hyaluronan to CD44 stimulates ROK phosphorylation of NHE1 in CD44-containing lipid rafts. ROK promotes Na^+/H^+ exchange activity, induces lysosomal pH changes and extracellular acidification leading to a concomitant activation of at least two low pH-dependent enzymes, hyaluronidase-2 and cathepsin B, that are required for ECM degradation, hyaluronan modification, and tumour cell invasion.

(Bourguignon et al, 2004). Moreover, synthesis of hyaluronan is upregulated by extracellular lactate accumulated in hypoxic regions.

Another hallmark of invasion is restructuring of ECM in terms of matrix stiffness. Lactate transported from tumour cells through hypoxia-induced monocarboxylate cotransporter MCT4 up-regulates synthesis of collagen type I, which is the major structural part of the ECM in solid tumours. An increased amount and crosslinking of collagen increases matrix stiffness and promotes tumour invasion. Extracellular matrix protein lysyl oxidase (LOX), another HIF-1 target, is responsible for covalent cross-linking of collagen I and profoundly affects mechanical properties of tissue (Postovit et al, 2008). This higher rigidity of ECM is sensed through integrins, which activate focal adhesion kinase and PI3K/Akt pathways that are strongly implicated in cancer cell migration and invasion (Ng et al, 2009). It is established that hypoxia induces LOX in many cancers and modulates tumour invasion by activation of integrins through elevation of fibrillar collagen and ECM stiffness (Erler et al, 2009, Levental et al, 2009).

Hypoxia and tumour cell migration

Many hypoxia-regulated proteins play important roles in cell migration, including c-Met tyrosine kinase receptor c-Met, phosphoglucose isomerase/autocrine motility factor (PGI/AMF) or pH regulators such as sodium-hydrogen exchanger (NHE1), sodium-bicarbonate co-transporter (NBCe1), carbonic anhydrase IX (CA IX) and monoclarboxylate cotransporter (MCT-4). For example, activation of AMF receptor leads to AMFR-phosphorylation, inositol production and PKC activation, which promotes cell locomotion (Funasaka et al., 2005). Interestingly, overexpression of AMF and AMFR correlates with progression of malignant tumours and a poor prognosis in non-small cell lung cancer, kidney and gastrointestinal cancer (Takanami et al., 2001, Baumann et al., 1990).

Binding of hepatocyte growth factor (HGF), a stromal cell-derived cytokine, to its receptor c-Met induces motility, proliferation, invasiveness, and angiogenesis (Otsuka et al., 1998, You et al., 2008). Interaction between HGF and c-Met can lead to activation of effector signalling pathways that initiate and regulate migration, such as PI3K/Akt, Ras/MEK, Src/FAK and p120/STAT3 (You et al., 2008, Benvenuti et al., 2007). In many tumours, expression of the c-Met oncoprotein is regulated by an autocrine loop via HGF (Otsuka et al., 1998).

Both c-Met signalling and hypoxia are connected with changes in the expression and topographic localisation of cadherins. These changes lead to reduction of cell-cell adhesion that represents an initial stage of migration (Sullivan et al., 2007). Destabilization of intercellular contacts can be regulated not only on genetic and epigenetic levels, but also via functional interference. We demonstrated that the ectopic expression of hypoxia-related CA IX protein weakens intercellular adhesion and leads to increased cell dissociation by reducing E-cadherin interaction with β-catenin (Svastova et al, 2003). Other tumour-associated proteins, such as IQGAP1 or MUC1, also function by a similar mechanism (Li et al., 2001, Fukata et al., 1999). In colorectal carcinoma, IQGAP1 expression is connected with an invasive front (Nabeshima et al., 2002). In stomach tumours, CA IX expression was confirmed in cells infiltrating lymfatic nodes as well as in lymfatic metastases (Chen et al., 2005).

pH regulators as promoters of tumour cell migration and invasion

Migration of tumour cells requires cell dissociation, dynamic cytoskeleton reorganisation and extracellular matrix degradation. All these processes depend on extracellular and intracellular pH, determined by local ion and water transport across the membrane (Sullivan et al., 2007). Pericellular pH (pHe) is more acidic at the cell front than at the rear end of migrating cells while the intracellular pH (pHi) slope is reversed. Such pH gradient is important for the migratory cycle composed of lamellipodium extension, formation of stable attachments near the leading edge, release of adhesions and retraction at the cell rear end (Webb et al., 2002). Active pH regulation in the migrating cell is facilitated by ion channels/transporters (including anion exchanger AE2 and Na^+/HCO_3^- co-transporter NBCe1), which are redistributed from their original basolateral position to the leading edge, where they intensify ion transport across the front plasma membrane (Klein et al., 2000). These exchangers ensure the local transport of H^+ ions outside and HCO_3^- inside by their simultaneous action, creating a necessary pH gradient (Stock and Schwab, 2009). The direct interaction and functional cooperation between CA IX and AE2 or NBCe1 could maximise HCO_3^- gradient across the plasma membrane and thereby optimise the buffering of pHi. In turn, CA IX-mediated extracellular accumulation of

H^+ increases pHe acidification (Svastova et al, 2004), and in this way CA IX can contribute to the activation of matrix metalloproteinases and potentiate tumour cell metastasis. In support of this concept we recently demonstrated the physical interaction of CA IX with bicarbonate transporters NBCe1 and AE2 in lamellipodia of the migrating tumour cells (Svastova et al., 2011). Hypoxia and associated acidosis also induce/activate additional tumour-related regulators of pH such as MCT4, and NHE1 that re-localize to the leading edge of migrating cells and facilitate migration (Ullah et al., 2006, Shimoda et al., 2006, Gallagher et al., 2008), see Figure 10.1.

pH gradient also affects focal adhesion assembly and disassembly. Larger focal adhesions at the leading edge of ARPE-19 cells were observed following MCT4 silencing (Gallagher et al., 2008). In addition, disruption of ion translocation activity of NHE1 alone impairs de-adhesion at the front and the rear part of migrating cells. The larger and more abundant focal adhesions at the front likely inhibit lamellipodial retraction while increased focal adhesions at the rear likely impair de-adhesion, resulting in a decreased rate of migration (Denker et al., 2002). Noteworthy, membrane recruitment of Akt, a downstream target of PI3K, was completely abolished with loss of transport activity of NHE1 and impaired cell polarity. Moreover, ion transport of NHE1 stimulated by integrins is connected with reorganisation of actin filaments and focal adhesions. Disruption of NHE1 binding to actin cytoskeleton through ERM proteins results in loss of cell polarity, inhibition of phosphatidylinositol signalling and decreased cell migration. Therefore, the two functions of NHE1 act cooperatively to enhance migration through focal adhesion turnover, regulation of pHe and pHi gradient and cytoskeletal anchoring (Denker et al., 2002). Moreover, NHE1 plays an important role in lamellipodia formation and migration via leading edge swelling directed by Na+ import (Schwab A, 2001).

Tumour cell motility and ivasion in vivo is asssociated with pseudopodia formation. Analysis of isolated pseudopodia from transformed MDCK cells as well as from glioma cells revealed the presence of β-actin and glycolytic enzyme glyceraldehyde-3-phosphate dehydrogenase GAPDH (Nguyen et al., 2000, Beckner et al., 2005). These results demonstrate the necessary role of glycolysis at sites of active polymerization of actin filaments, which serve as a driving force for lamellipodia extension and migration. It was shown that glycolysis, which is associated with cancer phenotype and is induced by hypoxia, is the primary energy source for tumour cell motility. Inhibition of glycolysis with 2-deoxyglucose resulted in the disruprion of β-actin-rich pseudopodia. Pseudopodia and lamellipodia are mitochondria- and organelle-free spaces. Interaction between actin and glycolytic enzymes may

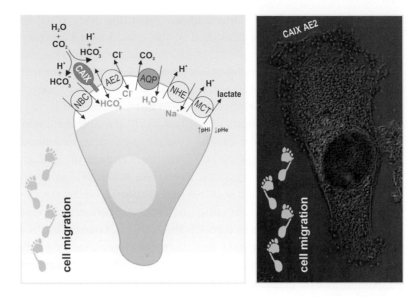

Figure 10.1 _ Regulators of pH in the lamellipodium of migrating cell. Left side shows schematic illustration of the selected components of the pH regulatory machinery that mediate intense ion transport and generate pH gradient facilitating cell migration, including carbonic anhydrase IX (CA IX), sodium-bicarbonate co-transporter NBCe1 (NBC), anion exchanger 2 (AE), aquaporins (AQP), sodium-hydrogen exchanger NHE1 (NHE), and monocarboxylate transporter (MCT4). These molecules extrude lactate and protons and import bicarbonate ions produced by CA IX thereby contributing to acidic extracellular pH ($\downarrow$pHe) and neutral-alkaline intracellular pH ($\uparrow$pHi). Right side shows image of migrating cell with the lamellipodium containing red signal that represents CA IX and AE2 interaction detected by proximity ligation assay (Svastova et al, 2012).

therefore provide an immediate and localised energy supply for the active assembly and disassembly of actin filaments, which drive pseudopodial protrusion (Nguyen et al., 2000).

The proteins identified in pseudopod proteome from transformed MDCK cells were classed into major families including cytoskeletal proteins (e.g. β-actin, myosin, ezrin, radixin, calpain, VASP), adhesion proteins (e.g. vinculin, talin, β1 integrin), glycolytic enzymes (e.g. GAPDH, PGI, LDH1, pyruvate kinase 3, phosphofructokinase), protein chaperones, and translation-associated proteins (Jia et al., 2005). Interestingly, almost all proteins enriched in the aforementioned proteome were also detected in U87 glioma cell pseudopodia. Moreover, HGF and c-Met as well as a number of their downstream signalling proteins including FAK, Raf1, MEK, Akt1, RhoGDI, ROCK etc. were identified in the pseudopod proteome (Jia et al., 2005, Beckner et al., 2005).

Specific conditions in hypoxic tumours with characteristic nutrient and oxygen deprivation and extracellular acidosis need different mechanisms directing cellular processes than in normal cells. Altered regulatory response to serum deprivation by activation of PKA and induction of migration contributes to "invasive switch". Reshkin et al. (2000) demonstrated that activation of NHE1 in response to serum deprivation of tumour cells and normal cells is completely opposite. In tumour cells, NHE activity is up-regulated by serum deprivation and this stimulation of NHE activity increases with an increasing neoplastic state. Serum deprivation induces formation of leading edge pseudopodia through the NHE1 activation by PKA and consequently increased migratory and invasive capacities of human breast carcinoma cells. Integrin-mediated activation of PKA is an early step in directional cell migration and localises activated PKA to lamellipodia (Lim et al., 2008). Furthermore, blocking PKA inhibits membrane protrusion and cell migration (Howe et al., 2005).

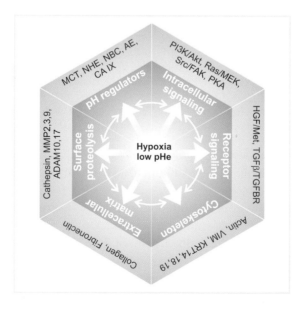

Figure 10. 2 _ Model of the central role of hypoxia and extracellular acidosis in activation of pathways and processes associated with cell migration.

PKA phosphorylates and also activates bicarbonate ion channels and transporters, such as NBCe1 and AE2, which are regulated by the VHL/ HIF pathway (Stock et al., 2009, Karumanchi et al., 2001). PKA-mediated phosphorylation of NBCe1 results in a transport stochiometry favorable for bicarbonate import (Gross et al., 2002). This mode is compatible with intracellular neutralisation activated in cells exposed to hypoxia/acidosis. We found that CA IX, which participates in bicarbonate metabolon, is directly phosphorylated by PKA and co-localises with NBCe1 as well as with phosphorylated PKA substrates. Phosphorylation of Thr443 by PKA is essential for CA IX-mediated pH regulation in hypoxic cells (Ditte et al., 2011).

This overview of events and molecules suggests that hypoxia and acidosis significantly contribute to tumour cell migration and invasion and thus represent important microenvironmental factors driving the metastatic cascade (Figure 10.2).

Acknowledgments _ The authors are supported by the EU 7th Framework program project METOXIA (FP7-HEALTH-2007-222741), by the Research and Development Support Agency projects (APVV-DORP-0017-09, APVV-0658-11, APVV-0893-11) and by the Slovak Scientific Grant Agency projects (VEGA-2/0130/11, VEGA-2/0129/11).

References

Beckner ME, Chen X, An J, Day BW, Pollack IF (2005). Proteomic characterization of harvested pseudopodia with differential gel electrophoresis and specific antibodies. Laboratory Investigation 85:316-327.

Benvenuti S, Comoglio PM (2007). The MET receptor tyrosine kinase in invasion and metastasis. J Cell Physiol 213(2):316-25.

Bourguignon LYW, Singleton PA, Diedrich F, Stern R, Gilad E (2004). CD44 Interaction with Na+-H+ Exchanger (NHE1) Creates Acidic Microenvironments Leading to Hyaluronidase-2 and Cathepsin B Activation and Breast Tumour Cell Invasion. J Biol Chem 279:26991-27007.

Christiansen JJ, Rajasekaran AK (2006). Reassessing Epithelial to Mesenchymal Transition as a Prerequisite for Carcinoma Invasion and Metastasis. Cancer Res 66: (17): 8319-8326.

Crawford SE, Stellmach V, Murphy-Ullrich JE, Ribeiro SM, Lawler J, Hynes RO, Boivin GP, Bouck N. (1998). Thrombospondin-1 is a major activator of TGF-beta1 in vivo. Cell 93(7):1159-70.

Denker SP, Barber DL (2002). Cell migration requires both ion translocation and cytoskeletal anchoring by the Na-H exchanger NHE1. Journal of Cell Biology 159(6): 1087-1096.

Ditte P, Dequiedt F, Svastova E, Hulikova A, Ohradanova-Repic A, Zatovicova M, Csaderova L, Kopacek J, Supuran CT, Pastorekova S, Pastorek J (2011). Phosphorylation of Carbonic Anhydrase IX Controls Its Ability to Mediate Extracellular Acidification in Hypoxic Tumours. Cancer Res 71(24):7558-67.

Erler JT, Weaver VM (2009). Three-dimensional context regulation of metastasis. Clin.
Exp. Metastasis 26, 35–49.

Funasaka T, Raz A (2007). The role of autocrine motility factor in tumour and tumour
microenvironment. Cancer Metastasis Rev 26:725–735

Gallagher SM, Castorino JJ, Philip NJ (2009). Interaction of monocarboxylate transporter 4 with β1-integrin and its role in cell migration. Am J Physiol Cell Physiol
296:C414-C421.

Gao Y, Xiao Q, Ma HM, Li L, Liu J, Feng Y, Fang Z, Wu J, Han X, Zhang J, Sun Y, Wu
G, Padera R, Chen H, Wong KK, Ge G, Ji H (2010). LKB1 inhibits lung cancer
progression through lysyl oxidase and extracellular matrix remodeling. PNAS
107(44): 18892-18897.

Gross E, Kurtz I (2002). Structural determinants and significance of regulation of
electrogenic Na(+) – HCO(3)(-) cotransporter stoichiometry. Am J Physiol Renal
Physiol 283:F876-87

Holman CM, Kan CC, Gehring MR, Van Wart HE (1999). Role of His-224 in the anoma-
lous pH dependence of human stromelysin-1. Biochemistry 38(2):677-81.

Howe IK, Baldor LC , Hogan BP (2005). Spatial regulation of the cAMP-dependent
protein kinase during chemotactic cell migration. PNAS 102:14320-14325.

Iessi E, Marino ML, Lozupone F, Fais S, De Milito A (2008). Tumour acidity and malignancy: novel aspects in the design of anti-tumour therapy. Cancer Therapy 6:55-66.

Jia Z, Barbier L, Stuart H, Amraei M, Pellech S, Dennis JW, Metalnikov P, O`Donnell
P, Nabi IR (2005). Tumour Cell Pseudopodial Protrusions. J Biol Chem 280:30564-
30573.

Karumanchi SA, Jiang L, Knebelmann B, Stuart-Tilley AK, Alper SL, Sukhatme
VP (2001). VHL tumour suppressor regulates Cl-/HCO3- exchange and Na+/H+
exchange activities in renal carcinoma cells. Physiol Genomics 5:119-28.

Klein M, Seeger P, Schuricht B, Alper SL, Schwab A (2000). Polarization of Na+/H+
and Cl-/HCO 3- exchangers in migrating renal epithelial cells. J Gen Physiol 115,
599–608.

Krishnamachary B, Berg-Dixon S, Kelly B, Agani F, Feldser D, Ferreira G, Iyer N,
LaRusch J, Pak B, Taghavi P, Semenza GL (2003). Regulation of Colon Carcinoma
Cell Invasion by Hypoxia-inducible Factor 1. Cancer Res 63:1138-1143.

Levental KR, Yu H, Kass L, Lakins JN, Egeblad M, Erler JT, Fong SFT, Csiszar K,
Giaccia A, Weninger W, Yamauchi M, Gasser DL, Weaver WM (2009). Matrix
crosslinking forces tumour progression by enhancing integrin signalling. Cell
139, 891–906.

Lim CJ, Kain KH, Tkachenko E, Goldfinger LE, Gutierrez E, Allen MD, Groisman A,
Zhang J, Ginsberg MH (2008). Integrin-mediated Protein Kinase A Activation at
the Leading Edge of Migrating Cells. Moll Biol Cell 19:4930-4941.

Micalizzi DM, Farabaugh SM, Ford HL (2010). Epithelial-Mesenchymal Transition in Cancer: Parallels Between Normal Development and Tumour Progression. J Mammary Gland Biol Neoplasia 15:117–134.

Monaco S, Gioia M, Rodriguez J, Fasciglione GF, Di Pierro D, Lupidi G, Krippahl L, Marini S, Coletta M (2007). Modulation of the proteolytic activity of matrix metalloproteinase-2 (gelatinase A) on fibrinogen. Biochemical Journal 402:503-513.

Ng MR, Brugge JS (2009). A Stiff Blow from the Stroma: Collagen crosslinking drives tumour progression. Cancer Cell 16, 455-457.

Nguyen TN, Wang HJ, Zalzal S, Nanci A, Nabi IR (2000). Purification and Characterization of β-Actin-Rich Tumour Cell Pseudopodia: Role of Glycolysis. Exp Cell Res 258:171-183.

Osada-Oka M, Ikeda T, Akiba S, Sato T (2008). Hypoxia stimulates the autocrine regulation of migration of vascular smooth muscle cells via HIF-1α-dependent expression of thrombospondin-1. J Cellular Biochem 104(5):1918-1926.

Otsuka T, Takayama H, Sharp R, Celli G, LaRochelle WJ, Bottaro DP, Ellmore N, Vieira W, Owens JW, Anver M, Merlino G (1998). c-Met autocrine activation induces development of malignant melanoma and acquisition of the metastatic phenotype. Cancer Res. 58(22):5157-67.

Pennacchietti S, Michieli P, Galluzzo M, Mazzone M, Giordano S, Comoglio PM (2003). Hypoxia promotes invasive growth by transcriptional activation of the *met* protooncogene. Cancer Cell 3(4):347-61.

Phelan MW, Forman LW, Perrine SP, Faller DV (1998). Hypoxia increases thrombospondin-1 transcript and protein in cultured endothelial cells. J Lab Clin Med. 132(6):519-29.

Postovit LM, Abbott DE, Payne SL, Wheaton WW, Margaryan NV, Sullivan R, Jansen MK, Csiszar K, Hendrix MJ, Kirschmann DA (2008). Hypoxia/reoxygenation: a dynamic regulator of lysyl oxidase-facilitated breast cancer migration. J Cell Biochem 103, 1369–1378.

Reshkin SJ, Bellizzihttp A, Albarani V, Guerra L, Tommasino M, Paradiso A, Casavola V (2000) Phosphoinositide 3-Kinase Is Involved in the Tumour-specific Activation of Human Breast Cancer Cell Na$^+$/H$^+$Exchange, Motility, and Invasion Induced by Serum Deprivation. J Biol Chem 275:5361-5369.

Shimoda LA, Fallon M, Pisarcik S, Wang J, Semenza GL (2006). HIF-1 regulates hypoxic induction of NHE1 expression and alkalinisation of intracellular pH in pulmonary arterial myocytes. Am J Physiol Lung Cell Mol Physiol 291: L941–9

Stock C, Schwab A (2009). Proton make tumour cells move like a clockwork. Pflugers Arch 458:981-992.

Stock C, Mueller M, Kraehling H, Mally S, Noël J, Eder C, Schwab A (2007). pH nanoenvironment at the Surface of Single Melanoma Cells. Cell Physiol Biochem 20:679-686.

Sullivan R, Graham CH (2007). Hypoxia-driven selection of the metastatic phenotype. Cancer Metastasis Rev. 26(2):319-31.

Svastova E, Hulikova A, Rafajova M, Zatovicova M, Gibadulinova A, Casini A, Cecchi A, Scozzafava A, Supuran CT, Pastorek J, Pastorekova S (2004). Hypoxia activates the capacity of tumour-associated carbonic anhydrase IX to acidify extracellular pH. FEBS Lett. 577(3):439-45.

Svastova E, Zilka N, Zatovicova M, Gibadulinova A, Ciampor F, Pastorek J, Pastorekova S (2003). Carbonic anhydrase IX reduces E-cadherin-mediated adhesion of MDCK cells via interaction with beta-catenin. Exp Cell Res 290, 332-345.

Svastova E, Witarski W, Csaderova L, Kosik I, Skvarkova L, Hulikova A, Zatovicova M, Barathova M, Kopacek J, Pastorek J, Pastorekova S (2012). Carbonic anhydrase IX interacts with bicarbonate transporters in lamellipodia and increases cell migration via its catalytic domain. J Biol Chem. 287(5):3392-402.

Takanami I, Takeuchi K,Watanabe H, Yanagawa T, Takagishi K, Raz A (2001). Significance of autocrine motility factor receptor gene expression as a prognostic factor in non-small-cell lung cancer. International Journal of Cancer 95: 384–387.

Ullah MS, Davies AJ, Halestrap AP (2006). The plasma membrane lactate transporter MCT4, but not MCT1, is up-regulated by hypoxia through a HIF-1α-dependent mechanism. J Biol Chem 281:9030–7.

Webb DJ, Parsons JT, Horwitz AF (2002). Adhesion assembly, disassembly and turnover in migrating cells–over and over and over again. Nat Cell Biol 4, E97–100.

Wewer O, Mareel M (2003). Role of tissue stroma in cancer cell invasion. J Pathol 200: 429–447.

Wykoff CC, Beasley NJ, Watson PH, Turner KJ, Pastorek J, Sibtain A, Wilson GD, Turley H, Talks KL, Maxwell PH, Pugh CW, Ratcliffe PJ, Harris AL (2000). Hypoxia-inducible expression of tumour associated carbonic anhydrases. Cancer Res 60: 7075–83.

You WK, McDonald DM (2008). The hepatocyte growth factor/c-Met signalling pathway as a therapeutic target to inhibit angiogenesis. BMB Rep. 41(12):833-9.

Chapter 11

Reactive oxygen species and hypoxia signalling

Agnes Görlach [*]

[*]Author for correspondence:
Experimental and Molecular Pediatric Cardiology, German Heart Center Munich
at the TU Munich, 80636 Munich, Germany E-mail: goerlach@dhm.mhn.de

Contents

Key points

— Reactive oxygen species (ROS) can induce HIF-α.

— ROS regulate HIF-α by different mechanisms including NF-κB.

— NADPH oxidases and mitochondria are important sources of ROS to regulate HIF-α.

— NADPH oxidases and mitochondrial respiratory chain subunits are sensitive to hypoxia.

— HIF-α can regulate transcription of NADPH oxidase and mitochondrial respiratory chain subunits.

Superoxide and its derived reactive oxygen species (ROS) have been considered for a long time to be generated as toxic by-products of metabolic events. More recently, it has been acknowledged that ROS generated in low amounts are also able to act as signalling molecules in a variety of responses. One of the major pathways regulated by the ambient concentration of oxygen relies on the activity of hypoxia-inducible transcription factors (HIF). Although it was originally thought to be induced and activated only under hypoxia, accumulating evidence suggests that HIFs play a more general role in the response to a variety of cellular activators and stressors, many of which use ROS as signal transducers. Thereby, ROS can regulate HIF-α at the level of protein stability and transcriptionally. Conversely, HIF-α have recently been shown to directly regulate ROS-generating NADPH oxidases and some components of the mitochondrial respiratory chain. Thus, a tight regulatory circuit exists whereby HIF may act as an important modulator of ROS available under different stress conditions.

Introduction

The adequate supply of oxygen is mandatory for the function of diverse processes within all aerobic organisms. Therefore, an intricate signalling system has been evolved aiming to assure optimal adaptation to inadequate and insufficient oxygen availability (hypoxia). A key element in this adaptive response is a family of transcription factors termed hypoxia-inducible factors (HIFs) which are regulated by complex signalling mechanisms to allow expression of selected genes for adaptation of cells and organs to hypoxia.

Despite the requirements of O_2 for cell and organ function, O_2 can often be transformed into highly reactive derivates, termed reactive oxygen species (ROS). Initially, ROS generation was considered to cause oxidative stress, a status which can damage cellular proteins, RNA, DNA, and lipids. Physiologically, an overshoot in ROS production is counterbalanced by the endogenous antioxidant defence systems which are comprised of different superoxide dismutases (MnSOD, Cu/ZnSOD, EC-SOD), glutathione peroxidases (GPX), catalase, peroxiredoxins, thioredoxin and exogenously taken up micronutrients and vitamins.

However, it has been increasingly acknowledged that ROS in nontoxic concentrations can also act as important signalling molecules. This assumption has been supported by the numerous cellular systems, which are able to generate ROS. While ROS generation has been long considered to be derived as an (unwanted) product of aerobic respiration in the electron transport chain in mitochondria, there is now increasing evidence that mitochondrial ROS generation as well as enzymatic ROS production for example by NADPH oxidases can be regarded as a regulated process aimed to specifically affect cellular pathways. There is now compelling evidence that one of these ROS-regulated pathways is the HIF signalling cascade. Although initially considered counterintuitive, that a rather "oxidative" milieu would be also effective in regulating the central signalling mechanism for adaptation to hypoxia, a variety of studies now provide evidence that the HIF pathway is redox-sensitive and responds to hypoxia and ROS signalling cascades. These findings have brought new implications for the role of HIF transcription factors in the pathogenesis of disease states associated with enhanced ROS levels including inflammation, metabolic diseases, thrombosis, ischemia-reoxygenation, atherosclerosis and many others. The purpose of this chapter is to give a brief overview of the most important sources of ROS associated with HIF signalling, the mechanisms of how ROS affect HIF activity, and recent findings of the role of HIFs in regulating ROS-generating pathways.

Reactive oxygen species: Identity and sources

Transfer of one electron to O_2 results in the production of superoxide anion radicals ($O_2^-\bullet$) which are often the precursors for formation of other reactive species such as hydrogen peroxide (H_2O_2), hydroxyl radicals ($OH\bullet$), peroxynitrite ($ONOO^-$), hypochlorous acid ($HOCl$) and singlet oxygen ($^1O_2$), see Figure 11.1. Whereas $O_2^-\bullet$ is less likely to act as second messenger since it is not freely diffusible, its freely diffusible dismutation product H_2O_2 is more suitable to fulfil such a function. Excess H_2O_2 is usually degraded by GPX or by catalase, but it may, in the presence of Fe(II), undergo a Fenton reaction where hydroxyl anions and highly reactive hydroxyl radicals are produced which in turn can affect signalling proteins. In addition to the mitochondrial respiratory chain, a variety of systems are able to generate ROS, mostly $O_2^-\bullet$ or H_2O_2. Among them are the arachidonic acid pathway, the cytochrome P450 family, NADH or NADPH oxidases, glucose oxidase, amino acid oxidases, xanthine oxidase, or under certain conditions even

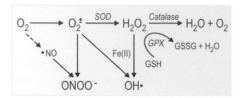

Figure 11.1 _ Formation of reactive oxygen species.

Electron transfer on molecular oxygen results in the formation of superoxide which can subsequently react to hydrogen peroxide catalyzed by superoxide dismutases.In the presence of nitric oxide formation of peroxynitrite is promoted. In the presence of FeII hydroxyl radical formation is promoted.

NO synthases. In particular NADPH oxidases have been gaining increasing interest over the past 15 years since they are specifically designed to generate $O_2 \cdot$ or H_2O_2.

NADPH Oxidases

Increasing evidence suggests that the family of NADPH oxidases is of great importance for regulated ROS generation in many cell types necessary for cell signalling. Although initially presumed to be an enzyme existing only in neutrophils, NADPH oxidases have also been identified in many if not all non-phagocytic cells including vascular cells and tumour cells (for review see Babior, 2004; Bedard and Krause, 2007; Brown and Griendling, 2009; Gorlach et al., 2002; Lambeth et al., 2007). NADPH oxidases are multi protein enzymes catalyzing the one electron reduction of oxygen to $O_2 \cdot$ using NADPH as an electron donor (Figure 11.2). In addition, they need FAD to perform the single electron reduction and two hemes in order to span the membrane since the site of NADPH binding and the site of reaction are oppositely located. The catalytic moieties are localised in a heterodimeric transmembrane complex forming a cytochrome b558, which consists of one out of several homologous NOX proteins and the p22phox protein. To date 5 homologous NOX proteins termed NOX1 to NOX5 have been identified. The catalytic NOX proteins carry all the cofactors needed for this reaction, and p22phox is believed to either assist in the proper folding of NOX or even to be part of the electron chain. In addition, a variety of cofactors are required for proper activation of some of these enzymes, in particular for NOX1, NOX2 and NOX3. The main function of these regulatory proteins is to bring NADPH in close proximity to FAD in order to facilitate the electron flow. This is accompanied by an internal refolding in order to transfer the electron from FAD to heme and later on to oxygen. In contrast, NOX4, although forming a complex with p22phox, which is required for functional activity, does not seem to require additional regulatory proteins to function. It is thus assumed that NOX4-dependent ROS generation is mainly regulated at the level of expression. Additionally, NOX5 does not seem to require p22phox for its function. Conversely, it contains a series of calcium binding EF hands at its N-terminus, which confer calcium sensitivity of this enzyme. Furthermore, two more distinct DUOX enzymes have additional putative peroxidase domains and seem to perform a two-electron reduction yielding H_2O_2 (Bedard and Krause, 2007; Lambeth et al., 2007).

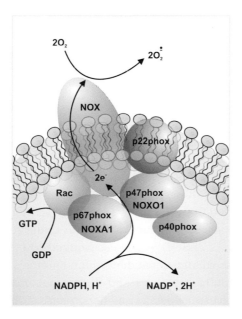

Figure 11.2 _ NADPH oxidases are important sources of cellular reactive oxygen species.

NADPH oxidases consist of a central catalytic core, the NOX protein, which contains FAD and heme to allow electron transfer from NADPH to molecular oxygen. Activity of NADPH oxidases can be controlled by regulatory proteins termed p47phox or its homologue NOXO1, p67phox or its homologue NOXA1, p40phox and the GTPase Rac.

Importantly, a variety of stimuli including growth factors, cytokines, hormones, vasoactive factors and coagulation factors have been shown to activate NADPH oxidases. Thus, ROS generated by NADPH oxidases have been considered part of the signalling pathways of many receptor-ligand interactions (Petry et al., 2010).

Mitochondrial ROS generation

Early evidence, mainly from studies using isolated mitochondria suggested that a small percentage of oxygen used by the electron transport chain is not completely reduced to water but is instead converted to $O_2^-\bullet$. In contrast to NADPH oxidases, mitochondrial ROS generation has only recently been related to receptor-ligand interactions; but has been mainly made dependent on oxygen consumption. Thus mitochondria have been related to hypoxic signalling for a long time although their role is still controversial (see below). ROS generation by mitochondria has been related to respiratory activity where a series of redox reactions occur along which electrons transferred from a donor molecule (NADH or QH2) to O_2, concluding at complex IV (cytochrome oxidase), where molecular O_2 is reduced to water. It has been suggested that formation of superoxide occurs upstream of complex IV, primarily by autooxidation of flavins in complex I, where superoxide can enter the matrix, and at complex III where superoxide is formed via the Q-cycle and can enter either the mitochondrial intermembrane space or the matrix, respectively (Rigoulet et al., 2011; Turrens, 2003). Once in the matrix, superoxide is converted first to H_2O_2 by MnSOD, and then to water by GPX. In the intermembrane space, superoxide can undergo multiple fates: it can be degraded by CuZnSOD, can be scavenged by cytochrome c or can enter the cytosol via voltage-dependent anion channels (Han et al., 2003). The relative contribution of complex I and III to superoxide generation appears to be cell and/or tissue specific and dependent on respiratory status.

Regulation of hypoxia-inducible transcription factors (HIF) by oxygen

The transcription factors of the HIF family represent key elements in cellular adaptation to hypoxia. These heterodimers consist of an α subunit and a β subunit. The latter is also known as arylhydrocarbon receptor-nuclear translocator ARNT (Hoffman et al., 1991), both basic helix-loop-helix and Per-ARNT-Sim (PAS) domain consisting proteins. Whereas the ARNT subunit is constitutively expressed, HIF-α proteins are tightly regulated by oxygen availability thus mediating the sensitivity towards environmental O_2 levels (reviewed by (Wenger, 2002)). The first identified HIF transcription factor was HIF-1 (Beck et al., 1993; Semenza and Wang, 1992) followed by HIF-2 (also termed EPAS-1) (Tian et al., 1997) and HIF-3 (Gu et al., 1998).

The predominant mode of HIF-α regulation appears to be posttranslational. This is brought about by the HIF-α oxygen-dependent degradation domain (ODD) (Huang et al., 1998) and two transactivation domains (TADs) referred to as amino-terminal (TADN) and carboxy-terminal (TADC) TAD (Jiang et al., 1997; Pugh et al., 1997). The ODD and the TADN partially overlap and are mainly responsible for HIF-α protein stability.

Normoxia thereby initiates hydroxylation of HIF-α on at least two proline residues within the ODD (Ivan et al., 2001, Jaakkola et al., 2001). This allows binding of the von Hippel-Lindau tumour suppressor protein (pVHL) which initiates ubiquitinylation and proteasomal degradation. To date, three prolylhydroxylase domain containing proteins (PHD-1, -2, -3,) also known as HIF-prolyl 4-hydroxylases (HIF-P4H), have been identified as being responsible for HIF-α hydroxylation. These enzymes vary in their subcellular localisation and target affinity (for review see Kaelin and Ratcliffe, 2008). A fourth enzyme, PHD4 or P4H-TM, is located in the endoplasmic reticulum, and seems to be more closely related to procollagen prolyl hydroxylases than the PHDs (Koivunen et al., 2007). By contrast, another hydroxylase named factor inhibiting HIF (FIH) hydroxylates an asparaginyl residue in the TADC which prevents the recruitment of the coactivator CREB binding protein (CBP)/p300 (Mahon et al., 2001). Interestingly, this domain is lacking in HIF-3α suggesting that HIF-3α may act differentially compared to the other HIF-α subunits. The fact that the activity of these enzymes has been considered to be strictly dependent on oxygen availability has made PHDs attractive elements in the oxygen-sensing cascade. However, in addition to oxygen, hydroxylase activity is also dependent on the presence of its cofactors Fe(II), 2-oxoglutarate and ascorbate (for review see (Kaelin and Ratcliffe, 2008)).

In addition to hydroxylation, and subsequent ubiquitinylation, other hydroxylase-independent post-translational modifications of HIF-α aimed to increase HIF-α levels under hypoxia have been recently described, among them, sumoylation (Bae et al., 2004), neddylation (Ryu et al., 2010) and acetylation/deacetylation by Sirt1 (Dioum et al., 2009).

While the synthesis of many proteins is reduced under hypoxic conditions, HIF-1α is able to escape this control thus allowing efficient translation under normoxic and hypoxic conditions (Gorlach et al., 2000b). The human HIF-1α gene has been shown to contain an internal ribosome entry site (IRES) which seems to be crucially involved in its translational maintenance (Lang et al., 2002). Although only limited data exists describing translational control of HIF-1α, it has been shown that polypyrimidine tract binding protein (PTB) can specifically interact with the HIF-1α IRES, and that this interaction is enhanced in hypoxic conditions (Schepens et al., 2005).

In addition to the regulation by protein stabilization and translation, HIF-1α has been shown to be regulated at the transcriptional level in response to hypoxia involving activation and binding of NF-κB to the HIF-1α promoter (Belaiba et al., 2007a; Rius et al., 2008).

Reactive oxygen species modulate hypoxia-inducible factors

The first evidence that HIF-1 is redox-sensitive came from studies in which treatment of purified HIF-1 with H_2O_2, diamide and N-ethyl-maleimide resulted in a loss in DNA-binding activity. This was counteracted by prior addition of dithiothreitol suggesting that HIF-1 DNA binding requires reducing conditions (Wang et al., 1995). Further, thioredoxin (Trx) was shown to enhance HIF-1α protein levels and this response was dependent on two redox-sensitive cysteines within the Trx protein (Huang et al., 1996; Welsh et al., 2002). Subsequently, the Trx effector Ref-1 was shown to bind to TADN and TADC. Also, this reaction seemed to be dependent on the redox state of cysteine 800 in HIF-1α and cysteine 848 in HIF-2α (Huang et al., 1996; Welsh et al., 2002); (Carrero et al., 2000; Ema et al., 1999) since mutation of cysteine 800 prevented the decrease in HIF-1α TADC activity in response to hydroxyl radicals (OH•) (Liu et al., 2004). Support of the view that H_2O_2 was the main ROS promoting HIF-α levels came from studies overexpressing Cu/ZnSOD. These cells had enhanced formation of H_2O_2 and increased HIF-1α levels (BelAiba et al., 2004). In addition, cell-permeable SOD mimetics enhanced

HIF-1α levels under normoxia in rat renal medullary interstitial cells and human cerebral vascular smooth muscle cells (Wellman et al., 2004). Furthermore, increased HIF-α protein levels were found in H_2O_2-treated artery smooth muscle cells (Bonello et al., 2007; Diebold et al., 2010a; Gorlach et al., 2001) and in Hep3B cells (Chandel et al., 2000). However, this effect seems to be cell type specific possibly related to the levels and activities of antioxidant enzymes present in a given cell. Subsequent evidence was provided, that HIF-α proteins are responsive to a variety of non-hypoxic stimuli in a ROS-dependent manner. Examples for such signalling pathways include insulin (Kietzmann et al., 2003; Treins et al., 2002), PDGF, TGF-β, IGF-1, EGF and HGF (Fukuda et al., 2003; Gorlach et al., 2001; Liu et al., 2006b; Richard et al., 2000; Tacchini et al., 2004), thrombin (Gorlach et al., 2001), angiotensin-II (Richard et al., 2000), cytokines (Stiehl et al., 2002), carbachol (Hirota et al., 2004), oxLDL (Shatrov et al., 2003), mechanical stress (Kim et al., 2002) as well as to the "hypoxic mimetic" $CoCl_2$ (BelAiba et al., 2004; Chandel et al., 2000).

Various studies identified NADPH oxidases as important sources of ROS in the regulation of HIF-α (Bonello et al., 2007; Diebold et al., 2008; Diebold et al., 2010a; Gorlach et al., 2001; Hirota et al., 2004; Kim et al., 2002). The findings that NADPH oxidases regulate HIF 1α were also substantiated by the *in vivo* observation that HIF-1α levels were elevated in carotid lesions of mice overexpressing p22phox in smooth muscle cells (Khatri et al., 2004). It appears that NOX4 may play an important role since depletion of NOX4 by siRNA diminished thrombin-induced HIF-1α levels (Bonello et al., 2007). NOX4 knockdown also decreased the levels of HIF-1α in ovarian cancer cells (Xia et al., 2007) while NOX1 mediated hyperthermia-induced up-regulation of HIF-1α in tumour cells (Moon et al., 2010). In line with this, depletion of NOX4 or NOX1 also decreased HIF-2α levels in VHL-deficient 786-O or RCC4 renal carcinoma cells suggesting that ROS may act via a VHL-dependent pathway (Block et al., 2007; Maranchie and Zhan, 2005). Additionally NOX4 was instrumental in regulating HIF-2α by thrombin in smooth muscle cells (Diebold et al., 2010a). LPS induced HIF-1α expression via NOX2 in microglia (Oh et al., 2008). Recent data indicates that NOX5 and NOX2, which seem to be important in endothelial ROS generation (BelAiba et al., 2007b; Gorlach et al., 2000a), also play a role in the regulation of HIF-1α (unpublished data). This data indicates that NADPH oxidases are important sources of ROS in a variety of non-hypoxic pathways, which result in HIF-α induction whereby the relative importance of NOX proteins in the regulation of HIF-α is most probably determined by the stimulus and the cell type involved.

Recently, some evidence has suggested that mitochondrial ROS generation may also contribute to stimulus-activated ROS levels under non-hypoxic conditions since induction of HIF-1α by angiotensin-II was repressed in smooth muscle cells upon application of a complex III inhibitor, by Rieske Fe-S protein siRNA, or by the mitochondrial-targeted antioxidant SkQ1 (Patten et al., 2010).

Mechanisms of HIF regulation by reactive oxygen species

Protein stability

There is now accumulating data that ROS can regulate HIF-α levels by different mechanisms. Evidence that ROS can affect HIF–α stability via interference with the PHD/pVHL pathway was provided by findings that thrombin and NOX4 increased HIF-2α TADN and TADC activity and this response was abolished upon mutation of the target prolines or asparagines, respectively (Diebold et al., 2010a). Similar observations were made with HIF-1α (unpublished data) indicating that ROS may mediate HIF-α stability by affecting hydroxylation and pVHL binding. In line, H_2O_2 decreased pVHL binding of HIF-2α (Diebold et al., 2010a) and HIF-1α (unpublished observation). However, since oxygen was not the limiting factor governing PHD activity under these circumstances, other mechanisms seemed to contribute to these observations.

Since ROS are known to be able to oxidize Fe(II) to Fe(III) it was reasonable to assume that the availability of Fe(II) may be disturbed under these conditions. In line with this assumption, in *junD*-deficient cells that exhibit chronic oxidative stress, it was shown that ROS interfered with Fe(II) availability in the HIF prolyl hydroxylase catalytic site possibly by a Fenton-type reaction thus diminishing HIF-1α hydroxylation and allowing its accumulation (Gerald et al., 2004). Interestingly, in thrombin-treated cells with NOX4-dependent increase in HIF-1α levels, the availability of Fe(II) was also decreased indicating that ROS generated by NADPH oxidases are able to diminish the pool of available Fe(II) (Diebold et al., 2010a). Conversely, it was shown that addition of iron to cultured human prostate adenocarcinoma cells stimulated HIF-1α degradation (Knowles et al., 2003) indicating that the balance between Fe(II) and Fe(III) is of major importance in controlling HIF-α levels.

In this context, it has been assumed that the major role of ascorbate, another cofactor of PHD/FIH hydroxylase activity is to maintain Fe(II) levels in the cell by providing a radical cycling system for regeneration of Fe(II) (Epstein et al., 2001). Although the mechanism is not entirely known yet, it is proposed that ascorbate reduces Fe(III) to Fe(II) within the enzyme active site thus rendering the enzyme active. Additionally, ascorbate might enhance the provision of Fe(II) from an intracellular pool such as ferritin by conversion of Fe(III) into Fe(II). In this case, it is proposed that superoxide ion, generated during the iron-promoted oxidation of ascorbate, acts as a reductant of ferritin iron (Boyer and McCleary, 1987).

In the cellular system, there is now ample evidence that ascorbate is an important factor regulating HIF-α levels under non-hypoxic conditions (BelAiba et al., 2004; Diebold et al., 2010a; Gorlach et al., 2001; Knowles et al., 2003; Page et al., 2008). Ascorbate was able to decrease induction of HIF-1α TADN and TADC activity by thrombin and H_2O_2, while it restored pVHL binding to HIF-2α in the presence of thrombin and H_2O_2 suggesting that in vivo activity of PHD and FIH is strongly dependent on ascorbate (Diebold et al., 2010a). Interestingly, thrombin and angiotensin-II decreased cellular ascorbate levels (Diebold et al., 2010a; Page et al., 2008), further confirming that ascorbate availability may provide an important mechanism in the regulation of HIF–α under non-hypoxic conditions. A further interesting point is that recent in vitro studies have suggested that other reducing agents such as glutathione and dithiothrcitol also promote HIF hydroxylase activity further indicating that the cellular redox state is important in controlling PHD activity (Flashman et al., 2010). In line, it was observed that the redox cycler DMNQ increased HIF-1α accumulation via reduction of pVHL binding suggesting that DMNQ was interfering with PHD activity (Kohl et al., 2006) while the same substance prevented accumulation of HIF-1α induced by TNF-α (Sandau et al., 2001) indicating that the current redox state is an essential determinant in regulation of HIFα stability via PHD activity. Such a notion may also explain the heterogeneous results observed on the role of ascorbate in regulating hypoxic HIF-α levels.

Transcription

In addition to regulation of HIF-α at the level of protein stability, non-hypoxic induction of HIF-1α has been described as being regulated by a transcriptional mechanism in a ROS-dependent manner (for review see Gorlach, 2009). Several studies have reported that cytokines, proinflammatory and prothrombotic factors, growth factors and vasoactive peptides including interleukin-1, HGF, angiotensin-II or lipopolysaccharides which are all known to increase ROS levels can induce HIF-1α mRNA levels in several cell types (Frede et al., 2006; Page et al., 2002; Tacchini et al., 2004).

Subsequently, it was shown that thrombin, NOX4 and H_2O_2 regulate HIF-1α transcription. This was mediated by ROS-sensitive activation of NF-κB, which bound to a specific consensus site in the HIF-1α promoter (Bonello et al., 2007; Gorlach and Bonello, 2008; Rius et al., 2008; van Uden et al., 2008). These findings indicate that transcriptional regulation of HIF-1α by ROS-sensitive activation of NF-κB may represent an important mechanism of how agonists can induce HIF-1α under non-hypoxic conditions and provide a pathophysiologically interesting link between these two important redox-sensitive transcription factors.

A role for ROS in increasing HIF-1α transcription was also shown in cells with a mutation in mitochondrial NADH dehydrogenase subunit 6 (ND6), and this pathway involved phosphatidylinositol 3-kinase (PI3K)-Akt, protein kinase C (PKC) and histone deacetylase (HDAC), although the specific transcription factor involved in this response has not been identified, yet (Koshikawa et al., 2009). In contrast to HIF-1α, only limited data is available on the regulation of HIF-2α mRNA and the contribution of ROS. It has been shown that NOX4 depletion decreased HIF-2α mRNA levels in RCC4 cells (Maranchie and Zhan, 2005) although the underlying mechanisms are not understood. Since the NF-κB binding site, which mediates transcriptional regulation of HIF-1α does not seem to be conserved in the HIF-2α promoter, this may be an important factor in determining non-redundant functions of HIF-1α and HIF-2α in hypoxic and non-hypoxic conditions.

Translation

In addition to this direct link between NF-κB and HIF-1α in response to ROS, it was proposed that the phosphatidylinositol 3-kinase (PI3K) pathway in conjunction with NF-κB may be involved in the translational regulation of HIF-1α in response to TNF-α (Zhou et al., 2004). Likewise, ROS-dependent activation of PI3K was also found to be involved in the increase in HIF-1α translation by angiotensin-II (Page et al., 2002). In addition, ROS-dependent but NF-κB-independent translation of HIF-1α was observed in human myeloid cells stimulated with lipopolysaccharide (LPS) (Nishi et al., 2008). However, the relative importance of ROS-dependent HIF-1α translational compared to transcriptional mechanisms and protein stabilization has not yet been clarified. The question of whether such a pathway is also important for ROS-dependent HIF-2α regulation has not been addressed either.

Other mechanisms of HIF–α regulation by ROS

Recent data has indicated that HIF-1α may also be regulated by neddylation involving Nedd8 (Ryu et al., 2010). This ubiquitin-like protein covalently
binds to its substrate proteins, and thus, regulates their stabilities and functions. Similar to the situation with ubiquitinylation, ROS prevented degradation of HIF-1α in the presence of NEDD8. It was also shown that the Sen-
trin/SUMO-specific protease 3 (SENP3) was stabilized by ROS resulting in
enhanced HIF-1 transactivation. This was brought about by SENP3-depend-
ent de-SUMOylation of the HIF coactivator p300 (Huang et al., 2009). Although
the relative importance of these pathways has not yet been clarified, these
findings further support the importance of ROS acting as versatile regulators of HIF-α under non-hypoxic conditions.

The reciprocal case: HIF regulation of ROS generating enzymes under normoxia and hypoxia

While evidence that ROS regulate HIF-α levels is compelling now under non-
hypoxic conditions, the role of ROS in the control of HIF-α under hypoxic conditions has been a matter of controversy for many years. Initial studies using
antioxidants observed a protective effect on HIF-1α stability under hypoxia-
reoxygenation conditions, while the effect on hypoxic HIF-1α was not clearly
evident (Haddad et al., 2000). Similarly, ascorbate treatment was unable to prevent hypoxic induction of HIF-1α (Knowles et al., 2003), and these results have been
observed by others in different cellular models (Brown and Nurse, 2008).

Conversely, the use of mitochondrial inhibitors and subsequently also
molecular approaches and mitochondria-depleted cells suggested that
ROS generated mainly by complex III of the mitochondria enhance HIF-
1α induction under hypoxic conditions (Chandel et al., 2000). These findings
seemed to be supported by studies showing that ROS levels increase under
hypoxic conditions, while this response was decreased upon inhibition
of mitochondrial complex III (Bell et al., 2007), complex II (Guzy et al., 2008) or
complex I (Agani et al., 2000). However, in contrast to these studies, hypoxic
induction of HIF-1α was not affected in mitochondria-depleted cells or
cells treated with mitochondrial inhibitors (Srinivas et al., 2001; Vaux et al., 2001).
In line with these observations, mitochondrial ROS production was also
reported to decrease under hypoxia (Archer and Michelakis, 2002).

In addition to mitochondrial ROS generation, NADPH oxidases have also been investigated with regard to their role in hypoxic ROS and HIF signalling using mostly in vivo models. In many cases, animals were exposed to acute or chronic hypoxia, and ROS levels were subsequently determined in isolated organs removed from these animals. This procedure resulted mostly in elevated ROS levels in wild type animals in response to hypoxia while ROS levels were often lower in knock out animals. For example, compared to wild type animals exposed to chronic hypoxia, ROS production was decreased in pulmonary arteries from NOX2 knock out mice, concomitant with decreased right ventricular hypertrophy and pulmonary vascular remodelling (Liu et al., 2006a). Similarly, hypoxia-induced ROS levels were reduced in p47phox-deficient carotid body cells (He et al., 2005).

On the other hand, in perfused lungs, $O_2^-\bullet$ release was decreased upon hypoxia in wild type animals as determined by EPR. Interestingly, p47phox deficiency already decreased $O_2^-\bullet$ levels under normoxia and this decrease was not further changed under hypoxic conditions (Weissmann et al., 2006). While no measurements of HIF-α levels have been performed in these studies, the discrepant findings in the regulation of ROS levels in response to hypoxia in particular in the in vivo situation might be explained by our observations that vessels exposed to hypoxia for longer time periods show decreased ROS generation when ROS measurements were performed under complete hypoxic conditions by EPR (unpublished observation). However, when ROS measurements were performed under normoxic conditions after exposure to hypoxia, ROS levels were increased. Similarly, ROS levels were elevated in vessels and organs derived from mice exposed to hypoxia for 2 weeks where sample preparation had to be performed under normoxic conditions (unpublished observation), suggesting that even short normoxic periods following exposure to hypoxia can exacerbate ROS release similar to reoxygenation.

Interestingly, it has been reported that hypoxia can increase the levels of several NADPH oxidase subunits, including NOX4 (Diebold et al., 2010b; Mittal et al., 2007). When ROS levels were determined under normoxia following a hypoxic incubation period maximizing NOX4 levels, ROS levels were elevated compared to normoxic conditions. This response was diminished when NOX4 was depleted by shRNA. However, when ROS levels were determined by the same method in cells exposed to short-term hypoxia not sufficient to induce NOX4, ROS levels were lower than in normoxic cells. However, overexpression of NOX4 restored ROS levels to normoxic values suggesting that induction of NOX4 and possibly other NADPH oxidase subunits under hypoxic conditions may be of importance to maintain ROS levels under hypoxia and to allow enhanced ROS generation under reoxygenation conditions (Diebold et al., 2010b). Strikingly, this adaptive response was regulated by HIF-α, since depletion of this transcription factor also prevented adaptive ROS production after hypoxia-reoxygenation similar to the situation with NOX4 depletion. Subsequent studies including site-directed mutagenesis of a putative HIF-binding site and chromatin immunoprecipitation revealed that NOX4 is a HIF target gene (Diebold et al., 2010b). Similarly, the regulatory NADPH oxidase protein Rac1 was also shown to be a HIF target gene (Diebold et al., 2008). These findings provide novel insights into the regulation of ROS production under hypoxic conditions. Since NADPH oxidases can increase HIF-α levels (see above), these findings may provide at least one explanation for the controversial data relating ROS, hypoxia and HIF- α.

In support of these findings it was reported that cells express the COX4-1 regulatory subunit of cytochrome c oxidase (complex IV) under aerobic conditions but switch to the COX4-2 subunit under hypoxic conditions, and this switch is transcriptionally regulated by HIF-1. Interestingly, COX4-2 was able to optimize electron flux under hypoxic conditions and did not promote ROS generation. Thus, it was suggested that under conditions of chronic hypoxia, complex IV can become a source of increased ROS production if the COX4 subunit switch does not occur (Fukuda et al., 2007).

Thus, an intricate link between hypoxia, HIF, ROS, mitochondria and NADPH oxidases is increasingly deciphered which provides intriguing

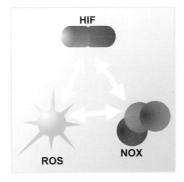

Figure 11.3 _ ROS, HIF and NOX – a reactive triangle

Reactive oxygen species (ROS) derived from NADPH oxidases (NOX) can induce HIF transcription factors. HIF on the other hand can induce NOX thus modulating ROS levels.

insights into the complex mechanisms of redox regulation of the HIF pathway under different conditions (Figure 11.3). Clearly, the HIF pathway is a central adaptive mechanism not only in response to hypoxia, but also as an effector of ROS-regulated signalling pathways under various stress conditions.

A c k n o w l e d g e m e n t s _ This work was supported by DFG GO709/4-4, the 7th European framework program (Metoxia) and Fondation Leducq.

References

Agani, F.H., Pichiule, P., Chavez, J.C., and LaManna, J.C. (2000). The role of mitochondria in the regulation of hypoxia-inducible factor 1 expression during hypoxia. J Biol Chem 275, 35863-35867.

Archer, S., and Michelakis, E. (2002). The mechanism(s) of hypoxic pulmonary vasoconstriction: potassium channels, redox O(2) sensors, and controversies. News Physiol Sci 17, 131-137.

Babior, B.M. (2004). NADPH oxidase. Curr Opin Immunol 16, 42-47.

Bae, S.H., Jeong, J.W., Park, J.A., Kim, S.H., Bae, M.K., Choi, S.J., and Kim, K.W. (2004). Sumoylation increases HIF-1alpha stability and its transcriptional activity. Biochem Biophys Res Commun 324, 394-400.

Beck, I., Weinmann, R., and Caro, J. (1993). Characterization of hypoxia-responsive enhancer in the human erythropoietin gene shows presence of hypoxia-inducible 120-Kd nuclear DNA-binding protein in erythropoietin-producing and nonproducing cells. Blood 82, 704-711.

Bedard, K., and Krause, K.H. (2007). The NOX family of ROS-generating NADPH oxidases: physiology and pathophysiology. Physiol Rev 87, 245-313.

Belaiba, R.S., Bonello, S., Zahringer, C., Schmidt, S., Hess, J., Kietzmann, T., and Gorlach, A. (2007a). Hypoxia up-regulates hypoxia-inducible factor-1alpha transcription by involving phosphatidylinositol 3-kinase and nuclear factor kappaB in pulmonary artery smooth muscle cells. Mol Biol Cell 18, 4691-4697.

BelAiba, R.S., Djordjevic, T., Bonello, S., Flugel, D., Hess, J., Kietzmann, T., and Gorlach, A. (2004). Redox-sensitive regulation of the HIF pathway under non-hypoxic conditions in pulmonary artery smooth muscle cells. Biol Chem 385, 249-257.

BelAiba, R.S., Djordjevic, T., Petry, A., Diemer, K., Bonello, S., Banfi, B., Hess, J., Pogrebniak, A., Bickel, C., and Gorlach, A. (2007b). NOX5 variants are functionally active in endothelial cells. Free Radic Biol Med 42, 446-459.

Bell, E.L., Klimova, T.A., Eisenbart, J., Moraes, C.T., Murphy, M.P., Budinger, G.R., and Chandel, N.S. (2007). The Qo site of the mitochondrial complex III is required for the transduction of hypoxic signalling via reactive oxygen species production. J Cell Biol 177, 1029-1036.

Bonello, S., Zahringer, C., BelAiba, R.S., Djordjevic, T., Hess, J., Michiels, C., Kietzmann, T., and Gorlach, A. (2007). Reactive oxygen species activate the HIF-1alpha promoter via a functional NFkappaB site. Arterioscler Thromb Vasc Biol 27, 755-761.

Boyer, R.F., and McCleary, C.J. (1987). Superoxide ion as a primary reductant in ascorbate-mediated ferritin iron release. Free Radic Biol Med 3, 389-395.

Brown, D.I., and Griendling, K.K. (2009). Nox proteins in signal transduction. Free Radic Biol Med 47, 1239-1253.

Brown, S.T., and Nurse, C.A. (2008). Induction of HIF-2alpha is dependent on mitochondrial O2 consumption in an O2-sensitive adrenomedullary chromaffin cell line. Am J Physiol Cell Physiol 294, C1305-1312.

Carrero, P., Okamoto, K., Coumailleau, P., O'Brien, S., Tanaka, H., and Poellinger, L. (2000). Redox-regulated recruitment of the transcriptional coactivators CREB-binding protein and SRC-1 to hypoxia-inducible factor 1alpha. Mol Cell Biol 20, 402-415.

Chandel, N.S., McClintock, D.S., Feliciano, C.E., Wood, T.M., Melendez, J.A., Rodriguez, A.M., and Schumacker, P.T. (2000). Reactive oxygen species generated at mitochondrial complex III stabilize hypoxia-inducible factor-1alpha during hypoxia: a mechanism of O2 sensing. J Biol Chem 275, 25130-25138.

Diebold, I., Djordjevic, T., Hess, J., and Gorlach, A. (2008). Rac-1 promotes pulmonary artery smooth muscle cell proliferation by upregulation of plasminogen activator inhibitor-1: role of NFkappaB-dependent hypoxia-inducible factor-1alpha transcription. Thromb Haemost 100, 1021-1028.

Diebold, I., Flugel, D., Becht, S., Belaiba, R.S., Bonello, S., Hess, J., Kietzmann, T., and Gorlach, A. (2010a). The hypoxia-inducible factor-2alpha is stabilized by oxidative stress involving NOX4. Antioxid Redox Signal 13, 425-436.

Diebold, I., Petry, A., Hess, J., and Gorlach, A. (2010b). The NADPH oxidase subunit NOX4 is a new target gene of the hypoxia-inducible factor-1. Mol Biol Cell 21, 2087-2096.

Dioum, E.M., Chen, R., Alexander, M.S., Zhang, Q., Hogg, R.T., Gerard, R.D., and Garcia, J.A. (2009). Regulation of hypoxia-inducible factor 2alpha signalling by the stress-responsive deacetylase sirtuin 1. Science 324, 1289-1293.

Ema, M., Hirota, K., Mimura, J., Abe, H., Yodoi, J., Sogawa, K., Poellinger, L., and Fujii-Kuriyama, Y. (1999). Molecular mechanisms of transcription activation by HLF and HIF1alpha in response to hypoxia: their stabilization and redox signal-induced interaction with CBP/p300. EMBO J 18, 1905-1914.

Epstein, A.C., Gleadle, J.M., McNeill, L.A., Hewitson, K.S., O'Rourke, J., Mole, D.R., Mukherji, M., Metzen, E., Wilson, M.I., Dhanda, A., et al. (2001). C. elegans EGL-9 and mammalian homologs define a family of dioxygenases that regulate HIF by prolyl hydroxylation. Cell 107, 43-54.

Flashman, E., Davies, S.L., Yeoh, K.K., and Schofield, C.J. (2010). Investigating the dependence of the hypoxia-inducible factor hydroxylases (factor inhibiting HIF and prolyl hydroxylase domain 2) on ascorbate and other reducing agents. Biochem J 427, 135-142.

Frede, S., Stockmann, C., Freitag, P., and Fandrey, J. (2006). Bacterial lipopolysaccharide induces HIF-1 activation in human monocytes via p44/42 MAPK and NF-kap-paB. Biochem J 396, 517-527.

Fukuda, R., Kelly, B., and Semenza, G.L. (2003). Vascular endothelial growth factor gene expression in colon cancer cells exposed to prostaglandin E2 is mediated by hypoxia-inducible factor 1. Cancer Res 63, 2330-2334.

Fukuda, R., Zhang, H., Kim, J.W., Shimoda, L., Dang, C.V., and Semenza, G.L. (2007). HIF-1 regulates cytochrome oxidase subunits to optimize efficiency of respiration in hypoxic cells. Cell 129, 111-122.

Gerald, D., Berra, E., Frapart, Y.M., Chan, D.A., Giaccia, A.J., Mansuy, D., Pouyssegur, J., Yaniv, M., and Mechta-Grigoriou, F. (2004). JunD reduces tumour angiogenesis by protecting cells from oxidative stress. Cell 118, 781-794.

Gorlach, A. (2009). Regulation of HIF-1 at the Transcriptional Level. Curr Pharm Des.

Gorlach, A., and Bonello, S. (2008). The cross-talk between NF-kappaB and HIF-1: further evidence for a significant liaison. Biochem J 412, e17-19.

Gorlach, A., Brandes, R.P., Nguyen, K., Amidi, M., Dehghani, F., and Busse, R. (2000a). A gp91phox containing NADPH oxidase selectively expressed in endothelial cells is a major source of oxygen radical generation in the arterial wall. Circ Res 87, 26-32.

Gorlach, A., Camenisch, G., Kvietikova, I., Vogt, L., Wenger, R.H., and Gassmann, M. (2000b). Efficient translation of mouse hypoxia-inducible factor-1alpha under normoxic and hypoxic conditions. Biochim Biophys Acta 1493, 125-134.

Gorlach, A., Diebold, I., Schini-Kerth, V.B., Berchner-Pfannschmidt, U., Roth, U., Brandes, R.P., Kietzmann, T., and Busse, R. (2001). Thrombin activates the hypoxia-inducible factor-1 signalling pathway in vascular smooth muscle cells: Role of the p22(phox)-containing NADPH oxidase. Circ Res 89, 47-54.

Gorlach, A., Kietzmann, T., and Hess, J. (2002). Redox signalling through NADPH oxidases: involvement in vascular proliferation and coagulation. Ann N Y Acad Sci 973, 505-507.

Gu, Y.Z., Moran, S.M., Hogenesch, J.B., Wartman, L., and Bradfield, C.A. (1998). Molecular characterization and chromosomal localization of a third alpha-class hypoxia inducible factor subunit, HIF3alpha. Gene Expr 7, 205-213.

Guzy, R.D., Sharma, B., Bell, E., Chandel, N.S., and Schumacker, P.T. (2008). Loss of the SdhB, but Not the SdhA, subunit of complex II triggers reactive oxygen species-dependent hypoxia-inducible factor activation and tumourigenesis. Mol Cell Biol 28, 718-731.

Haddad, J.J., Olver, R.E., and Land, S.C. (2000). Antioxidant/pro-oxidant equilibrium regulates HIF-1alpha and NF-kappa B redox sensitivity. Evidence for inhibition by glutathione oxidation in alveolar epithelial cells. J Biol Chem 275, 21130-21139.

Han, D., Antunes, F., Canali, R., Rettori, D., and Cadenas, E. (2003). Voltage-dependent anion channels control the release of the superoxide anion from mitochondria to cytosol. J Biol Chem 278, 5557-5563.

He, L., Dinger, B., Sanders, K., Hoidal, J., Obeso, A., Stensaas, L., Fidone, S., and Gonzalez, C. (2005). Effect of p47phox gene deletion on ROS production and oxygen sensing in mouse carotid body chemoreceptor cells. Am J Physiol Lung Cell Mol Physiol 289, L916-924.

Hirota, K., Fukuda, R., Takabuchi, S., Kizaka-Kondoh, S., Adachi, T., Fukuda, K., and Semenza, G.L. (2004). Induction of hypoxia-inducible factor 1 activity by muscarinic acetylcholine receptor signalling. J Biol Chem 279, 41521-41528.

Hoffman, E.C., Reyes, H., Chu, F.F., Sander, F., Conley, L.H., Brooks, B.A., and Hankinson, O. (1991). Cloning of a factor required for activity of the Ah (dioxin) receptor. Science 252, 954-958.

Huang, C., Han, Y., Wang, Y., Sun, X., Yan, S., Yeh, E.T., Chen, Y., Cang, H., Li, H., Shi, G., et al. (2009). SENP3 is responsible for HIF-1 transactivation under mild oxidative stress via p300 de-SUMOylation. EMBO J 28, 2748-2762.

Huang, L.E., Arany, Z., Livingston, D.M., and Bunn, H.F. (1996). Activation of hypoxia-inducible transcription factor depends primarily upon redox-sensitive stabilization of its alpha subunit. J Biol Chem 271, 32253-32259.

Huang, L.E., Gu, J., Schau, M., and Bunn, H.F. (1998). Regulation of hypoxia-inducible factor 1alpha is mediated by an O2-dependent degradation domain via the ubiquitin-proteasome pathway. Proc Natl Acad Sci U S A 95, 7987-7992.

Ivan, M., Kondo, K., Yang, H., Kim, W., Valiando, J., Ohh, M., Salic, A., Asara, J.M., Lane, W.S., and Kaelin, W.G., Jr. (2001). HIFalpha targeted for VHL-mediated destruction by proline hydroxylation: implications for O2 sensing. Science 292, 464-468.

Jaakkola, P., Mole, D.R., Tian, Y.M., Wilson, M.I., Gielbert, J., Gaskell, S.J., Kriegsheim, A., Hebestreit, H.F., Mukherji, M., Schofield, C.J., et al. (2001). Targeting of HIF-alpha to the von Hippel-Lindau ubiquitylation complex by O2-regulated prolyl hydroxylation. Science 292, 468-472.

Jiang, B.H., Zheng, J.Z., Leung, S.W., Roe, R., and Semenza, G.L. (1997). Transactivation and inhibitory domains of hypoxia-inducible factor 1alpha. Modulation of transcriptional activity by oxygen tension. J Biol Chem 272, 19253-19260.

Kaelin, W.G., Jr., and Ratcliffe, P.J. (2008). Oxygen sensing by metazoans: the central role of the HIF hydroxylase pathway. Mol Cell 30, 393-402.

Khatri, J.J., Johnson, C., Magid, R., Lessner, S.M., Laude, K.M., Dikalov, S.I., Harrison, D.G., Sung, H.J., Rong, Y., and Galis, Z.S. (2004). Vascular oxidant stress enhances progression and angiogenesis of experimental atheroma. Circulation 109, 520-525.

Kietzmann, T., Samoylenko, A., Roth, U., and Jungermann, K. (2003). Hypoxia-inducible factor-1 and hypoxia response elements mediate the induction of plasminogen activator inhibitor-1 gene expression by insulin in primary rat hepatocytes. Blood 101, 907-914.

Kim, H.H., Lee, S.E., Chung, W.J., Choi, Y., Kwack, K., Kim, S.W., Kim, M.S., Park, H., and Lee, Z.H. (2002). Stabilization of hypoxia-inducible factor-1alpha is involved in the hypoxic stimuli-induced expression of vascular endothelial growth factor in osteoblastic cells. Cytokine 17, 14-27.

Knowles, H.J., Raval, R.R., Harris, A.L., and Ratcliffe, P.J. (2003). Effect of ascorbate on the activity of hypoxia-inducible factor in cancer cells. Cancer Res 63, 1764-1768.

Kohl, R., Zhou, J., and Brune, B. (2006). Reactive oxygen species attenuate nitric-oxide-mediated hypoxia-inducible factor-1alpha stabilization. Free Radic Biol Med 40, 1430-1442.

Koivunen, P., Tiainen, P., Hyvarinen, J., Williams, K.E., Sormunen, R., Klaus, S.J.,

Kivirikko, K.I., and Myllyharju, J. (2007). An endoplasmic reticulum transmembrane prolyl 4-hydroxylase is induced by hypoxia and acts on hypoxia-inducible factor alpha. J Biol Chem 282, 30544-30552.

Koshikawa, N., Hayashi, J., Nakagawara, A., and Takenaga, K. (2009). Reactive oxygen species-generating mitochondrial DNA mutation up-regulates hypoxia-inducible factor-1alpha gene transcription via phosphatidylinositol 3-kinase-Akt/protein kinase C/histone deacetylase pathway. J Biol Chem 284, 33185-33194.

Lambeth, J.D., Kawahara, T., and Diebold, B. (2007). Regulation of Nox and Duox enzymatic activity and expression. Free Radic Biol Med 43, 319-331.

Lang, K.J., Kappel, A., and Goodall, G.J. (2002). Hypoxia-inducible factor-1alpha mRNA contains an internal ribosome entry site that allows efficient translation during normoxia and hypoxia. Mol Biol Cell 13, 1792-1801.

Liu, J.Q., Zelko, I.N., Erbynn, E.M., Sham, J.S., and Folz, R.J. (2006a). Hypoxic pulmonary hypertension: role of superoxide and NADPH oxidase (gp91phox). Am J Physiol Lung Cell Mol Physiol 290, L2-10.

Liu, L.Z., Hu, X.W., Xia, C., He, J., Zhou, Q., Shi, X., Fang, J., and Jiang, B.H. (2006b). Reactive oxygen species regulate epidermal growth factor-induced vascular endothelial growth factor and hypoxia-inducible factor-1alpha expression through activation of AKT and P70S6K1 in human ovarian cancer cells. Free Radic Biol Med 41, 1521-1533.

Liu, Q., Berchner-Pfannschmidt, U., Moller, U., Brecht, M., Wotzlaw, C., Acker, H., Jungermann, K., and Kietzmann, T. (2004). A Fenton reaction at the endoplasmic reticulum is involved in the redox control of hypoxia-inducible gene expression. Proc Natl Acad Sci U S A 101, 4302-4307.

Mahon, P.C., Hirota, K., and Semenza, G.L. (2001). FIH-1: a novel protein that interacts with HIF-1alpha and VHL to mediate repression of HIF-1 transcriptional activity. Genes Dev 15, 2675-2686.

Maranchie, J.K., and Zhan, Y. (2005). Nox4 is critical for hypoxia-inducible factor 2-alpha transcriptional activity in von Hippel-Lindau-deficient renal cell carcinoma. Cancer Res 65, 9190-9193.

Mittal, M., Roth, M., Konig, P., Hofmann, S., Dony, E., Goyal, P., Selbitz, A.C., Schermuly, R.T., Ghofrani, H.A., Kwapiszewska, G., et al. (2007). Hypoxia-dependent regulation of nonphagocytic NADPH oxidase subunit NOX4 in the pulmonary vasculature. Circ Res 101, 258-267.

Moon, E.J., Sonveaux, P., Porporato, P.E., Danhier, P., Gallez, B., Batinic-Haberle, I., Nien, Y.C., Schroeder, T., and Dewhirst, M.W. (2010). NADPH oxidase-mediated reactive oxygen species production activates hypoxia-inducible factor-1 (HIF-1) via the ERK pathway after hyperthermia treatment. Proc Natl Acad Sci U S A 107, 20477-20482.

Nishi, K., Oda, T., Takabuchi, S., Oda, S., Fukuda, K., Adachi, T., Semenza, G.L., Shingu, K., and Hirota, K. (2008). LPS induces hypoxia-inducible factor 1 activation in macrophage-differentiated cells in a reactive oxygen species-dependent manner. Antioxid Redox Signal 10, 983-995.

Oh, Y.T., Lee, J.Y., Yoon, H., Lee, E.H., Baik, H.H., Kim, S.S., Ha, J., Yoon, K.S., Choe, W., and Kang, I. (2008). Lipopolysaccharide induces hypoxia-inducible factor-1 alpha mRNA expression and activation via NADPH oxidase and Sp1-dependent pathway in BV2 murine microglial cells. Neurosci Lett 431, 155-160.

Page, E.L., Chan, D.A., Giaccia, A.J., Levine, M., and Richard, D.E. (2008). Hypoxia-inducible factor-1alpha stabilization in nonhypoxic conditions: role of oxidation and intracellular ascorbate depletion. Mol Biol Cell 19, 86-94.

Page, E.L., Robitaille, G.A., Pouyssegur, J., and Richard, D.E. (2002). Induction of hypoxia-inducible factor-1alpha by transcriptional and translational mechanisms. J Biol Chem 277, 48403-48409.

Patten, D.A., Lafleur, V.N., Robitaille, G.A., Chan, D.A., Giaccia, A.J., and Richard, D.E. (2010). Hypoxia-inducible factor-1 activation in nonhypoxic conditions: the essential role of mitochondrial-derived reactive oxygen species. Mol Biol Cell 21, 3247-3257.

Petry, A., Weitnauer, M., and Gorlach, A. (2010). Receptor activation of NADPH oxidases. Antioxid Redox Signal 13, 467-487.

Pugh, C.W., O'Rourke, J.F., Nagao, M., Gleadle, J.M., and Ratcliffe, P.J. (1997). Activation of hypoxia-inducible factor-1; definition of regulatory domains within the alpha subunit. J Biol Chem 272, 11205-11214.

Richard, D.E., Berra, E., and Pouyssegur, J. (2000). Nonhypoxic pathway mediates the induction of hypoxia-inducible factor 1alpha in vascular smooth muscle cells. J Biol Chem 275, 26765-26771.

Rigoulet, M., Yoboue, E.D., and Devin, A. (2011). Mitochondrial ROS generation and its regulation: mechanisms involved in $H(2)O(2)$ signalling. Antioxid Redox Signal 14, 459-468.

Rius, J., Guma, M., Schachtrup, C., Akassoglou, K., Zinkernagel, A.S., Nizet, V., Johnson, R.S., Haddad, G.G., and Karin, M. (2008). NF-kappaB links innate immunity to the hypoxic response through transcriptional regulation of HIF-1alpha. Nature 453, 807-811.

Ryu, J.H., Li, S.H., Park, H.S., Park, J.W., Lee, B., and Chun, Y.S. (2011). Hypoxia-inducible factor subunit stabilization by NEDD8 conjugation is reactive oxygen species-dependent. J Biol Chem. 286(9):6963-70.

Sandau, K.B., Zhou, J., Kietzmann, T., and Brune, B. (2001). Regulation of the hypoxia-inducible factor 1alpha by the inflammatory mediators nitric oxide and tumour necrosis factor-alpha in contrast to desferroxamine and phenylarsine oxide. J Biol Chem 276, 39805-39811.

Schepens, B., Tinton, S.A., Bruynooghe, Y., Beyaert, R., and Cornelis, S. (2005). The polypyrimidine tract-binding protein stimulates HIF-1alpha IRES-mediated translation during hypoxia. Nucleic Acids Res 33, 6884-6894.

Semenza, G.L., and Wang, G.L. (1992). A nuclear factor induced by hypoxia via de novo protein synthesis binds to the human erythropoietin gene enhancer at a site required for transcriptional activation. Mol Cell Biol 12, 5447-5454.

Shatrov, V.A., Sumbayev, V.V., Zhou, J., and Brune, B. (2003). Oxidized low-density lipoprotein (oxLDL) triggers hypoxia-inducible factor-1alpha (HIF-1alpha) accumulation via redox-dependent mechanisms. Blood 101, 4847-4849.

Srinivas, V., Leshchinsky, I., Sang, N., King, M.P., Minchenko, A., and Caro, J. (2001). Oxygen sensing and HIF-1 activation does not require an active mitochondrial respiratory chain electron-transfer pathway. J Biol Chem 276, 21995-21998.

Stiehl, D.P., Jelkmann, W., Wenger, R.H., and Hellwig-Burgel, T. (2002). Normoxic induction of the hypoxia-inducible factor 1alpha by insulin and interleukin-1beta involves the phosphatidylinositol 3-kinase pathway. FEBS Lett 512, 157-162.

Tacchini, L., De Ponti, C., Matteucci, E., Follis, R., and Desiderio, M.A. (2004). Hepatocyte growth factor-activated NF-kappaB regulates HIF-1 activity and ODC expression, implicated in survival, differently in different carcinoma cell lines. Carcinogenesis 25, 2089-2100.

Tian, H., McKnight, S.L., and Russell, D.W. (1997). Endothelial PAS domain protein 1 (EPAS1), a transcription factor selectively expressed in endothelial cells. Genes Dev 11, 72-82.

Treins, C., Giorgetti-Peraldi, S., Murdaca, J., Semenza, G.L., and Van Obberghen, E. (2002). Insulin stimulates hypoxia-inducible factor 1 through a phosphatidylinositol 3-kinase/target of rapamycin-dependent signalling pathway. J Biol Chem 277, 27975-27981.

Turrens, J.F. (2003). Mitochondrial formation of reactive oxygen species. J Physiol 552, 335-344.

van Uden, P., Kenneth, N.S., and Rocha, S. (2008). Regulation of hypoxia-inducible factor-1alpha by NF-kappaB. Biochem J 412, 477-484.

Vaux, E.C., Metzen, E., Yeates, K.M., and Ratcliffe, P.J. (2001). Regulation of hypoxia-inducible factor is preserved in the absence of a functioning mitochondrial respiratory chain. Blood 98, 296-302.

Weissmann, N., Zeller, S., Schafer, R.U., Turowski, C., Ay, M., Quanz, K., Ghofrani, H.A., Schermuly, R.T., Fink, L., Seeger, W., et al. (2006). Impact of mitochondria and NADPH oxidases on acute and sustained hypoxic pulmonary vasoconstriction. Am J Respir Cell Mol Biol 34, 505-513.

Welsh, S.J., Bellamy, W.T., Briehl, M.M., and Powis, G. (2002). The redox protein thioredoxin-1 (Trx-1) increases hypoxia-inducible factor 1alpha protein expression: Trx-1 overexpression results in increased vascular endothelial growth factor production and enhanced tumour angiogenesis. Cancer Res 62, 5089-5095.

Wenger, R.H. (2002). Cellular adaptation to hypoxia: O2-sensing protein hydroxylases, hypoxia-inducible transcription factors, and O2-regulated gene expression. FASEB J 16, 1151-1162.

Xia, C., Meng, Q., Liu, L.Z., Rojanasakul, Y., Wang, X.R., and Jiang, B.H. (2007). Reactive oxygen species regulate angiogenesis and tumour growth through vascular endothelial growth factor. Cancer Res 67, 10823-10830.

Zhou, J., Callapina, M., Goodall, G.J., and Brune, B. (2004). Functional integrity of nuclear factor kappaB, phosphatidylinositol 3'-kinase, and mitogen-activated protein kinase signalling allows tumour necrosis factor alpha-evoked Bcl-2 expression to provoke internal ribosome entry site-dependent translation of hypoxia-inducible factor 1alpha. Cancer Res 64, 9041-9048.

Chapter 12
Calcium transport in hypoxia

Olga Krizanova[*]

[*]Author for correspondence:
Institute of Molecular Physiology and Genetics, Slovak Academy of Sciences, Vlarska 5,
833 34 Bratislava, Slovak Republic, Phone: +4212 5477 2211, olga.krizanova@savba.sk

Contents

Key points

— Calcium as an important second messenger regulates a variety
of processes in its physiological and pathological state.

— Calcium transport systems are core regulators of the intracellular
calcium concentration.

— During hypoxia, intracellular calcium concentration is increased through
the upregulation of intracellular and extracellular calcium transporters.

— Severe hypoxia can induce mitochondrial apoptotic pathway, where
calcium release from the sarcoplasmic/endoplasmic reticulum plays
a pivotal role.

Introduction

Mechanisms that regulate cellular metabolism represent a fundamental requirement of all cells. Among them, calcium as a second messenger plays a crucial role in a variety of cellular processes, e.g. excitation-contraction coupling, cell proliferation and growth, apoptosis, etc.

The specific Ca^{2+} signalling information is likely to be encoded in a calcium code as the amplitude, duration, frequency, waveform or timing of Ca^{2+} oscillations and decoded again at a later stage. Since calcium is such an important ion, mutations causing drastic functional changes in intracel-

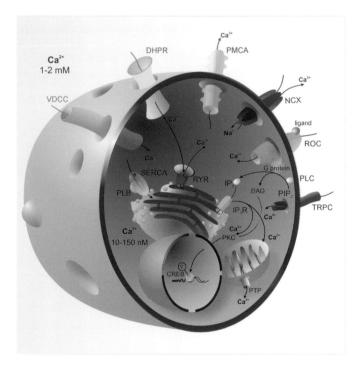

Figure 12.1 _ Calcium transport systems in cells. VDCC – voltage-dependent calcium channel, DHPR –dihydropyridine receptor, PMCA – plasma membrane Ca^{2+}-ATPase, AC – adenylyl cyclase, ROC – receptor operated channel, NCX – sodium-calcium exchanger, TRPC – transient receptor potential channel, RyR – ryanodine receptor, IP_3 – inositol 1,4,5-trisphosphate, IP_3R- IP_3 receptor, SERCA – sarco/endoplasmic reticulum Ca^{2+}-ATPase, PLB – phospholamban, DAG – diacylglycerol, PKC – protein kinase C, PTP – permeability transition pore.

lular calcium homeostasis are less likely to be compatible with life (Missiaen et al., 2000).

Calcium ions that control the activity of cells can be supplied to the cytosol from the extracellular space, or from intracellular calcium stores (Figure 12.1). The relative importance of both sources depends on the cell type.

Calcium transport systems

Many excitable cells express voltage gated calcium channels that translate electrical signals into the increase of $[Ca^{2+}]i$. Ligand operated cation channels are directly gated by binding of an extracellular agonist to the channel protein. In equilibrium conditions, the influx of extracellular calcium must be balanced by calcium extrusion by the plasma membrane calcium ATPase (PMCA) and by the Na^+/Ca^{2+} exchangers. Na^+/Ca^{2+} exchanger plays a crucial role in cardiac excitation-contraction coupling. It is interesting that the Na^+/Ca^{2+} exchanger can transport calcium in either direction across the cell membrane and possibly sometimes mediate Ca^{2+} influx. The direction of net Ca^{2+} transport is determined by three factors: the Na^+ gradient, the Ca^{2+} gradient and the membrane potential. During the early phases of the action potential, for example, depolarization favors reversal of the exchanger into the Ca^{2+} influx mode. On the other hand, Ca^{2+} will be rising rapidly at this time as a result of channel openings and sarcoplasmic reticulum (SR) Ca^{2+} release. An increased intracellular calcium level will push the exchanger back into the Ca^{2+} efflux mode (Philipson, 2002).

The sarcoplasmic reticulum in muscle and the endoplasmic reticulum (ER) in non-muscle cells are the major intracellular calcium stores. In steady-state conditions, the intracellular calcium stores must re-accumulate the same amount of Ca^{2+} as they release. Calcium is loaded to the reticulum through the sarco-/endoplasmic reticulum Ca^{2+}-ATPase (SERCA). Up to now, three isoforms of SERCA have been detected. The associated protein phospholamban modulates the activity of some SERCA isoforms (for review see Missiaen et al., 2000). Calcium ions are released from reticulum through IP_3 receptors (IP_3Rs) and ryanodine receptors (RyRs). Three IP_3 receptor isoforms (type 1, 2 and 3) have been cloned and splice variants have been described in both animal and human cells. The IP_3 receptors are tetramers composed of four subunits, which leads to the possibility that heteromultimeric channels are assembled with distinctive properties relating to their subunit content (Tran et al., 2000).

Mitochondria can rapidly accumulate and release calcium upon cell stimulation (Rizzuto, 2003). While it was originally thought that mitochondria took up calcium only when cells were damaged or became exposed to very high $[Ca^{2+}]i$ we now know that mitochondria in the vicinity of calcium channels become exposed to much higher calcium concentrations than the bulk $[Ca^{2+}]i$ and will temporarily store some calcium and release it when $[Ca^{2+}]i$ is lowered. Mitochondria transport Ca^{2+} through a complex system consisting of two modes of influx and two of efflux. The most thoroughly studied Ca^{2+} influx mechanism is the uniporter, which transports calcium down its electrochemical gradient without coupling the transport to any other ion or molecule (Gunter et al., 2000). Later, another mode of Ca^{2+} influx into mitochondria was discovered, permitting calcium to cross the inner membrane for brief periods at least hundreds of times faster than influx via the uniporter (Gunter et al., 2000). The primary efflux pathway of heart, brain, skeletal muscle, parotid gland, brown fat and most tumour mitochondria is the Na^+-dependent mechanism (Crompton et al., 1978; Murphy and Fiskum, 1988), while in liver, kidney, lung and smooth muscle of the Na^+ independent mechanism (Crompton et al, 1978, Fiskum and Lehninger, 1979). Excess of calcium accumulation in mitochondria activates a large conductance pore, also called the permeability transition pore (PTP). PTP, opened by an increase of $[Ca^{2+}]$ in the matrix above a given threshold and by a series of other toxic insults, including oxidative stress, could lead to mitochondrial swelling, breaking of the outer membrane, and loss to the outer medium of proteins, such as cytochrome c contained in the intermembrane space (Bernardi, 1999). Thus, mitochondria represent a sort of decoding station: they can sense different environmental conditions or receive diverse signals and integrate them all together, finally producing an outcome that can decide the fate of the cell (Rimessi et al., 2008).

Evidence in support of independent regulation of nuclear calcium (Leite et al., 2003) has centered on the existence of a mechanism for generating calcium signals in the nucleus. It was already shown that nucleus contains independent IP_3 receptors, which can activate nuclear PLC-γ1 (Malviya and Klein, 2006). Upon some specific stimuli, such as induction of the apoptosis, IP_3 receptors can translocate from endoplasmic reticulum to the nuclei (Ondrias et al., 2011).

Pathology related to calcium transporters

Variety of diseases is caused by mutations or abnormalities in Ca^{2+}-transport proteins. Mutations in RyR1 cause malignant hyperthermia – genetic predisposition of clinically otherwise normal individuals to react abnormally to volatile anesthetics like halothane or enflurane. Deletion of RyR3 results in specific changes in intracellular processes underlying spatial learning and hippocampal synaptic plasticity (Balshun et al., 1999). Increased IP3Rs of type1 were found in cerebella of patients suffering from ataxia. Using IP3R1 knock-out mice it was found, that they often die *in utero*. Those mice born alive exhibited ataxia, developed epilepsy and opisthotonos at day 20 and died very soon afterwards. Patients with Brody disease complain of exercise-induced impairment of skeletal-muscle relaxation. This autosomal recessive form is caused by mutations in the gene encoding SERCA1 in fast twitch skeletal muscle. SERCA2 is mutated in patients with Darier disease, an autosomal dominant skin disorder. These patients often have neurological and psychiatric symptoms, including mood disorders, epilepsy, mental retardation, etc. (Ruiz-Perez et al., 1999).

Familial hypokalemic periodic paralysis is an autosomal dominant disorder characterized by periodic attacks of muscle weakness and paralysis of the trunk and limbs. Three different mutations in the α1-subunit of the dihydropyridine receptor have been described. The site of mutation determines severity of the attacks.

Various abnormalities in Ca^{2+} handling proteins have been described in heart during ageing, hypertrophy, heart failure and during treatment with immunosuppressive drugs and in diabetes mellitus (for review see Missiaen et al., 2000).

Hypoxia, acidosis and calcium signalling

Hypoxia is a state of reduced oxygen supply to the tissue below physiological levels despite adequate perfusion of the tissue by blood. Depending on the duration and force of the hypoxia, it results in the failure of energy balance, excitotoxicity, free radical damage, inflammation and immune system overactivation and delayed cell death (Bickler and Fahlmann, 2004). One of the constant early responses to hypoxia in almost all cell types is an increase in intracellular Ca^{2+}. For example, the $[Ca^{2+}]i$ in rat cortical brain slices is approximately 150 nM under resting conditions and increased to 1000 nM within 10 min of hypoxia (Bickler and Hansen, 1994). The hypoxic increase in the intracellular calcium may result from extracellular calcium influx due to the inhibition of voltage-dependent K^+ channels, in addition to Ca^{2+} release from the sarcoplasmic reticulum through ryanodine receptors (Rathore et al., 2008). Also, hypoxia increased gene expression and protein levels of the type 1 and 2 IP_3 receptors in cerebellar granular cells. This increase was probably caused by reactive oxygen species, since antioxidant quercetin completely abolished the hypoxia-induced IP_3 receptors in cerebellar granular cells (Jurkovicova et al., 2007). It was shown that pharmacological and genetic inhibition of NADPH oxidases diminish hypoxic increase in the intracellular calcium in pulmonary artery smooth muscle cells (Rathore et al., 2008).

Rapidly declining oxygen levels lead to consequent switch to anaerobic metabolism, to maintain ATP production, resulting in increased generation of metabolic acid (Henrich and Buckler, 2009). This culminates in a rapidly developing tissue acidosis. Acidosis triggered a sustained Ca^{2+} release from internal stores. Depletion of endoplasmic reticulum by SERCA inhibitor and also by caffeine significantly reduced the sustained rise in the intracellular calcium levels. Depletion of mitochondrial calcium stores did not influence the sustained rise in the intracellular calcium evoked by pH 6.8 (Henrich and Buckler, 2009).

Two transcription factors are known to be affected by hypoxia – HIF and NF-κB. Calcium per se does not change NF-κB binding (Glazner et al., 2001). The transcription factor hypoxia-inducible factor-1 (HIF-1) constitutes a central component in coordinating adaptive responses to low oxygen availability. Microarray experiments indicate that far more than 200 HIF target genes might exist. HIF-1 is a heterodimer composed of the 120 kDa HIF-1α a 91-94 kDa HIF-1β. In pancreatic β-cells, blocking of Ca^{2+} flux through RyRs or IP_3Rs increased the expression of HIF-1β (Dror et al., 2008). SERCA pumps are not involved in this regulation. On the other hand, two reports provided evidence that lowering intracellular calcium by BAPTA-AM activates HIF-1 by attenuating hydroxylation of HIF-1α (Berchner-Pfannschmidt et al., 2004, Liu et al., 2004). Lowering calcium may not only block prolyl hydroxylase (PHD) activity but also attenuate calpain and both actions may synergize in stabilizing HIF-1α. However, on the basis of current information one would not assume a simple role of calcium as several reports noticed the involvement of calcium and/or calmodulin in signal transduction pathways, e.g. ERK activation, leading to enhanced HIF-1 transcriptional activity (Yuan et al., 2004, Zhou et al., 2006). Nevertheless, the role of calcium in supporting or antagonizing hypoxic responses is not yet fully defined and variables, such as calcium concentrations, calcium compartments and cell type-specific effects need to be sorted out.

Degradation of HIF-1α requires association of the von Hippel Lindau protein (pVHL) to provoke ubiquitination followed by proteasome digestion. Zhou et al. (2006) found that calpain participated in destruction of HIF-1α, supporting the notion for a role of calcium in affecting expression of hypoxia inducible genes. Thus, chelating intracellular calcium attenuated HIF-1α destruction by DETA-NO (donor NO), whereas a calcium increase was sufficient to lower the amount of HIF-1α even under hypoxia.

Calcium is proposed to play a role also in the adaptation to hypoxia and/or anoxia. Because increases in calcium are associated with surviving anoxia in hypoxia-tolerant neurons, moderate increases in calcium might be protective. Bickler (2004) showed that treating the hippocampal slice culture with ionophores to increase $[Ca^{2+}]i$ produces impressive resistance to subsequent oxygen and glucose deprivation. The mechanisms of this protective effect involve the activation of several recognized neuroprotective signalling cascades, like MAPK, ERK1/2, Akt or protein kinase B (Bickler and Fahlman, 2004).

Calcium signalling and cancer

In normal cells, Ca^{2+} regulates several processes as diverse as energy transduction, secretions, apoptosis, muscle contraction, chemotaxis and neuronal synaptic plasticity in learning and memory (Berridge, 2009). Nevertheless, Ca^{2+} mediated signalling pathways have been shown to play important roles in cancer initiation, tumour formation, tumour progression, metastasis, invasion and angiogenesis (Block et al., 2010; Saidak et al., 2009). Ca^{2+} signalling pathways are remodeled or deregulated in cancer that result in changes in their physiology and distinguish them from non-malignant cells. Remodeling or deregulation of Ca^{2+} signalling pathways can provide means by which cancer cells can overcome systemic anticancer defense mechanisms. The altered Ca^{2+} signalling pathways can also lead to genetic diversity found in cancerous tissues thereby providing effective cellular strategies to the selection pressure to acquire specific traits (Parkash and Asotra, 2010).

The role of intracellular and also plasma calcium transporters have not yet been studied in detail during carcinogenesis. Nevertheless, few observations already point to the importance of this field. For example, IP_3

receptor (IP_3R) inhibitors caffeine, 2-APB and xestospongin C inhibited the growth of the estrogen-dependent human breast cancer epithelial cell line MCF-7 stimulated by 5% fetal calf serum or 10 nM 17beta-estradiol (Szatkowski et al., 2010). Also, in cancer cells, the altered expression of Ca^{2+} channels and pumps cause alterations in Ca^{2+} wave characteristics resulting in a modified calcium code. Therefore, one can target these Ca^{2+} channels and pumps as therapeutic options to decrease cancer cell proliferation and increase calcium cell apoptosis (Parkash and Asorta, 2010).

To investigate the molecules that regulate the acquisition of cis- diamminedichloro-platinum (II) (cisplatin) resistance, Tsunoda and coworkers (2005) performed cDNA microarrays using two pairs of parental and cisplatin-resistant bladder cancer cell lines. They found a markedly reduced expression of IP_3 receptor type 1 (IP_3R1), endoplasmic reticulum membrane protein, in cisplatin-resistant cells. The suppression of IP_3R1 expression using small interfering RNA in parental cells prevented apoptosis and resulted in decreased sensitivity to cisplatin. Contrarily, overexpression of IP_3R1 in resistant cells induced apoptosis and increased sensitivity to cisplatin. These results suggest that cisplatin-induced downregulation of IP_3R1 expression was closely associated with the acquisition of cisplatin resistance in bladder cancer cells.

Since Ca^{2+} channels or pumps involved in regulating Ca^{2+} signalling pathways show altered expression in cancer, one can target these Ca^{2+} channels and pumps as therapeutic options to decrease proliferation of cancer cells and to promote their apoptosis.

Calcium and apoptosis

Mitochondria fulfills variety of functions in cellular physiology, such as energy production, free radical production, regulation of cytosolic Ca^{2+} signalling pathways and apoptosis (Duchen, 2004). There is a general agreement in the literature on this topic that calcium efflux from the endoplasmic reticulum and calcium accumulation into the mitochondria is linked to the effects of various apoptotic stimuli. Some classic death ligands, such as tumour necrosis factor α (TNFα) or Fas, can promote IP_3 generation in some, but not in all cells. Yet other apoptotic stimuli, such as ceramide, cytotoxic drugs and cisplatin, or manipulations such as withdrawal of trophic factors can also cause ER calcium release.

It has been postulated that activation of the inositol 1,4,5-trisphosphate receptors (IP$_3$Rs) signalling pathway could release Ca^{2+} from the endoplasmic/sarcoplasmic reticulum (ER/SR) to increase the microdomain Ca^{2+} concentration at focal contacts (known as mitochondria-associated ER membranes) between the ER and mitochondria, and then activate a low-affinity Ca^{2+} uniporter at mitochondrial membranes (Belmonte and Morad, 2008; Lu et al., 2010). The experimental evidence for an involvement of IP$_3$Rs in apoptosis has predominantly come from experiments, in which the expression level of the receptor protein has been manipulated. There is evidence that stable knockdown of the type I IP$_3$R in Jurkat T-lymphocytes can inhibit responsiveness to different apoptotic stimuli (Jayaraman and Marks, 1997). Similarly, DT40 cells (a chicken B lymphoma cell line) in which IP$_3$ receptor expression was prevented were not only deficient in IP$_3$-mediated Ca^{2+} signalling, but also substantially resistant to the apoptosis normally induced in response to B-cell receptor activation (Sugawara et al., 1997).

At present, it is not clear whether different IP$_3$ receptor isoforms have an equivalent role in apoptosis. In the studies using DT40 cells, there appeared to be redundancy between different IP$_3$ receptor isoforms. Cells where all three isoforms were knocked out showed the least death compared to cells missing either a single isoform or pairs of isoforms. In contrast to this, some studies have shown that reduction of either type 1 or type 3 IP$_3$ receptors abrogates apoptosis (Hanson et al., 2004).

In addition to the direct role of IP$_3$Rs in the initiation of apoptosis by providing a conduit for ER-to-mitochondria Ca^{2+} transfer, there are several additional feedback mechanisms that have been proposed which allow IP$_3$Rs to play a role in amplifying calcium dependent apoptotic pathways (Joseph and Hajnoczky, 2007). These include the cleavage of the receptor by caspases, which is proposed to provide an enhanced ER leak pathway, and the direct binding and regulation of the IP$_3$R calcium channel by several key players in apoptosis including cytochrome c and the anti-apoptotic proteins Bcl-2 and Bcl-xL. Moreover, the IP$_3$R can be directly phosphorylated by Akt kinase.

During [Ca^{2+}]c oscillations, mitochondrial Ca^{2+} uptake is closely coupled to the IP$_3$ dependent calcium release that is driven by the [Ca^{2+}] gradient between the ER lumen and the cytosol. Studies evaluating the connection between the ER calcium storage and cell survival have reported that fluctuations of ER luminal [Ca^{2+}] in a narrow range (approx 30%) cause massive changes in apoptosis (Joseph and Hajnoczky, 2007). A clue to the mechanism of this effect is that in cells where the apoptotic agents or Bcl-2 family proteins induced moderate differences in the [Ca^{2+}]$_{ER}$ and the IP$_3$-linked cytosolic calcium rise, relatively large changes occurred in the mitochondrial calcium signal.

Besides IP_3 receptors, some other calcium channels were also assigned to involvement in the process of apoptosis in various cells and tissues. Several other types of channel are known to transport Ca^{2+} and promote apoptosis. Yagami and colleagues (2010) demonstrated that fibroblast growth factor 2 caused apoptosis via L-type voltage-sensitive Ca^{2+} channel in the early neuronal culture. It has been confirmed that the Ca^{2+}ATPases on the plasma membrane are cleaved by caspases, thus preventing normal homeostasis and consequently causing Ca^{2+} elevation (Schwab et al., 2002).

It was already shown that transient receptor potential vanilloid 2 (TRPV2) channel proteins in human urothelial carcinoma (UC) cells are calcium-permeable and the regulation of calcium influx through these channels leads directly to the death of UC cells. TRPV2 channels in UC cells may be a potentially new therapeutic target, especially in higher-grade UC cells (Yamada et al., 2010). Moreover, menthol can induce mitochondrial membrane depolarization via the transient receptor potential melastatin 8 (TRPM8) channel (which appears to function as a plasmalemmal Ca^{2+} channel and an intracellular Ca^{2+} release channel) in cells of the human bladder cancer cell line T24, resulting in cell death (Li et al., 2009).

Nevertheless, in some cells, calcium can be involved in processes with antiapoptotic effect. For example, NF-κB signalling is known to induce the expression of antiapoptotic and proinflammatory genes in endothelial cells (ECs). Thippegowda and colleagues (2010) have shown that Ca^{2+} influx through canonical transient receptor potential (TRPC) channels activates NF-κB in ECs. Ca^{2+} influx via TRPC channels plays a critical role in the mechanism of cell survival signalling through A20 expression in ECs.

A considerable redundancy is apparent in apoptotic pathways and this has been a complicated feature of attempts to therapeutically modify this process in the treatment of diseases such as cancer or neurodegenerative disorders.

Conclusions

Calcium is known to play an incommutable role in the modulation of many metabolic pathways in physiological, but also in pathological conditions. Nevertheless, only limited information is available about the involvement of calcium in hypoxia and cancer, up to now. A body of evidence suggests that second messengers, such as modulations in the intracellular calcium concentration, could be involved in the beneficial effects shown by anti-cancer drugs (Florea and Busselberg, 2009). Discovering the role of calcium in the process of hypoxia and/of cancer will contribute significantly to understanding the mechanism of development of these processes. Calcium transport systems, which can alter intracellular calcium concentration, can serve as potential therapeutic targets in preventing and/or treatment of these diseases.

A c k n o w l e d g e m e n t s _ Author is supported by grants APVV-0045-11, VEGA 2/0049/10 and CEMAN.

References

Balschun D, Wolfer DP, Bertocchini F, Barone V, Conti A, Zuschratter W, Missiaen L, Lipp HP, Frey JU, Sorrentino V. Deletion of the ryanodine receptor type 3 (RyR3) impairs forms of synaptic plasticity and spatial learning. EMBO J. 1999 Oct 1;18(19):5264-73

Belmonte S, Morad M. Shear fluid-induced Ca^{3+} release and the role of mitochondria in rat cardiomyocytes. Ann NY Acad Sci. 2008;1123:58–63

Berchner-Pfannschmidt U, Petrat F, Doege K, Trinidad B, Freitag P, Metzen E, de Groot H, Fandrey J. Chelation of cellular calcium modulates hypoxia-inducible gene expression through activation of hypoxia-inducible factor-1alpha. J Biol Chem. 2004 Oct 22;279(43):44976-86

Bernardi P. Mitochondrial transport of cations: channels, exchangers, and permeability transition. Physiol Rev 1999;79:1127–1155.

Berridge MJ. Inositol trisphosphate and calcium signalling mechanisms. Biochim Biophys Acta. 2009 Jun;1793(6):933-40

Bickler PE. Clinical perspectives: neuroprotection lessons from hypoxia-tolerant organisms. J Exp Biol. 2004 Aug;207(Pt 18):3243-9

Bickler PE, Fahlman CS. Moderate increases in intracellular calcium activate neuroprotective signals in hippocampal neurons. Neuroscience. 2004;127(3):673-83

Bickler PE, Hansen BM. Causes of calcium accumulation in rat cortical brain slices during hypoxia and ischemia: role of ion channels and membrane damage. Brain Res. 1994 Dec 5;665(2):269-76

Crompton M, Moser R, Lüdi H, Carafoli E. The interrelations between the transport of sodium and calcium in mitochondria of various mammalian tissues. Eur J Biochem. 1978 Jan 2;82(1):25-31.

Dror V, Kalynyak TB, Bychkivska Y, Frey MH, Tee M, Jeffrey KD, Nguyen V, Luciani

DS, Johnson JD. Glucose and endoplasmic reticulum calcium channels regulate HIF-1beta via presenilin in pancreatic beta-cells. J Biol Chem. 2008 Apr 11;283(15):9909-16

Duchen MR. Mitochondria in health and disease: perspectives on a new mitochondrial biology. Mol Aspects Med. 2004;25:365–451

Fiskum G, Lehninger AL. Regulated release of Ca^{2+} from respiring mitochondria by $Ca^{2+}/2H^+$ antiport. J Biol Chem. 1979 Jul 25;254(14):6236-9

Florea AM, Büsselberg D. Anti-cancer drugs interfere with intracellular calcium signalling. Neurotoxicology. 2009 Sep;30(5):803-10

Glazner GW, Camandola S, Geiger JD, Mattson MP. Endoplasmic reticulum D-myo-inositol 1,4,5-trisphosphate-sensitive stores regulate nuclear factor-kappaB binding activity in a calcium-independent manner. J Biol Chem. 2001 Jun 22;276(25): 22461-7

Gunter TE, Buntinas L, Sparagna G, Eliseev R, Gunter K. Mitochondrial calcium transport: mechanisms and functions. Cell Calcium. 2000 Nov-Dec;28(5-6):285-96

Hanson CJ, Bootman MD, Roderick HL. Cell signalling : IP3 receptors channel calcium into cell death. Curr Biol. 2004 Nov 9;14(21):R933-5

Henrich M, Buckler KJ. Acid-evoked Ca2+ signalling in rat sensory neurones: effects of anoxia and aglycaemia. Pflugers Arch. 2009 Nov;459(1):159-81

Jayaraman T, Marks AR. T cells deficient in inositol 1,4,5-trisphosphate receptor are resistant to apoptosis. Mol Cell Biol. 1997 Jun;17(6):3005-12

Joseph SK, Hajnóczky G. IP3 receptors in cell survival and apoptosis: Ca^{2+} release and beyond. Apoptosis. 2007 May;12(5):951-68

Jurkovicova D, Kopacek J, Stefanik P, Kubovcakova L, Zahradnikova A Jr, Zahradnikova A, Pastorekova S, Krizanova O. Hypoxia modulates gene expression of IP_3 receptors in rodent cerebellum. Pflugers Arch. 2007 Jun;454(3):415-25

Leite MF, Thrower EC, Echevarria W, Koulen P, Hirata K, Bennett AM, Ehrlich BE, Nathanson MH. Nuclear and cytosolic calcium are regulated independently. Proc Natl Acad Sci U S A. 2003 Mar 4;100(5):2975-80

Li Q, Wang X, Yang Z, Wang B, Li S. Menthol Induces Cell Death via the TRPM8 Channel in the Human Bladder Cancer Cell Line T24. Oncology 2009;77:335–341

Liu Q, Berchner-Pfannschmidt U, Möller U, Brecht M, Wotzlaw C, Acker H, Jungermann K, Kietzmann T. A Fenton reaction at the endoplasmic reticulum is involved in the redox control of hypoxia-inducible gene expression. Proc Natl Acad Sci U S A. 2004 Mar 23;101(12):4302-7

Lu FH, Tian Z, Zhang WH, Zhao YJ, Li HL, Ren H, Zheng HS, Liu C, Hu GX, Tian Y, Yang BF, Wang R, Xu CQ. Calcium-sensing receptors regulate cardiomyocyte Ca^{2+} signalling via the sarcoplasmic reticulum-mitochondrion interface during hypoxia/reoxygenation. J Biomed Sci. 2010 Jun 17;17:50

Malviya AN, Klein C. Mechanism regulating nuclear calcium signalling. Can J Physiol Pharmacol. 2006 Mar-Apr;84(3-4):403-22.

Mammucari C, Rizzuto R. Signalling pathways in mitochondrial dysfunction and aging. Mech Ageing Dev. 2010 Jul-Aug;131(7-8):536-43

Missiaen L, Robberecht W, van den Bosch L, Callewaert G, Parys JB, Wuytack F,

Raeymaekers L, Nilius B, Eggermont J, De Smedt H. Abnormal intracellular Ca(2+)homeostasis and disease. Cell Calcium. 2000 Jul;28(1):1-21.

Murphy AN, Fiskum G. Abnormal Ca2+ transport characteristics of hepatoma mitochondria and endoplasmic reticulum. Adv Exp Med Biol. 1988;232:139-50.

Ondrias K, Lencesova L, Sirova M, Labudova M, Pastorekova S, Kopacek J, Krizanova O. Apoptosis induced clustering of IP$_3$R1 in nuclei of nondifferentiated PC12 cells. J Cell Physiol. 2011 (in press)

Parkash J, Asotra K. Calcium wave signalling in cancer cells. Life Sci. 2010 Nov 20;87(19-22):587-95

Philipson KD, Nicoll DA, Ottolia M, Quednau BD, Reuter H, John S, Qiu Z. The Na$^+$/Ca^{2+} exchange molecule: an overview. Ann N Y Acad Sci. 2002 Nov;976:1-10

Rathore R, Zheng YM, Niu CF, Liu QH, Korde A, Ho YS, Wang YX. Hypoxia activates NADPH oxidase to increase [ROS]i and [Ca^{2+}]i through the mitochondrial ROS-PKCepsilon signalling axis in pulmonary artery smooth muscle cells. Free Radic Biol Med. 2008 Nov 1;45(9):1223-31

Rimessi A, Giorgi C, Pinton P, Rizzuto R. The versatility of mitochondrial calcium signals: from stimulation of cell metabolism to induction of cell death Biochim Biophys Acta. 2008 ; 1777(7-8): 808–816

Ruiz-Perez VL, Carter SA, Healy E, Todd C, Rees JL, Steijlen PM, Carmichael AJ, Lewis HM, Hohl D, Itin P, Vahlquist A, Gobello T, Mazzanti C, Reggazini R, Nagy G, Munro CS, Strachan T. ATP2A2 mutations in Darier's disease: variant cutaneous phenotypes are associated with missense mutations, but neuropsychiatric features are independent of mutation class. Hum Mol Genet. 1999 Sep; 8(9):1621-30

Saidak Z, Mentaverri R, Brown EM. The role of the calcium-sensing receptor in the development and progression of cancer. Endocr Rev. 2009 Apr;30(2):178-95

Schwab, B.L., Guerini, D., Didszun, C., Bano, D., Ferrando-May, E., Fava, E., Tam, J., Xu, D., Xanthoudakis, S., Nicholson, D.W., Carafoli, E., Nicotera, P. Cleavage of plasma membrane calcium pumps by caspases: a link between apoptosis and necrosis. Cell Death Differ. 2002; 9, 818-831.

Sugawara, H., Kurosaki, M., Takata, M., and Kurosaki, T. Genetic evidence for involvement of type 1, type 2 and type 3 inositol 1,4,5-trisphosphate receptors in signal transduction through the Bcell antigen receptor. EMBO J. 1997; 16, 3078-3088.

Szatkowski C, Parys JB, Ouadid-Ahidouch H, Matifat F. Inositol 1,4,5-trisphosphate-induced Ca^{2+} signalling is involved in estradiol-induced breast cancer epithelial cell growth. Mol Cancer. 2010 Jun 21;9:156.

Thippegowda PB, Singh V, Sundivakkam PC, Xue J, Malik AB, Tiruppathi C. Ca^{2+} influx via TRPC channels induces NF-kappaB-dependent A20 expression to prevent thrombin-induced apoptosis in endothelial cells. Am J Physiol Cell Physiol. 2010 Mar;298(3):C656-64

Tran QK, Ohashi K, Watanabe H. Calcium signalling in endothelial cells. Cardiovasc Res. 2000 Oct;48(1):13-22

Tsunoda T, Koga H, Yokomizo A, Tatsugami K, Eto M, Inokuchi J, Hirata A, Masuda K, Okumura K, Naito S. Inositol 1,4,5-trisphosphate (IP3) receptor type1 (IP3R1) modulates the acquisition of cisplatin resistance in bladder cancer cell lines. Oncogene. 2005 Feb 17;24(8):1396-402

Yagami T, Takase K, Yamamoto Y, Ueda K, Takasu N, Okamura N, Sakaeda T, Fujimoto M. Fibroblast growth factor 2 induces apoptosis in the early primary culture of rat cortical neurons. Exp Cell Res. 2010 Aug 15;316(14):2278-90

Yamada T, Ueda T, Shibata Y, Ikegami Y, Saito M, Ishida Y, Ugawa S, Kohri K, Shimada S. TRPV2 activation induces apoptotic cell death in human T24 bladder cancer cells: a potential therapeutic target for bladder cancer. Urology. 2010 Aug;76(2):509.e1-7

Yuan G, Nanduri J, Bhasker CR, Semenza GL, Prabhakar NR. Ca2+/calmodulin kinase-dependent activation of hypoxia inducible factor 1 transcriptional activity in cells subjected to intermittent hypoxia. J Biol Chem. 2005 Feb 11;280(6):4321-8. Epub 2004 Nov 29.

Zhou J, Köhl R, Herr B, Frank R, Brüne B. Calpain mediates a von Hippel-Lindau protein-independent destruction of hypoxia-inducible factor-1alpha. Mol Biol Cell. 2006 Apr;17(4):1549-58

Chapter 13

HIF and Inflammation

Sandra Winning and Joachim Fandrey[*]

[*]Author for correspondence:
Institut für Physiologie, Universität Duisburg-Essen, Essen, D-45147; Germany,
Phone/Fax:–49-201-723 4608/4648, E-mail: joachim.fandrey@uni-due.de

Contents

Key points

—   HIF regulation occurs at levels other than the posttranslational level.

Classic HIF regulation describes the oxygen-dependent degradation of HIF-αs. Inflammatory mediators modulate HIF expression at the transcriptional, translational, and posttranslational levels.

—   Interaction of HIF-1 and NF-κB.

Both pathways are highly linked because both transcription factors are induced by hypoxia and inflammation, share regulating enzymes, and influence each other.

—   Contribution of HIF-2 to inflammatory settings.

The role of HIF-2 in inflammatory settings has recently been analyzed but is still unclear.

Introduction

Sites of inflammation are not only characterized by high expression of inflammatory cytokines, such as TNF-α or IL-1β, but also show low oxygen tension and restricted availability of nutrients (Cramer et al., 2003, Karhausen et al., 2005). The reasons for these characteristics are twofold: Extensive inflammation leads to vasculopathy, including blood vessel stenosis or micro-thrombosis, and therefore results in poor perfusion and subsequently in a decrease in the supply of oxygen to the area of inflamed tissue. Furthermore, increased interstitial pressure may reduce vascular diameter (Wakefield et al., 1989, Hatoum et al., 2003, Taylor, 2008), and the gradient of highly expressed inflammatory mediators and decreasing nutrients attracts effector cells of the innate and adaptive immune systems (Murdoch et al., 2005, Sitkovsky et Lukashev, 2005). The effectors cells' immense metabolic activity and oxygen consumption further decrease oxygen tension at the inflammatory site. Still, the immune cells must function properly if they are to fight infection, especially because many common bacterial pathogens proliferate well under anaerobic conditions. This proper function includes the ability to generate adenosine triphosphate (ATP) despite a low oxygen tension, an ability that can be achieved only by a switch from oxidative phosphorylation to anaerobic glycolysis.

The central transcription factors that adapt cells to these conditions are hypoxia-inducible factor HIF-1 and HIF-2 (Semenza et al., 1997, Ema et al., 1997, Wiesener et al., 1998). Recently, the importance of HIF-1 in inflammatory settings has increasingly come into the spotlight of current research, but in contrast very little is known about the contribution of HIF-2. Because the process of inflammation is indispensably connected with hypoxia, it is very likely that these transcription factors play a role in such situations. Both transcription factors share a common constitutively expressed β-subunit, HIF-1β or aryl hydrocarbon nuclear translocator (ARNT), whereas the α-subunits (HIF-1α and HIF-2α) are regulated according to actual oxygen tension (Fandrey et al., 2006). Elevations in HIF-1α levels have been detected in the inflamed joints of patients with rheumatoid arthritis (Hollander et al., 2001) and in inflammatory cells of healing wounds (Albina et al., 2001). Of course, these *in vivo* settings reflect activation of HIF-1α via inflammatory and hypoxic stimulation.

To clearly elucidate the effects of inflammatory mediators and to discriminate those effects from hypoxic regulation with respect to the HIF system, *in vitro* experiments were necessary. Several studies have found that various inflammatory stimuli, such as pro-inflammatory cytokines, bacterial lipopolysaccharides (LPS), or synthetic viral stimuli such as Poly(I:C), can induce the HIF system under normoxic conditions (Zhou et al. 2003, Frede et al., 2005, Frede et al., 2006, Paone et al., 2010). These findings have subsequently been confirmed in a wide range of cell types. After exposure to inflammatory stimuli, not only cells of the innate immune system but also tumour cells accumulate HIF-1α (Frede et al., 2005, Metzen et al., 2003, Hellwig-Bürgel et al., 1999). Epithelial cells (Sandau et al., 2001), and vascular smooth muscle cells (Richard et al., 2000) show marked upregulation of HIF-1 target gene expression in inflammatory settings. All of these findings indicate that HIF-1 plays an important role in the initiation, regulation, and coordination of cell responses during inflammatory processes.

Cramer et al. (2003) were the first to show that the proper function of leukocytes lacking HIF-1α is considerably restricted at sites of inflammatory lesions. Cramer and colleagues used Cre-*LoxP* recombination to establish a lineage-specific deletion of HIF-1α in all cells of myeloid origin. After engineering a mouse line containing two *LoxP* sites flanking the exon 2 of the *hif-1a* gene, they crossed these mice with animals in which the lysozyme M promoter drives Cre recombinase expression specifically in cells of the myeloid lineage. The resulting mice showed markedly diminished expression of functionally active HIF-1α in myeloid cells (because exon 2 contains the DNA binding domain of the protein, the expressed shortened isoform cannot induce gene expression) and no aberrant phenotype under normal conditions. In contrast, these mice showed markedly impaired inflammatory responses when treated with chemical irritants to the skin or subjected to a collagen-induced arthritis model.

In addition, significantly fewer leukocytes migrated to sites of inflammation in these mice, a finding indicating that HIF-1α plays a pivotal role in leukocyte recruitment (Cramer et al., 2003). This finding was further supported by Kong and co-workers, who found that the β_2 integrins CD18, CD11a, and CD11d, adhesion molecules that are crucial for the process of leukocyte extravasation, are HIF-1 target genes in U937 cells and in primary human monocytes (Kong et al., 2004, Kong et al., 2007). Furthermore, monocytes and neutrophils deficient in HIF-1α exhibited normal phagocytic capacity, but their ability to kill phagocytosed bacteria was significantly reduced (Peyssonnaux et al., 2004). Strikingly, this finding leads to the conclusion that the phagocytic capability of myeloid cells is increased under hypoxic conditions. Even more surprising is the finding that bacteria seem to be a more potent inducer of HIF-1α protein stabilization than is hypoxia itself (Peyssonnaux et al., 2004, Frede at al., 2006). The close interaction between the HIF system and the inflammatory transcription factor family nuclear factor (NF)-κB could be identified as one molecular explanation for this finding (Frede at al., 2006, BelAiba et al., 2007, van Uden et al., 2008, Culver et al., 2010).

Above all, HIF-1α also modulates the response of dendritic cells to bacterial stimuli by markedly increasing the release of proinflammatory cytokines and the expression of costimulatory molecules by murine dendritic cells (DCs) (Jantsch et al., 2008). This finding confirms that this transcription factor plays an important role in bridging innate and adaptive immunity (Nizet and Johnson, 2009). Recently, it was postulated that HIF-1α plays an important anti-inflammatory and tissue-protective role with respect to its activation in T lymphocytes. Lukashev et al. (2006) found that deletion of the alternative HIF-1α mRNA isoform I.1 in T cells results in significant upregulation of the production of inflammatory cytokines.

However, the enhanced expression of HIF-1α protein and, therefore, of HIF-1 target genes at sites of bacterial inflammation has some undesirable effects. The induction of vascular endothelial growth factor (VEGF), for example, results in increased vascular leakage, improved tumour vascularisation, or metastasis (Schoch et al., 2002, Pollard, 2004). Therefore, it is necessary to further understand the beneficial or counterproductive effects of HIF-1 induction at sites of inflammation. One strategy for addressing this question is to further elucidate the mechanisms leading to non-hypoxic induction of the transcription factor. The hypoxic regulation of the transcription factor is well known: HIF-1α is believed to be constitutively transcribed and translated. As long as oxygen is available, three enzymes containing prolyl hydroxylase domains (PHDs 1-3) and one asparaginyl hydroxylase (factor inhibiting HIF-1, or FIH-1) immediately hydroxylate specific residues within the α-subunit (Jaakola et al., 2001, Sang et al., 2002, Lando et al., 2002). Hydroxylation of the prolyl residues mediates contact to the von Hippel-Lindau (VHL) tumour suppressor protein and subsequent proteasomal degradation. The hydroxylation of the asparagyl residue prevents the recruitment of cofactors to the active transcription factor complex HIF-1. Under hypoxic conditions, all hydroxylases are inhibited. Therefore, the α-subunit accumulates in the cytosol of cells, translocates into the nucleus, and dimerizes with HIF-1β (Semenza et al., 1997). After recruitment of cofactors for DNA binding, transcription of HIF-1 target genes can begin (Arany et al., 1996, Kallio et al., 1998, Fandrey et al., 2006). It has recently become obvious that inflammatory regulation of the HIF system occurs at levels other than the posttranslational level. The variety of inflammatory mediators present at sites of inflammation also opens the possibility that the expression of HIF-1α can be modified in several ways, including regulation at the transcriptional and translational levels.

Regulation of HIF-1α by inflammatory cytokines

As mentioned above, sites of inflammation are characterized by high levels of proinflammatory cytokines such as IL-1β and TNF-α. Many cell types can produce these mediators and therefore create an environment in which inflammatory mediators may induce HIF-1α expression cooperatively with hypoxia via paracrine or autocrine pathways. The regulation of HIF-1α by IL-1β and TNF-α has been the subject of important research during recent years. It is known that in ovarian carcinoma cells IL-1β induces the translation of HIF-1α mRNA but leaves the degradation of the protein unaffected (Frede et al., 2005). Very similar results were obtained by Zhou and coworkers (2003), who treated human embryonic kidney cells (HEK cells) and proximal tubular cells with TNF-α. They found that the interaction between HIF-1α and the VHL protein was intact but that HIF-1α protein levels were still elevated because of increased synthesis of the protein.

In rheumatoid synovial fibroblasts, both IL-1β and TNF-α induce the expression of HIF-1α protein but also stimulate HIF-1α mRNA (Westra et al., 2007). Similarly, Thornton et al. (2000) found that both HIF-1α mRNA expression and HIF-1 DNA binding were increased after stimulation with IL-1. An increase in HIF-1 DNA binding was also observed by Hellwig-Bürgel et al. (1999), who analyzed the human hepatoma cell line HepG2 after stimulation with TNF-α or IL-1β under normoxic and hypoxic conditions. Both cytokines induced a moderate increase in HIF-1 DNA binding under normoxic conditions and achieved a much more prominent effect under hypoxic conditions. Only IL-1β led to an increase in HIF-1α protein expression by HepG2 cells, and none of the cytokines affected HIF-1α mRNA.

A recent study found that the expression of both TNF-α and IL-1β is significantly enhanced in macrophages that lack the HIF-1αI.1 mRNA isoform (Ramanathan et al., 2009). These findings indicate a negative feedback mechanism between HIF-1α and the expression of proinflammatory cytokines. In addition, the findings also illustrate an intimate signalling crosstalk between cytokines and the HIF system, a crosstalk that contributes to the concise adaptation of cells to hypoxic inflammatory conditions.

Regulation of HIF-1 by nitric oxide

Nitric oxide (NO) is an inflammatory mediator that can be found under conditions of inflammation, ischemia-reperfusion, or hypoxia. It modulates a variety of intracellular signalling pathways, including the activation of NF-κB, p38 mitogen-activated protein kinase (MAPK), and c-jun (Lander et al., 1996), and thus participates in the adjustment of the acute response to inflammatory stimulation. Biological effects of NO are often alluded to "reactive nitrogen intermediates" (RNI) rather than to the radical itself. RNIs include various oxidative states and adducts of the products of the NO synthase, e.g. $NO^{.}$, NO^{+}, NO^{-}, NO_2, or NO_3^{-} (Brüne and Zhou, 2007). Regarding the HIF system, NO indirectly influences HIF-1α stability. Most likely, NO replaces molecular oxygen in the active centre of the PHDs under normoxic conditions because of its structural similarity to oxygen and the fact that NO is an electron-donating complex ligand for the central iron atom of the PHDs. Because oxygen can no longer bind to the central iron atom, hydroxylation cannot be performed. This inhibition of the enzymes results in normoxic stabilization of the HIF-1α protein and transcriptional activation of HIF-1 target gene expression (Kimura et al., 2000, Sandau et al., 2001, Zhou et al., 2003, Metzen et al., 2003).

However, under hypoxic conditions, some NO donors exhibit the opposite effect and destabilize HIF-1α protein rather than inducing its stability and activity (Liu et al., 1998, Sogawa et al., 1998, Huang et al., 1999). Currently, several approaches are being discussed as explanations for this effect. First, NO-derived species such as peroxynitrite ($ONOO^{-}$) and other reactive oxygen species (ROS) such as the superoxide anion (O_2^{-}) could reactivate the PHD enzymes under hypoxic conditions and therefore shorten the half-life of the HIF-1α protein under hypoxic conditions (Wellman et al., 2003, Callapina et al., 2005, Köhl et al., 2006). Agani et al. (2002) obtained very similar results in studies of Hep3B and PC12 cells. Furthermore, they proposed that mitochondria are involved in NO-regulated HIF-1 expression under hypoxic conditions.

NO is known to inhibit cytochromes in the respiratory chain, and this inhibition results in a marked reduction of oxygen consumption by the mitochondria. In this setting, Hagen et al. (2003) found that oxygen is redistributed within the cell toward nonrespiratory oxygen-dependent targets such as the prolyl hydroxylases. As a consequence, oxygen-dependent hydroxylation of the HIF-1α protein is re-induced and, therefore, the hypoxic stability of the protein is diminished. However, under these conditions the cell may fail to sensitize surrounding oxygen concentrations.

One can speculate whether this scenario may depict a feedback system that limits unrestricted HIF signalling under the induction by NO (Brüne and Zhou, 2007). This hypothesis of a negative feedback mechanism would agree with the findings of Berchner-Pfannschmidt et al. (2007), who identified NO as a putative modulator of the HIF-1α–PHD2 autoregulatory loop. They observed that NO exerts a biphasic effect on the HIF system: HIF-1α protein levels increased soon after hypoxic NO treatment because of the inhibitory impact of NO on PHD activity, but this increase was followed by a later decrease in HIF-1α protein levels. This decrease was explained by the fact that the PHD2 itself is a HIF-1 target gene. Therefore, the high levels of HIF-1α protein at early time points led directly to an induction of PHD2 mRNA and later resulted in elevated PHD2 protein levels, which degraded HIF-1α.

Other stimuli affecting the HIF system

Insulin is known to play a central role in regulating metabolic pathways associated with energy storage and utilization. Because of the striking overlap of genes that are induced both by insulin and hypoxic stress, Zelzer et al. (1998) found that these stimulants shared HIF-1 as a common transcription factor complex. Therefore, insulin is one of the first stimuli other than hypoxia to be proved to induce HIF-1 under normoxic conditions. Stiehl et al. (2003) further widened our knowledge about insulin-induced stimulation of the HIF-1 pathway by research showing that this induction is phosphatidyl inositol kinase (PI3K) dependent. Currently, many stimuli have been shown to induce HIF-1α accumulation under normoxic conditions. Among these are thrombin, transforming growth factor β (TGF-β), ROS, and inflammatory mediators. It has been known for nearly a decade that thrombin, platelet-derived growth factor-AB (PDGF-AB), and TGF-β1 can upregulate HIF-1α protein in cultured and native vascular smooth muscle cells (VSMCs; Görlach et al., 2001). Thereby, the induction of thrombin and PDGFs by HIF-1α is attenuated by antioxidant treatment.

Further experiments revealed that p22(phox), a subunit of a membrane-bound nicotinamide adenine dinucleotide phosphate (NADPH) oxidase, p38 MAPK, and the PI3K pathway play a crucial role in thrombin- and growth factor–mediated HIF-1α induction; this finding indicates that ROS play a pivotal role in this setting. The main site of intracellular production of ROS is the mitochondrion, although many sources of intracellular ROS exist (Cash et al., 2007). Recent reports show that only about 0.15% of the electron flow on the electron transfer chain results in ROS production (St-Pierre et al., 2002). The high concentration of mitochondrial superoxide dismutase (SOD) ensures immediate generation of H_2O_2 from $O_2^{\cdot-}$. H_2O_2 is much more stable and can diffuse through biological membranes. Therefore, it has the potential to act as a low-range signalling molecule. However, many sources of intracellular ROS exist besides the mitochondria, e.g., the endoplasmatic reticulum with resident cytochrome P-450, plasma membrane–associated NADPH oxidases, which achieve local microbicidal functions in phagosomes, and H_2O_2-generating enzymes in peroxisomes (Cash et al., 2007).

The impact of ROS on cellular oxygen sensing and therefore on HIF regulation is intensely discussed but is still incompletely understood. Various reports describe a stabilization of HIF-1α protein because of the production of ROS (Chandel et al., 1998, Chandel et al., 2000, Görlach et al., 2001, Acker et al., 2006). Intracellular signalling pathways involved in ROS-dependent HIF-1α stabilization have been shown to involve p38 MAPK (Görlach et al., 2001, Emerling et al., 2005), but ROS also seem to modulate PHD activity. The effects of ROS on PHDs may be concentration dependent, because high doses of ROS block PHD activity and therefore stabilize HIF-1α protein, whereas low-dose ROS can induce PHD activity (Callapina et al., 2005). Furthermore, ROS may affect co-factor concentrations needed for PHD function. Oxidation of ferrous iron (Knowles et al., 2003) or increased levels of fumarate and succinate (Isaacs et al., 2005, Selak et al., 2005), both members of the mitochondrial Krebs cycle and therefore likely to be affected by ROS production, have been shown to inhibit PHD activity, thus providing an additional mechanism by which ROS may block PHD activity (Acker et al., 2006).

Very recently, our understanding of the impact of ROS on cellular oxygen sensing has been extended by findings demonstrating that ROS-mediated induction of HIF-1α can mediate either the stabilization or destabilization of ROS. In UT-7/TPO cells, HIF-1α activation attenuates the overproduction of thrombopoietin (TPO)-induced ROS via transcriptional induction of pyruvate dehydrogenase kinase (PDK)-1 (Kirito et al., 2009). In contrast, Diebold et al. (2010) identified the NADPH oxidase subunit NOX4 as a HIF-1α target gene. Induction of NOX4 by HIF-1α under hypoxic conditions has been shown to contribute to the maintenance of ROS levels beyond incubation and to hypoxia-induced proliferation of pulmonary artery smooth muscle cells. In conclusion, the crosstalk between ROS and the HIF system seems to be complex and highly dependent on cell type. Further studies will be needed to elucidate the cellular structures involved.

Hypoxia and NF-κB

Whereas HIF-1 is the central transcription factor regulating the cellular response to hypoxia (Semenza, 2007), NF-κB has been shown to be one of the master regulators of cellular adaptation to inflammatory conditions (Barnes and Karin, 1997, Rius et al., 2008). The NF-κB family consists of five members: Rel (c-Rel), RelA (p65), RelB, NF-κB1 (p50/p105), and NF-κB2 (p52/p100). One or two family members form homodimers or heterodimers that recognize a common DNA consensus sequence and therefore regulate a large number of target genes that are associated, for example, with the response to inflammation, stress, or injury (Brown et al., 2008). NF-κB activation generally follows two principal signalling pathways: the classical/canonical NF-κB activation pathway and the alternative/noncanonical pathway. The classical signalling cascade involves phosphorylation and degradation of inhibitor of NF-κB (IκB) proteins and most commonly results in the activation of the heterodimer of p65/p50. The alternative pathway includes phosphorylation and proteolytic processing of NF-κB2 (p100) and most commonly results in the activation of RelB/p52. Classical NF-κB signalling occurs after the stimulation of various cell membrane receptors, such as TNF receptor, IL-1 receptor, Toll-like receptors (TLRs), T-cell receptor (TCR), and B cell receptor (BCR). Stimulation leads to phosphorylation, ubiquitination, and subsequent degradation of IκB proteins (Li and Verma, 2002, Hayden and Ghosh, 2004, Brown et al., 2008). The initial phosphorylation step is catalyzed by IκB kinases (IKK), of which IKKβ is the one predominantly involved in the classical NF-κB pathway. All in all, the classical NF-κB activation pathway can be called essential at multiple stages of normal development, but especially in the function of the immune system (Brown et al., 2008).

The alternative NF-κB activation pathway depends on IKKα rather than on IKKβ. IKKα phosphorylates the carboxyl-terminus of NF-κB2/p100, and this phosphorylation results in proteolytic cleavage of the carboxyl-terminal half of the NF-κB protein. Upon this cleavage, p52 is released, dimerizes with RelB, and translocates into the nucleus, where it develops transcriptional activity (Hayden and Ghosh, 2004, Brown et al., 2008). The alternative NF-κB signalling pathway, among others, is activated by stimulation of the lymphotoxin receptor (LTβR), B-cell activating factor receptor (BAFFR), and CD40 (Hayden and Ghosh, 2004). The alternative NF-κB pathway exerts important functions during the development, selection, and survival of B and T lymphocytes and in the differentiation of antigen-presenting cells (e.g., dendritic cells). Thus, this pathway plays a pivotal role in the regulation of immune central and peripheral tolerance (Brown et al., 2008).

Hypoxia has been shown to influence the NF-κB pathways in various ways. The first findings demonstrated that hypoxia enhances NF-κB activation in various settings. In macrophages, Lo et al. (1998) found that hypoxia further increases eicosanoid production (prostaglandin E$_2$), which is driven by hypoxic activation of NF-κB. Compared with normoxic, endotoxin-treated cells, hypoxic endothelial cells exhibit a significantly enhanced upregulation of the NF-κB target gene intercellular adhesion molecule (ICAM)-1 in response to LPS (Zünd et al., 1997). Similar observations were made by Chakrabarti et al. (2009), who found that the interaction between endothelial cells and the human monocytic cell line THP-1 via CD40-CD40L was higher after hypoxic stimulation with LPS than after LPS stimulation under normoxic conditions. Studying the effects of hypoxia alone, Koong et al. (1994) were the first to observe an induction in NF-κB binding activity in Jurkat T cells under severe hypoxic conditions (0.02% O$_2$ in cell culture medium). They found that a hypoxia-mediated degradation of the IκBα protein resulted in a corresponding accumulation of nuclear p65 and increasing NF-κB DNA binding activity after 3 to 4 hours of hypoxia.

More recently, researchers noted a novel role for the HIF-regulating prolyl hydroxylases. Under hypoxic conditions, PHD1 in particular not only hydroxylates specific prolyl residues of the HIF-α proteins but can also recognize a specific LXXLAP motif of the IKK-β protein. Hydroxylation reduces IKK activity; therefore, hypoxia and subsequent PHD1 inhibition can induce NF-κB activation and DNA binding under hypoxic conditions (Cummins et al., 2006). To be more precise, coimmunoprecipitation revealed that both PHD1 and pVHL interact with IKK-β in normoxic HeLa cells. Cummins and coworkers identified a prolyl residue that is very likely to be recognized by the PHD enzyme, although direct evidence for the hydroxylation has not yet been found. Cummins and associates postulated that this hydroxylation subsequently inhibits the phosphorylation of the IKK-β at two specific serine sites. This phosphorylation in turn is crucial for activation of the kinase. Therefore, the downstream molecule IκB is not marked for degradation, and NF-κB homodimers and heterodimers remain inactively in the cytosol. Blocking the hydroxylation step under hypoxic conditions would therefore explain the induction of NF-κB activity. In contrast, Chan et al. (2009) recently demonstrated that the classical NF-κB pathway is significantly induced after knockdown of PHD2, but their findings also suggested a PHD2-mediated regulation of NF-κB independent of hydroxylation. The findings of our group seem to support the findings of Cummins and coworkers. We analyzed the effects of acute and severe hypoxia on leukocyte adhesion to endothelial cells. Coculturing monocytic cells with endothelial cells under nearly anoxic conditions (0.1% ambient O_2) resulted in an induction of monocyte adherence that was more than 50-fold higher than that in normoxic coculture (Winning et al., 2010). This adherent effect was very fast and short-lived; it began after 1 hour and had already decreased after 6 hours. In contrast to the findings of Kong et al. (2004), who found that the leukocyte adhesion molecules CD11a, CD11d, and CD18 were induced in an HIF-1 dependent fashion at later time points under milder conditions of hypoxia (3% O_2), we found that none of those molecules was affected in the acute, severe setting. Furthermore, knock-down of either HIF-1α or HIF-2α did not affect monocytic adherence under hypoxic conditions. Instead, we found a very rapid activation of the monocytic NF-κB system, and this activation resulted in elevated expression of the monocytic intercellular adhesion molecule (ICAM)-1. This molecule was crucially involved in induced adhesion under hypoxic conditions because its knock-down by a siRNA approach completely abrogated the effect. Furthermore, blocking classical NF-κB activation with the proteasomal inhibitor bortezomib also prevented the adherence of monocytes under hypoxia. Incubating the cocultured cells with the pan-hydroxylase inhibitor dimethyloxalylglycine (DMOG) induced monocyte adherence under normoxic conditions; this finding demonstrated that prolyl hydroxylases play an important role in the activation of NF-κB. Further experiments also showed that PHD1 is probably the enzyme that exerts the greatest effect on the monocytic NF-κB system. Elevated levels of nuclear p65 could be detected after hypoxia or treatment with DMOG. All in all, these findings demonstrate a functionally important hypoxic activation of the classic NF-κB signalling pathway in human THP-1 cells. How PHD enzymes are able to regulate the HIF and NF-κB pathways is summarized in Figure 13.1.

The induction of monocyte adherence caused by severe hypoxia in our setting is comparable to or even more pronounced than stimulation with high-dose LPS for the same duration (Figure 13.2). Adherent monocytes could only be detected on top of or in very close proximity to endothelial cells (63x magnification, Figure 13.2) indicating a direct cell-cell-interaction.

Hypoxia-mediated activation is PHD dependent but HIF-1 independent and can be completely abrogated by the NF-κB inhibitor bortezomib. This finding may open new therapeutic approaches in situations in which an overwhelming number of monocytes is recruited to hypoxic sites of inflammation (Winning et al., 2010).

Analyzing various cancer cell lines for their transcriptional activation under hypoxic conditions, Culver et al. (2010) also found a rapid but persis-

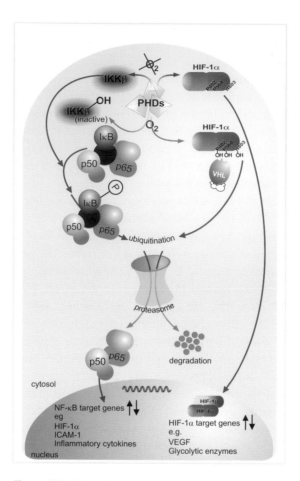

Figure 13.1 _ Prolyl hydroxylases as central regulators of the transcription factors HIF-1 and NF-κB.

Under normoxic conditions, prolyl hydroxylases are active and hydroxylate the HIF-1α subunit (right panel). Hydroxylation targets the protein for proteasomal degradation and therefore prevents activation of the transcription factor HIF-1. In addition, PHDs can also hydroxylate the IKK-β subunit of the IKK complex. Hydroxylation in this case renders the enzyme inactive. Therefore phosphorylation of the IκBs as well as their subsequent degradation is inhibited and the NF-κB subunits p65/p50 remain in the cytosol. Hypoxia reduces PHD activity, HIF-1α accumulates in the cytosol and translocates into the nucleus. After dimerization with HIF-1β gene expression of HIF-1 target genes (e.g. VEGF, glycolytic enzymes) is initiated. Less hydroxylation of the IKK complex results in phosphorylation of IκBs. The inhibitor proteins get degraded by the proteasome and NF-κB subunits is released. After translocation into the nucleus NF-κB-mediated gene transcription of e.g. *HIF-1α*, inflammatory cytokines, or adhesion molecules, such as *ICAM-1*, is induced.

tent activation of the NF-κB system. They demonstrated a marked induction of nuclear p65 levels after 1 hour of hypoxic incubation. Furthermore,
an increased DNA binding of the subunits p65, p50, and p52 was detected
after 30 minutes at 1% O_2. The authors found this effect to be IKK dependent but did not observe any effects after knock-down of PHD1, PHD2, or
PHD3. Instead, they proposed a mechanism of IKK activation via Ca^{2+}
release and calcium/calmodulin–dependent kinase 2 (CaMK2) activation
under hypoxic conditions. This mechanism was found to be crucial for the
activation of transforming growth factor-β–activated kinase 1 (TAK1). This
kinase in turn could be identified as a key upstream kinase of the IKK complex, and this kinase is required for hypoxic activation of NF-κB. In addition
to these findings, Fang et al. (2009) analyzed the hypoxic gene expression
pattern of isolated monocytes from buffy coats that were differentiated

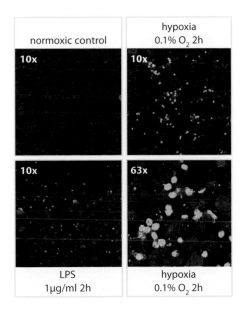

Figure 13.2 _ Induction of monocyte adhesion after LPS treatment and severe
hypoxia.

Human THP-1 (stained green) cells were cocultured with human umbilical vein
cord endothelial cells (HUVEC, red). Coculturing under severe hypoxia (0.1% O_2,
2h) results in a dramatic increase in monocyte adherence to the endothelium.
The effect is even more pronounced than the induction in adhesion after stimulation with high-dose LPS (1 μg/mL, 2h). Adherent monocytes can only be found
on top of or in close proximity to the endothelial cells (63x magnification).

into macrophages *in vitro*. The cells were incubated under severe hypoxic conditions (0.1% O_2 for 18 hours) and showed upregulated mRNA levels of IKKβ and γ, IκBα, p65, and p50, as well as of a plethora of NF-κB target genes.

HIF-1α and the classical NF-κB pathway: various possibilities for interactions

In recent years, the interdependence of hypoxic and innate immune responses has become a topic of intensive scientific research (reviewed in Nizet and Johnson, 2009). Because acute foci of tissue inflammation show hypoxia or near anoxia in addition to high expression levels of inflammatory mediators, a crosstalk between the two primary transcription factors that adapt cells to either hypoxic or inflammatory challenges, HIF-1 and NF-κB, seems more than likely. Indeed, there is evidence for a strictly regulated crosstalk between the two signalling pathways. The upregulation of NF-κB signalling under hypoxic conditions within the involvement of HIF-regulating prolyl hydroxylases, as demonstrated by Cummins and coworkers (2006), is an elegant example of the synergistic action of both transcription factors, although they do not interact directly.

In addition to this, a multitude of scientific studies have provided evidence of a direct induction of the HIF-1 pathway by NF-κB. Frede et al. (2006) were the first to postulate an active NF-κB binding site within the HIF-1α promoter region. They demonstrated that the stimulation of human monocytes and macrophages with bacterial LPS resulted in a significant induction of HIF-1α mRNA expression via activation of this NF-κB binding site. The signalling cascade also involved p44/42 MAPK and caused increased HIF-1α target gene expression under normoxic conditions. Further evidence of the induction of HIF-1α mRNA by NF-κB was provided by BelAiba et al. (2007) in experiments with pulmonary artery smooth muscle cells. The hypoxic induction of HIF-1α mRNA in these cells was shown to be dependent on the binding of the NF-κB family members p65 and p50 to the HIF-1α promoter. Hypoxic induction of NF-κB involved the PI3K/AKT pathway.

These findings were recently extended by analyses of the regulation of HIF-1α mRNA expression in HEK 293 cells (van Uden et al., 2008). All NF-κB family members –p65, RelB, c-Rel, p52, and p50 –were shown to be able to activate a HIF-1α promoter construct expressing a NF-κB binding site. Furthermore, all family members bound to the κB binding site within the HIF-1α promoter in HEK 293 cells. Subsequent knock-down of each NF-κB member demonstrated that basal HIF-1α mRNA levels were decreased by the silencing of p65, RelB, or p52. Interestingly, TNF-α stimulation can increase HIF-1α mRNA levels in HEK cells; this finding further indicates that the effects of inflammatory cytokines on the HIF system are highly dependent on the analyzed cell type. Van Uden et al. explained this effect by the activation of NF-κB, which subsequently induces HIF-α mRNA. In all analyzed settings, HIF-1β mRNA expression remains stable in HEK 293 cells. Very recently, Culver et al. (2010) found that the hypoxic accumulation of HIF-1α in U2OS cells depends on the activation of the NF-κB family members p65 and p100. All of these findings provide sufficient hints to allow us to further understand the hypoxic induction of HIF-1α mRNA, as exhibited in hypoxic lung tissue (Palmer et al., 1998) and in tissue from mice and rats in several *in vivo* studies when the animals were exposed to hypoxia (Wiener et al., 1996, Semenza et al., 1997).

Additionally, recent studies have demonstrated several effects of HIF-1α on the NF-κB system. Walmsley et al. (2005) were the first to describe a HIF-mediated induction of the NF-κB pathway. They found elevated hypoxic levels of p65 and IKK-α in neutrophils and revealed that the enhanced NF-κB activity was responsible for the survival of induced neutrophils under hypoxic and anoxic conditions. In comparing bone marrow–derived neutrophils from wild-type and constitutive HIF-1α knock-out mice they found that neutrophil survival was not increased under hypoxic conditions when HIF-1α was absent. Although the kinetics of p65 and IKK-α induction under hypoxic conditions were similar to those of typical HIF-1α target genes, Walmsley and coworkers did not provide evidence for a direct HIF-1α mediated regulation of p65. Further support for indirect and rather complex effects of the HIF system on the NF-κB pathway came from the analysis of the clear cell renal cell carcinoma (CCRCC) cell line 786-0 (An and Rettig, 2005). In these cells, the loss of VHL led to increased expression of both HIF-1α protein and HIF-2α protein. Via the participation of TGF-α and epidermal growth factor receptor (EGFR), the HIF system was able to activate the PI3K/AKT pathway. Finally, this activation caused an increased phosphorylation of IKK-α, which resulted in the induction of NF-κB activity. In addition, Kuhlicke et al. (2007) found hypoxia-responsive elements (HREs) in the promoters of TLRs 2 and 6 in murine DCs and in human DCs, macrophages, and endothelial cells. Prolonged hypoxia (24 h) induced the mRNA levels of TLRs 2 and 6 in a HIF-1α–dependent manner. In accordance with these findings, Shah et al. (2008) found increased TLR2 mRNA expression in VHL-depleted intestinal epithelial cells. Induced expression of the TLRs may lead to increased NF-κB activation and thus represents another example of HIF-mediated indirect modulation of NF-κB signalling.

In contrast to the reports of indirect but synergistic activation of both transcription factors, Thiel et al. (2007) demonstrated an antagonistic regulation in primary murine T cells. They found that NF-κB activation was induced after Cre/LoxP-mediated HIF-1α depletion. The NF-κB binding activity of p50 and p65 was significantly higher in T cells with depleted HIF-1α protein; furthermore, p50 mRNA was also significantly increased in these cells. However, Thiel and coworkers could not find a putative HRE in the promoter of the murine p50 gene and therefore proposed an indirect, HIF-mediated regulation.

Finally, Peyssonnaux et al. (2007) provided an example of two-sided interactions between the HIF system and the NF-κB system. In a murine sepsis model, LPS induced HIF-1α mRNA and protein levels in a TLR4–dependent manner that directly involved NF-κB. Afterward, the increased HIF-1α protein levels promoted the expression of NF-κB–related cytokines (e.g., TNF-α, IL-1β, IL-6, and IL-12). Depletion of HIF-1α is concordant with reduced amounts of released cytokines.

All in all, a close crosstalk between the HIF system and NF-κB activation exists in cells facing inflammatory processes (e.g., monocytes/macrophages, dendritic cells, T cells, and intestinal epithelial and endothelial cells). Fine tuning of this crosstalk ensures that the cells will function at sites of unique challenges, such as hypoxia and low delivery of nutrients in a setting of high concentrations of inflammatory cytokines.

HIF-1α and the alternative NF-κB pathway: relevance of endotoxin tolerance

The alternative NF-κB pathway has been described to be crucially involved in the establishment of endotoxin tolerance in macrophages and B cells (Frede et al., 2009, Wedel et al., 1999, Yoza et al., 2006). Endotoxin tolerance is defined as the reduced release of inflammatory cytokines in response to endotoxin challenge after prolonged pre-exposure to a first (low-dose) encounter of endotoxin. In vitro models of endotoxin tolerance have been of interest in recent years because they represent strategies for the further study of clinical diseases such as sepsis. Patients with sepsis exhibit features such as tissue injury, blood loss, hypoxia, bacterial translocation, and cell activation by microbial products; each of these features contributes to the inflammatory response and therefore modulates the quality of the patients' immune status. In addition, the immune status is affected by drugs such as opioids and anaesthetics, which often induce a depressed immune status.

These findings led Bone et al. (1997) to propose a two-sided model for the pathogenesis of the disease progress. If the inflammatory reactions prevail, sepsis as a systemic event (systemic inflammatory response syndrome, SIRS) results in organ dysfunction and cardiovascular compromise, which lead to shock. If, on the other hand, immune suppression predominates (compensatory anti-inflammatory response syndrome, CARS), anti-inflammatory responses associated with immune-suppressive effects are induced; these responses are also known as "immunoparalysis" (Cavaillon et al., 2004). The depressed immune status in those patients manifests itself in immune effector cells that show low expression of major histocompatibility complex II (MHCII) and, therefore, reduced antigen presentation, as well as diminished cellular cytotoxicity (Cavaillon et al., 2004). Whereas the first studies of endotoxin tolerance led to doubt as to whether leukocytes actually become tolerant to the applied endotoxin or whether rapid removal of the toxin by the reticuloendothelial system is responsible for the symptoms of tolerance (Cluff, 1953), it is now known that endotoxin tolerance affects immune cells directly (Matic and Simon, 1992, McCall et al., 1993). These findings have been fur-

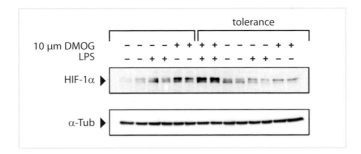

Figure 13.3 _ HIF-1α protein expression after establishment of endotoxin tolerance. Macrophage-like differentiated human THP-1 cells were made endotoxin tolerant as described previously (Frede et al., 2009). Naïve cells accumulate HIF-1α protein after stimulation with LPS, DMOG, or both. HIF-1α protein in tolerant cells is not induced by stimulation with LPS or DMOG. α-Tubulin serves as loading control (whole-cell lysates, 50 μg of protein lysate).

ther extended by the fact that the transfer of LPS-sensitive macrophages renders previously LPS-tolerant mice sensitive to sepsis (Freudenberg et al., 1986). Establishing LPS tolerance in a human macrophage model, Frede et al. (2009) demonstrated that endotoxin tolerance not only is induced via activation of the alternative NF-κB pathway but also affects the HIF system (Figure 13.3). The expression of HIF-1α mRNA and protein was significantly reduced in endotoxin-tolerant cells.

Incubation of the cells with the pan-hydroxylase inhibitor DMOG during the entire time of the experiment (establishment of tolerance + acute incubation) did not prevent the establishment of endotoxin tolerance. This finding showed that the reduction in the accumulation of HIF-1α protein after LPS stimulation was clearly independent of induced posttranslational degradation of the protein. Furthermore, incubation with DMOG alone cannot stabilize HIF-1α protein levels. This finding indicates that basal levels of the transcription factor subunit have been reduced. In additional experiments, Frede at al. (2009) found that activation of the alternative NF-κB was crucially involved in the establishment of endotoxin tolerance, because deletion of the p52 precursor p100 abrogated the establishment of tolerance. With respect to the HIF system, the researchers postulated that heterodimers of p52/RelB blocked functional NF-κB binding sites for p65/p50 within the HIF-1α promoter and therefore led to down-regulated HIF-1α mRNA expression in endotoxin-tolerant macrophages. This downregulation would result in reduced expression of the HIF-1α protein (Figure 13.4).

Very similar results could be obtained by using an *in vivo* model to induce endotoxin tolerance in C57/Bl6 mice. Isolated peritoneal macrophages were analyzed for their ability to accumulate HIF-1α protein under hypoxic conditions. Compared to macrophages from control mice treated with phosphate-buffered saline (PBS), macrophages from endotoxin-tolerant mice showed substantially lower expression of hypoxic HIF-1α protein, and this diminished expression resulted in decreased expression of HIF-1 target genes under hypoxic conditions. Furthermore, basal levels of HIF-1α mRNA were reduced. Functionally, endotoxin-tolerant and, therefore, HIF-1α deficient cells exhibited reduced viability under hypoxic conditions. In addition, these cells showed a diminished tendency to invade the extracellular matrix. All in all, the establishment of endotoxin tolerance is an elegant model for inducing a functional HIF-1α knockdown in immune effector cells, and this knockdown produces important consequences for cellular function under inflammatory and hypoxic conditions (Frede et al., 2009).

HIF-1α in bacterial infections

In the past decade, scientific research has increasingly gained insight into the importance of HIF-1α in inflammatory settings. Most findings could be obtained by analyzing bacterial infection processes such as sepsis, colitis, and rheumatoid arthritis. Sepsis is a serious medical condition characterized by a whole-body inflammatory state (a SIRS) and the presence of a known or suspected infection. It is the leading cause of death in intensive care units (Peyssonnaux et al.,2007). Recently, it has been shown that HIF-1α expression in cells of the myeloid lineage crucially affects the outcome of mice in a model of LPS-induced sepsis (Peyssonnaux et al., 2007). LPS increases HIF-1α expression in a TLR4-dependent fashion via both transcriptional and translational events. In line with Frede et al. (2006), the authors found an increase in HIF-1α mRNA after LPS treatment. In addition, peritoneal macrophages of mice expressing mutated TLR4 exhibit significantly reduced mRNA expression of PHD2 and PHD3. This effect could further enhance induced HIF-1α protein expression after LPS treatment.

In additional experiments Peyssonnaux et al. (2007) showed that HIF-1α deletion in cells of myeloid lineage results in a significantly better outcome in a model of LPS-induced sepsis. Mice deficient in HIF-1α exhibit a significantly reduced release of inflammatory cytokines, such as IL-1β, IL-6, TNF-α, and IL-12. Furthermore, LPS treatment of wild-type mice resulted in a dramatically higher mortality rate than did LPS treatment of HIF-1α myeloid-null mice. Observations by Schäfer et al. (unpublished) in our laboratory for the first time provide evidence that the induction of HIF-1α mRNA in patients with sepsis correlates with disease severity. It can be proved that the expression of procalcitonin, one crucial marker for the diagnosis of sepsis, was highest in patients with the most prominent induction of HIF-1α mRNA.

In addition, HIF-1α expression in T cells also seems to crucially contribute to the outcome in a murine sepsis model. T-cell targeted deletion of the HIF-1α gene results in much higher survival rates of the mice (Thiel et al., 2007). Survival rates were improved by reversing the HIF-1α–dependent inhibition of TCR-dependent T-cell responses. HIF-1α also seemed to indirectly inhibit the transcription of the NF-κB family member p50, and this inhibition resulted in suppression of the antibacterial function of the cells. All in all, inhibition of HIF-1 transcriptional activity in immune effector cells seems to be a potential target for novel therapeutic strategies in the clinical treatment of sepsis.

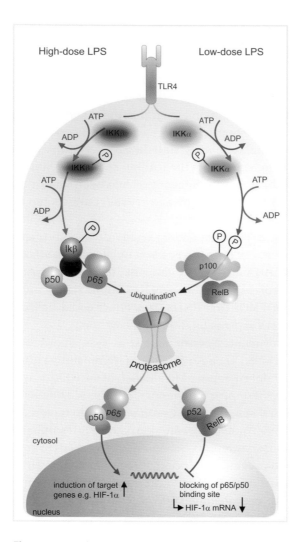

Figure 13.4 _ Classical and alternative NF-κB activation modulate the HIF-1 pathway.

Classical NF-κB activation involves TLR4 activation by high-dose LPS. Phosphorylation of IKK-β results in the phosphorylation and subsequent proteasomal degradation of the NF-κB inhibitor IκB. The heterodimer of p65/p50 gets released and translocates into the nucleus where NF-κB target genes (e.g. HIF-1α) are induced. Low-dose LPS can activate the alternative NF-κB pathway. This activation includes phosphorylation of IKK-α which afterwards phosphorylates p100. Proteolytical processing of p100/RelB results in the release of p52/RelB. After translocation into the nucleus, this heterodimer may block functional binding sites for p65/p50 and therefore reduce the expression of classical NF-κB target genes, such as _HIF-1α._

More than 300,000 people in Germany have chronic inflammatory bowel disease (IBD), the main forms of which are Crohn's disease and ulcerative colitis. The incidence and prevalence of IBD have been increasing during the past decade (Baumgart, 2009). This increase is surely one reason that numerous analyses have been performed to further elucidate the role of HIF-1α in murine colitis. However, the results have been quite contradictory. Karhausen and coworkers (2004) found that epithelial HIF-1α was protective in a murine dextran sulfate sodium (DSS) colitis model. Compared with wild-type mice, mice with a conditional knockout of HIF-1α in epithelial cells showed a much more severe clinical outcome, with an increase in clinical symptoms such as rectal bleeding, diarrhea, and weight loss and a decrease in colon length. In contrast, stabilization of HIF-1α in mice with the corresponding conditional knockout of the VHL gene resulted in less-severe symptoms. This finding was due to the fact that HIF-1α can directly increase the transcription of various genes inducing mucosal barrier function (e.g., multidrug resistance gene-1, intestinal trefoil factor). In addition, a more recent publication by the same group (Robinson et al., 2008) reported that pharmacological stabilization of HIF-1α by PHD inhibitors can improve the outcome *in vivo*. These researchers subjected wild-type mice and mice with a conditional HIF-1α knockout in the crypt cells to a trinitrobenzene sulfuric acid (TNBS) colitis model. Whereas the knockout mice again showed more severe disease symptoms, treatment of wild-type mice with PHD inhibitors significantly increased mucosal barrier function and improved clinical outcome. These findings were supported by Cummins and coworkers (2008), who described a protective role of DMOG in DSS-induced colitis. This pan-hydroxylase inhibitor induced the activation of both HIF-1α and NF-κB. This activation resulted in an anti-apoptotic phenotype of the epithelial cells accompanied by significantly reduced epithelial barrier dysfunction.

However, there are also some contradicting results. A study by Shah et al. (2008) showed that disruption of the VHL protein in the colon epithelium exacerbates DSS-induced colitis because of an increase in HIF signalling. Simultaneous knockdown of HIF-1β reverses this effect. Interestingly, knockdown of VHL in colon epithelial cells did not induce HIF-1α protein and significantly reduced HIF-1α mRNA. In contrast, a prominent induction of HIF-2α protein was detectable in these cells. Therefore, differences observed in the respective studies may be due to divergent roles of the two HIF-α isoforms in colon homeostasis (Shah et al., 2008).

The role of HIF-1α in colitis remains controversial, as is demonstrated by the findings obtained with models of colitis not induced pharmacologically. On the one hand, HIF activation was protective, as shown by the analysis of Peyer's patches after orogastric infection with *Yersinia enterolytica*. In this setting, the outcome of animals with HIF-1α knockout in epithelial cells was significantly worse; therefore, bacteria-induced activation of HIF-1α seemed to represent a host defense mechanism (Hartmann et al., 2008). Mechanistically, HIF activation probably occurred via inhibition of prolyl hydroxylase activity and was abolished upon infection with bacteria deficient in siderophore uptake. Siderophores are low-molecular-weight iron-chelating compounds that are secreted by bacteria and taken up again after iron chelation. Therefore, these small molecules can modulate the labile iron pool of the infected cell. In addition, deletion of intestinal epithelial HIF-1α resulted in a more severe outcome of *Clostridium difficile*–mediated colitis, whereas DMOG attenuated toxin-induced injury and inflammation. The induction of HIF-1α target genes sustained mucosal barrier function, whereas the release of proinflammatory molecules was reduced after HIF-1α inhibition (Hirota et al., 2010). On the other hand, HIF-1α silencing could prevent a switch from epithelial to mesenchymal marker expression in Afa/Dr diffusely adhering *E. coli* infection. This finding underlined an important role of HIF in angiogenesis and inflammation and may therefore link inflammation with the early onset of cancer (Cane et al., 2010).

Rheumatoid arthritis (RA) is a chronic systemic inflammatory disease affecting approximately 1% of the population worldwide (Muz et al., 2009). With regard to RA, it has long been known that the environment in the inflamed joint is characterized by a low partial pressure of oxygen (Lund-Olesen, 1970). RA synovium is hypoxic and expresses elevated levels of inflammatory cytokines; therefore, it is likely to induce the HIF system. Indeed, therapeutic manipulation of HIF-1α expression is increasingly a focus of RA treatment. Whereas overexpression of HIF-1α in murine lymphocytes resulted in a significant reduction in plaque size (Ben-Shoshan et al., 2009) and reduced the expression of IFN-γ in CD4[+] spleen-derived lymphocytes, the inflammatory-driven induction of HIF-1α in macrophages led to a more severe clinical outcome (Westra et al., 2010). HIF-1α activation in synovial joints results in the expression of angiogenic factors (e.g., VEGF, PDGF, fibroblast growth factor [FGF], EGFR, and hepatocyte growth factor [HGF]), which aggravates disease. Therefore, inhibition of the HIF system is considered to be clinically helpful and has become a subject of intensive research (Westra et al., 2010).

HIF-1α in allergy

Noninfectious allergic inflammation is considered to be a pathological key feature of a number of disorders, such as allergic asthma or allergic rhinitis (Sumbayev and Nicholas, 2010). Because VEGF, as a typical HIF-1 target gene, has been shown to be abnormally induced in allergic asthma (Lee et al., 2002), the role of the HIF system in allergic airway inflammation has been extensively studied in recent years. The key effector cells in allergic responses are mast cells and basophils. Both cell types are granulated cells fulfilling complex and overlapping functions in both innate and adaptive immunity. They are activated in an IgE-dependent manner and, upon activation, release Th2 cytokines, such as IL-4, IL-5, IL-9, and IL-13 (Sumbayev and Nicholas, 2010). Jeong et al. (2003) were the first to show that the release of inflammatory cytokines IL-8 and TNF-α by mast cells was HIF-1 and NF-κB dependent. Furthermore, it could be shown that the levels of HIF-1α mRNA and protein are significantly increased in hypoxic mast cells (Walczak-Drzewiecka et al., 2006).

Similarly, primary human basophils showed upregulated HIF-1α protein levels after IgE stimulation (Sumbayev et al., 2009). The effect depended on the activation of extracellular signal-regulated kinase (ERK) and p38 MAPK, and the knockdown of HIF-1α significantly reduced VEGF mRNA expression and protein release. HIF-1α protein altered IgE-induced ATP depletion and therefore promoted production of the proallergic cytokine IL-4. Allergy-mediated induction of VEGF in mast cells could also be shown to be HIF-1 dependent (Lee et al., 2008). Current knowledge indicates that released VEGF is one of the main inducers of asthma (Lee et al., 2002). It markedly increases vascular permeability and leads to airway inflammation. Thus, the inhibition of the HIF pathway and, therefore, the release of VEGF may be a good therapeutic strategy (Lee et al., 2008) for allergic airway disease.

Role of HIF-2α in inflammatory settings

Despite their extensive sequence homology, HIF-1α and HIF-2α also play non-overlapping and sometimes even opposing roles (Imtiyaz et al., 2010). Although the role of HIF-1α in inflammatory settings has been extensively studied (Cramer et al., 2003, Peyssonneaux et al., 2004 and 2007, Frede et al., 2006 and

2009), very little is known about the regulation of HIF-2α under those conditions. Only very recently have the first findings been published about the contribution of the HIF-1α homologue in inflammatory settings. Fang et al. (2009) analyzed the differing contributions of HIF-1α and HIF-2α to the hypoxic gene expression profile of macrophages. They found that both transcription factors were essential for metabolic adaptation of the cells to hypoxic challenge.

Interestingly, the hypoxic induction of mRNA and protein levels of the inflammatory cytokine IL-1β was attenuated by knockdown of either HIF-1α or HIF-2α. Furthermore, the knockdown of one or the other homologue attenuated hypoxic phosphorylation of the NF-κB family member p65. These findings suggest that HIF-1α and HIF-2α play similar roles in the adaptation of macrophages to hypoxic conditions and with respect to the induction of inflammatory genes. Additionally, despite the similarities in target gene induction, knockdown of one HIF-α isoform could not be compensated for by the other. The authors suggest that HIF-1 and HIF-2 may bind to different HREs within the promoter region of the target gene and that the cooperation of both bound transcription factors is necessary for maximal gene transcription (Fang et al., 2009). Whether or not this is really the case, remains to be clarified.

The first researchers to provide direct evidence for a pivotal role of HIF-2α in inflammation were Takeda et al. (2010), who analyzed NO homeostasis in macrophages after stimulation with either Th1 or Th2 cytokines. In short, they found that HIF-1α was upregulated by Th1 cytokines, such as IFN-γ, and by LPS challenge. These conditions are likely to be involved in macrophage M1 polarization. HIF-2α, on the other hand, was shown to be reduced during the M1 response but induced by Th2 cytokines (which are involved in M2 priming) with a markedly delayed time course. Upregulation of HIF-1α resulted in transcriptional induction of the target gene inducible NO synthase (iNOS), thereby increasing the generation of intracellular NO levels and facilitating the defence against pathogens. Later upregulation of HIF-2α, in contrast, induced transcription of the HIF-2α target gene arginase-1. Activation of this enzyme reduced intracellular NO levels thereby restoring preinflammatory conditions.

Imtiyaz et al. (2010) analyzed conditional HIF-2α knockout mice with a depletion of the transcription factor in cells of the myeloid lineage. They found those mice to be more resistant to LPS-induced endotoxemia. These mice with the myeloid cell–specific knockout exhibited significantly less-elevated plasma levels of various proinflammatory cytokines, such as IL-1β, TNF-α, and IL-12, than wild type mice. In addition to that, they exhibited higher plasma levels of the anti-inflammatory cytokine IL-10. Because LPS-induced hypothermia was significantly less pronounced in the knockout than in wild type animals, Imtiyaz and coworkers concluded that mice lacking HIF-2α in cells of the myeloid lineage were more resistant to LPS-induced endotoxemia than wild type animals. This conclusion could be further supported by their finding that myeloid HIF-2α deficiency partly protected the mice from LPS-induced cardiac impairment. Administering a neutralizing IL-10 antibody before LPS treatment significantly decreased the protective effect.

In further experiments, Imtiyaz et al. (2010) also found that neutrophil migration to inflammatory joints was attenuated by the loss of HIF-2α. They concluded that HIF-2α is an important immune regulator in neutrophils and macrophages.

All of these studies demonstrate that the homologous transcription factors HIF-1α and HIF-2α can perform similar and complementary roles in hypoxic and inflammatory gene transcription. In addition, they can also perform antagonistic functions. However, their antiphase regulation with delayed induction of the HIF-2 pathway still allows them to coordinate gene transcription to act jointly in adapting the cellular response.

A c k n o w l e d g m e n t s _ The work was supported by a grant from the Deutsche Forschungsgemeinschaft (TRR60 Project A3) and the COST Action TD0901 Hypoxi aNet. We thank Flo Witte, Bluegrass Editorial Services Team, LLC, Winchester, KY, for language editing of this manuscript. The authors declare no conflict of interest.

References

Acker T, Fandrey J, Acker H (2006). The good, the bad and the ugly in oxygen-sensing: ROS, cytochromes and prolyl-hydroxylases. Cardiovasc Res 71(2):195-207.

Agani FH, Puchowicz M, Chavez JC, Pichiule P, LaManna J (2002). Role of nitric oxide in the regulation of HIF-1alpha expression during hypoxia. Am J Physiol Cell Physiol 283(1):C178-186.

Albina JE, Mastrofrancesco B, Vessella JA, Louis CA, Henry WL Jr, Reichner JS (2001). HIF-1 expression in healing wounds: HIF-1alpha induction in primary inflammatory cells by TNF-alpha. Am J Physiol Cell Physiol 281(6):C1971-C1977.

Arany Z, Huang LE, Eckner R, Bhattacharya S, Jiang C, Goldberg MA, Bunn HF, Livingston DM (1996). An essential role for p300/CBP in the cellular response to hypoxia. Proc Natl Acad Sci U S A 93(23):12969-12973.

Baumgart DC (2009). The diagnosis and treatment of Crohn's disease and ulcerative colitis. Dtsch Arztebl Int 106(8):123-133.

Belaiba RS, Bonello S, Zähringer C, Schmidt S, Hess J, Kietzmann T, Görlach A (2007). Hypoxia up-regulates hypoxia-inducible factor-1alpha transcription by involving phosphatidylinositol 3-kinase and nuclear factor kappaB in pulmonary artery smooth muscle cells. Mol Biol Cell 18(12):4691-4697.

Berchner-Pfannschmidt U, Yamac H, Trinidad B, Fandrey J (2007). Nitric oxide modulates oxygen sensing by hypoxia-inducible factor 1-dependent induction of prolyl hydroxylase 2. J Biol Chem 282(3):1788-1796.

Brüne B, Zhou J (2007). Hypoxia-inducible factor-1alpha under the control of nitric oxide. Methods Enzymol 435:463-478.

Callapina M, Zhou J, Schmid T, Köhl R, Brüne B (2005). NO restores HIF-1alpha hydroxylation during hypoxia: role of reactive oxygen species. Free Radic Biol Med 39(7):925-936.

Cash TP, Pan Y, Simon MC (2007). Reactive oxygen species and cellular oxygen sensing. Free Radic Biol Med 43(9):1219-1225.

Chakrabarti S, Rizvi M, Pathak D, Kirber MT, Freedman JE (2009). Hypoxia influences CD40-CD40L mediated inflammation in endothelial and monocytic cells. Immunol Lett 122(2):170-184.

Chandel NS, Maltepe E, Goldwasser E, Mathieu CE, Simon MC, Schumacker PT (1998). Mitochondrial reactive oxygen species trigger hypoxia-induced transcription. Proc Natl Acad Sci U S A 95(20):11715-11720.

Chandel NS, McClintock DS, Feliciano CE, Wood TM, Melendez JA, Rodriguez AM, Schumacker PT (2000). Reactive oxygen species generated at mitochondrial complex III stabilize hypoxia-inducible factor-1alpha during hypoxia: a mechanism of O2 sensing. J Biol Chem 275(33):25130-25138.

Cluff LE (1953). Studies of the effect bacterial endotoxins on rabbit leucocytes. II. Development of acquired resistance. J Exp Med 98(4):349-364.

Cramer T, Yamanishi Y, Clausen BE, Förster I, Pawlinski R, Mackman N, Haase VH, Jaenisch R, Corr M, Nizet V, Firestein GS, Gerber HP, Ferrara N, Johnson RS (2003). HIF-1alpha is essential for myeloid cell-mediated inflammation. Cell 112(5):645-657 [erratum 2003;113:419].

Cramer T, Johnson RS (2003). A novel role for the hypoxia inducible transcription factor HIF-1alpha: critical regulation of inflammatory cell function. Cell Cycle 2(3):192-193.

Culver C, Sundqvist A, Mudie S, Melvin A, Xirodimas D, Rocha S (2010). Mechanism of hypoxia-induced NF-kappaB. Mol Cell Biol 30(20):4901-4921.

Cummins EP, Berra E, Comerford KM, Ginouves A, Fitzgerald KT, Seeballuck F, Godson C, Nielsen JE, Moynagh P, Pouyssegur J, Taylor CT (2006). Prolyl hydroxylase-1 negatively regulates IκB kinase-β, giving insight into hypoxia-induced NF-κB activity. Proc Natl Acad Sci U S A 103(48):18154-18159.

Diebold I, Petry A, Hess J, Görlach A (2010). The NADPH oxidase subunit NOX4 is a new target gene of the hypoxia-inducible factor-1. Mol Biol Cell 21(12):2087-2096.

Ema M, Taya S, Yokotani N, Sogawa K, Matsuda Y, Fujii-Kuriyama Y (1997). A novel bHLH-PAS factor with close sequence similarity to hypoxia-inducible factor 1alpha regulates the VEGF expression and is potentially involved in lung and vascular development. Proc Natl Acad Sci U S A 94(9):4273-4278.

Emerling BM, Platanias LC, Black E, Nebreda AR, Davis RJ, Chandel NS (2005). Mitochondrial reactive oxygen species activation of p38 mitogen-activated protein kinase is required for hypoxia signalling. Mol Cell Biol 25(12):4853-4862.

Fandrey J, Gorr TA, Gassmann M (2006). Regulating cellular oxygen sensing by hydroxylation. Cardiovasc Res 71:642-651.

Fang HY, Hughes R, Murdoch C, Coffelt SB, Biswas SK, Harris AL, Johnson RS, Imityaz HZ, Simon MC, Fredlund E, Greten FR, Rius J, Lewis CE (2009). Hypoxia-inducible factors 1 and 2 are important transcriptional effectors in primary macrophages experiencing hypoxia. Blood 114(4):844-859.

Frede S, Freitag P, Otto T, Heilmaier C, Fandrey J (2005). The proinflammatory cytokine interleukin 1beta and hypoxia cooperatively induce the expression of adrenomedullin in ovarian carcinoma cells through hypoxia inducible factor 1 activation. Cancer Res 65(11):4690-4697.

Frede S, Stockmann C, Freitag P, Fandrey J (2006). Bacterial lipopolysaccharide induces HIF-1 activation in human monocytes via p44/42 MAPK and NF-kappaB. Biochem J 396:517-527.

Frede S, Stockmann C, Winning S, Freitag P, Fandrey J (2009). Hypoxia-inducible factor (HIF) 1alpha accumulation and HIF target gene expression are impaired after induction of endotoxin tolerance. J Immunol 182(10):6470-6476.

Görlach A, Diebold I, Schini-Kerth VB, Berchner-Pfannschmidt U, Roth U, Brandes RP, Kietzmann T, Busse R (2001). Thrombin activates the hypoxia-inducible factor-1 signalling pathway in vascular smooth muscle cells: Role of the p22(phox)-containing NADPH oxidase. Circ Res 89(1):47-54.

Hagen T, Taylor CT, Lam F, Moncada S (2003). Redistribution of intracellular oxygen in hypoxia by nitric oxide: effect on HIF1alpha. Science 302(5652):1975-1978.

Hatoum OA, Miura H, Binion DG (2003). The vascular contribution in the pathogenesis of inflammatory bowel disease. Am J Physiol Heart Circ Physiol 285(5): H1791-H1796.

Hayden MS, Ghosh S (2004). Signalling to NF-kappaB. Genes Dev 18(18):2195-2224.

Hellwig-Bürgel T, Rutkowski K, Metzen E, Fandrey J, Jelkmann W (1999). Interleukin-1beta and tumour necrosis factor-alpha stimulate DNA binding of hypoxia-inducible factor-1. Blood 94(5):1561-1567.

Hollander AP, Corke KP, Freemont AJ, Lewis CE (2001). Expression of hypoxia-inducible factor 1alpha by macrophages in the rheumatoid synovium: implications for targeting of therapeutic genes to the inflamed joint. Arthritis Rheum 44(7):1540-1544.

Huang LE, Willmore WG, Gu J, Goldberg MA, Bunn HF (1999). Inhibition of hypoxia-inducible factor 1 activation by carbon monoxide and nitric oxide. Implications for oxygen sensing and signalling. J Biol Chem 274(13):9038-9044.

Imtiyaz HZ, Williams EP, Hickey MM, Patel SA, Durham AC, Yuan LJ, Hammond R, Gimotty PA, Keith B, Simon MC (2010). Hypoxia-inducible factor 2alpha regulates macrophage function in mouse models of acute and tumour inflammation. J Clin Invest 120(8):2699-2714.

Isaacs JS, Jung YJ, Mole DR, Lee S, Torres-Cabala C, Chung YL, Merino M, Trepel J, Zbar B, Toro J, Ratcliffe PJ, Linehan WM, Neckers L (2005). HIF overexpression correlates with biallelic loss of fumarate hydratase in renal cancer: novel role of fumarate in regulation of HIF stability. Cancer Cell 8(2):143-153.

Jaakkola P, Mole DR, Tian YM, Wilson MI, Gielbert J, Gaskell SJ, Kriegsheim Av, Hebestreit HF, Mukherji M, Schofield CJ, Maxwell PH, Pugh CW, Ratcliffe PJ (2001). Targeting of HIF-alpha to the von Hippel-Lindau ubiquitylation complex by O2-regulated prolyl hydroxylation. Science 292(5516):468-472.

Jantsch J, Chakravortty D, Turza N, Prechtel AT, Buchholz B, Gerlach RG, Volke M, Gläsner J, Warnecke C, Wiesener MS, Eckardt KU, Steinkasserer A, Hensel M, Willam C (2008). Hypoxia and hypoxia-inducible factor-1 alpha modulate lipopolysaccharide-induced dendritic cell activation and function. J Immunol 180(7):4697-4705.

Jung SN, Yang WK, Kim J, Kim HS, Kim EJ, Yun H, Park H, Kim SS, Choe W, Kang I, Ha J (2008). Reactive oxygen species stabilize hypoxia-inducible factor-1 alpha protein and stimulate transcriptional activity via AMP-activated protein kinase in DU145 human prostate cancer cells. Carcinogenesis 29(4):713-721.

Kallio PJ, Okamoto K, O'Brien S, Carrero P, Makino Y, Tanaka H, Poellinger L (1998). Signal transduction in hypoxic cells: inducible nuclear translocation and recruitment of the CBP/p300 coactivator by the hypoxia-inducible factor-1alpha. EMBO J 17(22):6573-6586.

Karhausen J, Haase VH, Colgan SP (2005). Inflammatory hypoxia: role of hypoxia-inducible factor. Cell Cycle 4(2):256-258.

Kimura H, Weisz A, Kurashima Y, Hashimoto K, Ogura T, D'Acquisto F, Addeo R, Makuuchi M, Esumi H (2000). Hypoxia response element of the human vascular endothelial growth factor gene mediates transcriptional regulation by nitric oxide: control of hypoxia-inducible factor-1 activity by nitric oxide. Blood 95(1):189-197.

Kirito K, Hu Y, Komatsu N (2009). HIF-1 prevents the overproduction of mitochondrial ROS after cytokine stimulation through induction of PDK-1. Cell Cycle 8(17):2844-2849.

Knowles HJ, Raval RR, Harris AL, Ratcliffe PJ (2003). Effect of ascorbate on the activity of hypoxia-inducible factor in cancer cells. Cancer Res 63(8):1764-1768.

Köhl R, Zhou J, Brüne B (2006). Reactive oxygen species attenuate nitric-oxide-mediated hypoxia-inducible factor-1alpha stabilization. Free Radic Biol Med 40(8):1430-1442.

Kong T, Eltzschig HK, Karhausen J, Colgan SP, Shelley CS (2004). Leukocyte adhesion during hypoxia is mediated by HIF-1-dependent induction of β_2 integrin gene expression. Proc Natl Acad Sci U S A 101(289:10440-10445.

Kong T, Scully M, Shelley CS, Colgan SP (2007). Identification of Pur α as a new hypoxia response factor responsible for coordinated induction of the β_2 integrin family. J Immunol 179:1934-1941.

Koong AC, Chen EY, Giaccia AJ (1994). Hypoxia causes the activation of nuclear factor kappa B through the phosphorylation of I kappa B alpha on tyrosine residues. Cancer Res 54(6):1425-1430.

Kuhlicke J, Frick JS, Morote-Garcia JC, Rosenberger P, Eltzschig HK (2007). Hypoxia inducible factor (HIF)-1 coordinates induction of Toll-like receptors TLR2 and TLR6 during hypoxia. PLoS One 2(12):e1364.

Lander HM, Jacovina AT, Davis RJ, Tauras JM (1996). Differential activation of mitogen-activated protein kinases by nitric oxide-related species. J Biol Chem. 271(33):19705-19709.

Lando D, Peet DJ, Gorman JJ, Whelan DA, Whitelaw ML, Bruick RK (2002). FIH-1 is an asparaginyl hydroxylase enzyme that regulates the transcriptional activity of hypoxia-inducible factor. Genes Dev 16(12):1466-1471.

Lee KS, Kim SR, Park SJ, Min KH, Lee KY, Choe YH, Park SY, Chai OH, Zhang X, Song CH, Lee YC (2008). Mast cells can mediate vascular permeability through regulation of the PI3K-HIF-1alpha-VEGF axis. Am J Respir Crit Care Med 178(8):787-797.

Lee YC, Kwak YG, Song CH (2002). Contribution of vascular endothelial growth factor to airway hyperresponsiveness and inflammation in a murine model of toluene diisocyanate-induced asthma. J Immunol 168(7):3595-3600.

Li Q, Verma IM (2002). NF-kappaB regulation in the immune system. Nat Rev Immunol 2(10):725-734.

Liu Y, Christou H, Morita T, Laughner E, Semenza GL, Kourembanas S (1998). Carbon monoxide and nitric oxide suppress the hypoxic induction of vascular endothelial growth factor gene via the 5' enhancer. J Biol Chem 273(24):15257-15262.

Lo CJ, Cryer HG, Fu M, Lo FR (1998). Regulation of macrophage eicosanoid generation is dependent on nuclear factor kappaB. J Trauma 45(1):19-24.

Lukashev D, Klebanov B, Kojima H, Grinberg A, Ohta A, Berenfeld L, Wenger RH, Ohta A, Sitkovsky M (2006). Cutting edge: hypoxia-inducible factor 1alpha and its activation-inducible short isoform I.1 negatively regulate functions of CD4+ and CD8+ T lymphocytes. J Immunol 177(8):4962-4965.

Matic M, Simon SR (1992). Effects of gamma interferon on release of tumour necrosis factor alpha from lipopolysaccharide-tolerant human monocyte-derived macrophages. Infect Immun 60(9):3756-3762.

McCall CE, Grosso-Wilmoth LM, LaRue K, Guzman RN, Cousart SL (1993). Tolerance to endotoxin-induced expression of the interleukin-1 beta gene in blood neutrophils of humans with the sepsis syndrome. J Clin Invest 91(3):853-861.

Metzen E, Zhou J, Jelkmann W, Fandrey J, Brüne B (2003). Nitric oxide impairs normoxic degradation of HIF-1alpha by inhibition of prolyl hydroxylases. Mol Biol Cell 14(8):3470-3481.

Murdoch C, Muthana M, Lewis CE (2005). Hypoxia regulates macrophage functions in inflammation. J Immunol 175(10):6257-6263.

Muz B, Khan MN, Kiriakidis S, Paleolog EM (2009). Hypoxia. The role of hypoxia and HIF-dependent signalling events in rheumatoid arthritis. Arthritis Res Ther 11(1):201.

Nizet V, Johnson RS (2009). Interdependence of hypoxic and innate immune responses. Nat Rev Immunol 9(9):609-617.

Oliver KM, Garvey JF, Ng CT, Veale DJ, Fearon U, Cummins EP, Taylor CT (2009). Hypoxia activates NF-κB-dependent gene expression through the canonical signalling pathway. Antioxid Redox Signal 11(9):2057-2064.

Palmer LA, Semenza GL, Stoler MH, Johns RA (1998). Hypoxia induces type II NOS gene expression in pulmonary artery endothelial cells via HIF-1. Am J Physiol 274(2 Pt 1):L212-L219.

Paone A, Galli R, Gabellini C, Lukashev D, Starace D, Gorlach A, De Cesaris P, Ziparo E, Del Bufalo D, Sitkovsky MV, Filippini A, Riccioli A (2010). Toll-like receptor 3 regulates angiogenesis and apoptosis in prostate cancer cell lines through hypoxia-inducible factor 1 alpha. Neoplasia 12(7):539-549.

Peyssonnaux C, Cejudo-Martin P, Doedens A, Zinkernagel AS, Johnson RS, Nizet V (2007). Cutting edge: Essential role of hypoxia inducible factor-1alpha in development of lipopolysaccharide-induced sepsis. J Immunol 178(12):7516-7519.

Peyssonnaux C, Nizet V, Johnson RS (2008). Role of the hypoxia inducible factors HIF in iron metabolism. Cell Cycle 7(1):28-32.

Pollard JW (2004). Tumour-educated macrophages promote tumour progression and metastasis. Nat Rev Cancer 4(1):71-78.

Ramanathan M, Luo W, Csóka B, Haskó G, Lukashev D, Sitkovsky MV, Leibovich SJ (2009). Differential regulation of HIF-1alpha isoforms in murine macrophages by TLR4 and adenosine A(2A) receptor agonists. J Leukoc Biol 86(3):681-689.

Richard DE, Berra E, Pouyssegur J (2000). Nonhypoxic pathway mediates the induction of hypoxia-inducible factor 1alpha in vascular smooth muscle cells. J Biol Chem. 275(35):26765-26771.

Robinson A, Keely S, Karhausen J, Gerich ME, Furuta GT, Colgan SP (2008). Mucosal protection by hypoxia-inducible factor prolyl hydroxylase inhibition. Gastroenterology 134(1):145-155.

Sandau KB, Fandrey J, Brüne B (2001). Accumulation of HIF-1alpha under the influence of nitric oxide. Blood 97(4):1009-1015.

Sang N, Fang J, Srinivas V, Leshchinsky I, Caro J (2002). Carboxyl-terminal transactivation activity of hypoxia-inducible factor 1 alpha is governed by a von Hippel-Lindau protein-independent, hydroxylation-regulated association with p300/CBP. Mol Cell Biol. 22(9):2984-2992.

Schoch HJ, Fischer S, Marti HH (2002). Hypoxia-induced vascular endothelial growth factor expression causes vascular leakage in the brain. Brain 125(Pt 11):2549-2557.

Selak MA, Armour SM, MacKenzie ED, Boulahbel H, Watson DG, Mansfield KD, Pan Y, Simon MC, Thompson CB, Gottlieb E (2005). Succinate links TCA cycle dysfunction to oncogenesis by inhibiting HIF-alpha prolyl hydroxylase. Cancer Cell 7(1):77-85.

Semenza GL, Agani F, Booth G, Forsythe J, Iyer N, Jiang BH, Leung S, Roe R, Wiener C, Yu A (1997). Structural and functional analysis of hypoxia-inducible factor 1. Kidney Int 51(2):553-555.

Sitkovsky M, Lukashev D (2005). Regulation of immune cells by local-tissue oxygen tension: HIF1 alpha and adenosine receptors. Nat Rev Immunol 5(9):712-721.

Sogawa K, Numayama-Tsuruta K, Ema M, Abe M, Abe H, Fujii-Kuriyama Y (1998).

Inhibition of hypoxia-inducible factor 1 activity by nitric oxide donors in hypoxia. Proc Natl Acad Sci U S A 95(13):7368-73.

Stiehl DP, Jelkmann W, Wenger RH, Hellwig-Bürgel T (2002). Normoxic induction of the hypoxia-inducible factor 1alpha by insulin and interleukin-1beta involves the phosphatidylinositol 3-kinase pathway. FEBS Lett 512(1-3):157-162.

St-Pierre J, Buckingham JA, Roebuck SJ, Brand MD (2002). Topology of superoxide production from different sites in the mitochondrial electron transport chain. J Biol Chem 277(47):44784-44790.

Takeda N, O'Dea EL, Doedens A, Kim JW, Weidemann A, Stockmann C, Asagiri M, Simon MC, Hoffmann A, Johnson RS (2010). Differential activation and antagonistic function of HIF-{alpha} isoforms in macrophages are essential for NO homeostasis. Genes Dev 24(5):491-501.

Taylor CT (2008). Interdependent roles for hypoxia-inducible factor and nuclear factor-κB in hypoxic inflammation. J Physiol 586:4055-4059.

Thornton RD, Lane P, Borghaei RC, Pease EA, Caro J, Mochan E (2000). Interleukin 1 induces hypoxia-inducible factor 1 in human gingival and synovial fibroblasts. Biochem J 350 Pt 1:307-312.

van Uden P, Kenneth NS, Rocha S (2008). Regulation of hypoxia-inducible factor-1alpha by NF-kappaB. Biochem J 412(3):477-484.

Wakefield AJ, Sawyerr AM, Dhillon AP, Pittilo RM, Rowles PM, Lewis AA, Pounder RE (1989). Pathogenesis of Crohn's disease: multifocal gastrointestinal infarction. Lancet 2(8671):1057-1062.

Walczak-Drzewiecka A, Ratajewski M, Wagner W, Dastych J (2008). HIF-1alpha is up-regulated in activated mast cells by a process that involves calcineurin and NFAT. J Immunol 181(3):1665-1672.

Wellman TL, Jenkins J, Penar PL, Tranmer B, Zahr R, Lounsbury KM (2004). Nitric oxide and reactive oxygen species exert opposing effects on the stability of hypoxia-inducible factor-1alpha (HIF-1alpha) in explants of human pial arteries. FASEB J 18(2):379-381.

Westra J, Brouwer E, Bos R, Posthumus MD, Doornbos-van der Meer B, Kallenberg CG, Limburg PC (2007). Regulation of cytokine-induced HIF-1alpha expression in rheumatoid synovial fibroblasts. Ann N Y Acad Sci 1108:340-348.

Wiener CM, Booth G, Semenza GL (1996). In vivo expression of mRNAs encoding hypoxia-inducible factor 1. Biochem Biophys Res Commun 225(2):485-488.

Wiesener MS, Turley H, Allen WE, Willam C, Eckardt KU, Talks KL, Wood SM, Gatter KC, Harris AL, Pugh CW, Ratcliffe PJ, Maxwell PH (1998). Induction of endothelial PAS domain protein-1 by hypoxia: characterization and comparison with hypoxia-inducible factor-1alpha. Blood 92(7):2260-2268.

Winning S, Splettstoesser F, Fandrey J, Frede S (2010). Acute hypoxia induces HIF-independent monocyte adhesion to endothelial cells through increased intercellular adhesion molecule-1 expression: the role of hypoxic inhibition of prolyl hydroxylase activity for the induction of NF-kappa B. J Immunol 185(3):1786-1793.

Yoza BK, Hu JY, Cousart SL, Forrest LM, McCall CE (2006). Induction of RelB participates in endotoxin tolerance. J Immunol 177(6):4080-4085.

Zarember KA, Malech HL (2005). HIF-1alpha: a master regulator of innate host defenses? J Clin Invest 115(7):1702-1704.

Zelzer E, Levy Y, Kahana C, Shilo BZ, Rubinstein M, Cohen B (1998). Insulin induces transcription of target genes through the hypoxia-inducible factor HIF-1alpha/ARNT. EMBO J 17(17):5085-5094.

Zhou J, Fandrey J, Schümann J, Tiegs G, Brüne B (2003). NO and TNF-alpha released from activated macrophages stabilize HIF-1alpha in resting tubular LLC-PK1 cells. Am J Physiol Cell Physiol 284(2):C439-C446.

Zinkernagel AS, Johnson RS, Nizet V (2007). Hypoxia inducible factor (HIF) function in innate immunity and infection. J Mol Med 85(12):1339-1346.

Zünd G, Dzus AL, McGuirk DK, Breuer C, Shinoka T, Mayer JE, Colgan SP (1996). Hypoxic stress alone does not modulate endothelial surface expression of bovine E-selectin and intercellular adhesion molecule-1 (ICAM-1). Swiss Surg Suppl Suppl 1:41-45.

Chapter 14

Interactions between HIF and oncogenic viruses

Martina Takacova, Tereza Goliasova
and Juraj Kopacek[*]

[*]Author for correspondence:
Department of Molecular Medicine, Institute of Virology, Slovak Academy of Sciences,
Dubravska cesta 9, 84505 Bratislava, Slovak Republic, Tel: + 4212 59302401,
Fax: + 4212 54774284, E-mail: virukopa@savba.sk

Contents

Key points

— Oncogenic viruses that actively participate in the process of tumour development are divided into RNA and DNA tumour viruses.

— RNA tumour viruses are able to capture and alter important cellular genes involved in the control of cellular proliferation and apoptosis.

— DNA tumour virus oncogenes differ by having viral origin and being essential for viral replication.

— Based on complex studies it is clear that the relationship between hypoxia and oncogenic viruses is reciprocal.

— The expression of HIF-1 can be influenced by several viral genes and vice versa.

Introduction

Viruses, as intracellular residents, often inhabit cells in tumour tissue. Based on their properties, they could be passively or in a worse case, actively involved in the process of tumour development. Viruses actively participating in this process are known as oncogenic viruses. The study of viral transformation mechanisms and oncogenesis extends far beyond virology and provides remarkable insights into the causes of cancer; e.g. by identification of oncogenes that are activated or captured by retroviruses (originally known as RNA tumour viruses), and viral proteins that inactivate tumour suppressor gene products.

Tumour viruses are divided into two general groups based on their genome, which is packaged into infectious viral particles. The differences between these two groups are also based on their oncogenic properties. A unique feature of RNA tumour viruses stems from their capacity to capture and alter important cellular genes involved in the control of cellular proliferation and apoptosis. On the contrary, DNA tumour virus oncogenes differ strikingly from those of RNA tumour viruses by having both a viral origin and an essential role in viral replication. Moreover, these oncogenes lack any recognizable sequence similarities to cellular genes.

In fact, current estimates suggest that approximately one fifth of all cases of human cancers are associated with viral infection. It is clear that during tumourigenesis, oncogenic viruses and their gene products are exposed to dramatic microenvironmental changes. One of the most profound phenomena of tumour growth is hypoxia as a result of insufficient oxygen supply of quickly proliferating tumour cells. Apart from hypoxia, there are viral proteins capable of stabilizing or transactivating hypoxia-inducible factor and promoting changes in the cells reminiscent of hypoxic conditions. In this chapter, we will introduce oncogenic viruses and the aspects of their interaction with the hypoxic signalling cascade.

Hypoxia and viruses

Initial studies of hypoxia-virus interactions were connected to oncolytic viruses that can possibly have a role in a viable and useful antitumour strategy (Bell et al, 2003). Oncolytic viruses have the ability to directly kill cancer cells and also the potential to stimulate production of cytokines with anticancer activity. Moreover, they may be utilized in gene therapy or as shuttle vectors that could carry various cytotoxic genes. Importantly, an oncolytic virus must be resistant to inhibition of DNA, RNA, and protein synthesis that occurs during hypoxia as an adaptive stress response. Vesicular stomatitis virus (VSV), an oncolytic RNA virus, is capable of replication under hypoxic conditions (Connor et al, 2004). In addition to oncolytic viruses, the influence of hypoxic conditions on the biology of viruses has been tested in a variety of different RNA and DNA viruses. So far, interplay between hypoxia and mammalian simian virus 40 (SV40), human neurotropic polyomavirus JC, human B19 erythrovirus, human respiratory syncytial virus (RSV) and lymphocytic choriomeningitis virus has been described (Haeberle et al, 2008; Pillet et al, 2004; Piña-Oviedo et al, 2009; Riedinger et al, 2001; Tomaskova et al, 2011).

The relevance of tumour viruses in viral carcinogenesis consists of two major roles. Firstly, oncogenic viruses serve as etiologic agents of human cancers and, secondly, they provide powerful tools for the discovery of fundamental molecular events crucial to cell signalling and growth control pathways. Importantly, all cases of human cancer caused by viruses are associated with infection with one of six viruses: Kaposi's sarcoma virus, Epstein-Barr virus, hepatitis B virus, hepatitis C virus, human T-cell leukemia virus type 1, and human papillomaviruses. In the following chapter, we will introduce the previously mentioned oncogenic viruses and the nature of their interaction with the hypoxia-signalling cascade.

Papillomaviruses

The first DNA virus to be associated with oncogenesis was a papillomavirus that causes warts (papillomas) in cottontail rabbits. Since then, a little over 100 human papillomaviruses (HPVs) and 20 animal papillomaviruses have been described and characterized (de Villiers et al, 2004). Papillomavirus infections are recognized as a major cause of human cancers. Fifteen different HPV types are associated with cervical cancer.

In general, encapsidated papillomavirus particles contain an approximately 8-kb double-stranded circular DNA genome, which is preferentially replicated in differentiating keratinocytes of squamous epithelia. This fact is in agreement with HPV-tropism for epithelial cells. Based on their tumourigenic potential, HPVs are classified into high- and low-risk. While low-risk HPVs are in general well known in the form of various lesions and warts, high-risk HPVs are known as etiological agents of several human cancers, out of which cervical cancer is most prevalent (zur Hausen, 2009). Significantly, two HPV types, HPV16 and HPV18, are now known to be responsible for ~70% of cervical cancers worldwide. One of the key events in HPV-induced carcinogenesis is the integration of the HPV genome into the host chromosome.

Regulation of viral gene expression involves several viral and cellular transcription factors and results in a time dependent production of only 10 viral proteins. Among these early genes, E6 and E7 and their protein products in high-risk HPV16 and 18 are demonstrably associated with malignant transformation of cervical cells (Kiyono et al, 1997; Liu et al, 1999; Munger, 1989). In the host genome, randomly integrated E6 and E7 are very well known as potent oncogenes with a broad range of effects on susceptible cells (Wentzensen et al, 2004). They can bind several important cellular proteins, and therefore contribute to chromosomal instability and malignant sensibility. The most prominent E6 protein feature is the binding to (indirectly through the cellular E6-AP protein) and subsequent degradation of p53 via the ubiquitin-proteasome pathway, which results in the loss of p53-dependent G1 arrest after DNA damage (Scheffner et al, 1990, Scheffner et al, 1993). A key function of E6 in HPV neoplasias is further highlighted by its ability to block apoptosis, activate telomerase, disrupt cell adhesion, polarity and epithelial differentiation, alter transcription and G-protein signalling and reduce immune recognition of HPV infected cells (Howie et al, 2009). Similarly to E6, E7 exerts its oncogenic potential by binding to the retinoblastoma tumour suppressor (pRb) and the related pocket proteins p107 and p130 (Dyson et al, 1992; Dyson et al, 1989; Munger et al, 1989). E7-pRb binding deregulates cell cycle restriction point by mimicking pRb phosphorylation, thus allowing the cell to enter the S phase without mitogenic signals. In addition to pRb binding and degradation, E7 has the ability to bind many cellular proteins (cell cycle regulators, metabolic enzymes) and transcription factors, and thus influence several important cellular pathways (McLaughlin-Drubin & Munger, 2009).

Carson and colleagues identified the differentially expressed transcription factors that specifically bind to HPV16 DNA, including the known promoter and regulatory regions (Carson and Khan, 2006). Hypoxia-inducible factor 1 (HIF-1) was discovered as one of 31 transcription factors with an increased binding to HPV16 regulatory regions during host cell differentiation. The fact that cervical tumours are highly vascular and have an increased expression of pro-angiogenic factors at a very early stage of premalignant lesions has pointed out the possible involvement of HPV gene products in the production of angiogenic factors (Clere et al, 2007; Smith-McCune et al, 1997). Small interfering RNAs (siRNAs) directed against HPV18 *E6* were able to reduce vascular endothelial growth factor (VEGF) expression in cell culture model (Clere et al, 2007). Since HIF-1 is a master transcription factor responsible for activation of the angiogenic pathway, a possible interaction between HIF-1α and HPV E6/E7 oncogenes was expected. Transient transfection of HPV E6/E7 increased HIF-1α protein and VEGF expression. Moreover, this effect was abrogated by the use of specific HIF-1α siRNAs or by blocking extracellular signal-regulated kinase 1/2 (ERK 1/2) and phosphatidylinositol 3-kinase (PI3K) (Tang et al, 2007). Hypoxia-specific stabilization of HIF-1α in E6/E7-expressing cell lines was demonstrated by Nakamura and colleagues (Nakamura et al, 2009). These results clearly demonstrate possible involvement and importance of papillomavirus oncogenes in the modulation of HIF-1α expression and stabilization by a so far unknown mechanism. Since HPV-infected cervical cells *in vivo* may activate angiogenic factors before the development of high-grade cancers, it is important to understand the details of this mechanism, and thus have the possibility of therapeutic intervention in the early stage of malignant progression.

Interestingly, Alarcon and colleagues demonstrated that the hypoxia-induced p53 accumulation occurs in HPV-infected cells through disruption of E6 and E6 AP interaction with p53, allowing for its nuclear accumulation (Alarcon et al, 1999). Moreover, hypoxia accelerates the selection of aggressive E6/E7 positive cells with a diminished apoptotic potential that could play an important role in human tumour progression (Kim et al, 1997).

Hepatitis B virus

Hepatitis B virus (HBV) belongs to an abundant family of Hepadnaviruses and is one of the most widely spread viruses around the globe. HBV infection results in an acute or chronic liver cell injury and inflammation (McMahon, 2010). Persistent HBV infection is strongly associated with human hepatocellular carcinoma (HCC), a typically fatal malignancy, which is highly vascularized (Ganem & Prince, 2004). Estimates indicate that HBV-induced HCC is associated with more than 300,000 deaths per year worldwide.

HBVs represent very small viruses, the viral particles of which are only 42 nm in size. Their phospholipid bilayer envelope contains surface antigens and encloses the nucleocapsid. HBV viral genome consists of partially double-stranded 3.2-kb long DNA (Okamoto et al, 1988). HBV genome has a coding capacity for only four overlapping open reading frames (ORFs), and their transcription results in the expression of surface (S), core (C), polymerase (P), and X genes. Among HBV proteins, the X-protein (HBx) consisting of 154 amino acids is indispensable for viral infectivity and represents a transcriptional co-activator (Tang et al, 2006). Moreover, HBx is the most frequently integrated portion of HBV DNA found in hepatocyte chromosomes during the development of HCC (Koike et al, 1994). HBx is a pleiotropic protein that modulates a variety of cellular processes by interacting with a wide range of viral and cellular factors (Murakami, 2001). Despite its binding promiscuity and transcriptional activities, the exact role of HBx in carcinogenesis is still not clearly elucidated.

Previously reported involvement of HBx in angiogenesis suggests that HBx may play a critical role in hypoxia-induced angiogenesis through transcriptional activation of VEGF during early stages of hepatocarcinogenesis (Lee et al, 2000). Furthermore, hypoxia up-regulates the expression of HBx by transactivating HBx enhancer 1 (HBx Enh1). HBx is predominantly detected in the cytoplasm but as co-activator, it can also be detected in the nucleus. The link to hypoxia signalling is demonstrated by several data. HBx is able to increase the transcriptional activity and the protein level of HIF-1α under normoxic as well as hypoxic conditions. Moreover, HBx inhibits the interaction of tumour suppressor von Hippel Lindau protein (pVHL) with HIF-1α and blocks its ubiquitin-dependent degradation (Moon et al, 2004). The carboxy-terminus of HBx binds the basic helix-loop-helix/PER-ARNT-SIM (bHLH/PAS), C-terminal oxygen-dependent degradation domain (ODDD), and C-terminal transactivation domain (C-TAD) of HIF-1α (Yoo et al, 2004). By binding to bHLH/PAS, HBx could potentiate HIF-1 interaction with hypoxia response elements (HREs) within target promoters. Through the C-TAD domain, HBx could block the association of factor inhibiting HIF-1 (FIH-1) with HIF-1α and inhibit Asn[803] hydroxylation, thus facilitating p300/CBP co-activator binding. As a potent modulator, HBx also activates the mitogen-activated protein kinase (MAPK) signalling pathway that induces transcriptional activation and nuclear translocation of HIF-1α (Yoo et al, 2003). Consequently, the crosstalk between HBx and HIF-1α stimulates transcriptional activation of HIF-1α target genes, which may play a critical role in hepatocarcinogenesis. Recently, Holotnakova and colleagues have shown that HBx increases the expression of carbonic anhydrase IX (CA IX), via HIF-1 and a functional HRE located -10/-3 bp upstream of the *CA9* transcription initiation site (Holotnakova et al, 2010).

Hepatitis C virus

Involvement of Hepatitis C virus (HCV), another human virus linked to HCC, in the stabilization of HIF-1α under normoxia, has been reported recently. In contrast to HBV, HCV belongs to the family of Flaviviruses, which possesses positive-sense single stranded RNA genome of about 9.6 kb. Previously mentioned stabilization of HIF-1α could be mediated in part by oxidative stress induced by HCV gene expression accompanied by activation of several different pathways, all of which could lead to up-regulation of VEGF expression (Nasimuzzaman et al, 2007). The activation of nuclear factor kappa-light-chain-enhancer of activated B cells (NF-κB), signal transducer and activator of transcription 3 (Stat 3), PI3K/Akt, and MAPK was necessary for HIF-1α stabilization. Moreover, HCV stabilization of HIF-1α leads to the induction of glycolytic enzymes as a result of HCV-mediated depression of mitochondrial oxidative phosphorylation (Ripoli et al, 2010). Importantly, this observation was confirmed in liver biopsy specimens from HCV-infected patients suffering from chronic hepatitis C, the progression of which very often evolves into hepatocellular carcinoma.

Epstein-Barr virus

Epstein-Barr virus (EBV, also called Human Herpesvirus 4, HHV-4) is a member of an ancient family of Herpesviruses. Based on its lymphotropism, EBV belongs to the Gammaherpesvirus subfamily. EBV was isolated from a patient with Burkitt's lymphoma as the first human tumour virus. Unexpectedly, subsequent epidemiologic studies showed that majority of the population was positive for serum antibodies, and this fact revealed the prevalence of EBV infection without developing any signs of the disease. The most common disease symptom connected to the primary infection is known as infectious mononucleosis. Primary targets of EBV are B-lymphocytes where the virus persists for the duration of life (Carter & Saunders, 2007).

In general, Herpesviruses are large enveloped DNA viruses. The EBV genome is a linear, double-stranded 184 kb DNA, which encodes close to one hundred proteins expressed during lytic infection. On the contrary, only a very limited number of genes are expressed in latently infected cells (Young et al, 1989). A close correlation between viral DNA persistence and human cancer has been confirmed in biopsies not only from Burkitt's lymphomas but also from several others, such as nasopharyngeal carcinoma, gastric carcinoma, T-cell lymphomas and Hodgkin's disease (Young & Murray, 2003). Exclusively, gene products produced in latently infected cells are of particular interest in relationship to oncogenic properties of EBV. Most of these genes mimic or bind a number of cellular genes involved in processes such as apoptosis, cytokine production or cell signalling pathways. These interactions result in an increased sensibility of host cells to oncogenic transformation (Rezk & Weiss, 2007). Among EBV genes, latent membrane protein 1 (LMP1) was the first recognized latent gene able to induce oncogenic transformation in cell lines. LMP1 is a transmembrane protein, the C-terminal cytoplasmic region of which is composed of three activation domains involved in different signalling pathways (Kilger et al, 1998; Kondo et al, 2005). Moreover, there are other latently expressed genes critical for effective B-lymphocytes growth transformation, such as EBV nuclear antigens 3A and 3C (EBNA3A and EBNA3C) (Tomkinson et al, 1993).

The idea of a crosstalk between hypoxia and EBV infection originates from the finding that HIF-1α expression is increased in EBV-infected cell lines, which express LMP1 and other EBV latent proteins. Deeper insight into this phenomenon showed that LMP1 was able to increase HIF-1α activity through p42/p44- and H_2O_2-dependent mechanisms (Wakisaka et al, 2004). Kondo and colleagues disclosed the mechanism of HIF-1α stabilization by LMP1 in human epithelial cells. LMP1 up-regulates Siah1 E3 ubiquitin ligase by enhancing its stability, which subsequently induces degradation of prolyl hydroxylase 1 and 3 (PHD1 and PHD3), thus allowing HIF-1α to escape pVHL recognition and proteosomal degradation (Kondo et al, 2006). Very recently however, Benders and colleagues have failed to find correlation between LMP1 and HIF-1α expression in naturally EBV-infected nasal carcinomas (Benders et al, 2009). It should also be noted that in this study, expression of HIF-1α did not correlate with vessel density, which was very variable among carcinomas. Finally, it is likely that the relationship between LMP1 and HIF-1α is only dependent on specific stages of malignancy. LMP1, as a potent oncogene certainly has different biological properties at various stages of cell transformation and may potentially induce additional factors that contribute to angiogenesis (Ren et al, 2004).

The ability of reactivation from latent state to lytic replication by various extra- or intra-cellular stimuli is one of the characteristic hallmarks of herpesviruses. EBV is no exception and treatment with 12-0-tetradecanyolphorbol-13-acetate (TPA), transforming growth factor beta 1 (TGF-β1), or Ca^{2+} ionophores could potentially reactivate the virus from latency in lymphoid and epithelial cells. This reactivation is connected to activation of the promoter of the immediate-early gene *BZLF1* (also known as *Zta*), which is a potent viral transactivator (Lieberman et al, 1990). Thus, the result of Zta expression is the activation of a whole battery of viral genes and the switch to viral replication. EBV as a herpesvirus has a large genome coding the viral DNA polymerase and several DNA modifying genes, which allows the virus to be less dependent on the host cell (O'Nions & Allday, 2004). This replication independency allows the virus to escape when the cells are exposed to various stimuli leading to stress and eventually to cell death. Prolonged hypoxia represents one of the potential stresses for cells and by hypoxia-dependent Zta activation, EBV could escape from the hostile microenvironment (Jiang et al, 2006). However, mechanism and pathways involved in this reactivation are yet unknown.

Kaposi's sarcoma-associated herpesvirus

Kaposi's sarcoma-associated herpesvirus (KSHV, also called HHV-8) is the most recently discovered human herpesvirus bearing tumourigenic properties. KSHV was first identified in AIDS patients suffering from Kaposi's sarcoma (KS), a highly vascularized tumour predominately made up of cells of endothelial origin (Dupin et al, 1999). Additionally, KSHV infection is associated with two lymphoproliferative disorders, primary effusion lymphoma (PEL) and multicentric Castleman's disease. Similarly to EBV, KSHV can establish a latent infection of B-lymphocytes (Carter & Saunders, 2007).

The KSHV genome is a double-stranded linear DNA of about 170 kb in size (Renne et al, 1996). During lytic infection, more than 90 viral genes are expressed. KSHV is also able to persist in the host cell in latent form. The hallmark of latently infected cells is the maintenance of the entire viral genome without producing viral particles. Similarly to EBV, only a limited set of viral genes is expressed and a switch to lytic replication can by induced by different stimuli. The ORF 73 product, which is named latency-associated nuclear antigen (LANA, LNA, or LNA1), is expressed in every cell type undergoing latency (Kedes et al, 1997). LANA is a multifunctional protein, and the best-characterized function of LANA is the establishment and maintenance of the viral episomal genomes in the cell nucleus (Ballestas et al, 1999). Evidence additionally indicates that LANA exerts its tumourigenic effect via interacting with multiple viral and cellular proteins (Radkov et al,

2000). Thus, LANA may contribute to KSHV-induced oncogenesis by target-ing the tumour suppressor Rb or interaction with p53.

In spite of the fact that KSHV represents the most recently discov-ered oncogenic herpesvirus, its relationship to hypoxia has been studied the most extensively out of all viruses. Subsequent findings indicate that this connection between hypoxia and KSHV is rather mutual (Figure 14.1). Carroll and colleagues reported that KSHV infection of endothelial cells led to increased expression of HIF-1α and HIF-2α. Consequently, elevated activity of both factors was demonstrated by vascular endothelial growth factor receptor 1 (VEGFR1) induction. This increased protein expression of HIF-1α, HIF-2α, and VEGFR1 upon KSHV infection was blocked by Src kinase inhibitor (SU6656) (Carroll et al, 2006). Furthermore, additional studies revealed that even LANA was able to bind HIF-1α and enhance its transcrip-tional activity. In fact, LANA directly functions as a component of the EC_5S ubiquitin complex targeting the tumour suppressor pVHL for degradation, and thus enhances the stabilization of HIF-1α (Cai et al, 2006b). Besides pVHL, the same ubiquitin-mediated degradation down-regulates p53. This implies that LANA ability to modify tumour suppressor properties contributes to changes in the cell microenvironment and to the tumourigenic vulnerabil-ity of KSHV infected cells.

Another latency-associated protein possesses the capability to interact with HIF-1α. KSHV viral interferon regulatory factor 3 (vIFR3) exhibits homology to cellular IRF4, and its main function is to block cellular immu-nity in response to KSHV infection (Offermann, 2007). Recently discovered evidence indicates that vIFR3, through its central double α-helix motifs, is able to bind HIF-1α. This interaction prevents HIF-1α protein degradation and also increases its transcriptional activity in normoxia, and thus helps modulate cellular pathways to favor viral survival (Shin et al, 2008). Just like LMP1 in EBV, the KSHV lytic gene ORF 74, which encodes viral G-protein-coupled receptor (vGPCR), can also lead to HIF-1α activation (Sodhi et al, 2000). Consequently, induction of HIF-1α activates VEGF transcription. Sodhi and colleagues demonstrated that stimulation of VEGF by vGPCR occurs through MAPK and p38 pathways acting on HIF-1α.

It is clear that viruses have evolutionally developed strategies to escape and thereafter infect healthy cells, when infected cells are exposed to stress conditions. In KSHV, LANA represents a double-edged sword, which is able to mediate HIF-1α-dependent reactivation of KSHV from latency. Func-tional assays demonstrate that this occurs via enhanced binding of the LANA protein to putative HRE elements in the promoter region of the *Rta* gene. Importantly, the RTA protein, encoded by ORF 50, is both necessary

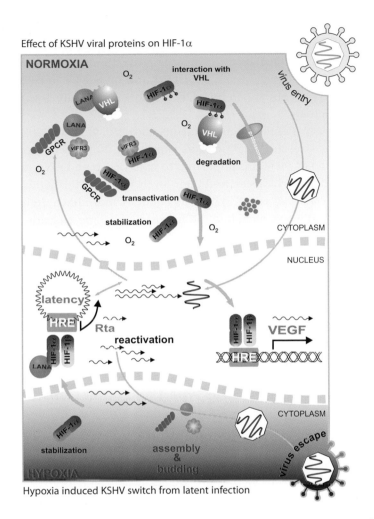

Effect of KSHV viral proteins on HIF-1α

Hypoxia induced KSHV switch from latent infection

Figure 14.1 _ Schematic illustration of the cross-talk between hypoxia and latent KSHV, which results in stabilization and transactivation of HIF-1α on one hand, and reactivation of the lytic KSHV infection on the other.

and sufficient for inducing KSHV lytic replication (Cai et al, 2006a). Cai and colleagues discovered six potential HREs in the *Rta* gene promoter, three of which were identified as functional. Viral escape from latency under hypoxia is further secured by another mechanism, which involves transcription factor X-box binding protein 1 (XBP-1). Hypoxia-activated form of XBP-1 transactivates the *Rta* promoter through an ACGT core sequence containing the XBP-1 response element, which has been previously identified as HRE4 (Dalton-Griffin et al, 2009). In addition to the *Rta* promoter, the promoter region of ORF 34 also contains a functional HRE, and thus can be activated by increased levels of HIF-1α and/or HIF-2α in cells exposed to hypoxia (Haque et al, 2003). In fact, ORF 34 codes for a late lytic protein of unknown function.

All previously mentioned mechanisms allow the virus to start lytic replication under stressful conditions, as represented by low oxygen tension. To have a complex view, it is important to note that both LANA and HIF-1α are expressed in KS biopsies, and their levels increase throughout tumour progression (Long et al, 2009). KSHV in its latent form is able to influence several cellular pathways including the hypoxic signalling cascade, and thus contributes to alteration of the cell microenvironment and disease progression. On the other hand, the virus itself has developed sophisticated mechanisms allowing the switch to lytic replication and an escape from dying cells. A similar strategy has been reported for Murine herpesvirus 4 whose ORF 50, a crucial gene responsible for viral reactivation from latency, is also up-regulated in response to hypoxia (Polcicova et al, 2008).

Human T-cell leukemia virus type 1 and other retroviruses

Oncogenic retroviruses were discovered almost 100 years ago as the first infectious agents able to transmit cancer from one individual to another. At the present time, retroviruses are generally accepted as viruses with the highest tumourigenic potential and a lot of fundamental knowledge regarding cancer, molecular biology, pathology etc. originates from the studies of this class of viruses. In fact, the most prominent feature of retroviruses stems from their unique capability to transcribe viral genomic RNA into a DNA copy by the medium of viral reverse transcriptase enzyme (Carter & Saunders, 2007).

In general, rctroviruses represent a large family of ancient viruses, which are enveloped viral particles of different shape. Viral envelope is composed of 8 to 9 structural proteins. Genetic material inside the capsid contains two molecules of linear single-stranded RNA from 7 up to 13 kb in length. Commonly, viral genomic RNA encodes capsid proteins (*gag*), envelope glycoproteins (*env*) and RNA polymerase (*pol*) genes, which are bound by 5' and 3' end terminal repetition regions (LTR). LTRs are crucial mediators of integration into the host genome where retroviruses are inserted in the form of a provirus.

Depending on the mechanism of tumour induction and their genome structure, oncogenic retroviruses are divided into two groups. The first group of retroviruses contains viral homologues of cellular proto-oncogenes in their genome, the v-oncogenes. Cell transformation is a result of their expression with direct influence on the biology of infected cells. The second group of retroviruses does not possess sequence coding for any viral oncogenes in their genome. Rather, the transcription of proto-oncogenes is inappropriately activated as a consequence of their integration into the host cell genome (Uren et al, 2005). In contrast to other oncogenic viruses, retroviruses carrying oncogenes are able to induce tumour formation within a period of a few weeks. Over 30 retroviral oncogenes originating from different animal species and humans have been identified (Butel, 2000). The first identified retroviral oncogene was v-*Src* encoded by the Rous sarcoma virus (RSV). This oncogene was derived from a closely related cellular proto-oncogene c-*Src* (Takeya & Hanafusa, 1983). c-Src is a non-receptor tyrosine kinase, and its function is in regulation of growth factor signalling, cell migration and adhesion. Despite its low transformation potential, c-Src is over-expressed in a wide variety of human cancers, mainly of breast and colon origin (Frame, 2002). v-Src, its viral counterpart, differs from c-Src on the basis of structural distinctions in the regulatory C-terminal region, which is responsible for kinase activity regulation, and therefore v-Src is constitutively active with a high cellular transformation potential (Brown and Cooper, 1996). Because Src affects essential cellular events, deregulation of its activity may lead to transformation in the target cellular genes with an impact on relevant signalling pathways. The effect of Src on the oxygen-sensing pathway seems to be mediated at least in part by a pVHL-independent mechanism (Chan et al, 2002), involving the up-regulation of HIF-1α protein synthesis (Karni et al, 2002). Chan and colleagues revealed that stabilization of HIF-1α is achieved by inhibition of Pro[564] hydroxylation. Consequently, induction of HIF-1α transcription factor up-regulates target gene expression. Consistent with this, a recent study revealed Src-mediated induction of CA IX expression, which was critically dependent on HIF-1α activity (Takacova et al, 2010).

Another retroviral oncogene with an enhancing effect on HIF-1α transcriptional activity under normoxia is Tax, an oncogene of human T-cell leukemia virus type 1 (HTLV-1). In fact, HTLV-1 is an etiologic agent of adult T-cell leukaemia (ATL), which is an aggressive malignancy of T lymphocytes recognized mainly in elderly people (Poiesz et al, 1980, Gallo et al, 1982).

Interestingly, HTLV-1 was the first identified human retrovirus, and it still represents the only known human retrovirus linked directly to a specific malignancy. Tax protein plays a crucial role in T-lymphocyte transformation and leukemogenesis. Thus, Tax acts as a transactivator protein, which modulates the expression of various transcription factors including CREB/ATF family, AP1, and NF-κB (Adya et al, 1994, Sun and Yamaoka, 2005). Additionally, the transforming properties of Tax seem to involve interference with cell cycle regulators, repression of tumour suppressor p53 or genetic alterations (Grassmann et al, 2005). Moreover, enhanced HIF-1α protein expression and DNA-binding activity were exhibited in HTLV-1-infected T-cell lines. Tomita and colleagues revealed that activation of the PI3K/Akt signalling pathway induced by Tax leads to HIF-1 activation. Moreover, knockdown of HIF-1α by siRNA suppresses the growth and VEGF expression of HTLV-1-infected T-cell lines (Tomita at al, 2007).

Table 14.1 _ The effect of human oncogenic viruses on HIF-1α.

Virus family	Virus	Viral oncoprotein	Impact on HIF-1α
Flaviviridae	HCV	unknown	Stabilization of HIF-1α
Hepadnaviridae	HBV	HBx	Increased HIF-1α protein level
			Increased transactivation of HIF-1α
			Decreased HIF-1α degradation
Herpesviridae	EBV	LMP1	Increased HIF-1α protein level
			Decreased HIF-1α degradation
	KSHV	LANA	Increased HIF-1α protein level
			Increased transactivation of HIF-1α
			Decreased HIF-1α degradation
		vGPCR	Increased transactivation of HIF-1α
		vIFR3	Increased transactivation of HIF-1α
			Decreased HIF-1α degradation
Papillomaviridae	HPV*	E6/E7	Increased HIF-1α protein level
Retroviridae	HTLV-1	Tax	Increased HIF-1α protein level
			Increased transactivation of HIF-1α

HCV –hepatitis C virus, HBV –hepatitis B virus, HBx –hepatitis B virus X protein, EBV –Epstein-Barr virus, LMP1 –latent membrane protein 1, KSHV –Kaposi's sarcoma-associated herpesvirus, LANA –latency-associated nuclear antigen, vGPCR –viral G-protein-coupled receptor, vIFR3 –viral interferon regulatory factor 3, HPV * –human papilloma virus high-risk types, HTLV-1 –human T-cell leukemia virus type 1.

In summary, the previously described interaction mechanisms between hypoxia and oncogenic viruses (summarized in Table 14.1) have clarified an interesting fact that HIF-1 plays a crucial role in tumour progression but it also represents a critical segment in the molecular events that contribute to viral oncogenesis. Therefore, the solution to this molecular jigsaw puzzle of reciprocal virus-cell interactions is attractive for the development of effective therapeutic strategies against viral oncogenesis.

A c k n o w l e d g e m e n t s _ We would like to thank members of the Department of Molecular Medicine for helpful suggestions and comments. The Department of Molecular Medicine is supported by EU 7th Framework Program of the European Commission (project METOXIA FR7-HEALTH-2007-222741), and by the EU Structural Funds (project BIOMAKRO 2, ITMS 26240120027).

References

Adya N, Zhao LJ, Huang W, Boros I, Giam CZ (1994) Expansion of CREB's DNA recognition specificity by Tax results from interaction with Ala-Ala-Arg at positions 282-284 near the conserved DNA-binding domain of CREB. Proc Natl Acad Sci U S A 91(12): 5642-5646

Alarcon R, Koumenis C, Geyer RK, Maki CG, Giaccia AJ (1999) Hypoxia induces p53 accumulation through MDM2 down-regulation and inhibition of E6-mediated degradation. Cancer Res 59(24): 6046-6051

Ballestas ME, Chatis PA, Kaye KM (1999) Efficient persistence of extrachromosomal KSHV DNA mediated by latency-associated nuclear antigen. Science 284(5414): 641-644

Benders AA, Tang W, Middeldorp JM, Greijer AE, Thorne LB, Funkhouser WK, Rathmell WK, Gulley ML (2009) Epstein-Barr virus latent membrane protein 1 is not associated with vessel density nor with hypoxia inducible factor 1 alpha expression in nasopharyngeal carcinoma tissue. Head Neck Pathol 3(4): 276-282

Brott BK, Decker S, Shafer J, Gibbs JB, Jove R (1991) GTPase-activating protein interactions with the viral and cellular Src kinases. Proc Natl Acad Sci U S A 88(3): 755-759

Cai Q, Lan K, Verma SC, Si H, Lin D, Robertson ES (2006a) Kaposi's sarcoma-associated herpesvirus latent protein LANA interacts with HIF-1 alpha to upregulate RTA expression during hypoxia: Latency control under low oxygen conditions. J Virol 80(16): 7965-7975

Cai QL, Knight JS, Verma SC, Zald P, Robertson ES (2006b) EC5S ubiquitin complex is recruited by KSHV latent antigen LANA for degradation of the VHL and p53 tumour suppressors. PLoS Pathog 2(10): e116

Carroll PA, Kenerson HL, Yeung RS, Lagunoff M (2006) Latent Kaposi's sarcoma-associated herpesvirus infection of endothelial cells activates hypoxia-induced factors. J Virol 80(21): 10802-10812

Clere N, Bermont L, Fauconnet S, Lascombe I, Saunier M, Vettoretti L, Plissonnier ML, Mougin C (2007) The human papillomavirus type 18 E6 oncoprotein induces Vascular Endothelial Growth Factor 121 (VEGF121) transcription from the promoter through a p53-independent mechanism. Exp Cell Res 313(15): 3239-3250

Dalton-Griffin L, Wilson SJ, Kellam P (2009) X-box binding protein 1 contributes to induction of the Kaposi's sarcoma-associated herpesvirus lytic cycle under hypoxic conditions. J Virol 83(14): 7202-7209

de Villiers EM, Fauquet C, Broker TR, Bernard HU, zur Hausen H (2004) Classification of papillomaviruses. Virology 324(1): 17-27

Dupin N, Fisher C, Kellam P, Ariad S, Tulliez M, Franck N, van Marck E, Salmon D, Gorin I, Escande JP, Weiss RA, Alitalo K, Boshoff C (1999) Distribution of human herpesvirus-8 latently infected cells in Kaposi's sarcoma, multicentric Castleman's disease, and primary effusion lymphoma. Proc Natl Acad Sci U S A 96(8): 4546-4551

Dyson N, Guida P, Munger K, Harlow E (1992) Homologous sequences in adenovirus E1A and human papillomavirus E7 proteins mediate interaction with the same set of cellular proteins. J Virol 66(12): 6893-6902

Dyson N, Howley PM, Munger K, Harlow E (1989) The human papilloma virus-16 E7 oncoprotein is able to bind to the retinoblastoma gene product. Science 243(4893): 934-937

Ganem D, Prince AM (2004) Hepatitis B virus infection–natural history and clinical consequences. N Engl J Med 350(11): 1118-1129

Giatromanolaki A, Harris AL (2001) Tumour hypoxia, hypoxia signalling pathways and hypoxia inducible factor expression in human cancer. Anticancer Res 21(6B): 4317-4324

Holotnakova T, Tylkova L, Takacova M, Kopacek J, Petrik J, Pastorekova S, Pastorek J Role of the HBx oncoprotein in carbonic anhydrase 9 induction. J Med Virol 82(1): 32-40

Howie HL, Katzenellenbogen RA, Galloway DA (2009) Papillomavirus E6 proteins. Virology 384(2): 324-334

Chan DA, Sutphin PD, Denko NC, Giaccia AJ (2002) Role of prolyl hydroxylation in oncogenically stabilized hypoxia-inducible factor-1alpha. J Biol Chem 277(42): 40112-40117

Jiang JH, Wang N, Li A, Liao WT, Pan ZG, Mai SJ, Li DJ, Zeng MS, Wen JM, Zeng YX (2006) Hypoxia can contribute to the induction of the Epstein-Barr virus (EBV) lytic cycle. J Clin Virol 37(2): 98-103

Kedes DH, Lagunoff M, Renne R, Ganem D (1997) Identification of the gene encoding the major latency-associated nuclear antigen of the Kaposi's sarcoma-associated herpesvirus. J Clin Invest 100(10): 2606-2610

Kilger E, Kieser A, Baumann M, Hammerschmidt W (1998) Epstein-Barr virus-mediated B-cell proliferation is dependent upon latent membrane protein 1, which simulates an activated CD40 receptor. EMBO J 17(6): 1700-1709

Kim CY, Tsai MH, Osmanian C, Graeber TG, Lee JE, Giffard RG, DiPaolo JA, Peehl DM, Giaccia AJ (1997) Selection of human cervical epithelial cells that possess reduced apoptotic potential to low-oxygen conditions. Cancer Res 57(19): 4200-4204

Kiyono T, Hiraiwa A, Fujita M, Hayashi Y, Akiyama T, Ishibashi M (1997) Binding of high-risk human papillomavirus E6 oncoproteins to the human homologue of the Drosophila discs large tumour suppressor protein. Proc Natl Acad Sci U S A 94(21): 11612-11616

Kondo S, Seo SY, Yoshizaki T, Wakisaka N, Furukawa M, Joab I, Jang KL, Pagano JS (2006) EBV latent membrane protein 1 up-regulates hypoxia-inducible factor 1alpha through Siah1-mediated down-regulation of prolyl hydroxylases 1 and 3 in nasopharyngeal epithelial cells. Cancer Res 66(20): 9870-9877

Kondo S, Wakisaka N, Schell MJ, Horikawa T, Sheen TS, Sato H, Furukawa M, Pagano JS, Yoshizaki T (2005) Epstein-Barr virus latent membrane protein 1 induces the matrix metalloproteinase-1 promoter via an Ets binding site formed by a single nucleotide polymorphism: enhanced susceptibility to nasopharyngeal carcinoma. Int J Cancer 115(3): 368-376

Lee SW, Lee YM, Bae SK, Murakami S, Yun Y, Kim KW (2000) Human hepatitis B virus X protein is a possible mediator of hypoxia-induced angiogenesis in hepato-carcinogenesis. Biochem Biophys Res Commun 268(2): 456-461

Lieberman PM, Hardwick JM, Sample J, Hayward GS, Hayward SD (1990) The zta transactivator involved in induction of lytic cycle gene expression in Epstein-Barr virus-infected lymphocytes binds to both AP-1 and ZRE sites in target promoter and enhancer regions. J Virol 64(3): 1143-1155

Liu Y, Chen JJ, Gao Q, Dalal S, Hong Y, Mansur CP, Band V, Androphy EJ (1999) Multiple functions of human papillomavirus type 16 E6 contribute to the immortalization of mammary epithelial cells. J Virol 73(9): 7297-7307

Long E, Ilie M, Hofman V, Havet K, Selva E, Butori C, Lacour JP, Nelson AM, Cathomas G, Hofman P (2009) LANA-1, Bcl-2, Mcl-1 and HIF-1alpha protein expression in HIV-associated Kaposi sarcoma. Virchows Arch 455(2): 159-170

McLaughlin-Drubin ME, Munger K (2009) The human papillomavirus E7 oncoprotein. Virology 384(2): 335-344

McMahon BJ Natural history of chronic hepatitis B. Clin Liver Dis 14(3): 381-396

Moon EJ, Jeong CH, Jeong JW, Kim KR, Yu DY, Murakami S, Kim CW, Kim KW (2004) Hepatitis B virus X protein induces angiogenesis by stabilizing hypoxia-inducible factor-1alpha. FASEB J 18(2): 382-384

Munger CB (1989) Child day-care programs. A must, says MSMS Committee on Concerns of Women Physicians. Mich Med 88(6): 35-36

Munger K, Werness BA, Dyson N, Phelps WC, Harlow E, Howley PM (1989) Complex formation of human papillomavirus E7 proteins with the retinoblastoma tumour suppressor gene product. EMBO J 8(13): 4099-4105

Murakami S (2001) Hepatitis B virus X protein: a multifunctional viral regulator. J Gastroenterol 36(10): 651-660

Nakamura M, Bodily JM, Beglin M, Kyo S, Inoue M, Laimins LA (2009) Hypoxia-specific stabilization of HIF-1alpha by human papillomaviruses. Virology 387(2): 442-448

Nasimuzzaman M, Waris G, Mikolon D, Stupack DG, Siddiqui A (2007) Hepatitis C virus stabilizes hypoxia-inducible factor 1alpha and stimulates the synthesis of vascular endothelial growth factor. J Virol 81(19): 10249-10257

O'Nions J, Allday MJ (2004) Deregulation of the cell cycle by the Epstein-Barr virus. Adv Cancer Res 92: 119-186

Offermann MK (2007) Kaposi sarcoma herpesvirus-encoded interferon regulator factors. Curr Top Microbiol Immunol 312: 185-209

Okamoto H, Tsuda F, Sakugawa H, Sastrosoewignjo RI, Imai M, Miyakawa Y, Mayumi M (1988) Typing hepatitis B virus by homology in nucleotide sequence: comparison of surface antigen subtypes. J Gen Virol 69 (Pt 10): 2575-2583

Pahl HL (1999) Activators and target genes of Rel/NF-kappaB transcription factors. Oncogene 18(49): 6853-6866

Poiesz BJ, Ruscetti FW, Gazdar AF, Bunn PA, Minna JD, Gallo RC (1980) Detection and isolation of type C retrovirus particles from fresh and cultured lymphocytes of a patient with cutaneous T-cell lymphoma. Proc Natl Acad Sci U S A 77(12): 7415-7419

Polcicova K, Hrabovska Z, Mistrikova J, Tomaskova J, Pastorek J, Pastorekova S, Kopacek J (2008) Up-regulation of Murid herpesvirus 4 ORF50 by hypoxia: possible implication for virus reactivation from latency. Virus Res 132(1-2): 257-262

Radkov SA, Kellam P, Boshoff C (2000) The latent nuclear antigen of Kaposi sarcoma-associated herpesvirus targets the retinoblastoma-E2F pathway and with the oncogene Hras transforms primary rat cells. Nat Med 6(10): 1121-1127

Ren Q, Sato H, Murono S, Furukawa M, Yoshizaki T (2004) Epstein-Barr virus (EBV) latent membrane protein 1 induces interleukin-8 through the nuclear factor-kappa B signalling pathway in EBV-infected nasopharyngeal carcinoma cell line. Laryngoscope 114(5): 855-859

Renne R, Lagunoff M, Zhong W, Ganem D (1996) The size and conformation of Kaposi's sarcoma-associated herpesvirus (human herpesvirus 8) DNA in infected cells and virions. J Virol 70(11): 8151-8154

Rezk SA, Weiss LM (2007) Epstein-Barr virus-associated lymphoproliferative disorders. Hum Pathol 38(9): 1293-1304

Ripoli M, D'Aprile A, Quarato G, Sarasin-Filipowicz M, Gouttenoire J, Scrima R, Cela O, Boffoli D, Heim MH, Moradpour D, Capitanio N, Piccoli C Hepatitis C virus-linked mitochondrial dysfunction promotes hypoxia-inducible factor 1 alpha-mediated glycolytic adaptation. J Virol 84(1): 647-660

Shin YC, Joo CH, Gack MU, Lee HR, Jung JU (2008) Kaposi's sarcoma-associated herpesvirus viral IFN regulatory factor 3 stabilizes hypoxia-inducible factor-1 alpha to induce vascular endothelial growth factor expression. Cancer Res 68(6): 1751-1759

Scheffner M, Werness BA, Huibregtse JM, Levine AJ, Howley PM (1990) The E6 oncoprotein encoded by human papillomavirus types 16 and 18 promotes the degradation of p53. Cell 63(6): 1129-1136

Smith-McCune K, Zhu YH, Hanahan D, Arbeit J (1997) Cross-species comparison of angiogenesis during the premalignant stages of squamous carcinogenesis in the human cervix and K14-HPV16 transgenic mice. Cancer Res 57(7): 1294-1300

Takacova M, Holotnakova T, Barathova M, Pastorekova S, Kopacek J, Pastorek J Src induces expression of carbonic anhydrase IX via hypoxia-inducible factor 1. Oncol Rep 23(3): 869-874

Takeya T, Hanafusa H (1983) Structure and sequence of the cellular gene homologous to the RSV src gene and the mechanism for generating the transforming virus. Cell 32(3): 881-890

Tang H, Oishi N, Kaneko S, Murakami S (2006) Molecular functions and biological roles of hepatitis B virus x protein. Cancer Sci 97(10): 977-983

Tang X, Zhang Q, Nishitani J, Brown J, Shi S, Le AD (2007) Overexpression of human papillomavirus type 16 oncoproteins enhances hypoxia-inducible factor 1 alpha protein accumulation and vascular endothelial growth factor expression in human cervical carcinoma cells. Clin Cancer Res 13(9): 2568-2576

Tomaskova J, Oveckova I, Labudova M, Lukacikova L, Laposova K, Kopacek J, Pastorekova S, Pastorek J (2011) Hypoxia induces the gene expression and extracellular transmission of persistent lymphocytic choriomeningitis virus. J Virol 85(24): 13069-76

Tomkinson B, Robertson E, Kieff E (1993) Epstein-Barr virus nuclear proteins EBNA-3A and EBNA-3C are essential for B-lymphocyte growth transformation. J Virol 67(4): 2014-2025

Torgeman A, Ben-Aroya Z, Grunspan A, Zelin E, Butovsky E, Hallak M, Lochelt M, Flugel RM, Livneh E, Wolfson M, Kedar I, Aboud M (2001) Activation of HTLV-I long terminal repeat by stress-inducing agents and protection of HTLV-I-infected T-cells from apoptosis by the viral tax protein. Exp Cell Res 271(1): 169-179

Uren AG, Kool J, Berns A, van Lohuizen M (2005) Retroviral insertional mutagenesis: past, present and future. Oncogene 24(52): 7656-7672

Wakisaka N, Kondo S, Yoshizaki T, Murono S, Furukawa M, Pagano JS (2004) Epstein-Barr virus latent membrane protein 1 induces synthesis of hypoxia-inducible factor 1 alpha. Mol Cell Biol 24(12). 5223-5234

Wentzensen N, Vinokurova S, von Knebel Doeberitz M (2004) Systematic review of genomic integration sites of human papillomavirus genomes in epithelial dysplasia and invasive cancer of the female lower genital tract. Cancer Res 64(11): 3878-3884

Yeatman TJ (2004) A renaissance for SRC. Nat Rev Cancer 4(6): 470-480

Yoo YG, Cho S, Park S, Lee MO (2004) The carboxy-terminus of the hepatitis B virus X protein is necessary and sufficient for the activation of hypoxia-inducible factor-1alpha. FEBS Lett 577(1-2): 121-126

Yoo YG, Oh SH, Park ES, Cho H, Lee N, Park H, Kim DK, Yu DY, Seong JK, Lee MO (2003) Hepatitis B virus X protein enhances transcriptional activity of hypoxia-inducible factor-1alpha through activation of mitogen-activated protein kinase pathway. J Biol Chem 278(40): 39076-39084

Young L, Alfieri C, Hennessy K, Evans H, O'Hara C, Anderson KC, Ritz J, Shapiro RS, Rickinson A, Kieff E, et al. (1989) Expression of Epstein-Barr virus transformation-associated genes in tissues of patients with EBV lymphoproliferative disease. N Engl J Med 321(16): 1080-1085

Young LS, Murray PG (2003) Epstein-Barr virus and oncogenesis: from latent genes to tumours. Oncogene 22(33): 5108-5121

zur Hausen H (2009) Papillomaviruses in the causation of human cancers –a brief historical account. Virology 384(2): 260-265

Part III

Medical aspects of hypoxia

Chapter 15

Noninvasive hypoxia imaging

Sarah Peeters, Philippe Lambin and Ludwig Dubois[*]

[*]Author for correspondence:
Department of Radiation Oncology (MaastRO Lab), GROW – School for Oncology
and Developmental Biology, Maastricht University Medical Centre, UNS 50/23 PO Box 616,
6200 MD Maastricht, The Netherlands, Phone: +31 (0)43 388 2909 – Fax: +31 (0)43 388 4540 –
Email: ludwig.dubois@maastrichtuniversity.nl

Contents

Key points

— Imaging tumour hypoxia will lead to improved treatment planning since low oxygen concentrations negatively influence treatment response and outcome.

— Repeatable noninvasive imaging techniques, applicable to all solid tumours, give a direct representative three-dimensional image of the tumour.

— New PET hypoxia markers with optimized pharmacokinetic and clearance properties are under continuous development.

— SPECT, BOLD-MRI and ^{19}F-MRS evaluation of tumour hypoxia are gaining attention and might be good alternatives.

— Visualizing the hypoxia-dependent pathways will increase the success of molecular cancer therapeutics targeting hypoxic responses.

Introduction

Visualization of hypoxic regions within tumours is gaining more importance in daily clinical practice. Hypoxia, deprivation of oxygen, is a very common event in solid tumours, caused by the rapid growth and the impaired development of blood vessels. It is known that cells exposed to low oxygen concentrations are less sensitive to conventional anticancer therapies (Brizel et al, 1996; Brown, 2000; Hockel et al, 1996) and that the prognosis of these patients is worse (Kaanders et al, 2002; Nordsmark & Overgaard, 2000). Therefore, hypoxia imaging of tumours can contribute to better treatment planning and follow-up.

Several methodologies exist to quantify the amount of hypoxia from which polarographic oxygen electrodes and antibody-based detection of exogenous hypoxia markers are considered as 'standard' (Davda & Bezabeh, 2006) (see Figure 15.1). Immunohistological assays based on staining of bioreductive 2-nitroimidazoles, such as pimonidazole, are performed on tumour resections or after taking a biopsy. These markers demonstrate an irreversible accumulation in hypoxic cells after systemic injection and can be visualized by the binding of an antibody on a tissue slice. On the other hand, oxygen electrodes are able to monitor tumour oxygenation in vivo by inserting cathode electrodes into the tumour (Brurberg et al, 2003). Although these methods enable tumour oxygenation measurements they are limited by practical challenges such as invasiveness and tumour accessibility. Furthermore, a global picture of tumour oxygenation status of the whole tumour is lacking, since the availability of small tumour specimen after biopsy is limited or measurement of oxygen occurs only at certain points (Padhani et al, 2007).

This illustrates that there is a need for alternatives to measure tumour oxygenation. These alternatives should be applicable to all solid tumours, give a direct representative three-dimensional image of the whole tumour, be easy repeatable, and should not be invasive for the patient (see Figure 15.1). The optimal non-invasive method for imaging hypoxia has not yet been found, however, several non-invasive techniques are capable of measuring the amount and location of hypoxia in tumours. In this chapter we will discuss the imaging modalities that look the most promising.

PET

Positron emission tomography (PET) is one of the most used techniques to visualize tumours and makes use of tracers labelled with radioactive isotopes injected and distributed throughout the body. These unstable isotopes emit positrons, a type of beta decay, which leads upon annihilation with an electron to the emission of two photons in opposite directions. When detected by the scintillators in the detector ring, a signal is transduced to photomultiplier tubes and coincidence is determined in order to reconstruct images, which visualize the difference in tracer uptake in different regions of the body (Jones, 1996).

PET Tracers

Different tumour microenvironmental characteristics, such as proliferation, hypoxia, glucose metabolism, protein synthesis, apoptosis, etc., can be visualized using a range of specific PET markers for each individual process (Bussink *et al*, 2010). More specifically, PET tracers to visualize hypoxic regions can be roughly divided into nitroimidazole and non-nitroimidazole groups. In addition, hypoxia response can also be evaluated using radioactive labelled antibodies against endogenous proteins up-regulated under hypoxic conditions, such as carbonic anhydrase IX.

Nitroimidazoles

All tracers based on nitroimidazoles consist of a NO_2 group combined with a rest group (R). The compound RNO_2 can freely diffuse into cells where it is reduced to RNO_2^- only in viable cells by intracellular electron reductases. In the presence of oxygen, an oxidation reaction occurs and the compound can diffuse again out of the cell. However, when oxygen concentrations are low, RNO_2^- is further reduced into reactive intermediary metabolites, which bind to thiol groups of macromolecules in the cell. Since this is an irreversible phenomenon, the tracer gets trapped in the hypoxic cell. In dead cells like necrotic regions, no reduction occurs due to a lack of enzymatic activity and therefore the compound can diffuse freely in and out the cell (Lee & Scott, 2007; Padhani *et al*, 2007). When radiolabelling these nitroimidazoles with a PET radioisotope, these compounds can be detected by PET imaging.

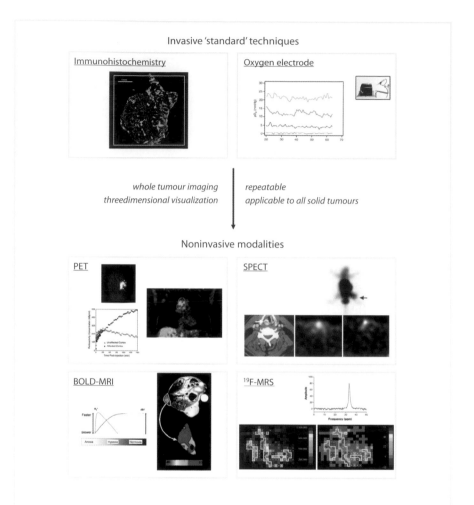

Figure 15.1 _ Hypoxia evaluation. For the invasive 'standard' techniques, immunohisto-chemical staining and oxygen electrode measurements are demonstrated. An immuno-fluorescent staining for pimonidazole (green), blood vessels (light blue) and proliferat-ing cells (red) is shown for a laryngeal carcinoma biopsy. An example of pO$_2$ traces recorded with oxygen electrodes is shown for different regions in a human melanoma tumour-bearing mouse. Several limitations are associated with the above invasive tech-niques, illustrating the need for noninvasive monitoring of tumour oxygenation. These modalities can be based on nuclear or magnetic resonance imaging. Typical [^{18}F]-FMISO-PET uptake patterns are shown for low oxygen regions in a rat stroke model compared with the uptake in the well-oxygenated surrounding tissues. Heterogeneous [^{18}F]-HX4-PET accumulation is found in a NSCLC patient (GTV depicted in pink). SPECT imaging, although with lower sensitivity, can also be used for evaluation of hypoxia, as seen by the tumour uptake in a lung tumour (black arrow) bearing mouse and a patient

with head and neck cancer (tumour indicated by the arrow). An increase in BOLD-MRI signal (R_2*) has been demonstrated with lowered oxygen concentration and this seems to be influenced by the blood volume (rBV) information. Microscopic hypoxic regions (blue) are depicted using BOLD-MRI in an A253 tumour bearing mouse (red delineation on MRI image). Areas with high microvessel density are shown in green, while necrotic areas are indicated in purple. A typical ^{19}F spectrum, intensity map and correlated oxygen map are shown for a large Dunning prostate R3327-HI tumour in rats. Figure is composed of parts adapted from (Bhattacharya *et al*, 2004; Brurberg *et al*, 2003; Bussink *et al*, 2010; Hoebers *et al*, 2002; Hoskin *et al*, 2007; Lee *et al*, 2008a; Seddon *et al*, 2003; Takasawa *et al*, 2007; van Loon *et al*, 2010; Zhao *et al*, 2003).

[^{18}F]-FMISO

The first and most extensively studied hypoxia PET tracer based on 2-nitro-imidazoles is [^{18}F]-Fluoromisonidazole ([^{18}F]-FMISO). Its delivery to tumours is not hampered by perfusion and the degree of hypoxia is identified by increased uptake of [^{18}F]-FMISO. Due to its relatively hydrophilic charac-ter and its partition coefficient nearly to unity, the molecule diffuses eas-ily across the extracellular membrane of all cells. When the compound enters hypoxic cells, a second electron reduction occurs and [^{18}F]-FMISO becomes trapped. Over time, free circulating compound within the body will be cleared and the trapped molecule in the hypoxic cells can be bet-ter visualized as a result of the decreasing background signal (see Fig-ure 15.1) (Takasawa *et al*, 2007). Metabolization of [^{18}F]-FMISO occurs via the liver and excretion through the kidneys and the bladder, resulting in high [^{18}F]-FMISO signals within these organs. Furthermore, higher uptake in the intestine is observed, while tissues with a low uptake and subsequently with a low background signal are the blood, spleen, heart, lung, muscle, bone and the brain (Lee & Scott, 2007).

The feasibility of measuring hypoxia using [^{18}F]-FMISO-PET was observed in mice bearing mammary carcinomas. Upon modulation of hypoxia in the tumours, a significant change was obtained in the [^{18}F]-FMISO uptake (Bentzen *et al*, 2002; Gronroos *et al*, 2004). A homogeneous distribution of [^{18}F]-FMISO in viable C6 glioma brain tumour tissue of rats was found with a significantly higher uptake in the tumour compared to the normal brain (Tochon-Danguy *et al*, 2002). The first clinical study demonstrating the feasibil-ity of [^{18}F]-FMISO-PET proved that the amount of hypoxia varied markedly between tumours with the same histology, indicating that hypoxia was heterogeneously distributed within a single tumour, and that the hypoxic fraction did not correlate with tumour size (Rasey et al, 1996). Furthermore, a clinical study in eight non-small cell lung cancer patients revealed the possibility of detecting hypoxia by using [^{18}F]-FMISO-PET (Gagel et al, 2006) and similar results were obtained in 73 head and neck cancer patients in which [^{18}F]-FMISO was able to visualize the hypoxic fraction in the tumours (Rajendran et al, 2006).

Several studies have established the feasibility and utility of [^{18}F]-FMISO-PET in the noninvasive evaluation of tumour hypoxia by comparison with 'standard' oxygen measurements. Measuring hypoxia in pig livers revealed a correlation between [^{18}F]-FMISO accumulation and the tissue oxygenation as detected by oxygen electrodes (Piert et al, 1999; Piert et al, 2000). However, no correlation could be found comparing tumour hypoxia measurements of the oxygen electrode method with [^{18}F]-FMISO-PET uptake in mice bearing mammary carcinomas (Bentzen et al, 2002). Comparison between [^{18}F]-FMISO uptake and the oxygen status of 22 head and neck cancer patients detected by CT-guided oxygen electrode polarography demonstrated a moderate correlation (Zimny et al, 2006). A similar study revealed only a slight correlation in 36 patients (Gagel et al, 2006). Differences observed in comparative studies can be explained by the difference of the two techniques in measuring hypoxia. Oxygen electrode polarography measures extracellular oxygen tension (Zimny et al, 2006) and does not discriminate between severe hypoxic and necrotic regions (Jenkins et al, 2000) and can therefore overestimate the extent of tumour hypoxia.

Comparison between the hypoxic volumes assessed with [^{18}F]-FMISO-PET imaging and with immunohistochemical evaluation using pimonidazole in a rat rhabdomyosarcoma tumour model resulted in a significant correlation (Dubois et al, 2004). This was confirmed in a [^{18}F]-FMISO autoradiography study, where a pixel-to-pixel comparison was performed with pimonidazole staining in mice bearing different human tumour lines (Troost et al, 2006). A significant correlation was observed in two of the three cell lines between the mean pimonidazole and the mean [^{18}F]-FMISO signal intensity. Clamping in order to reduce the amount of oxygen in the tumour resulted in a significant increase of the mean signal intensities for both hypoxia markers. Carbogen breathing, which increases the amount of oxygen in the tumour, lead to a significant reduction in mean pimonidazole intensity, but only a marginal effect was seen for the mean [^{18}F]-FMISO signal intensity, probably related to the intra-tumoural trapping of unbound marker (Troost et al, 2006). Furthermore, the degree of correlation between the two hypoxia markers was influenced by the microregional distribution pattern of hypoxia within the tumour (Troost et al, 2008). Only for ribbon-like patterns of hypoxia, a high significant relationship between mean signal intensity of [18F]-FMISO and pimonidazole was found. In patchy patterns of hypoxia, the binding characteristics of pimonidazole and [18F]-FMISO could be more different, explaining the lower correlation.

In mice bearing human colorectal HT-29 tumours, the uptake of [18F]-FMISO was compared with the hypoxia-inducible dual reporter herpes simplex virus type 1 thymidine kinase and enhanced green fluorescence protein (HSV1-TKeGFP) under the control of hypoxia responsive elements (9HRE). Upon production of the gene product under hypoxic conditions, TK is able to phosphorylate substrates such as [124I]-FIAU, which is consequently trapped inside the tumour cell. A comparable heterogeneous spatial distribution of [124I]-FIAU and [18F]-FMISO was observed within the same tumour, which co-localized with pimonidazole staining (He et al, 2008).

Although [18F]-FMISO is the most studied PET tracer for imaging tumour hypoxia, the clinical potential of [18F]-FMISO-PET imaging might be limited. There are some concerns about the stability of the fluorine-18 linkage and the formation of metabolites in blood and urine (Rasey et al, 1999). Furthermore, only modest signal to noise ratios are obtained due to the relative low uptake into tumour tissues and the slow clearance from oxygen-rich tissues resulting in high background signals (Krohn et al, 2008). Therefore, the development of other hypoxia PET tracers has continued and second generation 2-nitroimidazoles have been designed with slightly different characteristics in relation to water solubility and degradation.

[18F]-FAZA

One of these second generation 2-nitroimidazoles is [18F]-Fluoroazomycin arabinoside ([18F]-FAZA), a nitroimidazole coupled to an arabinose sugar. The compound is more hydrophilic than [18F]-FMISO, which should result in better tumour to background contrast. [18F]-FAZA uptake was found to be increased in vitro upon exposure to conditions without oxygen, although this increase was variable between cells of different tumours (Busk et al, 2008). Although tumour to muscle ratios are similar 1 hour after injection, uptake of [18F]-FAZA in the tumour is lower compared to the uptake of [18F]-FMISO, as shown in an animal study. A possible explanation was given by the faster clearance of [18F]-FAZA (Sorger et al, 2003). However, a different study on mice demonstrated that imaging as late as possible is advisable to obtain higher tumour to muscle and tumour to blood ratios (Piert et al, 2005). Another mice study revealed no differences in uptake between [18F]-FAZA and [^{18}F]-FMISO after 180 minutes. However, [^{18}F]-FAZA uptake was significantly faster with superior biokinetics because of its better clearance from background tissues, resulting in higher tumour to background ratios compared to [^{18}F]-FMISO (Reischl et al, 2007). A large variation among different animal studies was observed, probably due to the different tumour models used, indicating that the uptake of [^{18}F]-FAZA is dependent on the tumour type. [^{18}F]-FAZA clinical studies on patients with cancers at different sites show adequate image quality with high uptake and acceptable tumour to blood ratios, suggesting its feasibility and potential as a hypoxia imaging agent (Postema et al, 2009; Souvatzoglou et al, 2007).

[^{18}F]-FETNIM

Another interesting second generation 2-nitroimidazole is [^{18}F]-Fluoro-erythronitroimidazole ([18F]-FETNIM). Higher tumour to background ratios can be obtained using [^{18}F]-FETNIM, since it is more hydrophilic compared with [^{18}F]-FMISO and therefore it can be easier eliminated from the well oxygenated tissues (Gronroos et al, 2001). Despite having a slow peripheral metabolism and little defluorination, uptake correlated with the oxygenation status in tumours. Comparative studies with [^{18}F]-FMISO in mice bearing mammary carcinomas demonstrated no significant differences in intratumoural uptake between the two markers (Gronroos et al, 2004). However, a high uptake in the bladder wall was detected, making it essential to adequately hydrate the patients and to follow a voiding schedule in order to dilute the activity in the bladder and to decrease the risk of damage (Tolvanen et al, 2002). Recently, the clinical value of [^{18}F]-FETNIM has been demonstrated in NSCLC patients, since in a multivariate survival analysis its maximum tumour to blood ratios were found to be an independent prognostic factor (Li et al, 2010).

[^{18}F]-EF1, [^{18}F]-EF3 and [^{18}F]-EF5

As the high hydrophilicity of the previous compounds limits the diffusion into tumours, a new class of more lipophilic, fluorinated etanidazole compounds (such as EF1, EF3 and EF5) is of potential interest. These tracers are characterized by the same side chains (similar to etanidazole) but differ in the number of fluorine atoms, what determines the lipophilicity of the compound (Evans et al, 2000); the higher the number of fluorine atoms, the more lipophilic. Preliminary animal experiments indicated more homogeneous distribution in normal tissues together with tracer elimination through the kidneys and tracer accumulation in hypoxic tumours (Busch et al, 2000; Evans et al, 2000; Koch, 2002). [^{18}F]-EF1 imaging was proved to be an excellent noninvasive hypoxia marker in two rat tumour types, a study which was mainly focused on the optimization of the drug's biodistribution (Evans et al, 2000). EF3 was recently radiolabeled with fluorine-18 and has been demonstrated to be a good alternative for [^{18}F]-FMISO, based on ex vivo pharmacokinetics and biodistribution of both tracers in mice studies (Josse et al, 2001; Mahy et al, 2004). No major differences in tracer delivery were observed even though [^{18}F]-FMISO is more hydrophilic and expected to show a faster body clearance (Mahy et al, 2008a). Quantitative comparison between [^{18}F]-EF3 and [^{18}F]-FMISO in a rat tumour model showed that the [^{18}F]-EF3 uptake was significantly lower at 2 hours post injection, but similar 4 hours after injection, compared with [^{18}F]-FMISO uptake at 2 hours post injection. They concluded that [^{18}F]-EF3 appears to be a potential in vivo tracer for the noninvasive detection and evaluation of tumour hypoxia, yet without being superior over [^{18}F]-FMISO (Dubois et al, 2009a). In a phase I study on 10 head and neck cancer patients the tracer was demonstrated to be safe in relation to toxicity. However, from an imaging point of view the results were disappointing, since only one patient showed distinguishable [^{18}F]-EF3 uptake in tumours known to be hypoxic where other tracers have shown uptake in hypoxic regions (Mahy et al, 2008b). EF5 was first developed as a hypoxic marker to be visualized by fluorescence microscopy after binding to an EF5 specific antibody (Evans et al, 1995). Later on the compound was labelled with fluorine-18 and used for hypoxia imaging by PET. [^{18}F]-EF5 is the most lipophilic compound of the three and therefore has the most homogenous distribution in normal tissue (Koch, 2002). Both preclinical and clinical studies show that [^{18}F]-EF5 is potentially a good tracer for hypoxia imaging (Komar et al, 2008; Ziemer et al, 2003). In rats bearing early passage 9L glioma or Morris 7777 (Q7) hepatoma, tumours were easily visible 60 minutes after injection only when the final tumour to muscle ratios 3 hours after injection were greater than 2. However, neither the less hypoxic 9L nor the smaller Q7 tumours were visible on the PET images, indicating that [^{18}F]-EF5 is only suited for imaging of large and highly hypoxic tumours (Ziemer et al, 2003). A recent study demonstrated the potential of [^{18}F]-EF5 to detect hypoxia in HNSCC patients. However, further development and evaluation is warranted, since only low tumour to muscle ratios were obtained 3 hours after injection in this tumour model (Komar et al, 2008). Recently, although observations were only made on three patients, the uptake of the PET hypoxia marker [^{18}F]-EF5 has been confirmed by immunohistochemistry staining using the EF5 antibody demonstrating high staining in high uptake regions (Koch *et al*, 2010).

[^{18}F]-HX4

Another alternative 3-[^{18}F]Fluoro-2-(4-((2-nitro-1H-imidazol-1-yl)methyl)-1H-1,2,3-triazol-1-yl)propan-1-ol ([^{18}F]-HX4), which overcomes some of the limitations associated with previously described tracers, has been developed and evaluated as a noninvasive hypoxia marker. It represents a new, click chemistry-based generation of 2-nitroimidazole derivatives in which structure-activity relationships have been used to design an agent with preferred pharmacokinetics and clearance properties (Kolb *et al*, 2001). Biodistribution and dosimetry studies in monkeys and humans demonstrated that the amount of unmetabolized [^{18}F]-HX4 in blood and urine samples decreased slowly from 97% at 5 minutes to 83% at 120 minutes after injection. Furthermore, the highest uptake of [^{18}F]-HX4 was found in the urinary bladder, indicating an excretion primarily through the kidneys. Therefore, the bladder wall is considered to be the critical organ and patients should be encouraged to maintain adequate hydration and void frequently (Doss *et al*, 2010). Evaluation of [^{18}F]-HX4 as a noninvasive hypoxia imaging agent has been performed in rat and mice tumour models and data indeed indicates a faster clearance from the non-specific uptake regions compared to [^{18}F]-FMISO and [^{18}F]-FAZA. Accumulation of [^{18}F]-HX4 has been found to be hypoxia specific, since increasing the oxygen concentration using a combination of nicotinamide and carbogen breathing resulted in a significantly decreased uptake. On the other hand, pretreatment with 7% oxygen breathing caused a significant increase in [^{18}F]-HX4 uptake. Furthermore, [^{18}F]-HX4 has been validated as a noninvasive hypoxia marker based on a significant correlation between the percentage [^{18}F]-HX4 and pimonidazole positivity (Dubois *et al*, 2011). The clinical applicability of [^{18}F]-HX4 has recently been demonstrated in a phase 1 study in NSCLC patients with no obvious toxicity. Furthermore, a heterogeneous [^{18}F]-HX4 accumulation was observed (see Figure 15.1) with a substantial increase in tumour to muscle ratios in the second hour after injection (van Loon *et al*, 2010).

Non-nitroimidazole tracers

Cu-ATSM

The most important non-nitroimidazole hypoxia marker is based on the reduction of Copper^{2+}, namely Cu-ATSM (diacetyl-2,3-bis(N(4)-methyl-3-thio-semicarbazone). Cu-ATSM is a low molecular weight compound with a lipo-philic character, making it highly membrane permeable allowing it to diffuse easily from the bloodstream into the surrounding cells. When Cu^{2+}-ATSM diffuses into cell it reacts with thiol groups or redox-active proteins with NADH as a required cofactor and is consequently reduced to Cu^{1+}-ATSM. The reduced, charged form is less lipophilic, but this process is reversible when oxygen is present. Protonation of the reduced form will lead to disso-ciation of the complex and copper will be irreversibly trapped in the hypoxic cell (Dearling & Packard, 2010). To visualize this trapping, different copper iso topes exist, all with varying half lives: [^{60}Cu] $t_{1/2}$ = 23.7 min, [^{61}Cu] $t_{1/2}$ = 3.35 hours, [^{62}Cu] $t_{1/2}$ = 9.74 min, [^{64}Cu] $t_{1/2}$ = 12.7 hours and [^{67}Cu] $t_{1/2}$ = 61.9 hours (Vavere & Lewis, 2007). It has been shown that Cu-ATSM is selective for hypoxia in several tumour types; however, in one animal study using fibrosarcomas-bearing mice, uptake of [^{64}Cu]-ATSM was observed in well-perfused areas of the tumour, indicating a correlation between [^{64}Cu]-ATSM uptake and vascular perfusion irrespective of to hypoxia. Furthermore, breathing car-bogen did not result in a decreased [^{64}Cu-ATSM] uptake, indicating some other retention mechanisms, as opposed to hypoxia, are involved in this type of tumour (Yuan et al, 2006). In 9L tumour-bearing rats, an excellent cor-relation was observed between [^{64}Cu]-ATSM] and [^{18}F]-FMISO uptake, while regional comparisons between [^{64}Cu-ATSM and [^{18}F]-FDG resulted in a very poor relationship (Dence et al, 2008). Clinical data obtained from non-small cell lung cancer patients demonstrated the feasibility of [^{60}Cu]-ATSM imaging. Also, a significant lower tumour to muscle ratio was found in patients with a good response to the treatment (Dehdashti et al, 2003). Similar results were obtained in patients with cervical cancer, where a low [^{60}Cu]-ATSM uptake in the tumour related to progression free survival (Dehdashti et al, 2008). Initially only [^{60}Cu]-ATSM was used in clinical studies because of its short half life (23.7 min), while animal experiments were mainly performed using [^{64}Cu]-ATSM. Recently, the image quality and tumour uptake of [^{60}Cu]-ATSM and [^{64}Cu]-ATSM were compared in 10 patients with cervical carcinoma. [^{64}Cu]-ATSM was reported to be safe and can be used to obtain high-quality images of tumour hypoxia in human cancers, based on an improved imaging quality due to lower noise (Lewis et al, 2008).

[^{18}F]-FDG imaging

[^{18}F]-FDG (Fluorodeoxyglucose) is often used in the clinic for the imaging of tumours and has been postulated as a surrogate marker for tumour hypoxia. FDG has the same structure as glucose, except for one hydroxyl group which is replaced by fluor. It is known that regions of hypoxia are characterized by an increased glycolysis. Due to the lack of oxygen there is an impairment of the process which delivers the most energy, the oxidative phosphorylation. This leads to a reduction of the available energy, while there is still a huge need for it. In order to produce a sufficient amount of energy, the anaerobic glycolysis is upregulated. [^{18}F]-FDG is taken up by the cell in a similar way as glucose and enters the glycolysis where it is converted like any other glucose molecule. However, due to the fluor replacement, the molecule cannot proceed in this irreversible process and gets trapped (Oriuchi *et al*, 2006). According to this theory, [^{18}F]-FDG uptake should correlate with the amount of hypoxia in the tumour. Incubation of cells under low oxygen concentration or in the absence of oxygen has indeed been shown to have increased [^{18}F]-FDG uptake (Dierckx & Van de Wiele, 2008). When [^{18}F]-FDG uptake by tumours grown in rat or mice are compared to uptake by [^{18}F]-FMISO in preclinical settings, the pattern of normoxic and hypoxic regions within the xenografts, as imaged by [^{18}F]-FMISO, largely correlated with glucose metabolism although minor locoregional differences could not be excluded (Dierckx & Van de Wiele, 2008). In 10 different xenografts in nude mice, a positive correlation was observed for the spatial patterns of [^{18}F]-FDG and [^{18}F]-FMISO (Wyss *et al*, 2006). Similar results were obtained in rat tumour models, although subtle but possibly significant differences in intratumoural distribution were observed (Zanzonico *et al*, 2006). However, several clinical studies have shown that [^{18}F]-FDG is not correlated or associated with other hypoxia markers. A study in head and neck cancer patients comparing [^{18}F]-FDG and [^{18}F]-FMISO uptake could not demonstrate a voxel-to-voxel relationship between the two markers, concluding that the two tracers provide independent information (Thorwarth *et al*, 2006). Investigation of [^{18}F]-FMISO and [^{18}F]-FDG uptake in non-small cell lung cancer patients showed that [^{18}F]-FMISO uptake was significantly lower than [^{18}F]-FDG uptake and that there was no correlation between the two (Cherk *et al*, 2006; Gagel *et al*, 2006). Therefore, further evaluation of [^{18}F]-FDG uptake in relation to intrinsic (CA IX) and/or bioreductive ([^{18}F]-FMISO etc.) markers of hypoxia is needed to fully assess its possibilities as a marker of hypoxia in clinical settings.

Imaging hypoxia response

Substantial evidence associates hypoxia with tumour development, growth, metastasis and poor response to therapy (Brizel et al, 1996; Hockel et al, 1996) and it has been shown that this tumour phenotype is due to hypoxia-dependent signalling pathways which regulate the expression of many genes important for the development and growth of solid tumours (Brown, 2000). It is important to understand these pathways in order to increase the success of recently developed molecular cancer therapeutics targeting hypoxic responses. Therefore, noninvasive evaluation of these pathways can be a potentially important tool for treatment guidance and patient selection. Tumour-associated carbonic anhydrase IX (CA IX) is such a protein upregulated and activated under hypoxic conditions (Dubois et al, 2007) in most solid tumours, while in normal healthy tissue CA IX is only expressed in a limited number of tissues (Potter & Harris, 2004). Because of the upregulation and activation upon low oxygen concentrations, CA IX could be an endogenous marker for the hypoxic response. Antibodies raised against the extracellular part can be used to detect the protein and visualization can be done by labelling these antibodies. The choice of radioactive isotope to be coupled to the antibodies is based on the biological half life and the accumulation time of the antibodies. In general it takes several days before maximum antibody accumulation is reached, which makes fast decaying positron emitters like [^{18}F] or [^{64}Cu] unsuitable for labelling. Zirconium-89 [^{89}Zr] and Iodine-124 [^{124}I], with a respective half-life of 78 and 100 hours, better match the relative slow pharmacokinetics of monoclonal antibodies (Brouwers et al, 2004). Labelling of cG250, a CA IX specific monoclonal antibody, with the radioactive isotope [^{89}Zr] was shown to be stable, did not affect the immunoreactivity of the antibody and demonstrated most optimal images after 72 hours post injection in a nude rat bearing renal cell tumours (Brouwers et al, 2004). Although it has been shown that the presence of CA IX can be detected by [^{124}I]-cG250 using PET scan in renal cell carcinoma bearing mice, [^{124}I]-cG250 uptake was not correlated with oxygen tension measurements, supporting the hypothesis that cell lines may subvert known hypoxia mechanisms in hypoxic environments (Lawrentschuk et al, 2009). A phase 1 clinical trial demonstrated that [^{124}I] labelled cG250 can be used to detect renal cell carcinomas very accurately, but the correlation with hypoxic regions has not been investigated (Divgi et al, 2007). Because of the large molecular size of antibodies, F(ab')$_2$ fragments are developed by enzymatic degradation of the intact antibody. These F(ab')$_2$ fragments show a much faster accumulation than intact antibodies, but are still able to bind the target protein CA IX and are shown to accurately localize with hypoxic regions at microscopic level. Furthermore the feasibility of detecting [^{89}Zr] labelled cG250-F(ab')$_2$ using PET has been demonstrated (Hoeben *et al*, 2010). However since antibody binding also occurs upon reoxygenation, no discrimination can be made between hypoxic and aerobic cells expressing CA IX, indicating the inability to reveal periodic or cycling areas of tumour oxygenation. Recently, high CA IX affinity fluorescent sulfonamides were developed which exclusively bind CA IX during hypoxia, a condition in which CA IX has to be in an open conformational state (Dubois *et al*, 2007; Supuran, 2008). Furthermore, it has been demonstrated that the in vivo accumulation of these sulfonamides occurred in delineated areas of the tumour in a hypoxia dependent manner (Dubois *et al*, 2009b), suggesting that it will be interesting to pursue further clinical development of sulfonamides for imaging and therapy purposes.

Applications in the clinic

PET imaging is often used for the evaluation of tumour characteristics such as metabolism, proliferation, and hypoxia in patients. Combined with the anatomical information obtained by computed tomography (CT), the site of the tumour and the hypoxic regions within the tumour can be localized (Vikram *et al*, 2007). Phase 1 clinical trials are focused on determining the possible toxicity of the new candidate compound and often imaging quality will be analyzed in relation to the dose used. Additionally, radiation dosimetry will be performed to assess the absorbed dose for different organs in order to determine the critical organ and to take precautions when carrying out imaging. When the tracer passes these phase 1 requirements, the use for treatment planning and monitoring treatment response can be evaluated. A high amount of hypoxia is known to be associated with a bad patient prognosis (Kaanders *et al*, 2002; Nordsmark & Overgaard, 2000), but is it possible to make this prediction based on PET images? Or is it possible to investigate the effect of a therapy by measuring the hypoxic fraction before and after chemo- or radio- therapy? If so, this would contribute to an improved treatment outcome.

It has been shown that PET imaging with [^{18}F]-FMISO is predictive for treatment outcome. A group of advanced head and neck cancer or non-small cell lung cancer was subjected to [^{18}F]-FMISO-PET imaging before curative radiotherapy. Patients with local recurrence could be separated from disease-free patients, suggested by high [^{18}F]-FMISO uptake and high tumour to background ratios. Furthermore, qualitative analysis of time-activity curves revealed 3 curve types: rapid washout, intermediate delayed washout and accumulation. Only in the patients with a rapid wash-out curve could no recurrences be observed, making time-activity curve an interesting tool for patient selection (Eschmann et al, 2005). Another study in NSCLC patients demonstrated the possibility of using [^{18}F]-FMISO-PET for qualitative and quantitative definition of hypoxic sub-areas which may correspond to a localization of local recurrences. In addition, a decreased [^{18}F]-FMISO uptake after chemotherapy treatment resulted for most patients in a good tumour response while an increase or unchanged high tumour to background ratio corresponded to worse local tumour outcomes (Gagel et al, 2006).

Several clinical studies in head and neck cancer patients investigated the feasibility of dose painting of hypoxic regions within the tumour. In 10 head and neck patients, it was possible to deliver on average an additional dose of 20% to the hypoxic areas of the primary tumour without compromising normal tissue tolerance. The hypoxic regions were determined based on a [^{18}F]-FMISO-PET scan using a tumour to blood ratio threshold of 1.3, representing higher tumour to blood ratios as hypoxic. For two patients, an attempt was made to deliver an additional 50% dose on the primary tumour, but this succeeded in only one patient, since normal healthy tissue constraints were exceeded in the other patient (Lee et al, 2008b). While the previous study treatment plans were designed based on one [^{18}F]-FMISO-PET scan, a second study was performed in 7 head and neck cancer patients, where the treatment plans made based on a first [^{18}F]-FMISO scan and on a second scan 3 days later were compared (Lin et al, 2008). In 4 of the 7 patients the hypoxic volume within the tumour changed remarkably. However, although the importance of these changes must be recognized, the extra dose can still have a notable effect on the hypoxic volume (Lin et al, 2008). In a recent study, hypoxic regions were determined based on a tumour to cerebellum ratio of 1.3 as a threshold for [^{18}F]-FMISO-PET/CT. Dose-escalation to the hypoxic target volume without exceeding the normal tissue dose was feasible in six of eight head and neck cancer patients. Further acceptable dose escalation depended primarily on the primary tumour site and the extent of disease (Choi et al, 2010).

SPECT

Single photon emission computed tomography (SPECT) uses single photon emitting radionuclides ligated with hypoxia specific compounds that generate a signal from the hypoxic area of the tumour. SPECT data is acquired by collecting planar images at multiple angles around the patient using single-, dual- or triple-head scintillation cameras, typically equipped with parallel-hole collimators. SPECT images suffer from poor spatial resolution (typically > 1 cm) and often lack anatomic landmarks for precise determinations of location of areas of abnormal uptake (Patton & Turkington, 2008). However, the value of SPECT can be found in the detection of isotopes that cannot be visualized using other techniques.

For the detection of hypoxia, most SPECT tracers are based on the same structure as several PET tracers, nitroimidazoles. Iodine-123 [^{123}I] was the isotope initially used for this purpose. Nowadays, Technetium-99m [^{99m}Tc] is increasingly being used as it is less expensive and can be easily chelated to many different compounds and shows favourable biological half-life as compared to [^{123}I] (Davda & Bezabeh, 2006).

Nitroimidazoles

The SPECT nitroimidazoles are based on the same principle as the PET nitroimidazoles, namely on the reduction of the NO_2 group to NH_2 and the subsequent binding to intracellular macromolecules in the absence of oxygen, resulting in trapping inside the cell.

[^{123}I]-IAZA

Iodine-123 labelled iodoazomycin arabinoside ([^{123}I]-IAZA) has the same structure as the hypoxia PET tracer [^{18}F]-FAZA apart from the radioactive compound. In mice bearing EMT-6 tumours this tracer shows an optimal tumour to blood ratio eight hours after injection as observed in a biodistribution study (Parliament et al, 1992). A preliminary report of a clinical study in patients with advanced malignancies demonstrated that the use of [^{123}I]-IAZA is feasible and safe and although image quality varies between different types of cancer, it is adequate (Parliament et al, 1992). Nevertheless, in a larger patient cohort, highly inconsistent uptake was found in various tumours, with frequencies ranging from 60% in small cell lung cancer to 0% in malignant gliomas (Urtasun *et al*, 1996). Although pharmacokinetics and radiation dosimetry are suited for imaging, the major drawback of inconsistent uptake, prompted research towards modified iodinated azomycin arabinosides. Iodoazomycin pyranoside (IAZP), beta-D-iodinated azomycin galactopyranoside (IAZGP) and iodoazomycin xylopyranoside (IAZXP) have been developed and evaluated as hypoxia markers. In mice bearing FM3 mammary carcinoma tumours, a higher accumulation of [^{123}I]-IAZGP was observed in tumours than in normal tissue at 24 hours after administration (Saitoh *et al*, 2002).

[^{99m}Tc]-BMS-181321 and [^{99m}Tc]-BRU59-21

BMS-181321 was the first [^{99m}Tc] labelled 2-nitroimidazole which was investigated for its ability to visualize tumour hypoxia. Because of its high lipophylicity, instability, slow clearance from blood and high background levels in normal tissue, low tumour to blood ratios are obtained in biodistribution studies and therefore [^{99m}Tc]-BMS-181321 is not optimal for tumour hypoxia imaging (Ballinger *et al*, 1996). On the other hand, [^{99m}Tc]-BRU59-21 is more hydrophilic, has a greater stability in vitro and a faster clearance in vivo. The compound demonstrates a good retention in tumours compared to muscle and blood and has proven to be suitable for hypoxia imaging. However, tumour to blood ratios in mice studies remain very low (Melo *et al*, 2000). The safety and biodistribution of [^{99m}Tc]-BRU59-21 was investigated in a phase 1 clinical trial in patients with head and neck carcinomas. The study demonstrated that [^{99m}Tc]-BRU59-21 was safe to use in patients (see Figure 15.1). Furthermore, tumour to normal tissue ratios of the primary tumour correlated with the intensity of pimonidazole staining, although this was less reliable for the involved lymph nodes (Hoebers *et al*, 2002).

Non-nitroimidazoles

[^{99m}Tc]-HL91

The most investigated non-nitroimidazole hypoxia marker for SPECT imaging is Prognox ([^{99m}Tc]-HL91 also known as [^{99m}Tc]-BnAO). The mechanism of localization to hypoxic regions is not completely understood but it is thought to work in the same way as the PET tracer Cu-ATSM. [^{99m}Tc]-

HL91 has a more hydrophilic character than other SPECT tracers, such as [^{99m}Tc]-BRU59-21 and is thought to have better clearance resulting in higher tumour to background sensitivity (Zhang *et al*, 2001). Measurements in mice bearing KHT-C leg tumours demonstrated that [^{99m}Tc]-HL91 accumulation was selective in hypoxic versus normoxic cells (see Figure 15.1) and its tumour to blood ratios were shown to be five times higher compared to BMS-181321 (Zhang *et al*, 1998), making it a promising agent for clinical studies on tumour hypoxia. Furthermore, an excellent correlation between [^{99m}Tc]-HL91 and hypoxia, as measured by Eppendorf electrodes, was observed in different tumour models and a combination treatment of nicotinamide and carbogen significantly reduced its uptake (Honess *et al*, 1998). On the other hand, N2 breathing or hydralazine treatment significantly increased its uptake (Kinuya *et al*, 2002; Lee *et al*, 2008a). A patient study with non-small cell lung carcinomas demonstrated the ability of [^{99m}Tc]-HL91 to predict treatment outcome, when a tumour to normal tissue ratio of 1.47 was used to segregate patients (Li *et al*, 2006).

Magnetic resonance techniques

A widely used imaging technique to study anatomical details of tumours is magnetic resonance imaging (MRI). Magnetic resonance spectroscopy (MRS) is based on the same principle as MRI to visualize the biochemical interactions in the tumour.

BOLD-MRI

Specialized magnetic resonance imaging (MRI) techniques such as blood oxygen level dependence (BOLD) MRI are shown to have the potential to detect hypoxia in tumours. Instead of the amount of hydrogen used in regular MRI, BOLD-MRI utilizes the oxygen status of endogenous hemoglobin. Upon low oxygen exposure, hemoglobin is present in the blood as deoxyhemoglobin. Deoxyhemoglobin is paramagnetic and generates a local magnetic gradient that can interact with the external magnetic field passing through it (Ogawa *et al*, 1990). The transverse relaxation times R_2 and R_2^* of water in blood and in the surrounding tissues is enhanced with the presence of deoxyhemoglobin, indicating that well oxygenated regions have lower R_2 and R_2^* values (Padhani, 2010). Although it seems that BOLD-MRI is the ideal noninvasive method to measure the amount of hypoxia in a tumour, determination of the oxygen status is influenced by the distribution of blood flow and blood volume, since BOLD-MRI does not directly measure the absolute oxygen concentration in tissues (Bhattacharya et al, 2004; Howe et al, 2001). Applying corrections for the amount of blood volume will increase the sensitivity of the measurement (see Figure 15.1) as observed in a clinical study in prostate cancer patients (Hoskin et al, 2007). High R_2^* levels increased the probability of hypoxia as measured by pimonidazole staining (Hoskin et al, 2007) or by invasive polarographic oxygen electrode methods (Chopra et al, 2009). In agreement with the findings in prostate cancer, a study on rats bearing mammary cancers observed a relationship between a heterogeneous baseline R_2^* and hypoxia (McPhail & Robinson, 2010). Furthermore, carbogen breathing resulted in a more homogeneous lower R_2^*. Not only low oxygen conditions, but also the necrotic areas of tumours can contribute to increases in deoxyhemoglobin contrast. Besides blood flow and blood volume, the hematocrite concentration, the pH and the temperature are known to change the fraction of deoxyhemoglobin levels and with that the R_2^* values (McPhail & Robinson, 2010). This indicates that BOLD-MRI is able to provide information on the tissue oxygen status, but that interpretation of the result has to be done with some caution.

^{19}F magnetic resonance spectrocopy

The MRS method most extensively investigated to detect hypoxia is fluorine MRS using perfluorocarbon (PFC) emulsions or fluorinated nitroimidazoles. Perfluorocarbons are hydrocarbons whose protons are replaced by fluorine atoms, making them sensitive for tissue oxygen tension. Molecular oxygen dissolves in the PFCs and this proportionally increases the relaxation rates of PFCs in MR analysis (Duong et al, 2001). A linear relationship between R_1 of the ^{19}F signal and the oxygen concentration is observed when PFCs are injected intravenously or directly into the tumour (Krohn et al, 2008). The combination a ^{19}F MRS with an anatomical ^{1}H MRI makes it possible to detect the origin of the signal (Robinson & Griffiths, 2004). PFCs are selected based on a reliable R_1 response, a good distribution throughout the body and tissue, and on the ability to form a stable emulsion. Several PFCs have been tried, but only two PFCs are commonly used for the measurement of hypoxia (Robinson & Griffiths, 2004). An important limitation for the use of PFCs is the temperature dependent relaxation time of the ^{19}F spins.

Perfluoro-15-crown-5-ether

Perfluoro-15-crown-5-ether (15C5), reflected in R_1, is shown to be dependent of oxygen tension, since a linear increase in longitudinal relaxation rate $1/T1$ (=R_1) was observed with increasing oxygen concentrations (Parhami & Fung, 1983). PFC uptake in mice bearing glioma xenografts was observed in perfused regions of the tumour where the mean R_1 values corresponded with the mean oxygen electrode values. Furthermore, the average R_1 values increased upon carbogen breathing (van der Sanden et al, 1999). Upon intravenous injection, a major part of 15C5 is sequestered in the liver and spleen, and only a small amount is taken up by the tumour, often not sufficient for determination of R_1 values by ^{19}F-MRS. To overcome this problem, PFCs (perfluorotributylamine) can be administrated encapsulated in a semipermeable hydrogel formed from an alginate solution with Ba^{2+} ions. Recently it was demonstrated that this method could be used to assess tumour hypoxia. Carbogen and hydralazine, but not nicotinamide was able to influence oxygen concentration measurements (Noth et al, 2004).

Hexafluorobenzene

Hexafluorobenzene (HFB, C_6F_6) is the second commonly used PFC for evaluation of tumour hypoxia. In Dunning prostate rat tumours (R3327-AT1) HFB was injected directly into the tumour to obtain more sensitive and precise maps of regional tumour oxygenation (see Figure 15.1) (Zhao et al, 2003). For larger tumours, a significantly lower baseline oxygenation was observed compared to smaller tumours with a more heterogeneous baseline. Both tumour sizes however responded to respiratory challenges with carbogen, but the rate was generally faster in initially well-oxygenated regions (Hunjan et al, 2001).

Fluorinated 2-nitroimidazoles

Other probes for detection of tumour hypoxia by ^{19}F-MRS are based on fluorinated 2-nitroimidazoles, such as hexafluoromisonidazole (CCI-103F), EF5 and SR-4554 (Davda & Bezabeh, 2006). The best results are obtained using SR-4554. In mice bearing C3H mammary, RIF-1 or SCCVII tumours, although no linear relationship was observed between ^{19}F retention parameters and Eppendorf electrode oxygen tension, substantial retention of

SR-4554 was associated with low oxygen concentrations (Aboagye *et al*, 1998). Patients with histologically proven solid malignancies underwent in a phase 1 clinical trial unlocalized ^{19}F-MRS, providing a global index of oxygenation rather than spatial distribution of oxygen tension. However, the increased tracer accumulation in the tumour could be due to increased blood flow, and so further investigation is needed to look at tracer concentration at prolonged time points until all unbound drug is washed out (Seddon *et al*, 2003).

Conclusion & future applications

Since the presence of hypoxia in tumours is associated with worse prognosis, there is a need for noninvasive evaluation of tumour oxygenation to predict treatment outcome and identify cancer patients who would benefit from appropriate treatments. In this chapter an overview was given of several investigated markers and imaging techniques which are able to detect these hypoxic regions. However, each marker and imaging modality has its own pros and cons and a particular technique or compound may be best suited for one tumour type, grade or stage. The ideal marker for hypoxia imaging should primarily be hypoxia specific and capable of discriminating normoxia, hypoxia/anoxia and necrosis with sufficient sensitivity and resolution. Furthermore, it should be able to discriminate between perfusion- and diffusion-limited hypoxia. Also, it should be lipophilic enough to ensure homogeneous distribution in all tissues, including tumours, but at the same time should be hydrophilic enough to ensure fast clearance resulting in high tumour-to-background ratios. Lastly, it should be easily available, cost-effective, non-toxic, easy to perform and have minimal hypoxia-independent degradation and metabolite formation. We can conclude that although currently no hypoxic marker completely corresponds with these requirements, a lot of potentially good hypoxia tracers are under development and investigation.

Acknowledgements _ This work has been funded with the support of the EU 7th framework Program (Metoxia Project Ref. 2008-222741) and the Center for Translational Molecular Medicine (www.ctmm.nl) (AIRFORCE Project Ref. 030-103). The authors declare no conflict of interest.

References

Aboagye EO, Maxwell RJ, Horsman MR, Lewis AD, Workman P, Tracy M, Griffiths JR (1998) The relationship between tumour oxygenation determined by oxygen electrode measurements and magnetic resonance spectroscopy of the fluorinated 2-nitroimidazole SR-4554. Br J Cancer 77: 65-70

Ballinger JR, Kee JW, Rauth AM (1996) In vitro and in vivo evaluation of a technetium-99m-labeled 2-nitroimidazole (BMS181321) as a marker of tumour hypoxia. J Nucl Med 37: 1023-31

Bentzen L, Keiding S, Horsman MR, Gronroos T, Hansen SB, Overgaard J (2002) Assessment of hypoxia in experimental mice tumours by [18F]fluoromisonidazole PET and pO2 electrode measurements. Influence of tumour volume and carbogen breathing. Acta Oncol 41: 304-12

Bhattacharya A, Toth K, Mazurchuk R, Spernyak JA, Slocum HK, Pendyala L, Azrak R, Cao S, Durrani FA, Rustum YM (2004) Lack of microvessels in well-differentiated regions of human head and neck squamous cell carcinoma A253 associated with functional magnetic resonance imaging detectable hypoxia, limited drug delivery, and resistance to irinotecan therapy. Clin Cancer Res 10: 8005-17

Brizel DM, Scully SP, Harrelson JM, Layfield LJ, Bean JM, Prosnitz LR, Dewhirst MW (1996) Tumour oxygenation predicts for the likelihood of distant metastases in human soft tissue sarcoma. Cancer Res 56: 941-3

Brouwers A, Verel I, Van Eerd J, Visser G, Steffens M, Oosterwijk E, Corstens F, Oyen W, Van Dongen G, Boerman O (2004) PET radioimmunoscintigraphy of renal cell cancer using 89Zr-labeled cG250 monoclonal antibody in nude rats. Cancer Biother Radiopharm 19: 155-63

Brown JM (2000) Exploiting the hypoxic cancer cell: mechanisms and therapeutic strategies. Mol Med Today 6: 157-62

Brurberg KG, Graff BA, Rofstad EK (2003) Temporal heterogeneity in oxygen tension in human melanoma xenografts. Br J Cancer 89: 350-6

Busch TM, Hahn SM, Evans SM, Koch CJ (2000) Depletion of tumour oxygenation during photodynamic therapy: detection by the hypoxia marker EF3 [2-(2-nitroimidazol-1[H]-yl)-N-(3,3,3-trifluoropropyl)acetamide]. Cancer Res 60: 2636-42

Busk M, Horsman MR, Jakobsen S, Bussink J, van der Kogel A, Overgaard J (2008) Cellular uptake of PET tracers of glucose metabolism and hypoxia and their linkage. Eur J Nucl Med Mol Imaging 35: 2294-303

Bussink J, van Herpen CM, Kaanders JH, Oyen WJ (2010) PET-CT for response assessment and treatment adaptation in head and neck cancer. Lancet Oncol 11: 661-9

Cherk MH, Foo SS, Poon AM, Knight SR, Murone C, Papenfuss AT, Sachinidis JI, Saunder TH, O'Keefe GJ, Scott AM (2006) Lack of correlation of hypoxic cell fraction and angiogenesis with glucose metabolic rate in non-small cell lung cancer assessed by 18F-Fluoromisonidazole and 18F-FDG PET. J Nucl Med 47: 1921-6

Choi W, Lee SW, Park SH, Ryu JS, Oh SJ, Im KC, Choi EK, Kim JH, Jung SH, Kim S,

Ahn SD (2010) Planning study for available dose of hypoxic tumour volume using fluorine-18-labeled fluoromisonidazole positron emission tomography for treatment of the head and neck cancer. Radiother Oncol 97(2):176-82.

Chopra S, Foltz WD, Milosevic MF, Toi A, Bristow RG, Menard C, Haider MA (2009) Comparing oxygen-sensitive MRI (BOLD R2*) with oxygen electrode measurements: a pilot study in men with prostate cancer. Int J Radiat Biol 85: 805-13

Davda S, Bezabeh T (2006) Advances in methods for assessing tumour hypoxia in vivo: implications for treatment planning. Cancer Metastasis Rev 25: 469-80

Dearling JL, Packard AB (2010) Some thoughts on the mechanism of cellular trapping of Cu(II)-ATSM. Nucl Med Biol 37: 237-43

Dehdashti F, Grigsby PW, Lewis JS, Laforest R, Siegel BA, Welch MJ (2008) Assessing tumour hypoxia in cervical cancer by PET with 60Cu-labeled diacetyl-bis(N4-methylthiosemicarbazone). J Nucl Med 49: 201-5

Dehdashti F, Mintun MA, Lewis JS, Bradley J, Govindan R, Laforest R, Welch MJ, Siegel BA (2003) In vivo assessment of tumour hypoxia in lung cancer with 60Cu-ATSM. Eur J Nucl Med Mol Imaging 30: 844-50

Dence CS, Ponde DE, Welch MJ, Lewis JS (2008) Autoradiographic and small-animal PET comparisons between (18)F-FMISO, (18)F-FDG, (18)F-FLT and the hypoxic selective (64)Cu-ATSM in a rodent model of cancer. Nucl Med Biol 35: 713-20

Dierckx RA, Van de Wiele C (2008) FDG uptake, a surrogate of tumour hypoxia? Eur J Nucl Med Mol Imaging 35: 1544-9

Divgi CR, Pandit-Taskar N, Jungbluth AA, Reuter VE, Gonen M, Ruan S, Pierre C, Nagel A, Pryma DA, Humm J, Larson SM, Old LJ, Russo P (2007) Preoperative characterization of clear-cell renal carcinoma using iodine-124-labelled antibody chimeric G250 (124I-cG250) and PET in patients with renal masses: a phase I trial. Lancet Oncol 8: 304-10

Doss M, Zhang JJ, Belanger MJ, Stubbs JB, Hostetler ED, Alpaugh K, Kolb HC, Yu JQ (2010) Biodistribution and radiation dosimetry of the hypoxia marker 18F-HX4 in monkeys and humans determined by using whole-body PET/CT. Nucl Med Commun 31(12):1016-24.

Dubois L, Douma K, Supuran CT, Chiu RK, van Zandvoort MA, Pastorekova S, Scozzafava A, Wouters BG, Lambin P (2007) Imaging the hypoxia surrogate marker CA IX requires expression and catalytic activity for binding fluorescent sulfonamide inhibitors. Radiother Oncol 83: 367-73

Dubois L, Landuyt W, Cloetens L, Bol A, Bormans G, Haustermans K, Labar D, Nuyts J, Gregoire V, Mortelmans L (2009a) [18F]EF3 is not superior to [18F]FMISO for PET-based hypoxia evaluation as measured in a rat rhabdomyosarcoma tumour model. Eur J Nucl Med Mol Imaging 36: 209-18

Dubois L, Landuyt W, Haustermans K, Dupont P, Bormans G, Vermaelen P, Flamen P, Verbeken E, Mortelmans L (2004) Evaluation of hypoxia in an experimental rat tumour model by [(18)F]fluoromisonidazole PET and immunohistochemistry. Br J Cancer 91: 1947-54.

Dubois LJ, Lieuwes NG, Janssen MH, Peeters WJ, Windhorst AD, Walsh JC, Kolb HC, Ollers MC, Bussink J, van Dongen GA, van der Kogel A, Lambin P. (2011) Preclinical evaluation and validation of [18F]HX4, a promising hypoxia marker for PET imaging. Proc Natl Acad Sci U S A. 2011 Aug 30;108(35):14620-5. Epub 2011 Aug 23.

Dubois L, Lieuwes NG, Maresca A, Thiry A, Supuran CT, Scozzafava A, Wouters BG, Lambin P (2009b) Imaging of CA IX with fluorescent labelled sulfonamides distinguishes hypoxic and (re)-oxygenated cells in a xenograft tumour model. Radiother Oncol 92: 423-8

Duong TQ, Iadecola C, Kim SG (2001) Effect of hyperoxia, hypercapnia, and hypoxia on cerebral interstitial oxygen tension and cerebral blood flow. Magn Reson Med 45: 61-70

Eschmann SM, Paulsen F, Reimold M, Dittmann H, Welz S, Reischl G, Machulla HJ, Bares R (2005) Prognostic impact of hypoxia imaging with 18F-misonidazole PET in non-small cell lung cancer and head and neck cancer before radiotherapy. J Nucl Med 46: 253-60

Evans SM, Joiner B, Jenkins WT, Laughlin KM, Lord EM, Koch CJ (1995) Identification of hypoxia in cells and tissues of epigastric 9L rat glioma using EF5 [2-(2-nitro-1H-imidazol-1-yl)-N-(2,2,3,3,3-pentafluoropropyl) acetamide]. Br J Cancer 72: 875-82

Evans SM, Kachur AV, Shiue CY, Hustinx R, Jenkins WT, Shive GG, Karp JS, Alavi A, Lord EM, Dolbier WR, Jr., Koch CJ (2000) Noninvasive detection of tumour hypoxia using the 2-nitroimidazole [18F]EF1. J Nucl Med 41: 327-36

Gagel B, Reinartz P, Demirel C, Kaiser HJ, Zimny M, Piroth M, Pinkawa M, Stanzel S, Asadpour B, Hamacher K, Coenen HH, Buell U, Eble MJ (2006) [18F] fluoromisonidazole and [18F] fluorodeoxyglucose positron emission tomography in response evaluation after chemo-/radiotherapy of non-small-cell lung cancer: a feasibility study. BMC Cancer 6: 51

Gronroos T, Bentzen L, Marjamaki P, Murata R, Horsman MR, Keiding S, Eskola O, Haaparanta M, Minn H, Solin O (2004) Comparison of the biodistribution of two hypoxia markers [18F]FETNIM and [18F]FMISO in an experimental mammary carcinoma. Eur J Nucl Med Mol Imaging 31: 513-20

Gronroos T, Eskola O, Lehtio K, Minn H, Marjamaki P, Bergman J, Haaparanta M, Forsback S, Solin O (2001) Pharmacokinetics of [18F]FETNIM: a potential marker for PET. J Nucl Med 42: 1397-404

He F, Deng X, Wen B, Liu Y, Sun X, Xing L, Minami A, Huang Y, Chen Q, Zanzonico PB, Ling CC, Li GC (2008) Noninvasive molecular imaging of hypoxia in human xenografts: comparing hypoxia-induced gene expression with endogenous and exogenous hypoxia markers. Cancer Res 68: 8597-606

Hockel M, Schlenger K, Aral B, Mitze M, Schaffer U, Vaupel P (1996) Association between tumour hypoxia and malignant progression in advanced cancer of the uterine cervix. Cancer Res 56: 4509-15

Hoeben BA, Kaanders JH, Franssen GM, Troost EG, Rijken PF, Oosterwijk E, van Dongen GA, Oyen WJ, Boerman OC, Bussink J (2010) PET of hypoxia with 89Zr-labeled cG250-F(ab')2 in head and neck tumours. J Nucl Med 51: 1076-83

Hoebers FJ, Janssen HL, Olmos AV, Sprong D, Nunn AD, Balm AJ, Hoefnagel CA, Begg AC, Haustermans KM (2002) Phase 1 study to identify tumour hypoxia in patients with head and neck cancer using technetium-99m BRU 59-21. Eur J Nucl Med Mol Imaging 29: 1206-11

Honess DJ, Hill SA, Collingridge DR, Edwards B, Brauers G, Powell NA, Chaplin DJ (1998) Preclinical evaluation of the novel hypoxic marker 99mTc-HL91 (Prognox) in murine and xenograft systems in vivo. Int J Radiat Oncol Biol Phys 42: 731-5

Hoskin PJ, Carnell DM, Taylor NJ, Smith RE, Stirling JJ, Daley FM, Saunders MI, Bentzen SM, Collins DJ, d'Arcy JA, Padhani AP (2007) Hypoxia in prostate cancer: correlation of BOLD-MRI with pimonidazole immunohistochemistry-initial observations. Int J Radiat Oncol Biol Phys 68: 1065-71

Howe FA, Robinson SP, McIntyre DJ, Stubbs M, Griffiths JR (2001) Issues in flow and oxygenation dependent contrast (FLOOD) imaging of tumours. NMR Biomed 14: 497-506

Hunjan S, Zhao D, Constantinescu A, Hahn EW, Antich PP, Mason RP (2001) Tumour oximetry: demonstration of an enhanced dynamic mapping procedure using fluorine-19 echo planar magnetic resonance imaging in the Dunning prostate R3327-AT1 rat tumour. Int J Radiat Oncol Biol Phys 49: 1097-108

Jenkins WT, Evans SM, Koch CJ (2000) Hypoxia and necrosis in rat 9L glioma and Morris 7777 hepatoma tumours: comparative measurements using EF5 binding and the Eppendorf needle electrode. Int J Radiat Oncol Biol Phys 46: 1005-17

Jones T (1996) The imaging science of positron emission tomography. Eur J Nucl Med 23: 807-13

Josse O, Labar D, Georges B, Gregoire V, Marchand-Brynaert J (2001) Synthesis of [18F]-labelled EF3 [2-(2-nitroimidazol-1-yl)-N-(3,3,3-trifluoropropyl)-acetamide], a marker for PET detection of hypoxia. Bioorg Med Chem 9: 665-75

Kaanders JH, Wijffels KI, Marres HA, Ljungkvist AS, Pop LA, van den Hoogen FJ, de Wilde PC, Bussink J, Raleigh JA, van der Kogel AJ (2002) Pimonidazole binding and tumour vascularity predict for treatment outcome in head and neck cancer. Cancer Res 62: 7066-74

Kinuya S, Yokoyama K, Li XF, Bai J, Watanabe N, Shuke N, Takayama T, Bunko H, Michigishi T, Tonami N (2002) Hypoxia-induced alteration of tracer accumulation in cultured cancer cells and xenografts in mice: implications for pre-therapeutic prediction of treatment outcomes with (99m)Tc-sestamibi, (201)Tl chloride and (99m)Tc-HL91. Eur J Nucl Med Mol Imaging 29: 1006-11

Koch CJ (2002) Measurement of absolute oxygen levels in cells and tissues using oxygen sensors and 2-nitroimidazole EF5. Methods Enzymol 352: 3-31

Koch CJ, Scheuermann JS, Divgi C, Judy KD, Kachur AV, Freifelder R, Reddin JS, Karp J, Stubbs JB, Hahn SM, Driesbaugh J, Smith D, Prendergast S, Evans SM (2010) Biodistribution and dosimetry of (18)F-EF5 in cancer patients with preliminary comparison of (18)F-EF5 uptake versus EF5 binding in human glioblastoma. Eur J Nucl Med Mol Imaging 37: 2048-59

Kolb HC, Finn MG, Sharpless KB (2001) Click Chemistry: Diverse Chemical Function from a Few Good Reactions. Angew Chem Int Ed Engl 40: 2004-2021

Komar G, Seppanen M, Eskola O, Lindholm P, Gronroos TJ, Forsback S, Sipila H,

Evans SM, Solin O, Minn H (2008) 18F-EF5: a new PET tracer for imaging hypoxia in head and neck cancer. J Nucl Med 49: 1944-51

Krohn KA, Link JM, Mason RP (2008) Molecular imaging of hypoxia. J Nucl Med 49 Suppl 2: 129S-48S

Lawrentschuk N, Lee FT, Jones G, Rigopoulos A, Mountain A, O'Keefe G, Papenfuss AT, Bolton DM, Davis ID, Scott AM (2011) Investigation of hypoxia and carbonic anhydrase IX expression in a renal cell carcinoma xenograft model with oxygen tension measurements and (124)I-cG250 PET/CT. Urol Oncol 29(4):411-20.

Lee BF, Chiu NT, Hsia CC, Shen LH (2008a) Accumulation of Tc-99m HL91 in tumour hypoxia: in vitro cell culture and in vivo tumour model. Kaohsiung J Med Sci 24: 461-72

Lee NY, Mechalakos JG, Nehmeh S, Lin Z, Squire OD, Cai S, Chan K, Zanzonico PB, Greco C, Ling CC, Humm JL, Schoder H (2008b) Fluorine-18-labeled fluoromisoni-dazole positron emission and computed tomography-guided intensity-modulated radiotherapy for head and neck cancer: a feasibility study. Int J Radiat Oncol Biol Phys 70: 2-13

Lee ST, Scott AM (2007) Hypoxia positron emission tomography imaging with 18f-fluo-romisonidazole. Semin Nucl Med 37: 451-61

Lewis JS, Laforest R, Dehdashti F, Grigsby PW, Welch MJ, Siegel BA (2008) An imaging comparison of 64Cu-ATSM and 60Cu-ATSM in cancer of the uterine cervix. J Nucl Med 49: 1177-82

Li L, Hu M, Zhu H, Zhao W, Yang G, Yu J (2010) Comparison of 18F-Fluoroerythronitro-imidazole and 18F-fluorodeoxyglucose positron emission tomography and prognostic value in locally advanced non-small-cell lung cancer. Clin Lung Cancer 11: 335-40

Li L, Yu J, Xing L, Ma K, Zhu H, Guo H, Sun X, Li J, Yang G, Li W, Yue J, Li B (2006) Serial hypoxia imaging with 99mTc-HL91 SPECT to predict radiotherapy response in nonsmall cell lung cancer. Am J Clin Oncol 29: 628-33

Lin Z, Mechalakos J, Nehmeh S, Schoder H, Lee N, Humm J, Ling CC (2008) The influence of changes in tumour hypoxia on dose-painting treatment plans based on 18F-FMISO positron emission tomography. Int J Radiat Oncol Biol Phys 70: 1219-28

Mahy P, De Bast M, de Groot T, Cheguillaume A, Gillart J, Haustermans K, Labar D, Gregoire V (2008a) Comparative pharmacokinetics, biodistribution, metabolism and hypoxia-dependent uptake of [18F]-EF3 and [18F]-MISO in rodent tumour models. Radiother Oncol 89: 353-60

Mahy P, De Bast M, Leveque PH, Gillart J, Labar D, Marchand J, Gregoire V (2004) Preclinical validation of the hypoxia tracer 2-(2-nitroimidazol-1-yl)- N-(3,3,3-[(18)F] trifluoropropyl)acetamide, [(18)F]EF3. Eur J Nucl Med Mol Imaging 31: 1263-72

Mahy P, Geets X, Lonneux M, Leveque P, Christian N, De Bast M, Gillart J, Labar D, Lee J, Gregoire V (2008b) Determination of tumour hypoxia with [18F]EF3 in patients with head and neck tumours: a phase I study to assess the tracer pharmacokinetics, biodistribution and metabolism. Eur J Nucl Med Mol Imaging 35: 1282-9

McPhail LD, Robinson SP (2010) Intrinsic susceptibility MR imaging of chemically induced rat mammary tumours: relationship to histologic assessment of hypoxia and fibrosis. Radiology 254: 110-8

Melo T, Duncan J, Ballinger JR, Rauth AM (2000) BRU59-21, a second-generation 99mTc-labeled 2-nitroimidazole for imaging hypoxia in tumours. J Nucl Med 41: 169-76

Nordsmark M, Overgaard J (2000) A confirmatory prognostic study on oxygenation status and loco-regional control in advanced head and neck squamous cell carcinoma treated by radiation therapy. Radiother Oncol 57: 39-43

Noth U, Rodrigues LM, Robinson SP, Jork A, Zimmermann U, Newell B, Griffiths JR (2004) In vivo determination of tumour oxygenation during growth and in response to carbogen breathing using 15C5-loaded alginate capsules as fluorine-19 magnetic resonance imaging oxygen sensors. Int J Radiat Oncol Biol Phys 60: 909-19

Ogawa S, Lee TM, Nayak AS, Glynn P (1990) Oxygenation-sensitive contrast in magnetic resonance image of rodent brain at high magnetic fields. Magn Reson Med 14: 68-78

Oriuchi N, Higuchi T, Ishikita T, Miyakubo M, Hanaoka H, Iida Y, Endo K (2006) Present role and future prospects of positron emission tomography in clinical oncology. Cancer Sci 97: 1291-7

Padhani A (2010) Science to practice: what does MR oxygenation imaging tell us about human breast cancer hypoxia? Radiology 254: 1-3

Padhani AR, Krohn KA, Lewis JS, Alber M (2007) Imaging oxygenation of human tumours. Eur Radiol 17: 861-72

Parhami P, Fung BM (1983) Fluorine-19 relaxation study of perfluoro chemicals as oxygen carriers. The Journal of Physical Chemistry 87: 1928-1931

Parliament MB, Chapman JD, Urtasun RC, McEwan AJ, Golberg L, Mercer JR, Mannan RH, Wiebe LI (1992) Non-invasive assessment of human tumour hypoxia with 123I-iodoazomycin arabinoside: preliminary report of a clinical study. Br J Cancer 65: 90-5

Patton JA, Turkington TG (2008) SPECT/CT physical principles and attenuation correction. J Nucl Med Technol 36: 1-10

Piert M, Machulla H, Becker G, Stahlschmidt A, Patt M, Aldinger P, Dissmann PD, Fischer H, Bares R, Becker HD, Lauchart W (1999) Introducing fluorine-18 fluoromisonidazole positron emission tomography for the localisation and quantification of pig liver hypoxia. Eur J Nucl Med 26: 95-109

Piert M, Machulla HJ, Becker G, Aldinger P, Winter E, Bares R (2000) Dependency of the [18F]fluoromisonidazole uptake on oxygen delivery and tissue oxygenation in the porcine liver. Nucl Med Biol 27: 693-700

Piert M, Machulla HJ, Picchio M, Reischl G, Ziegler S, Kumar P, Wester HJ, Beck R, McEwan AJ, Wiebe LI, Schwaiger M (2005) Hypoxia-specific tumour imaging with 18F-fluoroazomycin arabinoside. J Nucl Med 46: 106-13

Postema EJ, McEwan AJ, Riauka TA, Kumar P, Richmond DA, Abrams DN, Wiebe LI (2009) Initial results of hypoxia imaging using 1-alpha-D: -(5-deoxy-5-[18F]-fluoroarabinofuranosyl)-2-nitroimidazole (18F-FAZA). Eur J Nucl Med Mol Imaging 36: 1565-73

Potter C, Harris AL (2004) Hypoxia inducible carbonic anhydrase IX, marker of tumour hypoxia, survival pathway and therapy target. Cell Cycle 3: 164-7

Rajendran JG, Schwartz DL, O'Sullivan J, Peterson LM, Ng P, Scharnhorst J, Grierson JR, Krohn KA (2006) Tumour hypoxia imaging with [F-18] fluoromisonidazole positron emission tomography in head and neck cancer. Clin Cancer Res 12: 5435-41

Rasey JS, Hofstrand PD, Chin LK, Tewson TJ (1999) Characterization of [18F]fluoroetanidazole, a new radiopharmaceutical for detecting tumour hypoxia. J Nucl Med 40: 1072-9

Rasey JS, Koh WJ, Evans ML, Peterson LM, Lewellen TK, Graham MM, Krohn KA (1996) Quantifying regional hypoxia in human tumours with positron emission tomography of [18F]fluoromisonidazole: a pretherapy study of 37 patients. Int J Radiat Oncol Biol Phys 36: 417-28

Reischl G, Dorow DS, Cullinane C, Katsifis A, Roselt P, Binns D, Hicks RJ (2007) Imaging of tumour hypoxia with [124I]IAZA in comparison with [18F]FMISO and [18F] FAZA–first small animal PET results. J Pharm Pharm Sci 10: 203-11

Robinson SP, Griffiths JR (2004) Current issues in the utility of 19F nuclear magnetic resonance methodologies for the assessment of tumour hypoxia. Philos Trans R Soc Lond B Biol Sci 359: 987-96

Saitoh J, Sakurai H, Suzuki Y, Muramatsu H, Ishikawa H, Kitamoto Y, Akimoto T, Hasegawa M, Mitsuhashi N, Nakano T (2002) Correlations between in vivo tumour weight, oxygen pressure, 31P NMR spectroscopy, hypoxic microenvironment marking by beta-D-iodinated azomycin galactopyranoside (beta-D-IAZGP), and radiation sensitivity. Int J Radiat Oncol Biol Phys 54: 903-9

Seddon BM, Payne GS, Simmons L, Ruddle R, Grimshaw R, Tan S, Turner A, Raynaud F, Halbert G, Leach MO, Judson I, Workman P (2003) A phase I study of SR-4554 via intravenous administration for noninvasive investigation of tumour hypoxia by magnetic resonance spectroscopy in patients with malignancy. Clin Cancer Res 9: 5101-12

Sorger D, Patt M, Kumar P, Wiebe LI, Barthel H, Seese A, Dannenberg C, Tannapfel A, Kluge R, Sabri O (2003) [18F]Fluoroazomycinarabinofuranoside (18FAZA) and [18F]Fluoromisonidazole (18FMISO): a comparative study of their selective uptake in hypoxic cells and PET imaging in experimental rat tumours. Nucl Med Biol 30: 317-26

Souvatzoglou M, Grosu AL, Roper B, Krause BJ, Beck R, Reischl G, Picchio M, Machulla HJ, Wester HJ, Piert M (2007) Tumour hypoxia imaging with [18F]FAZA PET in head and neck cancer patients: a pilot study. Eur J Nucl Med Mol Imaging 34: 1566-75

Supuran CT (2008) Carbonic anhydrases: novel therapeutic applications for inhibitors and activators. Nat Rev Drug Discov 7: 168-81

Takasawa M, Beech JS, Fryer TD, Hong YT, Hughes JL, Igase K, Jones PS, Smith R, Aigbirhio FI, Menon DK, Clark JC, Baron JC (2007) Imaging of brain hypoxia in permanent and temporary middle cerebral artery occlusion in the rat using 18F-fluoromisonidazole and positron emission tomography: a pilot study. J Cereb Blood Flow Metab 27: 679-89

Thorwarth D, Eschmann SM, Holzner F, Paulsen F, Alber M (2006) Combined uptake of [18F]FDG and [18F]FMISO correlates with radiation therapy outcome in head-and-neck cancer patients. Radiother Oncol 80: 151-6

Tochon-Danguy HJ, Sachinidis JI, Chan F, Chan JG, Hall C, Cher L, Stylli S, Hill J, Kaye A, Scott AM (2002) Imaging and quantitation of the hypoxic cell fraction of viable tumour in an animal model of intracerebral high grade glioma using [18F] fluoromisonidazole (FMISO). Nucl Med Biol 29: 191-7

Tolvanen T, Lehtio K, Kulmala J, Oikonen V, Eskola O, Bergman J, Minn H (2002) 18F-Fluoroerythronitroimidazole radiation dosimetry in cancer studies. J Nucl Med 43: 1674-80

Troost EG, Laverman P, Kaanders JH, Philippens M, Lok J, Oyen WJ, van der Kogel AJ, Boerman OC, Bussink J (2006) Imaging hypoxia after oxygenation-modification: comparing [18F]FMISO autoradiography with pimonidazole immunohisto-chemistry in human xenograft tumours. Radiother Oncol 80: 157-64

Troost EG, Laverman P, Philippens ME, Lok J, van der Kogel AJ, Oyen WJ, Boerman OC, Kaanders JH, Bussink J (2008) Correlation of [18F]FMISO autoradiography and pimonidazole [corrected] immunohistochemistry in human head and neck carcinoma xenografts. Eur J Nucl Med Mol Imaging 35: 1803-11

Urtasun RC, Parliament MB, McEwan AJ, Mercer JR, Mannan RH, Wiebe LI, Morin C, Chapman JD (1996) Measurement of hypoxia in human tumours by non-invasive spect imaging of iodoazomycin arabinoside. Br J Cancer Suppl 27: S209-12

van der Sanden BP, Heerschap A, Simonetti AW, Rijken PF, Peters HP, Stuben G, van der Kogel AJ (1999) Characterization and validation of noninvasive oxygen tension measurements in human glioma xenografts by 19F-MR relaxometry. Int J Radiat Oncol Biol Phys 44: 649-58

van Loon J, Janssen MH, Ollers M, Aerts HJ, Dubois L, Hochstenbag M, Dingemans AM, Lalisang R, Brans B, Windhorst B, van Dongen GA, Kolb H, Zhang J, De Ruysscher D, Lambin P (2010) PET imaging of hypoxia using [18F]HX4: a phase I trial. Eur J Nucl Med Mol Imaging 37: 1663-8

Vavere AL, Lewis JS (2007) Cu-ATSM: a radiopharmaceutical for the PET imaging of hypoxia. Dalton Trans: 4893-902

Vikram DS, Zweier JL, Kuppusamy P (2007) Methods for noninvasive imaging of tissue hypoxia. Antioxid Redox Signal 9: 1745-56

Wyss MT, Honer M, Schubiger PA, Ametamey SM (2006) NanoPET imaging of [(18)F] fluoromisonidazole uptake in experimental mouse tumours. Eur J Nucl Med Mol Imaging 33: 311-8

Yuan H, Schroeder T, Bowsher JE, Hedlund LW, Wong T, Dewhirst MW (2006) Inter-tumoural differences in hypoxia selectivity of the PET imaging agent 64Cu(II)-diacetyl-bis(N4-methylthiosemicarbazone). J Nucl Med 47: 989-98

Zanzonico P, Campa J, Polycarpe-Holman D, Forster G, Finn R, Larson S, Humm J, Ling C (2006) Animal-specific positioning molds for registration of repeat imaging studies: comparative microPET imaging of F18-labeled fluoro-deoxyglucose and fluoro-misonidazole in rodent tumours. Nucl Med Biol 33: 65-70

Zhang X, Melo T, Ballinger JR, Rauth AM (1998) Studies of 99mTc-BnAO (HL-91): a non-nitroaromatic compound for hypoxic cell detection. Int J Radiat Oncol Biol Phys 42: 737-40

Zhang X, Melo T, Rauth AM, Ballinger JR (2001) Cellular accumulation and retention of the technetium-99m-labelled hypoxia markers BRU59-21 and butylene amine oxime. Nucl Med Biol 28: 949-57

Zhao D, Constantinescu A, Chang CH, Hahn EW, Mason RP (2003) Correlation of tumour oxygen dynamics with radiation response of the dunning prostate R3327-HI tumour. Radiat Res 159: 621-31

Ziemer LS, Evans SM, Kachur AV, Shuman AL, Cardi CA, Jenkins WT, Karp JS, Alavi A, Dolbier WR, Jr., Koch CJ (2003) Noninvasive imaging of tumour hypoxia in rats using the 2-nitroimidazole 18F-EF5. Eur J Nucl Med Mol Imaging 30: 259-66

Zimny M, Gagel B, DiMartino E, Hamacher K, Coenen HH, Westhofen M, Eble M, Buell U, Reinartz P (2006) FDG–a marker of tumour hypoxia? A comparison with [18F]fluoromisonidazole and pO2-polarography in metastatic head and neck cancer. Eur J Nucl Med Mol Imaging 33: 1426-31

Chapter 16

Hypoxia, hypoxia response and conventional anti-cancer therapy

Bart Reymen[*] and Philippe Lambin

[*]Author for correspondence:
Department of Radiotherapy, Maastricht University Medical Center/University Maastricht/
MAASTRO clinic/ GROW/ Maastricht 6229 ET, The Netherlands
Phone: 0031/884455666, E-mail: bart.reymen@maastro.nl

Contents

Key points

— Hypoxia and hypoxia response are not synonyms.

— Both the presence of hypoxia and the cellular response to hypoxia impact tumour control and survival after conventional anti-cancer treatment.

— The "hypoxic cellular response" is neither exclusive nor specific to the presence of hypoxia in tumours. The perfect hypoxic biomarker does not yet exist.

— In studies using hypoxia or "hypoxic biomarkers" as a surrogate for hypoxia, prognostic significance is often lost in multi-variate analysis. This emphasizes the reciprocal relationship of hypoxia and tumour phenotype.

Introduction

It has been known since the mid 1950`s that tumours display a varying amount of hypoxia. Depending on the histology, in up to almost 70 % of malignant tumours a certain degree of hypoxia can be found (Chapman 1991). Under hypoxic conditions tumour cells have been demonstrated *in vitro* and *in vivo* to exhibit greater therapy resistance than in normoxic conditions.

Not only radioresistance, but also chemoresistance and resistance to anti-hormonal therapy have been demonstrated (Gray et al. 1953; Dewey 1960; Gray 1961; Teicher et al. 1981). The mechanisms by which hypoxic cells become resistant to therapy are multifold and intertwined and therefore difficult to unravel.

Malignant tumours are hampered in their development by nutrient supply, which is diffusion limited. In order to fulfil their metabolic needs, neo-angiogenesis is initiated by up-regulation of genes encoding products like VEGF, PDGF, Notch etc, resulting in a chaotic and typically deficient vasculature still leaving areas of the tumour underperfused. This lack of perfusion not only renders cells in these areas hypoxic, but apart from less oxygen and other nutrients reaching the tumour cells, also chemotherapy or anti-hormonal therapy is less likely to reach these cells in lethal concentrations.

Moreover, a typical defence mechanism of cells, which lack nutrients, is to slow-down their cell cycle, making them less susceptible to DNA damage by conventional cancer therapy. (Liu et al., 2010) Furthermore, cells which are in metabolic jeopardy rely on mechanisms such as autophagy to remove cell organelles damaged by therapy, thereby creating a win-win situation for themselves: using damage by anti-cancer therapy otherwise leading to cell death as a source of energy (Degenhardt et al. 2006).

A lack of oxygen also means the following: radiotherapy is hypothesized to deliver indirect damage to cell DNA by free radicals caused by the ionisation of oxygen in well-oxygenated areas. Obviously, in hypoxic conditions this type of damage is less likely to occur (Rockwell et al. 2009).

In response to hypoxia, numerous genes are up-regulated or mutated to ensure survival of cancer cells like Hif-1α, which regulates numerous gene products such as multi-drug resistance (MDR) genes, ensuring an increased efflux of cytotoxic drugs from the cells, giving yet another explanation for the influence of hypoxia on chemoresistance. Other factors activated by hypoxia include Snail, which has also been linked to chemoresistance through upregulated DNA repair (Hsu et al. 2010).

Furthermore, hypoxia drives cells towards an epithelial-to-mesenchymal transition (EMT), resulting in a more aggressive, metastasis-prone phenotype, which inevitably impacts the metastasis-free and overall survival rate of patients solely treated locally. (Klymkowsky and Savagner 2009)

In the following chapter we will briefly describe the current evidence in humans for the main tumour types, which have been studied over the past decades.

One of the main problems researchers investigating tumour hypoxia are facing is the difficulty in demonstrating their subject of study. The electrode measurements pioneered in the 1980's are widely considered as the gold standard as they are the only way of directly measuring hypoxia and are able to demonstrate regional differences in oxygenation of the tumour. However, these instruments are not suited to map the incredible variation in oxygenation which can occur over extremely small distances (Helmlinger et al. 1997). Furthermore, due to the invasive nature of the technique, not every tumour-bearing site is apt for these kinds of measurements. Therefore, surrogate techniques have been sought, mainly aiming at visualizing the hypoxic response of cells.

When confronted with changes in the microenvironment, tumour cells exhibit a response characterized by the upregulation of certain genes and the activation of numerous survival pathways. The most intensively studied of these pathways were discussed more extensively earlier on in this book. The gene products related to this stress response can either be demonstrated immunohistochemically or can be retrieved in the blood. Examples are the HIF-1α pathway, CA IX, osteopontin and GLUT-1.

We will refer to these products as "biomarkers" in this chapter, recognizing the fact that none of the products mentioned are truly specific for hypoxia, as numerous genes interfere with these pathways or can also be upregulated in normoxic conditions.

Finally, another way of demonstrating the hypoxic response is by using non-invasive imaging modalities of which the nitroimidazoles are the most known and most studied option. The basic principle of all these imaging compounds is the coupling of a radio-active PET-tracer to a molecule which is preferably taken up by the tumour cells in hypoxic circumstances. The downside to these tracers is the fact that the pathways which regulate the uptake of the tracers are also activated in conditions other than hypoxia.

Bearing these limitations of the different techniques in mind, distinction will be made according to the way hypoxia (direct measurement of pO_2) or the molecular response to hypoxia (indirect evidence of hypoxia) was evaluated.

Breast cancer

In the past decade, evidence for an adverse prognostic impact of hypoxia present in breast cancer has been accumulating.

Direct measurements of pO_2

Already in 1991 Vaupel et al performed polarographic measurements on breast tissue and demonstrated the presence of hypoxia in 40 % of breast cancer sites. (Vaupel et al. 1991). However, due to methodological issues, consequent doubts on the accuracy and reproducibility of these measurements and the invasive nature of the technique, large- scale investigations on the impact of hypoxia have not been performed in breast cancer using Eppendorf electrodes. Thus the largest body of evidence on the impact of hypoxia in breast cancer comes from measurement of hypoxic biomarkers.

Biomarker evidence

HIF-1α

The expression of transcription factor HIF-1α is one of the most widely investigated depictors of hypoxia in breast cancer. In all studies cited, the stabilization of HIF-1α is a negative prognostic factor for treatment response and survival. One of the first groups to study this effect was Schindl et al who investigated the histological samples of 206 patients with node positive breast cancer. Dividing the samples into 4 groups according to the magnitude of HIF-1 expression, they found a clear correlation between HIF-1 and overall survival which held up in multivariate analysis. (Schindl et al. 2002).

Bos et al. investigated the prognostic value of HIF-1α in a group of 150 patients with early stage breast cancer. HIF-1α expression in > 1% of cells was found in 75% of breast carcinomas and in node negative patients a staining level of > 5% of cells was found to correlate with significantly worse overall and disease free survival. This correlation was not found in node positive patients.(Bos et al. 2003).

In another study by Gruber et al HIF-1α overexpression was an unfavourable prognostic factor in T1 and T2 node positive breast cancer and had a negative impact on disease free survival and distant metastases free survival. In a small group of T3/4 patients this correlation was not found (Gruber et al. 2004). In the largest series of unselected breast cancer patients examined for HIF overexpression (>10 % of cells), Dales et al confirmed the negative impact on overall survival, disease free survival and metastasis free survival. However the HIF-1α prognostic significance in terms of over-all survival in the node-negative subset of patients reported by Bos et al could not be found. Interestingly, they showed that HIF-1α overexpression correlated strongly with early relapse (local relapse and distant metasta-sis) in all patients, including the node-negative subset. They also observed that HIF-1α expression was predictive of metastasis risk in all patients, including the node negative subgroup, which could help identify patients in need of a more intensive systemic treatment schedule who are passed by the current criteria for adjuvant therapy (Dales et al. 2005).

Vleugel et al stained 200 samples of unselected patients with invasive breast cancer and found a significantly worse disease free survival for patients with positive (>1% of cells) HIF-1α overexpression. Patients with diffuse staining fared better than patients with perinecrotic staining pat-terns. HIF-1α staining also correlated significantly with a more aggressive phenotype, CA IX and GLUT-1 expression (Vleugel et al. 2005).

Lastly, Trastour et al investigated specimens of 132 unselected patients with invasive breast cancer. HIF 1α and CA IX staining was more promi-nent in high grade tumours and was strongly correlated with worse DMFS and DFS in multivariate analysis, but not overall survival in this series. Interestingly these investigators also investigated the effect of positive HIF-1α on the response to adjuvant therapy and found a significantly nega-tive impact on the response to radiotherapy as well as chemotherapy. The same could not be proven for CA IX expression (Trastour et al. 2007).

Carbonic Anhydrase (CA IX)

Being a downstream target gene of HIF-1α, numerous groups have investi-gated the impact of an upregulation of CA IX on treatment results for breast cancer. Chia et al were the first to demonstrate CA IX expression to be asso-ciated with worse relapse-free survival and overall survival in an unselected cohort of 106 patients with invasive breast carcinoma (Figure 16.1). On multi-variate analysis CA IX expression and positive lymph node status were the only significant factors influencing survival, in the case of CA IX staining decreasing overall survival with a hazard ratio of 2.61 (Chia et al. 2001).

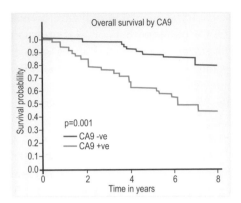

Figure 16.1 _ Adopted from Chia et al. 2001). Overall survival according to CA IX positivity of breast cancer.

Vleugel et al (2005), as mentioned above, also stained their tumour samples for CA IX and found positive staining in 12.5% of cases, mostly in the perinecrotic areas. Brennan et al investigated the expression of CA IX in a cohort of premenopausal breast cancer patients with stage II disease randomized between tamoxifen and placebo in a Swedish trial. They could not provide evidence for an effect of CA IX expression on tamoxifen response, possibly due to underpowerment. CA IX expression was associated with a worse disease free and overall survival however and was the only independent prognostic marker in patients with one to three positive lymph nodes, which led the authors to the assumption CA IX could be a putative marker for radiotherapy resistance as this was the only adjuvant treatment administered in these patients (Brennan et al. 2006).

Hussain et al investigated a cohort of 144 women with operable breast cancer of whom 37 were CA IX positive. CA IX positivity was an independent prognostic variable for 2 year overall survival, being 83 % vs 97% for CA IX negative patients. (Hussain et al. 2007). Tan et al did an interesting analysis of the material of 407 breast cancer patients, 49 of which were CA IX positive, showing that CA IX expression had a negative prognostic significance only in the group of patients treated with chemotherapy. In patients not treated with chemotherapy CA IX expression had no clear effect on survival (Tan et al. 2009). Kyndi et al performed a subgroup analysis on patients enrolled in the DBCG82b and c trials, evaluating CA IX expression on 945 surgical specimens of high-risk patients with breast cancer. Survival analysis showed that for the whole group CA IX expression was not predictive for survival and only in subgroup analyses did it infer a survival effect in premenopausal women with more than three positive lymph nodes, which contradicted the findings of Brennan et al. CA IX status did not have an effect on the results of post-mastectomy irradiation (Kyndi et al. 2008).

GLUT-1

GLUT-1 staining was first performed in 2002 on 100 unselected patients with breast cancer. On multivariate analysis disease free survival, but not overall survival was shown to be negatively influenced by GLUT-1 expression (Kang et al. 2002).

Vleugel et al also stained their aforementioned specimens for GLUT-1 and came to the conclusion that although GLUT-1, CA IX and HIF-1α were often present in the same cells, mainly in perinecrotic regions which was associated with a worse prognosis, the GLUT-1 overexpression also occurred frequently in a HIF-independent manner, showing GLUT-1 overexpression to also be regulated by other factors. Separate analyses on the influence of GLUT-1 on survival were not undertaken in this study (Vleugel et al. 2005).

Conclusion on breast cancer studies

Numerous studies have been performed on breast cancer patients, linking putative biomarkers for hypoxia to outcome after standard therapy (Table 16.1). Most of these studies have found a detrimental effect of the presence of hypoxic biomarkers in tissue samples of breast cancer patients. The major limitation of all of these studies is they are mainly retrospective, frequently apply subgroup analyses and the assays applied to the tissue are not standardized, which makes comparisons between different trials quite difficult.

However, be it subgroups of patients treated with surgery, chemotherapy, hormonal therapy or radiotherapy, a negative effect is found quite consistently. The main question to be answered remains the subgroups of patients for whom this effect exists and the magnitude of that effect.

Table 16.1 _ Overview of studies on breast cancer.

Authors	n	Therapy	Parameter	Prognostic significance (Univariate analysis)	Prognostic significance (Multivariate analysis)	Remarks
Schindl et al	206	Surgery + Tamoxifen +/- Chemo	HIF-1α	OS, DFS	OS, DFS	LN positive patients
Bos et al	150	Surgery	HIF-1α	OS, DFS	OS, DFS	valid for LN- patients only
Gruber et al	77	Surgery + Chemo + RT	HIF-1α	DFS, DMFS	DFS, DMFS	valid in sub-group of T1/T2
Dales et al	745	Surgery	HIF-1α	OS, MFS, LC	OS, MFS	Less pronounced in node negative patients
Vleugel et al	166	Surgery + Chemo	HIF-1α	DFS	Not performed	Diffuse pattern: better prognosis
Trastour et al	132	Surgery + RT /Chemo /Tamoxifen	HIF-1α	OS, DFS, DMFS	DFS, DMFS	Negative impact on adjuvant RT and CT
			CA IX	OS	DFS, DMFS	
Chia et al	103	Surgery + RT/ Chemo/Tamoxifen	CA IX	OS, RFS	OS	
Brennan et al	400	Surgery + RT /(chemo) /Tamoxifen	CA IX	OS, RFS, BCSS	BCSS	Only 2% chemotherapy, all pre-menopausal
						Subgroup analysis: 1-3 LN worse prognosis
Hussain et al	144	Surgery	CA IX	OS	OS	
Tan et al	407	Surgery	CA IX	DFS, OS	OS	Only in sub-group of pts treated with chemotherapy
Kyndi et al	945	Mastectomy + Chemotherapy +/- RT	CA IX	OS, DSS	Not significant	No effect on post-mastectomy irradiation

DFS, disease-free survival; OS, overall survival; DSS, disease-specific survival; DMFS, distant metastases-free survival; MFS, metastasis-free survival; BCSS, breast cancer-specific survival; RFS, relapse-free survival; RT, radiotherapy; CT, chemotherapy; LN, lymph nodes.

Lung cancer

Biomarker evidence

HIF-1α

In operable lung cancer patients, a lot of research has been done in examining the expression of HIF-α correlated with survival. Giatromanolaki et al examined specimens of 108 patients with operable lung cancer and 10 normal specimens operated for various reasons. HIF-1α and 2α staining in normal bronchial and alveolar epithelium was virtually absent, in contrast with cancer cells, which showed a wide variability of HIF-α expression. HIF-1α and 2α were significantly associated with the expression by cells of angiogenic factors (VEGF, PD-ECGF and bFGF) and with microvessel density (MVD) as a measure of angiogenic activity. In a multivariate analysis where all the examined factors were incorporated, only T-stage was associated with poorer survival, whereas HIF-1α and 2α were not, probably due to the strong association between all the examined factors, making it impossible to dissociate their effects. When considered separately, both HIF-2α and HIF-1α expression correlated to a worse prognosis (Giatromanolaki et al. 2001)

In their analysis of 84 specimens of operable lung cancer, Lee et al found different expression patterns of HIF-1α between squamous cell carcinoma (SCC) and adenocarcinoma (AC); HIF-1α being expressed in 66% of SCC versus 20% of AC. A prognostic value of HIF-1α expression could not be demonstrated in this series (Lee et al. 2003).

Kim et al collected a series of 74 resected stage I-II non-small cell lung cancers (NSCLC) and stained them for HIF-1α, CA IX, VEGF and MMP-9. They also evaluated the extent of tumour necrosis present. They showed a strong correlation of CA IX with HIF-1α and noticed a clear co-localization with CA IX in areas relative to the degree of necrosis present, showing strong expression of both markers in areas with moderate to severe tumour necrosis relative to areas with minimal necrosis. No significant relationship was found between VEGF-expression and MMP-9. On multivariate analysis only pathological stage and expression of CA IX above the median value inferred a worse prognosis (Kim et al. 2005).

Yohena et al used a PCR technique to examine the expression of mRNA coding for HIF-1α in tumour bearing tissue and adjacent tissue in 66 stage I, II or III resected NSCLC specimens. The expression level of HIF-1α mRNA was significantly higher in tumour tissue than in the adjacent lung tissue. In node-negative patients, high expression levels of HIF-1α mRNA in tumours were associated with a poor prognosis. This correlation was lost in the node-positive cases (Yohena et al. 2009).

Park et al retrospectively investigated the prognostic effect of HIF-1α overexpression relative to the EGFR status of NSCLC in 178 patients. In multivariate analysis only age group and stage were significantly associated with prognosis. However, when EGFR status was taken into account, HIF-1α expression along with age group and stage had a negative impact on prognosis, yet only in the EGFR-negative patients. The reasons for this association are as yet poorly understood (Park et al. 2011).

CA IX

In 2001 Giatromanolaki et al. examined the expression of CA IX in 107 samples of NSCLC. They showed that the staining of CA IX was mainly confined to areas of necrosis, was more common in cancers of squamous cell histology and advanced T-stage and was a prognostic factor independent of angiogenesis in multivariate analysis (Giatromanolaki et al. 2001).

Swinson et al investigated different patterns of CA IX expression in tissue samples of 175 patients with resected NSCLC. They found perinuclear (p) CA IX expression to be an independent prognostic variable, whereas membranous (m), cytoplasmic or stromal was not. pCA staining was only found in those cells with high mCA counts (Swinson et al. 2003).

Kim et al confirmed the negative prognostic impact of CA IX in resectable (stage I and II) NSCLC and found CA IX expression was higher in tumours with a higher proliferative index measured by Ki-67 expression and less micro-vessel density (Kim et al. 2004). Later on they established in a separate study that CA IX was a more reliable prognosticator than HIF-1α or MMP-9 in NSCLC (Kim et al. 2005).

A downside to CA IX expression was that it could only be assessed in operable patients. However, CA IX recently has been shown to be detectable in plasma. Therefore Ilie and colleagues assessed the prognostic value CA IX in plasma as well as in tissue samples of 209 patients with NSCLC and the plasma of 58 healthy individuals. The amount of CA IX found in plasma was significantly higher in the NSCLC patients and both tissue CA IX and plasma CA IX were independent prognostic variables for overall survival. The higher expression of CA IX in SCC reported by Kim et al was also confirmed in this series (Ilie et al. 2010).

Osteopontin (OPN)

Mack et al performed plasma testing for osteopontin in 172 NSCLC patients prior to the start of chemotherapy in the SWOG OO3 trial of carbopla-tin/paclitaxel with or without tirapazamine (TPZ) in stage IIIb or IV. OPN plasma level showed a highly significant association with both progression-free survival and overall survival, which was not the case for 2 other sampled markers, namely PA-I and VEGF. Interestingly, no significant association between the OPN plasma levels and immunohistochemically measured OPN tumour expression was found. The authors commented that this might be partly due to non-malignant cells (e.g. macrophages) contributing to plasma OPN concentrations (Mack et al. 2008).

Validation of these results was provided by Isa and colleagues who obtained samples from 67 patients prior to starting chemotherapy in a prospective randomized phase III trial investigating advanced non-small cell lung cancer comparing paclitaxel plus carboplatin versus vinorelbine, gemcitabine followed by docetaxel. Patients with low plasma levels of OPN (OPN levels below the median) showed significantly favourable OS and PFS (Isa et al. 2009).

Imaging: FETNIM/FDG/TC99/FMISO/Cu-ATSM

NSCLC is an interesting entity because of the large amount of patients unfit for surgery. This has prompted researchers to assess the presence of hypoxia with imaging instead of immunohistochemical analysis of tissue samples attained with difficulty. One of the earliest efforts to demonstrate hypoxia in NSCLC was made by Dehdasti et al., who investigated the feasibility of ^{60}Cu-ATSM PET scans to detect hypoxia in 19 patients with NSCLC. In all but one patient uptake was present in the tumour. They demonstrated a significantly lower tumour-to-muscle ratio in non-responders to therapy. The group also used ^{18}FDG-PET scans in the same population, but did not find a correlation between Cu-ATSM uptake and tumour SUV, nor between tumour SUV and response to therapy (Dehdashti et al. 2003).

These findings contrast with those of Van Baardwijk et al, who investigated the correlation between the uptake of ^{18}FDG and immunohistochemical staining for hypoxic markers GLUT-1, HIF-1α and CA IX in 102 patients with resected NSCLC stages I-III. Patients with a low SUV had a markedly better prognosis than those with a high SUV: 2-year survival of resp. 58.6% and 90.6% (p = 0.001), see Figure 16.2. Furthermore, a strong association

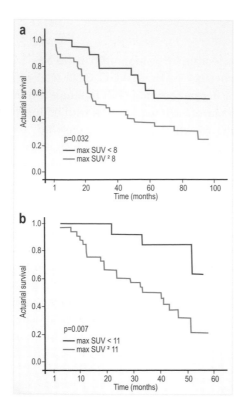

Figure 16.2 _ Actuarial survival curves for NSCLC with low vs high SUV (2 different centres using different cut-offs according to median SUV per centre). Taken from Van Baardwijk et al. (2007).

was found between expression of GLUT-1 and HIF-1α and SUV. Although a strong association was found between HIF-1α and CA IX, the association between CA IX and FDG-uptake was not significant (van Baardwijk et al. 2007).

Eschmann et al used [^{18}F]-FMISO PET scans to evaluate hypoxia in 14 patients with NSCLC. A tumour to mediastinum ratio of more than 2.0 proved predictive for tumour recurrence or progression after radiotherapy for NSCLC (Eschmann et al. 2005). An interesting study by Li et al used serial [^{99m}Tc]-HL91 SPECT scans to evaluate the evolution of the pattern of uptake during a radiotherapy course in 32 patients with stage IIIA and IIIB NSCLC. No concurrent chemotherapy was given; a subpopulation received either neo-adjuvant chemotherapy or adjuvant chemotherapy or a combination of both in a variety of schemes. Using a tumour/normal

(T/N) ratio of 1.47 to divide the group in a low-and high uptake cohort they found a significantly worse survival in the high uptake group with 1-year and 2-year survival rates of 87.5% and 18.7% in patients with T/N <1.47 compared with 68.8% and 6.2% in those with T/N >1.47. 13 patients underwent repeat scanning during and after radiotherapy. In all patients a decrease in T/N ratio could be demonstrated, however no significant difference in survival was shown in patients with a large decrease in uptake (Li et al. 2006).

Conclusion on NSCLC

The largest body of evidence in NSCLC on the effect of hypoxia comes from operable patients on which biomarker studies have been performed (Table 16.2). Whichever biomarker is studied, when considered separately their presence has a consistent negative effect on the prognosis. However, in multivariate analysis this negative effect is not often present when T-stage is included in the analysis. In non-operable patients the circulating hypoxic biomarkers such as OPN and the imaging studies have provided us with evidence of a detrimental effect of hypoxia on chemotherapy and chemo-radiotherapy.

Table 16.2 _ Overview of studies on hypoxia in lung cancer.

Authors	n	Therapy	Parameters	Prognostic significance (Univariate analysis)	Prognostic significance (Multivariate analysis)	Remarks
Giatro-manolaki et al	108	Surgery	HIF-1α	Not significant	Not Significant	T1-2 N0-1 NSCLC
Lee et al	84	Surgery	HIF-1α	Not significant	Not performed	
Kim et al	74	Surgery	HIF-1α	DFS	Not significant	
			CA IX	DFS	OS	
Kim et al	75	Surgery	CA IX	DFS	DFS, OS	
Yohena et al	66	Surgery	HIF-1α	OS	Not performed	Only applicable in N0 patients
Park et al	178	Surgery	HIF-1α	OS	OS	Only in EGFR negative patients
Giatro-manolaki et al	107	Surgery	CA IX	OS	OS	

Authors	n	Therapy	Parameters	Prognostic significance (Univariate analysis)	Prognostic significance (Multivariate analysis)	Remarks
Swinson et al	175	Surgery	CA IX	OS	OS	Only for pCA9, not mCA9, sCA9 or cCA9
Ilie et al	209	Surgery	plasma CA IX	OS, DSS	OS, DSS	Subgroup analysis: not valid for stage III/IV
			tissue CA IX	OS, DSS	DSS	Subgroup analysis: not valid for stage III/IV
Mack et al	172	Chemotherapy +/- Tirapazamine	Osteopontin plasma	PFS, OS, ORR	Not performed	Only stage IIIB or IV included
			Osteopontin tissue	Not significant	Not performed	
Isa et al	67	Chemotherapy	Osteopontin plasma	OS, PFS	Not performed	
Dehdasti et al	19	Radiotherapy and/ or chemotherapy	Cu-ATSM: T/M ratio	Response to therapy	Not performed	Not valid for SUV
Van Baardwijk et al	102	Surgery	18-FDG: SUVmax	OS	Not performed	Strong association between Hif-1α and SUV
Eschmann et al	16	Radiotherapy	18-Fmiso	LRC	Not performed	
Li et al	32	Radiotherapy +/- (neo-) adjuvant chemo	99mTc HL91 SPECT: T/N ratio	OS, Response to therapy	Not performed	Decrease during RT course not prognostic

Colorectal cancer

Biomarker evidence

Cu-ATSM

19 patients with distally located T2 to T4 or node-positive rectal cancer scheduled for induction radiochemotherapy followed by proctectomy were evaluated by Cu-ATSM scanning to demonstrate the presence of hypoxia

pre-radiotherapy. Overall and progression-free survival of patients with hypoxic tumours was significantly worse than non-hypoxic tumours (tumour-to-muscle activity ratio > or ≤2.6). Follow-up studies have as yet not been published (Dietz et al. 2008).

HIF-1α

Theodoropoulos et determined MVD, VEGF, p53, bcl-2 expression and HIF-1α upregulation and apoptotic index (AI) in tumour tissue samples from 92 patients with T3,4/N±. rectal cancer. HIF-1α presence correlated strongly with VEGF and MVD and was one of two factors correlating with diminished PFS and OS in multivariate analysis, the other being positive lymph node status (Theodoropoulos et al. 2006), see Figure 16.3.

Almost identical results were found in a similar, but smaller study of 30 rectal cancer tissue samples by Lu et al. The correlation between HIF-1α and VEGF was confirmed, as was the link between HIF-1α and a more advanced phenotype characterized by presence of lymph node metastases, higher Dukes stage and worse overall survival and local control (Lu et al. 2006).

While the former two studies focused on patients undergoing neo-adjuvant therapy, Rasheed et al investigated the samples of 90 patients who had undergone solely surgery for rectal adenocarcinoma. Staining was performed for HIF-1α as well as HIF-2α, yet only HIF-1α turned out to be strongly correlated with TNM stage and overall survival (Rasheed et al. 2009).

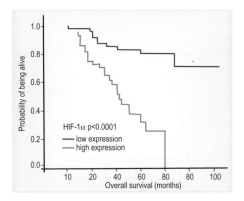

Figure 16.3 _ Overall survival of rectal cancer patients according to intensity of HIF-1α expression. Taken from Theodoropoulos et al, 2006.

Toiyama et al investigated the gene expression of VEGF, EGFR and HIF-1α in 40 patients with stage II-III rectal adenocarcinoma receiving neo-adjuvant 5-fluorouracil based chemoradiotherapy. In univariate analysis all three factors were associated with significantly worse disease free survival. Also, responders to neo-adjuvant treatment had significantly lower values of expression of these 3 genes. However, in multivariate analysis only VEGF remained significant, contrasting with findings of previous studies (Toiyama et al. 2010).

A large study by Korkeila et al was performed on a more heterogenous group of patients treated with surgery with/without neo-adjuvant radiotherapy with/without chemotherapy. Operative samples were present of 168 patients of which 79 also had pre-operative samples taken. Samples were positive for HIF-1α in 70% of the pre-treatment cases and in 40% of the post-radiotherapy operative specimens. In univariate analysis negative HIF-1α status was significantly associated with poor disease specific survival, this was however lost in multivariate analysis concerning preoperative treatment group, sex, age, preoperative T, number of metastatic lymph nodes and vessel invasion, in which the only significant predictor was the preoperative treatment received (Korkeila et al. 2010).

GLUT-1

Cooper et al retrospectively examined tissue specimens for GLUT-1 expression from 43 patients who underwent resection of a rectal adenocarcinoma. Only a minority (6) of patients had pre-operative radiotherapy with/without chemotherapy. 70% expressed GLUT-1. On multi-variate analysis only the GLUT-1 staining on the deep lying parts of the tumour was significant for overall survival (Cooper et al. 2003).

Brophy et al retrospectively reviewed the specimens of 69 patients with pre-operative biopsies and operative specimens of rectal cancer, stages T3/4 or N1, treated with pre-operative chemo-radiotherapy. Any positivity for GLUT-1 was significantly associated with diminished response to chemoradiotherapy. The higher the GLUT-1 expression, the lower the response. For GLUT-1 negative tumours a 70% probability of good response was found, compared to only 31% in GLUT-1 positive tumours. This association was not lost after including pathological T stage in the analysis (Brophy et al. 2009).

Osteopontin

In a small study of 30 patients with resected rectal cancer, all treated pre-operatively with 5 FU based radiochemotherapy, Debucquoy et al evaluated expression patterns of Cox-2, Ki-67 and plasma levels of osteopontin. Although follow-up was rather short, patients with elevated levels of osteopontin (10/30) had a significantly higher tendency to develop metastases (Debucquoy et al. 2006).

Conclusion on colorectal cancer

Rectal cancer is a particularly interesting pathology to study the influence of hypoxia on treatment results due to the various treatment approaches, which are available and the availability of pathologic validation (Table 16.3). Presence of hypoxia (demonstrated indirectly) consistently reveals a detrimental effect on the results of and response to chemotherapy, radiotherapy and surgery.

Table 16.3 _ Overview of studies on colorectal cancer.

Authors	n	Therapy	Parameters	Prognostic significance (Univariate analysis)	Prognostic significance (Multivariate analysis)	Remarks
Dietz et al	19	Radiochem-otherapy + Surgery	Cu-ATSM	PFS, OS, Response to RCT	Not performed	
Theodoro-poulos et al	92	Radiochem-otherapy + Surgery	HIF-1α	DFS, OS	DFS, OS	Stage T3-4N0-1
Lu et al	30	Radiochem-otherapy + Surgery	HIF-1α	LC, OS	Not performed	
Rasheed et al	90	Surgery	HIF-1α	CSS, DFS	CSS	
			HIF-2α	Not significant	Not significant	
Toiyama et al	40	Radiochem-otherapy + Surgery	HIF-1α	Response to RCT	Not significant	
Korkeila et al	168	Surgery +/- neo-adju-vant RT+/- chemo	HIF-1α	DFS	Not significant	

Authors	n	Therapy	Parameters	Prognostic significance (Univariate analysis)	Prognostic significance (Multivariate analysis)	Remarks
Cooper et al	43	Surgery	GLUT-1 ("strong" expression)	OS	OS	Minority radiotherapy+/- chemotherapy
						Valid for deep GLUT-1 staining
Brophy et al	69	Radiochem- otherapy + Surgery	GLUT-1	Response to RCT	Response to RCT	Survival not examined
Debucquoy	30	Surgery	Osteopon- tin	MFS	Not performed	Mainly T3/4 tumours

PFS, progression-free survival; OS, overall survival; DFS, disease-free survival; LC, local control; CSS, cancer-specific survival; RCT, radiochemotherapy; RT, radiotherapy; MFS, metastasis-free survival.

Cervical cancer

Direct measurements of pO$_2$

Hockel et al were the first to report on the detrimental effect of tumour hypoxia in cervical cancer. They first published the interim results of a study in 1993 on the influence of tumour hypoxia on outcome in 31 patients with cervical cancer treated with radiotherapy or combined modality therapy. A clear detrimental effect was shown for patients with a median pO$_2$ of <10 mmHg measured by Eppendorf electrode (Hockel et al. 1993).

The follow-up article in 1996 confirmed these results: 50 % of 103 patients with cervical cancer had hypoxic tumours pre-treatment. Next to FIGO stage the presence of hypoxia was the single most important factor predicting a worse survival outcome both in patients treated with radical radiotherapy and surgery, mainly because of poor locoregional control (Figure 16.4). Patients with hypoxic tumours also demonstrated more frequent parametrial and lympho-vascular extension when operated compared to well oxygenated specimens (Hockel et al. 1996). Knocke et al confirmed these results by duplicating the modus operandi of Hockel et al in 51 patients with cervical cancer treated solely with radiotherapy. Median tumour pO$_2$ had a significant impact on 3-year disease free survival, being 34% for patients with levels of ≤ 10 mm Hg compared to 69% for patients with higher median pO$_2$ levels (P=0:02) (Knocke et al. 1999).

In contrast, studying 30 patients with cervical cancer treated solely with radiotherapy, Suzuki et al did see a significant impact on local control of hypoxia. Patients with well oxygenated tumours ($pO_2 \geq 20$ mmHg) pre-treatment or after 9 Gy of radiotherapy fared significantly better than patients with hypoxic tumours or non-reoxygenated tumours. An effect on overall survival or metastases was not demonstrated (Suzuki et al. 2006).

Lyng and colleagues also investigated the tumoural pO_2 at 2 time points (before and during radiotherapy) and found not only the less oxygenated tumours to be less responsive to radiotherapy, but also demonstrated the pretreatment oxygenation of the tumour to have a greater impact on prognosis than the measurements after 2 weeks of treatment (Lyng et al. 2000).

A study of 106 patients treated with definitive radiotherapy by Fyles et al failed to demonstrate a significant impact of pre-therapy oxygen tension in multivariate analysis. However, excluding the limited number of patients with node positive disease, hypoxia gained significance as a prognostic factor, mainly due to an increased risk of distant metastases. In this study, local control was not influenced by the presence of hypoxia (Fyles et al. 2002).

In a study reported by Nordsmark et al 120 patients had either pimonidazole, Eppendorf measurements or a combination of both prior to treatment for cervical cancer. Treatment modalities were quite heterogenous: radiotherapy +/- chemotherapy +/- carbogen breathing or surgery or a combination. This multicenter prospective study is one of the only trials not to find a prognostic impact of hypoxia on outcome. The reason for this is unclear. The median pO_2 for the whole group was only 4 mmHg, which

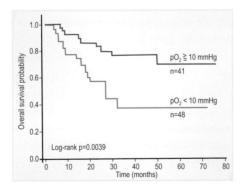

Figure 16.4 _ Overall survival curves for patients with cervical cancer with low vs high median pO2 measurements of the tumour. Taken from (Hockel et al. 1996)

is a lot less than the 10 mmHg found in the previously mentioned trials and makes it difficult to define an optimal cut-off for hypoxia. Also, the different diagnostic and therapeutic procedures in this trial might have scrambled their results (Nordsmark et al. 2006).

Biomarker evidence

HIF-1α

Birner et al immunohistochemically stained surgical specimens of 91 patients with cervical cancer stage pT1b for HIF-1α as a surrogate marker for hypoxia. Strong expression of HIF-1α was found in 22% of samples and this correlated both in univariate and multivariate analysis with a significantly worse overall survival and disease-free survival rate compared to patients with moderate to absent HIF-1α expression (Birner et al. 2000).

An interesting study by Haugland on specimens of 42 patients with locally advanced cervical carcinoma treated with radiotherapy did not find a correlation between HIF-1α status and disease free survival. They did however find a positive match between oxygenation status measured by Eppendorf electrode and the expression of HIF-1α (Haugland et al. 2002).

A similar analysis of the influence of HIF on the prognosis of 78 patients with locally advanced cervical cancer was performed by Burri et al. They found HIF-1α expression to be strongly correlated with overall survival, but the presence of lymph node metastases seemed prognostically more influential. A clear correlation between HIF-1α and the presence of lymph node metastases was not present in this study (Burri et al. 2003).

Bachtiary et al specifically looked at the response to radiotherapy of cervical cancer patients with locally advanced disease. In 47% of patients a moderate/strong expression of HIF-1α was found. These patients showed a significantly worse response to radiotherapy, had a shorter disease free survival and cervical cancer specific survival rate (Bachtiary et al. 2003).

Different results were obtained by Hutchison et al, who found a differential correlation in small vs large tumours: they demonstrated a significant correlation between HIF-1α expression and worse survival in small cervical cancers, whereas a high HIF-1α expression inferred a good prognosis in large tumours. They suggested this might be due to size-related changes in the genes upregulated by HIF-1α (Hutchison et al. 2004).

Mayer et al performed an analysis of HIF-1α expression and pO_2 in locally advanced cervical cancer patients. Their results did not suggest a correlation between pO_2 and HIF-1α, nor did HIF-1α expression or pO_2 influence survival (Mayer et al. 2004).

Conversely, Ishikawa et al investigated in a homogenous group of only stage IIIB cervical cancer patients all treated with EBRT and brachytherapy in whom a strong negative impact of strong HIF-1α expression on worse recurrence free survival, both locally and distant was observed. An effect on overall survival was not noted, despite the overall survival rate at 10 years in this series being quite high at 44 % (Ishikawa et al. 2004).

Dellas et al report similar findings in radiotherapeutically treated locally advanced cervical cancer, with HIF-1α expression correlating negatively with tumour related survival in multivariate analysis in 44 patients (Dellas et al. 2008).

GLUT-1

Airley et al investigated the use of GLUT-1 as a surrogate marker for hypoxia in locally advanced cervical cancer. In a pilot study they confirmed a slight, but significant correlation between GLUT-1 expression and HP2.5 as measured by Eppendorf electrode in 54 patients. Thereafter they retrospectively studied the outcomes of 121 patients with locally advanced cervical cancer from their database and found GLUT-1 staining to be associated with worse metastasis-free, but not disease free or local recurrence free survival (Airley et al. 2001).

Mayer et al evaluated GLUT-1 expression in a group of 47 patients with cervical cancer at various stages ranging from IB to IVB. Patients were treated preferably with surgery and radiotherapy was used for inoperable patients. Although GLUT-1 staining was associated with worse survival in univariate analysis, this association was lost in multivariate analysis using T-stage or N-stage, the latter being the only significant variable in multivariate analysis (Mayer et al. 2005).

CA IX

In a prospective trial performing Eppendorf measurements and staining for CA IX in 68 patients with locally advanced cervical cancer, a significant positive correlation was noted between the presence of tumour hypoxia (HP5) and the extent of CA IX expression by Loncaster et al. They further demonstrated in a consequent retrospective study of 130 squamous cell cervical carcinomas treated with radiotherapy that CA IX expression was a significant and independent prognostic indicator of overall and metastasis-free survival (Loncaster et al. 2001). In concordance with these results, Lee et al demonstrated a detrimental effect on disease free survival of upregulated CA IX in patients treated with radiotherapy for locally advanced cervical cancer (Lee et al. 2007).

In contrast, Hedley et al failed to reproduce these results in a similar study on 110 patients treated with radiotherapy or chemoradiotherapy for locally advanced cervical cancer. They did not demonstrate a correlation between pO2 measurements and CA IX staining of biopsies, nor did they find a predictive value of CA IX on outcome, which was the case for the Eppendorf measurements (Hedley et al. 2003). The lack of correlation between the 2 studies might have been due to a difference in sampling technique: Loncaster et al describe taking biopsies of the Eppendorf trajectories, while Hedley et al used punch biopsies, apparently not linked to the trajectory of the electrodes, leading to a possibly greater risk of sampling error. Finally on the specimens of 166 women enrolled on a study by the GOG, treated surgically for early stage cervical cancer and randomized between adjuvant radio-or radiochemotherapy for positive lymph nodes or incomplete resection, Liao et al. performed staining for CA IX. They demonstrated a lower progression free survival and an increased risk of death for the 21 % of patients in which a high level of CA IX expression was found. (Liao et al., 2010)

Conclusion on cervical cancer

In cervical cancer the presence of hypoxia almost invariably infers a negative response to both (chemo)-radiotherapy or surgery (Tab. 16.4). When considered in multivariate analysis the effect is sometimes lost due to the importance of T-stage and/or N-stage.

Table 16.4 _ Overview of studies on hypoxia in cervical cancer.

Authors	n	Therapy	Parameters	Prognostic significance (Univariate analysis)	Prognostic significance (Multivariate analysis)	Remarks
Hockel et al	31	Radio-therapy +/- chemo	Median $pO_2 < 10$ mmHg		OS, DFS	

Authors	n	Therapy	Parameters	Prognostic significance (Univariate analysis)	Prognostic significance (Multivariate analysis)	Remarks
Hockel et al	89	Surgery/ Radio- therapy	Median $pO_2 < 10$ mmHg		OS, DFS	50 % hypoxic tumours
Knocke et al	51	Radio- therapy +/- chemo	Median $pO_2 < 10$ mmHg		DFS	
Suzuki et al	30	Radio- therapy +/- chemo	Median $pO_2 < 20$ mmHg before RT	LC	Not signifi- cant	
			Median $pO_2 < 20$ mmHg after 9 Gy	LC	LC	
Fyles et al	106	Radio- therapy	Median $pO_2 < 5$ mmHg		PFS, DFS, DS	Only valid on N0 patients
Nordsmark et al	127	RT +/- Chemo +/- CO +/- Surgery	Median $pO_2 < 4$ mmHg	Not significant	Not significant	
Lyng et al	40	EBRT + brachy- therapy	HSV5 before RT	OS, DFS, LRC	OS, DFS, LRC	
			HSV5 after 2 weeks of RT	DFS	Not performed	
Birner et al	91	Surgery+/- radiother- apy	HIF-1α	OS, DFS	OS, DFS	Only stage T1b
Haugland et al	45	Radio- therapy	HIF-1α	Not significant	Not significant	Hif corre- lated sig- nificantly with pO2
Burri et al	78	Radio- therapy +/- chemo	HIF-1α	LPFS	OS	
Bachtiary et al	67	Radio- therapy	HIF-1α	PFS, CSS	PFS, CSS	
Hutchison et al	99	Radio- therapy	HIF-1α	Not significant	Not significant	Small tumours: HIF-1α associated with worse prognosis Large tumours: HIF-1α associated with good prognosis

Authors	n	Therapy	Parameters	Prognostic significance (Univariate analysis)	Prognostic significance (Multivariate analysis)	Remarks
Mayer et al	34	Surgery/radiotherapy	HIF-1α	Not significant	Not significant	Mainly locally advanced tumours
Ishikawa et al	38	Radiotherapy	HIF-1α	MFS, RFS	Not significant	Only stage IIIB
Dellas et al	44	Radiotherapy	HIF-1α	CSS, OS	CSS	Mainly locally advanced tumours
Airley et al	121	Radiotherapy	GLUT-1	MFS	MFS	
Mayer et al	42	Surgery/Radiotherapy +/- chemotherapy	GLUT-1	OS, RFS	Not significant	Stages IB to IVB
Loncaster et al	130	Radiotherapy	CA IX	DSS, MFS	OS, MFS	
Hedley	110	Radiotherapy +/- chemotherapy	CA IX	Not significant	Not significant	Locally advanced cervical cancer
Liao	166	Surgery + Radiotherapy/radiochemotherapy	CA IX	OS	PFS, OS	Early stage cervical cancer

OS, overall survival; DFS disease-free survival; LC, local control; PFS, progression-free survival; DF, distant failure; LRC, loco-regional control; CSS, cancer-specific survival; MFS, metastases-free survival; RFS, relapse- free survival.

Head and Neck

Direct measurements of pO$_2$

One of the first studies to evaluate the impact of tumour hypoxia on the response to radiotherapy was the trial by Brizel et al in which they evaluated pO$_2$ by Eppendorf electrodes in 26 patients with extensive head and neck squamous cell carcinoma (HNSCC) treated by radiotherapy with/

without neck dissection. The average tumour median pO_2 of tumours, which were not locally controlled by radiotherapy (4.1+/-1.2 mm Hg), was significantly lower than that of tumours, which did not recur (17.1+/-2.4 mm Hg; p=0.007). After a follow-up of only one year, highly oxygenated tumours had a significantly better overall survival (90%) than the poorly oxygenated tumours (40%), using a cut-off of 10 mmHg for median pO_2 (Brizel et al. 1997; Brizel et al. 1999).

Similar results were reported by Nordsmark and Overgaard: in 2 studies, the second being a confirmatory study of the first, they proved in 2 separate cohorts of respectively 35 and 31 patients the negative influence of hypoxia on locoregional control in patients with HNSCC (Nordsmark et al. 1996; Nordsmark and Overgaard 2000).

In a later study, using the same patient population plus 1 added patient, they subsequently showed the fraction of pO_2 values < or = 2.5 mmHg (HP2.5) not only to be a strong indicator of poor loco-regional control, but they also proved this to be independent of the hemoglobin level (Nordsmark and Overgaard 2004). In contrast Terris at al did not find a statistically significant influence of a low tumour pO2 on locoregional control after radiotherapy (Terris 2000).

Rudat et al obtained results similar to the previously mentioned trials by demonstrating the fraction of pO_2 values <2.5 mmHg as the only significant prognostic factor for survival in 41 patients and later in a follow-up

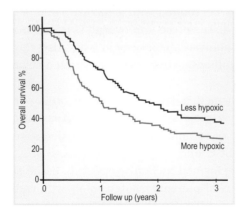

Figure 16.5 _ Actuarial survival curves for patients with less hypoxic (HP2.5≤19%) vs more hypoxic (HP2.5>19%) HNSCC tumours. Taken from Nordsmark et al (Nordsmark, Bentzen et al. 2005).

cohort of 134 patients with HNSCC treated by radiotherapy or radiochemotherapy (Rudat et al. 2000; Rudat et al. 2001).

All previously mentioned authors then joined forces to collect the largest dataset on HNSCC and polarographic measurements known to date. In 397 patients from seven centres with HNSCC median pO_2, HP2.5 and HP5 were evaluated at baseline. In multivariate analysis, stratified according to institution, HP2.5 was the strongest independent factor influencing survival (Nordsmark et al. 2005) see Figure 16.5.

Nordsmark et al also performed a study on 5 hypoxic markers (CA IX, plasma osteopontin, tumour osteopontin, HIF-1α, tumour pO_2) to check inter-marker correlations and their influence on locoregional control in patients with HNSCC treated with radiotherapy and nimorazole. There were no consistent relations between markers, only plasma osteopontin correlated inversely with median tumour pO2 and CA IX with HIF-1α. In multivariate analysis the HP2.5 the strongest variable to predict for locoregional tumour control remained, consistent with the results of their publication in 2005 (Nordsmark et al. 2007).

Biomarker evidence

HIF-1α

Aebersold et al investigated the presence of HIF-1α in biopsies of 98 patients treated with radiotherapy for oropharyngeal cancer. The degree of intensity of staining was inversely correlated with a hazard ratio of over 2 for local control rate as well as disease free and overall survival, maintaining significance in multivariate analysis (Aebersold et al. 2001). Also, the response rate to radiotherapy was significantly better in cases with a strong expression of HIF-1α.

Koukourakis et al performed a similar research on a series of 75 patients and confirmed these results: high HIF-1α expression correlates significantly to a low chance of complete response in patients treated with chemoradiotherapy for HNSCC and poor survival. (Beasley et al. 2002; Koukourakis et al. 2002). In a trial performed by Schrijvers et al, tissue samples of 91 T1-2 glottic SCC specimens of patients treated solely with radiotherapy staining was performed for GLUT-1, CA IX and HIF-1α. HIF-1α and CA IX correlated significantly with worse local control and OS by a hazard ratio of nearly 3. The authors proposed radiotherapy as single modality treatment ought to be replaced by surgery or complemented with hypoxic sensitizers for patients with high up-front HIF-1α or CA IX expression (Schrijvers et al. 2008). Finally, Koukourakis showed that the negative prognostic value of CA IX and HIF-1α in HNSCC are valid in hyperfractionated as well as hypofractionated cisplatin based radiochemotherapy for HNSCC (Koukourakis et al. 2008).

Beasley et al found similar results on overall survival and disease free survival in a series of 79 surgically treated patients: HIF-1α positive patients fared significantly worse (Beasley et al. 2002; Koukourakis et al. 2002). This finding correlates well with the results of Winter et al in 151 patients treated surgically with postoperative radiotherapy in the majority of their population. HIF-1α had a major impact on DSS and DFS in this series. (Kyzas et al. 2005; Winter et al. 2006).

CA IX

All previously mentioned radiotherapy trials used mostly conventional fractionation and radiosensitization by chemotherapy. In the ARCON trial an effort was made to overcome hypoxia using nicotinamide and CO inhalation. The negative connotation of CA IX (Kim et al. 2007) and GLUT-1 with respect to survival and local control found in other trials could not be confirmed by Jonathan et al in patients participating in this trial. As one of the only groups they even found a significantly positive result of CA IX positivity on local control and freedom from distant metastases after treatment with ARCON. Whether this can be an attributed to an actual radiosensitizing effect remains to be elucidated, but it seems probable (De Schutter et al. 2005; Jonathan et al. 2006).

Conclusion on head and neck cancer

The presence of hypoxia in HNSCC is widely investigated due to the accessibility of the tumours. Results are quite consistent when different trials are compared, revealing a detrimental effect of hypoxia on the results of radio(-chemo)therapy as well as in operated patients and a possible reversibility of this effect when measures are taken to overcome hypoxia (Table 16.5).

Table 16.5 _ Overview of studies on head and neck cancer.

Authors	n	Therapy	Parameter	Prognostic significance (Univariate analysis)	Prognostic significance (Multivariate analysis)	Remarks
Brizel et al	26	Radiotherapy +/- neck dissection	median $pO_2 < 10$ mmHg	DFS, OS	Not performed	
Brizel et al	63	Radiotherapy/ radiochemo- therapy	median $pO_2 < 10$ mmHg	LRC, DFS, OS	LC, OS	
Nordsmark	35	Radiotherapy +/- nimorazole	HP2,5	LC	LC	
Nordsmark	31	Radiotherapy +/- nimorazole	HP2,5	LC	LC	
Terris	63	Radiotherapy	median pO_2	Not significant	Not significant	
Rudat	41	Radiotherapy +/- chemotherapy	HP2,5	OS	OS	All stage IV
Rudat	134	Radiotherapy +/- chemotherapy	HP2,5	OS	OS	
Nordsmark	397	Surgery and/ or radiotherapy or radiochemo- therapy	HP2,5	OS	OS	
Aebersold	98	Radiotherapy	HIF-1α	LRC, DFS, OS	OS, DFS. LRC	Oropharyn- geal cancer
Koukourakis	75	Chemoradio- therapy	HIF-2α	OS, LRC	Not significant	HIF-2α Significant impact on OS multi- variate
Schrijvers	91	Radiotherapy	HIF-1α	LC, OS	LC, OS	T1-T2 glottic SCC
			GLUT-1	Not significant	Not significant	
			CA IX	LC, OS	LC	
Beasley	79	Surgery +/- radio- therapy	HIF-1α	OS, DFS	OS, DFS	
Winter	151	Surgery + Radio- therapy	HIF-1α	DFS, DSS	DFS, DSS	

DFS, disease-free survival; OS, overall survival; LRC, loco-regional control; LC, local control; DSS, disease-specific survival.

General conclusion and future prospects

The studies presented here grossly agree on the negative impact of hypoxia or the presence of the so-called "hypoxic response" on therapy in different pathologies. "Grossly" is albeit the correct wording, because although the laboratory data on hypoxia and treatment responses are quite robust, there is still a quite large heterogeneity in the results of the aforementioned trials.

There are indeed numerous difficulties in interpreting the results of trials investigating the prognostic impact of hypoxia. As mentioned in the introduction, the techniques used to demonstrate hypoxia in tumours have been quite extensively studied and linked to hypoxia in laboratory conditions, but are far from flawless when actually applied in patients. Not only can all described techniques not be used in all patients, but details on the implementation of one technique in the same patient population can differ between different centres, making results hard to compare. Standardization of the currently applied measuring techniques and essays is of utmost importance for accurately guiding research efforts in years and decades to come. Furthermore, a definite disadvantage of the current gold standard of hypoxia measurements in human tumours- the Eppendorf electrode –is its invasive nature, making it suitable only for easily reachable sites. For the large majority of patients, physicians and researchers will be forced to use biomarkers or imaging tools which are faced with the inherent property of not being specific enough for hypoxia targeting. Currently, each study performed using biomarkers can be criticized because their mechanism of action is influenced by factors other than hypoxia, inherently linked to the numerous changes in the micro-environment or the cellular metabolism caused by malignant transformation of human cells.

Imaging modalities used for hypoxia detection on the other hand are mainly radioactively labelled molecules used as PET-tracers, the most common example being the nitroimidazoles. Nitroimidazoles however have the disadvantage of not being taken up by areas of necrosis, thus not correlating in a 1/1 fashion with Eppendorf measurements. Another disadvantage of PET to be noted is the low resolution of images, making it difficult to evaluate small lesions.

Lastly, a large amount of the evidence presented in this chapter is based on the retrospective examination of tissue specimens gathered in patients treated with miscellaneous modalities of differing pathologies and stages on which sub-group analyses are performed. Large scale prospective data in homogenously treated and patient groups selected upfront are scarce and still need to be collected to provide us with definite answers to which subgroups of patients might really benefit from adaptive strategies to overcome the detrimental effects of hypoxia.

A c k n o w l e d g e m e n t s _ The authors declare no conflicts of interest. Part of this chapter was written in the context of the Metoxia Framework of the European Union.

References

Aebersold, D. M., P. Burri, et al. (2001). "Expression of hypoxia-inducible factor-1alpha: a novel predictive and prognostic parameter in the radiotherapy of oropharyngeal cancer." Cancer Res 61(7): 2911-6.

Airley, R., J. Loncaster, et al. (2001). "Glucose transporter glut-1 expression correlates with tumour hypoxia and predicts metastasis-free survival in advanced carcinoma of the cervix." Clin Cancer Res 7(4): 928-34.

Bachtiary, B., M. Schindl, et al. (2003). "Overexpression of hypoxia-inducible factor 1alpha indicates diminished response to radiotherapy and unfavourable prognosis in patients receiving radical radiotherapy for cervical cancer." Clin Cancer Res 9(6): 2234-40.

Beasley, N. J., R. Leek, et al. (2002). "Hypoxia-inducible factors HIF-1alpha and HIF-2alpha in head and neck cancer: relationship to tumour biology and treatment outcome in surgically resected patients." Cancer Res 62(9): 2493-7.

Birner, P., M. Schindl, et al. (2000). "Overexpression of hypoxia-inducible factor 1alpha is a marker for an unfavourable prognosis in early-stage invasive cervical cancer." Cancer Res 60(17): 4693-6.

Bos, R., P. van der Groep, et al. (2003). "Levels of hypoxia-inducible factor-1alpha independently predict prognosis in patients with lymph node negative breast carcinoma." Cancer 97(6): 1573-81.

Brennan, D. J., K. Jirstrom, et al. (2006). "CA IX is an independent prognostic marker in premenopausal breast cancer patients with one to three positive lymph nodes and a putative marker of radiation resistance." Clin Cancer Res 12(21): 6421-31.

Brizel, D. M., R. K. Dodge, et al. (1999). "Oxygenation of head and neck cancer: changes during radiotherapy and impact on treatment outcome." Radiother Oncol 53(2): 113-7.

Brizel, D. M., G. S. Sibley, et al. (1997). "Tumour hypoxia adversely affects the prognosis of carcinoma of the head and neck." Int J Radiat Oncol Biol Phys 38(2): 285-9.

Brophy, S., K. M. Sheehan, et al. (2009). "GLUT-1 expression and response to chemoradiotherapy in rectal cancer." Int J Cancer 125(12): 2778-82.

Burri, P., V. Djonov, et al. (2003). "Significant correlation of hypoxia-inducible factor-1alpha with treatment outcome in cervical cancer treated with radical radiotherapy." Int J Radiat Oncol Biol Phys 56(2): 494-501.

Chapman, J. D. (1991). "Measurement of tumour hypoxia by invasive and non-invasive procedures: a review of recent clinical studies." Radiother Oncol 20 Suppl 1: 13-9.

Chia, S. K., C. C. Wykoff, et al. (2001). "Prognostic significance of a novel hypoxia-regulated marker, carbonic anhydrase IX, in invasive breast carcinoma." J Clin Oncol 19(16): 3660-8.

Cooper, R., S. Sarioglu, et al. (2003). "Glucose transporter-1 (GLUT-1): a potential marker of prognosis in rectal carcinoma?" Br J Cancer 89(5): 870-6.

Dales, J. P., S. Garcia, et al. (2005). "Overexpression of hypoxia-inducible factor HIF-1alpha predicts early relapse in breast cancer: retrospective study in a series of 745 patients." Int J Cancer 116(5): 734-9.

De Schutter, H., W. Landuyt, et al. (2005). "The prognostic value of the hypoxia markers CA IX and GLUT 1 and the cytokines VEGF and IL 6 in head and neck squamous cell carcinoma treated by radiotherapy +/- chemotherapy." BMC Cancer 5: 42.

Debucquoy, A., L. Goethals, et al. (2006). "Molecular responses of rectal cancer to preoperative chemoradiation." Radiother Oncol 80(2): 172-7.

Degenhardt, K., R. Mathew, et al. (2006). "Autophagy promotes tumour cell survival and restricts necrosis, inflammation, and tumourigenesis." Cancer Cell 10(1): 51-64.

Dehdashti, F., M. A. Mintun, et al. (2003). "In vivo assessment of tumour hypoxia in lung cancer with 60Cu-ATSM." Eur J Nucl Med Mol Imaging 30(6): 844-50.

Dellas, K., M. Bache, et al. (2008). "Prognostic impact of HIF-1alpha expression in patients with definitive radiotherapy for cervical cancer." Strahlenther Onkol 184(3): 169-74.

Dewey, D. L. (1960). "Effect of oxygen and nitric oxide on the radio-sensitivity of human cells in tissue culture." Nature 186: 780-2.

Dietz, D. W., F. Dehdashti, et al. (2008). "Tumour hypoxia detected by positron emission tomography with 60Cu-ATSM as a predictor of response and survival in patients undergoing Neoadjuvant chemoradiotherapy for rectal carcinoma: a pilot study." Dis Colon Rectum 51(11): 1641-8.

Eschmann, S. M., F. Paulsen, et al. (2005). "Prognostic impact of hypoxia imaging with 18F-misonidazole PET in non-small cell lung cancer and head and neck cancer before radiotherapy." J Nucl Med 46(2): 253-60.

Fyles, A., M. Milosevic, et al. (2002). "Tumour hypoxia has independent predictor impact only in patients with node-negative cervix cancer." J Clin Oncol 20(3): 680-7.

Giatromanolaki, A., M. I. Koukourakis, et al. (2001). "Expression of hypoxia-inducible carbonic anhydrase-9 relates to angiogenic pathways and independently to poor outcome in non-small cell lung cancer." Cancer Res 61(21): 7992-8.

Giatromanolaki, A., M. I. Koukourakis, et al. (2001). "Relation of hypoxia inducible factor 1 alpha and 2 alpha in operable non-small cell lung cancer to angiogenic/molecular profile of tumours and survival." Br J Cancer 85(6): 881-90.

Gray, L. H. (1961). "Radiobiologic basis of oxygen as a modifying factor in radiation therapy." Am J Roentgenol Radium Ther Nucl Med 85: 803-15.

Gray, L. H., A. D. Conger, et al. (1953). "The concentration of oxygen dissolved in tissues at the time of irradiation as a factor in radiotherapy." Br J Radiol 26(312): 638-48.

Gruber, G., R. H. Greiner, et al. (2004). "Hypoxia-inducible factor 1 alpha in high-risk breast cancer: an independent prognostic parameter?" Breast Cancer Res 6(3): R191-8.

Haugland, H. K., V. Vukovic, et al. (2002). "Expression of hypoxia-inducible factor-1alpha in cervical carcinomas: correlation with tumour oxygenation." Int J Radiat Oncol Biol Phys 53(4): 854-61.

Hedley, D., M. Pintilie, et al. (2003). "Carbonic anhydrase IX expression, hypoxia, and prognosis in patients with uterine cervical carcinomas." Clin Cancer Res 9(15): 5666-74.

Helmlinger, G., F. Yuan, et al. (1997). "Interstitial pH and pO_2 gradients in solid tumours in vivo: high-resolution measurements reveal a lack of correlation." Nat Med 3(2): 177-82.

Hockel, M., C. Knoop, et al. (1993). "Intratumoural pO_2 predicts survival in advanced cancer of the uterine cervix." Radiother Oncol 26(1): 45-50.

Hockel, M., K. Schlenger, et al. (1996). "Association between tumour hypoxia and malignant progression in advanced cancer of the uterine cervix." Cancer Res 56(19): 4509-15.

Hsu, D. S., H. Y. Lan, et al. (2010) "Regulation of excision repair cross-complementation group 1 by Snail contributes to cisplatin resistance in head and neck cancer." Clin Cancer Res 16(18): 4561-71.

Hussain, S. A., R. Ganesan, et al. (2007). "Hypoxia-regulated carbonic anhydrase IX expression is associated with poor survival in patients with invasive breast cancer." Br J Cancer 96(1): 104-9.

Hutchison, G. J., H. R. Valentine, et al. (2004). "Hypoxia-inducible factor 1alpha expression as an intrinsic marker of hypoxia: correlation with tumour oxygen, pimonidazole measurements, and outcome in locally advanced carcinoma of the cervix." Clin Cancer Res 10(24): 8405-12.

Ilie, M., N. M. Mazure, et al. (2010) "High levels of carbonic anhydrase IX in tumour tissue and plasma are biomarkers of poor prognostic in patients with non-small cell lung cancer." Br J Cancer 102(11): 1627-35.

Isa, S., T. Kawaguchi, et al. (2009). "Serum osteopontin levels are highly prognostic for survival in advanced non-small cell lung cancer: results from JMTO LC 0004." J Thorac Oncol 4(9): 1104-10.

Ishikawa, H., H. Sakurai, et al. (2004). "Expression of hypoxic-inducible factor 1alpha predicts metastasis-free survival after radiation therapy alone in stage IIIB cervical squamous cell carcinoma." Int J Radiat Oncol Biol Phys 60(2): 513-21.

Jonathan, R. A., K. I. Wijffels, et al. (2006). "The prognostic value of endogenous hypoxia-related markers for head and neck squamous cell carcinomas treated with ARCON." Radiother Oncol 79(3): 288-97.

Kang, S. S., Y. K. Chun, et al. (2002). "Clinical significance of glucose transporter 1 (GLUT1) expression in human breast carcinoma." Jpn J Cancer Res 93(10): 1123-8.

Kim, S. J., Z. N. Rabbani, et al. (2005). "Expression of HIF-1alpha, CA IX, VEGF, and MMP-9 in surgically resected non-small cell lung cancer." Lung Cancer 49(3): 325-35.

Kim, S. J., Z. N. Rabbani, et al. (2004). "Carbonic anhydrase IX in early-stage non-small cell lung cancer." Clin Cancer Res 10(23): 7925-33.

Kim, S. J., H. J. Shin, et al. (2007). "Prognostic value of carbonic anhydrase IX and Ki-67 expression in squamous cell carcinoma of the tongue." Jpn J Clin Oncol 37(11): 812-9.

Klymkowsky, M. W. and P. Savagner (2009). "Epithelial-mesenchymal transition: a cancer researcher's conceptual friend and foe." Am J Pathol 174(5): 1588-93.

Knocke, T. H., H. D. Weitmann, et al. (1999). "Intratumoural pO2-measurements as predictive assay in the treatment of carcinoma of the uterine cervix." Radiother Oncol 53(2): 99-104.

Korkeila, E., P. M. Jaakkola, et al. (2010). "Preoperative radiotherapy downregulates the nuclear expression of hypoxia-inducible factor-1alpha in rectal cancer." Scand J Gastroenterol 45(3): 340-8.

Koukourakis, M. I., A. Giatromanolaki, et al. (2008). "Hypoxia inducible factor (HIf1alpha and HIF2alpha) and carbonic anhydrase 9 (CA9) expression and response of head-neck cancer to hypofractionated and accelerated radiotherapy." Int J Radiat Biol 84(1): 47-52.

Koukourakis, M. I., A. Giatromanolaki, et al. (2002). "Hypoxia-inducible factor (HIF1A and HIF2A), angiogenesis, and chemoradiotherapy outcome of squamous cell head-and-neck cancer." Int J Radiat Oncol Biol Phys 53(5): 1192-202.

Kyndi, M., F. B. Sorensen, et al. (2008). "Carbonic anhydrase IX and response to post-mastectomy radiotherapy in high-risk breast cancer: a subgroup analysis of the DBCG82 b and c trials." Breast Cancer Res 10(2): R24.

Kyzas, P. A., D. Stefanou, et al. (2005). "Hypoxia-induced tumour angiogenic pathway in head and neck cancer: an in vivo study." Cancer Lett 225(2): 297-304.

Lee, C. H., M. K. Lee, et al. (2003). "Differential expression of hypoxia inducible factor-1 alpha and tumour cell proliferation between squamous cell carcinomas and adenocarcinomas among operable non-small cell lung carcinomas." J Korean Med Sci 18(2): 196-203.

Lee, S., H. J. Shin, et al. (2007). "Tumour carbonic anhydrase 9 expression is associated with the presence of lymph node metastases in uterine cervical cancer." Cancer Sci 98(3): 329-33.

Li, L., J. Yu, et al. (2006). "Serial hypoxia imaging with 99mTc-HL91 SPECT to predict radiotherapy response in nonsmall cell lung cancer." Am J Clin Oncol 29(6): 628-33.

Liao, S. Y., K. M. Darcy, et al. (2010). "Prognostic relevance of carbonic anhydrase-IX in high-risk, early-stage cervical cancer: a Gynecologic Oncology Group study." Gynecol Oncol 116(3): 452-8.

Liu, Y., C. Laszlo, et al. (2010) "Regulation of G(1) arrest and apoptosis in hypoxia by PERK and GCN2-mediated eIF2alpha phosphorylation." Neoplasia 12(1): 61-8.

Loncaster, J. A., A. L. Harris, et al. (2001). "Carbonic anhydrase (CA IX) expression, a potential new intrinsic marker of hypoxia: correlations with tumour oxygen measurements and prognosis in locally advanced carcinoma of the cervix." Cancer Res 61(17): 6394-9.

Lu, X. G., C. G. Xing, et al. (2006). "Clinical significance of immunohistochemical expression of hypoxia-inducible factor-1alpha as a prognostic marker in rectal adenocarcinoma." Clin Colorectal Cancer 5(5): 350-3.

Lyng, H., K. Sundfor, et al. (2000). "Disease control of uterine cervical cancer: relationships to tumour oxygen tension, vascular density, cell density, and frequency of mitosis and apoptosis measured before treatment and during radiotherapy." Clin Cancer Res 6(3): 1104-12.

Mack, P. C., M. W. Redman, et al. (2008). "Lower osteopontin plasma levels are associated with superior outcomes in advanced non-small-cell lung cancer patients receiving platinum-based chemotherapy: SWOG Study S0003." J Clin Oncol 26(29): 4771-6.

Mayer, A., M. Hockel, et al. (2005). "Microregional expression of glucose transporter-1 and oxygenation status: lack of correlation in locally advanced cervical cancers." Clin Cancer Res 11(7): 2768-73.

Mayer, A., A. Wree, et al. (2004). "Lack of correlation between expression of HIF-1alpha protein and oxygenation status in identical tissue areas of squamous cell carcinomas of the uterine cervix." Cancer Res 64(16): 5876-81.

Nordsmark, M., S. M. Bentzen, et al. (2005). "Prognostic value of tumour oxygenation in 397 head and neck tumours after primary radiation therapy. An international multi-center study." Radiother Oncol 77(1): 18-24.

Nordsmark, M., J. G. Eriksen, et al. (2007). "Differential risk assessments from five hypoxia specific assays: The basis for biologically adapted individualized radiotherapy in advanced head and neck cancer patients." Radiother Oncol 83(3): 389-97.

Nordsmark, M., J. Loncaster, et al. (2006). "The prognostic value of pimonidazole and tumour pO2 in human cervix carcinomas after radiation therapy: a prospective international multi-center study." Radiother Oncol 80(2): 123-31.

Nordsmark, M. and J. Overgaard (2000). "A confirmatory prognostic study on oxygenation status and loco-regional control in advanced head and neck squamous cell carcinoma treated by radiation therapy." Radiother Oncol 57(1): 39-43.

Nordsmark, M. and J. Overgaard (2004). "Tumour hypoxia is independent of hemoglobin and prognostic for loco-regional tumour control after primary radiotherapy in advanced head and neck cancer." Acta Oncol 43(4): 396-403.

Nordsmark, M., M. Overgaard, et al. (1996). "Pretreatment oxygenation predicts radiation response in advanced squamous cell carcinoma of the head and neck." Radiother Oncol 41(1): 31-9.

Park, S., S. Y. Ha, et al. "Prognostic implications of hypoxia-inducible factor-1alpha in epidermal growth factor receptor-negative non-small cell lung cancer." Lung Cancer. 2011 Apr; 72(1):100-7

Rasheed, S., A. L. Harris, et al. (2009). "Hypoxia-inducible factor-1alpha and -2alpha are expressed in most rectal cancers but only hypoxia-inducible factor-1alpha is associated with prognosis." Br J Cancer 100(10): 1666-73.

Rockwell, S., I. T. Dobrucki, et al. (2009). "Hypoxia and radiation therapy: past history, ongoing research, and future promise." Curr Mol Med 9(4): 442-58.

Rudat, V., P. Stadler, et al. (2001). "Predictive value of the tumour oxygenation by means of pO2 histography in patients with advanced head and neck cancer." Strahlenther Onkol 177(9): 462-8.

Rudat, V., B. Vanselow, et al. (2000). "Repeatability and prognostic impact of the pre-treatment pO(2) histography in patients with advanced head and neck cancer." Radiother Oncol 57(1): 31-7.

Schindl, M., S. F. Schoppmann, et al. (2002). "Overexpression of hypoxia-inducible factor 1alpha is associated with an unfavourable prognosis in lymph node-positive breast cancer." Clin Cancer Res 8(6): 1831-7.

Schrijvers, M. L., B. F. van der Laan, et al. (2008). "Overexpression of intrinsic hypoxia markers HIF1alpha and CA-IX predict for local recurrence in stage T1-T2 glottic laryngeal carcinoma treated with radiotherapy." Int J Radiat Oncol Biol Phys 72(1): 161-9.

Suzuki, Y., T. Nakano, et al. (2006). "Oxygenated and reoxygenated tumours show better local control in radiation therapy for cervical cancer." Int J Gynecol Cancer 16(1): 306-11.

Swinson, D. E., J. L. Jones, et al. (2003). "Carbonic anhydrase IX expression, a novel surrogate marker of tumour hypoxia, is associated with a poor prognosis in non-small-cell lung cancer." J Clin Oncol 21(3): 473-82.

Tan, F. Y., M. Yan, et al. (2009). "The key hypoxia regulated gene CAIX is upregulated in basal-like breast tumours and is associated with resistance to chemotherapy." Br J Cancer 100(2): 405-11.

Teicher, B. A., J. S. Lazo, et al. (1981). "Classification of antineoplastic agents by their selective toxicities toward oxygenated and hypoxic tumour cells." Cancer Res 41(1): 73-81.

Terris, D. J. (2000). "Head and neck cancer: the importance of oxygen." Laryngoscope 110(5 Pt 1): 697-707.

Theodoropoulos, G. E., A. C. Lazaris, et al. (2006). "Hypoxia, angiogenesis and apoptosis markers in locally advanced rectal cancer." Int J Colorectal Dis 21(3): 248-57.

Toiyama, Y., Y. Inoue, et al. (2010). "Gene expression profiles of epidermal growth factor receptor, vascular endothelial growth factor and hypoxia-inducible factor-1 with special reference to local responsiveness to neoadjuvant chemoradiotherapy and disease recurrence after rectal cancer surgery." Clin Oncol (R Coll Radiol) 22(4): 272-80.

Trastour, C., E. Benizri, et al. (2007). "HIF-1alpha and CA IX staining in invasive breast carcinomas: prognosis and treatment outcome." Int J Cancer 120(7): 1451-8.

van Baardwijk, A., C. Dooms, et al. (2007). "The maximum uptake of (18)F-deoxyglucose on positron emission tomography scan correlates with survival, hypoxia inducible factor-1alpha and GLUT-1 in non-small cell lung cancer." Eur J Cancer 43(9): 1392-8.

Vaupel, P., K. Schlenger, et al. (1991). "Oxygenation of human tumours: evaluation of tissue oxygen distribution in breast cancers by computerized O2 tension measurements." Cancer Res 51(12): 3316-22.

Vleugel, M. M., A. E. Greijer, et al. (2005). "Differential prognostic impact of hypoxia induced and diffuse HIF-1alpha expression in invasive breast cancer." J Clin Pathol 58(2): 172-7.

Winter, S. C., K. A. Shah, et al. (2006). "The relation between hypoxia-inducible factor (HIF)-1alpha and HIF-2alpha expression with anaemia and outcome in surgically treated head and neck cancer." Cancer 107(4): 757-66.

Yohena, T., I. Yoshino, et al. (2009). "Upregulation of hypoxia-inducible factor-1alpha mRNA and its clinical significance in non-small cell lung cancer." J Thorac Oncol 4(3): 284-90.

Chapter 17

Targeting hypoxic cells with bioreductive prodrugs

Kaye J. Williams[1]* and Stephanie R. McKeown[2]

*Author for correspondence:
[1]Hypoxia and Therapeutics Group, School of Pharmacy and Pharmaceutical Sciences, University of Manchester, Oxford Road, Manchester, M13 9PT, [2]Director, Health and Rehabilitation Science Research Institute, School of Health Sciences, University of Ulster, Jordanstown, Newtownabbey, Northern Ireland BT37 OQB, E-mail: kaye.williams@manchester.ac.uk

Contents

Key points

—   Hypoxia is an exploitable difference between normal and neoplastic
    tissues.

—   "Bioreductive drugs" are effectively inert in tissues with normal levels
    of oxygenation, but activated specifically in hypoxic (tumour) tissues to
    generate a cytotoxic product.

—   Bioreductive agents are most likely to be beneficial in combination with
    standard treatments.

—   Identifying those patients who have tumours most likely to respond
    to bioreductives (and that are coincidentally those most likely to be
    refractory to standard treatments predominantly targeting oxygenated
    cells) is imperative to better interpret trial data.

Introduction

Hypoxia poses a significant challenge in cancer therapy. It is a recognised hallmark of solid tumours and is associated with both therapeutic resistance and poor prognosis. However, hypoxia is rare in normal tissues and is thereby an exploitable difference between normal and neoplastic tissues. Sartorelli and colleagues paved the way towards the development of therapies that selectively kill hypoxic cells (Lin et al 1973). They proposed the concept of "bioreductive drugs" that would be effectively inert in tissues with normal levels of oxygenation, but activated specifically in hypoxic (tumour) tissues to generate a cytotoxic product. At inception, the idea was to combine bioreductive drugs with other standard therapies (for example, radiation) where the presence of hypoxic cells within the target population was known to impair therapeutic outcome (Gray et al 1953, Thomlinson et al 1955). The physical-chemical mechanism by which oxygen enhances radiation response is well recognised (oxygen fixation theory) although in an *in vivo* situation it is likely that gene expression induced by hypoxia also contributes (Moeller et al 2005; Williams et al 2005). However for many chemotherapies, hypoxia similarly poses a challenge to effective treatment (Teicher 1994) through complex and as yet not fully understood mechanisms. Furthermore the prognostic significance of hypoxia lies not only in resistance to therapy, but also in the promotion of a more aggressive tumour phenotype, and a wealth of data links hypoxia to metastatic progression (reviewed by Lunt et al 2009). Taken together, an agent that selectively kills hypoxic cells whilst having little effect on oxygenated tissues would be a very attractive adjuvant to the majority of therapeutic approaches in clinical practice to improve both local control and disease free survival.

Early prototypes: the quinone, Mitomycin C (MMC) and the nitroaromatic, misonidazole

Bioreductive drugs are essentially pro-drugs that are activated in tumours as a consequence of the physiological difference in oxygenation between neoplastic and normal tissue. Bioreduction to the cytotoxic species is promoted by hypoxia and by the activity of specific reductase enzymes within the tissue. In the presence of oxygen, futile cycling is observed, whereby one-electron intermediaries of the reductive process are back-oxidised to the parent compound.

The first bioreductive agents developed belonged to two chemical classes, the quinones and the nitroaromatics. The prototypes in each class were the chemotherapeutic agent mitomycin C (MMC) and the hypoxic cell radiosensitiser misonidazole. MMC had already been used for over 30 years in the clinic when it was first recognised that its activation, and subsequent cytotoxicity could be enhanced in hypoxic conditions (Kennedy et al 1980; Rockwell et al 1986; Stratford et al 1989). The nitroaromatic misonidazole was developed in parallel with MMC and was found to have equivalent or greater hypoxia-selectivity. Hypoxic activation of both drugs occurs as a consequence of one electron reduction to yield cytotoxic products. The flavoenzyme NADPH/cytochrome p450 reductase (P450R) appears to play an important role in the one electron reduction of MMC to generate the semi-quinone radical anion that causes DNA cross-links. Activation of mis-onidazole occurs via the step-wise addition of up to 6-electrons by various one-electron reductases. The reactions after the addition of the first elec-tron are effectively irreversible. Reduction causes the fragmentation of the molecule leading to the generation of alkylating species (Raleigh and Liu 1984).

MMC and misonidazole were both important compounds in the initial validation of the bioreductive concept. However their activity was clearly not optimal. They generally showed only a 3-5 fold increase in potency against hypoxic versus aerobic cells that was deemed as being insufficient. Furthermore MMC is substrate of the oxygen-independent two-electron reducing enzyme NAD(P)H: quinone oxidoreductase (NQO1, also known as DT-diaphorase). NQO1 is commonly over-expressed in tumours (Malkin-son et al., 1992, Smitskamp Wilms et al., 1995, Marin et al., 1997, Li et al., 2001, Gan et al., 2001), resulting in aerobic bioactivation of MMC that significantly hampers evaluation of "hypoxic" sensitisation with this agent (Traver et al 1992; Gan et al 2001; Cowen et al 2003). However the agents solidified belief that better bioreductives could be achieved through exploitation of specific chemical classes- the original quinones and nitroaromatics, and subsequently devel-oped aliphatic N-oxides and heteroaromatic N-oxides- to generate clinically relevant agents.

Concept to clinic – development of bioreductive agents for clinical application

Potential clinical candidates have so far arisen from each of the four distinct chemical groups of bioreductive agents.

Quinones

Porfiromycin

The major confounds with MMC as a bioreductive agent were the poor hypoxia cytotoxicity ratio (HCR; ratio of drug concentration required to elicit equivalent toxicity against hypoxic versus aerobic cells) and aerobic bioactivation in the presence of the two-electron reducing enzyme NQO1. Consequently very few recent clinical trials have been designed/undertaken exploiting MMC as a true hypoxia-selective bioreductive (reviewed in McKeown et al 2007). However chemical approaches yielded MMC-derivatives with better bioreductive properties. A methylated analogue of MMC, porfiromycin, was developed that had a greater HCR than the parent compound (Fracasso and Sartorelli 1986) and showed preferential toxicity against hypoxic cells even in cell models where MMC failed to do so (Belcourt 1986). The improved HCR manifested as a result of a number of contributing factors; porfiromycin was a poorer substrate for NQO1 than MMC, showed preferential reduction via one-electron reductases and enhanced uptake in hypoxic conditions (Keyes 1987). Pre-clinical studies suggested that porfiromycin successfully targeted radioresistant hypoxic cells within tumour models yielding a supra-additive effect when combined with radiotherapy (Rockwell 1988) and yielded less systemic toxicity than MMC. A clinical study was initiated based on this data comparing porfiromycin or MMC in combination with standard radiotherapy in squamous cell carcinoma of the head and neck. Unfortunately the study showed that porfiromycin failed to provide any advantage over MMC (Haffty et al, 2005).

E09

Development within this chemical class then turned to indolequinones. A series of compounds were developed of which E09 (apaziquone) appeared most promising. Like pofiromycin, E09 showed a superior HCR compared with MMC (Robertson 1994, Saunders 2000). Hypoxic-bioactivation of the drug is linked with the one-electron reductase P450R, which leads to the generation of a DNA-damaging radical (Saunders 2000, Bailey 2001). However E09 is also an excellent substrate for 2-electron reduction via NQO1, which leads to a reduced hypoxic selectivity in cells with high NQO1 levels (Walton et al 1992, Robertson 1994, Plumb 1994). Combination with radiotherapy revealed promising data in pre-clinical tumour models (Stratford et al, 2003) prompting clinical studies. Phase I trials revealed proteinuria as the most substantive toxicity, with no effects on bone marrow. Rapid drug clearance was also reported (Schellens et al, 1994; McLeod et al, 1996). Phase II studies investigated single agent activity and were unsuccessful (Dirix et al, 1996; Pavlidis et al, 1996). One potential interpretation is that E09 may have shown efficacy against hypoxic tumour cells, but overall response was driven by the aerobic compartment. However E09 also exhibited very poor biodistribution which, coupled with a very short plasma half-life would compromise tumour cell exposure to the agent (Loadman et al 2002) when administered into the blood stream. A clever development towards trying to elucidate a clinical setting where the inherent characteristics of E09 would be less likely to impair efficacy has come with studies in superficial bladder cancer when E09 is delivered as an intravesical therapy. In two marker-tumour studies it was shown that E09 had the ability to eradicate the marker-tumour as effectively as MMC and with less toxicity than bacillus Calmette-Guerin (Puri et al 2006, van der Heijden et al 2006). This shows that when tumour cells come into direct contact with EO9, effective anti-tumour cytotoxicity can be obtained.

RH1

RH1 is a novel aziridinylbenzoquinone alkylating agent that shows very high selectivity towards NQO1 (Sharp et al 2000) and the related NRH:quinone oxidoreductase 2 (NQO2) (Yan et al 2008). In vivo studies have shown activity of RH-1 against NQO1 expressing tumours (Loadman et al 2000) and improved pharmacological properties in comparison with E09 (Loadman et al 2000). When screened against the NCI60 correlations were observed between NQO1 levels and cytotoxicity. In addition leukaemia and lymphoma cell lines appeared sensitive irrespective of NQO1 expression (Tudor et al 2005). This prompted initiation of a Phase I intervention study in advanced cancers and Non-Hogdkin's lymphoma in the US (NCT00558727 http://www.clinicaltrials.gov/) and a Phase I dose escalation study in the UK (Danson et al 2007). The trial in the US was terminated, but clinical interest has been maintained, particularly with recent observations of preclinical activity in paediatric tumour models in vitro and in vivo (Hussein et al 2009).

Nitroaromatics

RSU1069/RB6145

A drug development programme focused around derivatives of misonidazole. The first to show substantial activity was RSU1069; a 2-nitroimidazole that has an aziridine group in the N1 side-chain and fragments under hypoxic conditions to yield a bi-functional alkylating agent (Stratford et al 1986). One electron reduction via P450R appears important in the bioactivation of RSU1069 (Patterson et al 1997, Patterson et al, 2002). The hypoxia-selectivity of RSU1069 markedly improved upon that of misonidazole and the agent showed excellent radio-enhancing abilities in pre-clinical models (Stratford et al 1989b, 2003). The promising pre-clinical data prompted clinical evaluation of this compound. However gastrointestinal toxicity resulted in termination of these studies (Horwich et al 1986). A less toxic pro-drug of RSU1069 was developed (RB6145), but the R-enantiomer caused retinal toxicity in preclinical models which blocked further development (Brieder et al 1998).

TH-302

TH-302 is a prodrug in which a phosphoramide mustard group is attached to 2-nitroimidazole. Reduction of the nitro group under hypoxic conditions causes fragmentation of the molecule releasing the DNA-alkylating mustard bromo-isophosphoramide. It has been termed a HAP (hypoxia activated prodrug). Preclinical studies have shown good hypoxic selectivity, with a 270-fold increase in potency reported for H460 cells which express high levels of NQO1, thereby ruling out 2-electron reduction by this enzyme as a confounding factor in selectivity (Duan et al 2008). The compound was not sensitive to microsomal enzymes and showed significant single agent activity against orthotopic pancreatic xenografts (Duan et al 2008) and the murine 5T33MM model of multiple myeloma (Hu et al 2010), and synergistic interactions with gemcitabine (Duan et al 2008). Initial Phase I clinical studies aimed to establish dose limiting toxicity and maximum tolerated dose (MTD). 29 patients with advanced or metastatic solid tumours were evaluated. TH-302 was given on day 1, 8 and 15 of a 28 day cycle. Little haematological toxicity was observed, but adverse skin and mucosal events were observed at higher doses. The MTD was suggested as $575mg/m^2$ from this initial study. Despite primary objectives of toxicity, TH-302 demonstrated tumour responses (Bendell et al 2009), which were also observed in a follow up dose expansion trial in metastatic melanoma and lung cancer patients (Weber et al 2010). The latter study concluded that a dose of $480\ mg/m^2$ should be used in follow-up monotherapy studies to improve tolerability. The encouraging Phase I data has precipitated a series of Phase II trials investigating TH-302 in combination with a number of chemotherapies; doxorubicin in advanced soft tissue sarcoma (TH-CR-403, NCT00742963), gemcitabine in advanced pancreatic cancer (TH-CR-404, NCT01144455), gemcitabine or docetaxel or pemetrexed in advanced solid tumours (TH-CR-402, NCT00743379) and further Phase I studies as a monotherapy in advanced leukaemia (TH-CR-407, NCT01149915) and advanced solid tumours (TH-CR-401, NCT00495144; http://www.clinicaltrial.gov/).

NLCQ-1

NLCQ-1 (NSC 709257) is the lead agent from a rationale approach to develop nitroaromatics with weak DNA-intercalating properties that may improve drug biodistribution (reviewed by Papadopoulou and Bloomer 2003). The hypoxic selectivity ratio for this agent is up to 40-fold (Papadopolou 2000, Williams et al, unpublished). NLCQ-1 contains two reductive centres such that increased potency is observed when exposure time is increased (reviewed by Papadopoulou and Bloomer 2003). Activation occurs via one electron reduction with key roles implicated for P450R and cytochrome b_5 reductase. NLCQ-1 is a poor substrate for NQO1 such that overexpression of the enzyme does not influence NLCQ-1 activity (Williams and Cowen, unpublished). Preclinical studies using tumour xenografts have demonstrated that NLCQ-1 is a potent radiosensitiser and combines synergistically with a range of chemotherapies of differing modes of action (Papadopoulou et al 2001ab, 2002ab, 2006) without increasing normal tissue toxicity (Papadopoulou and Bloomer 2003). Very recent data also demonstrates that NLCQ-1 is an excellent adjuvant to radiotherapy in the control of metastatic disease (Lunt et al 2010). The clinical development of NLCQ-1 is currently being negotiated.

Dinitrobenzamide mustards: PR-104

A series of dinitrobenzamide mustards (DNBMs) have been developed that are analogues of the bioreductive agent CB1954. They are activated under severe hypoxia and provide for a bystander effect due to the formation of relatively stable cytotoxic metabolites. They were initially developed as analogues of the weak mono-functional alkylating agent CB1954 (Denny, 2010). This drug was found to have potent anti-tumour activity against the Walker rat carcinoma, associated with its reduction by rat DTD, which is present at high levels in this tumour model. CB1954 is reduced to the 4-hydroxylamino derivative, which undergoes further reaction with acetyl coenzyme A to produce a potent DNA inter-strand cross-linking agent. However, its therapeutic efficacy is limited in human tumours as CB1954 is not as good substrate for human DTD as it is for the rat isoform. CB1954 was subsequently found to be a substrate for nitroreductase and has been clinically developed in gene therapy protocols (see below). The first generation of DNBMs (e.g. SN 23862) had poor aqueous solubility and limited hypoxic selectivity leading to the more recent development of phosphate esters analogues. These have excellent solubility and formulation characteristics, and act as "pre-prodrugs"; the systemic phosphatase activity generates the corresponding alcohols (prodrugs) which are subsequently activated by nitroreductases. A lead compound, PR-104 (Proacta), has now been identified and recently completed in a Phase 1 trial in solid tumours designed to establish MTD (NCT00349167; http://www.clinicaltrial.gov/; Jameson et al 2010).

PR-104 (Proacta) is the lead compound of a series of dinitrobenzamide (DNBMs) mustards that are activated under severe hypoxia (Wilson et al 2004). A bystander effect is elicited as the cytotoxic metabolites are relatively stable. DNBMs were initially developed as analogues of the weak mono-functional alkylating agent CB1954. PR-104 is effectively a "pre-prodrug" in that it has been developed as a water-soluble phosphate ester that once administered, releases the corresponding alcohol via the action of systemic phosphatases. The alcohol (PR-104A) is then reduced via one electron reductases, including P450R to the corresponding hydroxylamine (PR-104-H) and amine (PR-104M; Patterson et al 2007, Guise et al 2007, Singleton et al 2009). Pre-clinical evaluations described excellent hypoxic selectivity in vitro. Further PR-104 exhibited single agent activity against a range of tumour xenografts and enhanced both radio- and chemotherapeutic outcome (Patterson et al 2007). Recent studies focusing upon the marked range in aerobic toxicity of the agent, which in combination with the substantial bystander effect of PR-104H may explain the single agent activity, identified that PR-104A is a substrate for the aerobic aldo-keto reductase 1C3 (Guise et al 2010). A recent Phase I clinical trial enrolled 29 patients with solid tumours that were refractory or not amenable to conventional treatment. 27 received PR-104 as an intravenous infusion every three weeks over the dose range 135 to 1400mg/m^2. Patients received a median of 2 cycles. Two were not administered PR-104 due to a change in their eligibility status. Cohort expansions were undertaken at the 135 and 1100mg/m^2 levels as a consequence of dose limiting toxicities (DLT) of Grade 3 dehydration (1 of 6 patients) and Grade 3 fatigue (1 of 6 patients) respectively. DLT were observed in 2/3 patients treated with the highest dose of 1400mg/m^2. The MTD was therefore established as 1100mg/m^2 for single agent studies, which was sufficient to yield plasma concentrations that exceeded those required for activity in xenograft models (Jameson et al 2010). Subsequent single agent and combined modality trials (with docetaxel or gemcitabine) are underway in patients with solid tumours (NCT00459836, http://www.clinicaltrials.gov/) in addition to Phase I/II in acute myeloid leukaemia.

Aliphatic N-Oxides

Banoxantrone (AQ4N)

Banoxantrone (previously known as AQ4N) is the lead compound in the aliphatic N-oxide class. It is activated under hypoxic conditions via 2 sequential 2-electron reductions, generating first the intermediate AQ4M and then the stable cytotoxin AQ4, which is an analogue of mitoxantrone (reviewed by Patterson and McKeown 2000). P450R is not implicated in the bioactivation. Instead cytochrome p450s (particular CYP1A1, CYP2B6 and CYP3A4) and the oxidoreductase protein nitric oxide synthase (NOS) appear to play important roles (Raleigh et al 1998; Patterson et al 1999; Fitzpatrick et al 2008 review; Nishida and Ortiz de Montellano 2008, Mehibel et al 2009). AQ4 has high DNA binding activity and is a potent inhibitor of topoisomerase II. Because AQ4 is a stable and persistent cytotoxin, there is potential for a bystander effect in which cytotoxicity is observed in cells other than those in which the drug was activated. Indeed recent studies have shown that activated macrophages can be used as a source of NOS to bioactivate AQ4N leading to cell death in co-cultured tumour cell populations (Mehibel et al 2009). Hypoxic selectivity ratios were initially challenging to determine for banoxantrone as the expression of the bioactivating cytochrome p450 enzymes is commonly down-regulated in cultured cells. However, supplementing cells with liver microsomes as a source of cytochrome enzymes enabled hypoxic selectivity to be observed (Patterson and McKeown, 2000). Pre-clinical studies demonstrated clear benefits of banoxantrone in combination with chemo, radio and chemoradiotherapy (McKeown et al 1995, 1996; Patterson et al 2000; Friery et al 2000; Gallager et al 2001; Williams et al 2009; Trèdan et al 2009) and impressive single agent activity in pancreatic models (Lalani et al 2007). Banoxantrone was devoid of normal tissue effects at doses that were effective in tumours and could be scheduled to avoid exacerbating toxicity associated with standard chemotherapy. The fluorescent nature of AQ4 (and banoxantrone) enables easy assessment of tissue biodistribution. Studies using multi-cellular in vitro culture models and tumour xenografts have exemplified that banoxantrone rapidly permeates aerobic tissue and accumulates in hypoxic regions (Trèdan et al 2009; Williams et al 2009). Given a clear aim to develop banoxantrone in the clinic, pre-clinical studies were also undertaken to identify hypoxic biomarkers that were co-incident with tumour-accumulation of AQ4 that could facilitate patient selection. To this end, expression of the hypoxia regulated protein glucose transporter-1 (GLUT-1) showed excellent co-registration with AQ4 accumulation in human tumour xenografts, suggesting that Glut-1 could be used as an endogenous marker of tumours that could potentially respond to treatment with banoxantrone (Williams et al 2009).

Clinical evaluation of banoxantrone started with a Phase I trial in oesophageal cancer. Patients received two doses of banoxantrone with a 2 week interval in between. The second dose was followed by palliative radiotherapy (5 x 4Gy). An MTD was not established. Banoxantrone was well tolerated in all patients, with no DLTs observed or any enhancement of radiotherapy reactions at the highest dose level administered (447 mg/m^2; Steward et al 2007). A follow up trial focused primarily on translational endpoints (drug activation and hypoxic selectivity) following a single administration of banoxantrone and subsequent surgery. Thirty-two patients (8 glioblastoma, 9 bladder, 8 head and neck, 6 breast, and 1 cervix) received banoxantrone at a single dose level of 200mg/m^2. 12 to 36h later, multiple biopsies of tumour and normal (where possible) tissue were surgically resected. Banaoxantrone and AQ4 were analysed by liquid chromatography-tandem mass spectrometry. AQ4 fluorescence was assessed in histological samples with respect to the expression of GLUT-1. AQ4 was detected in all tumours and in two thirds achieved levels greater than that required to elicit effects in preclinical studies. AQ4 co-localised with GLUT-1 and was detected at higher levels in tumour compared with adjacent normal tissue in 24/30 evaluable samples (Albertella et al 2008).

A Phase I dose escalation study has also been reported to establish an MTD for banoxantrone. 16 patients were enrolled with solid tumours refractory to standard therapy, or for which no therapy was suitable. Banoxantrone was administered i.v. on days 1, 8, and 15 of a 28 day treatment cycle. The starting dose was 12 mg/m^2. Dose was escalated by doubling until the first drug-related Grade 2 toxicity was observed, with one patient per dose to this point. Thereafter, the dose was increased by a maximum of 50% with a minimum of 3 patients per cohort. Single patients were evaluated at 12, 24, 48, 96, 192, and 384 mg/m^2, and five patients each were evaluated at doses of 768 and 1,200 mg/m^2. The median number of cycles was two. Two patients in the 1,200 mg/m^2 cohort exhibited dose limiting toxicity of Grade 3 fatigue and fatal Grade 5 respiratory failure that may have been attributed to extensive metastatic disease found within the heart and pulmonary organs upon post-mortem. No dose limiting toxicities were observed in the 768mg/m^2 cohort and this was established as the MTD. Although not a primary endpoint, stable disease was noted in 3 patients (Papadopoulos et al 2008). Further Phase I combination studies with cisplatin and Phase II with radiotherapy are ongoing in Europe, while a study of AQ4N, temozolomide and radiotherapy in glioblastoma is reportedly recruiting in the USA.

Heteroaromatic N-oxides

Tirapazamine

Tirapazamine is a heteroaromatic N-oxide that was first identified as a hypoxia selective agent in the late 1980s (Zeman et al, 1986) and has advanced through to Phase III clinical development. Tirapazamine is a substrate for one-electron reduction via cytochrome p450s, P450R and NOS (reviewed by Patterson et al 1998; Saunders et al 2000b; Chinje et al 2003; Cowen et al 2004). Under hypoxia, the reducing radical undergoes rearrangement to a DNA-targeting cytotoxic benzotriazinyl radical (Shinde et al 2004). In air, the one-electron reduction product is back-oxidised. The exceptionally high reactivity of the radical species means that tirapazamine has no bystander effect. However, tirapazamine shows marked hypoxia selectivity in vitro (HCR 50-200 fold) and significantly enhanced both radiation and chemotherapy response in xenograft studies, with little enhancement of normal tissue toxicities (reviewed by Brown 2002). Further tirpazamine appears able to control metastatic dissemination from murine tumours when administered as a neo-adjuvant to radiation treatment (Lunt et al 2005). An interesting property of tirapazamine is the relationship between observed cytotoxicity and oxygenation status. Whereas most bioreductive agents require very low oxygen conditions for bioactivation, tirapazamine becomes increasingly toxic as oxygen is depleted (Koch 1993). This means that tirapazamine can target cells at intermediate oxygen tensions that may be radioresistant, but not sufficiently hypoxic for targeting via other bioreductives. The control of tumour cells that reside at intermediate oxygen tensions is thought very important both in terms of local control and metastases (Lunt et al 2005). However a downside to tirapazamine is that it exhibits poor diffusion characteristics in studies using multi-cellular models that could impede its ability to target the full complement of hypoxic cells within a tissue (Hicks et al 2006).

Phase I clinical trials with tirapazamine suggested a dose range between 260mg/m^2 and 330mg/m^2 could be used in combination studies dependent upon schedule. The commonly reported adverse effects were neutropaenia, although this was deemed tolerable, with non-haematological toxicities of nausea, vomiting, diarrhoea and skin rash proving dose limiting (reviewed in McKeown et al 2007). Phase II trials enlisting over 1100 patients reported, in the majority of cases, clinical benefit when tirapazamine was combined with platinum-based chemotherapy and both radio- and chemoradiotherapy (reviewed in McKeown et al 2007). The earliest reported Phase III trial, however, did not match initial expectations. 367 patients with NSCLC received paclitaxel and carboplatin with or without tirapazamine. Interim analysis showed no difference in response rates or objective outcomes, and toxicity was enhanced in the tirapazamine-containing arm. The trial was closed early (Williamson et al 2005). The results of a Phase III study investigating tirapazamine, cisplatin, and radiation versus cisplatin and radiation in advanced head and neck squamous cell carcinoma (HNSCC; trial identifier TROG 02.02, HeadSTART) undertaken by the Trans-Tasman Radiation Oncology Group have been recently reported (Rischin et al 2010). The trial followed the group's encouraging randomised Phase II study reporting an 11% improvement in 3-year failure-free survival rates (55% versus 44%) and 18% improvement in 3-year locoregional failure-free rates (84% versus 66%) when tirapazamine was combined with chemo-radiotherapy in IINSCC (Rischin et al 2005). In the Phase III study 861 patients with previously untreated stage III or IV were accrued from 89 sites in 16 countries and were randomly assigned to receive definitive radiotherapy concurrently with either cisplatin or cisplatin plus tirapazamine. Disappointingly there was no significant difference in 2-year overall survival rates (65.7% for cisplatin and 66.2% for tirapazamine plus cisplatin), failure-free survival, time to locoregional failure, or quality of life in this patient population (Rischin et al

2010). However a major confounding factor to the trial outcome was revealed upon Quality Assurance analysis of the radiotherapy protocol. 12% of the accrued patients had deficiencies within their radiotherapy protocol that would be anticipated to have major impact on therapy outcome. For those that received 60 Gy or more, patients with noncompliant plans (n=87) had a 2 year overall survival rate of 50% compared with 70% in the 502 patients with compliant protocols. Noncompliance was significantly higher in centres that treated few patients (less than 5 patients, 29.8%; > or = 20 patients, 5.4%; P < .001; Peters et al 2010). These findings highlight the challenge in driving forward complex chemo-radiotherapy clinical trials in multiple centres with varying experience in patient management using standard of care protocols. Indeed additional trials with tirapazamine, which were on track to yield positive data (SWOG 0222; Le et al 2009), have been closed early due to reported toxicity in unrelated trials performed elsewhere, which may again point to inconsistencies in patient management and consequences thereof. Furthermore in none of these recently reported trials has the degree of tumour hypoxia been used to stratify patients. Where this has been previously undertaken in smaller cohorts of patients, the addition of tirapazamine to treatment protocols shows clear benefit in patients identified as having hypoxic tumours following positron emission tomography using an [18]F- fluorinated version of misonidazole (Rischin et al 2006).

Tirapazamine analogues

Clearly there are significant complexities in taking bioreductive cytotoxins through to late stage clinical evaluation. Trials with tirapazamine are still ongoing although it may be challenging to counter the lack of success so far reported in improving survival benefit. Further the observation remains that tirapazamine is not an ideal drug with respect to its diffusion properties (Hicks et al 2006). Denny, Wilson and co-workers have focused on a rational drug design programme around developing analogues of tirapazamine within the same benzotriazine di-N-oxide (BTO) class that have improved extravascular perfusion and reductive properties (Denny 2010; Hicks et al 2010). By measuring the transport parameters of tirapazamine in multicellular layer culture models they developed a spatially resolved pharmacokinetic / pharmacodynamic (SR-PKPD) model for tirapazamine. The model described the activity of tirapazamine as a function of relative position within a microvascular tissue network (Hicks et al 2006). The SR-PKPD model predicted well the relative in vivo activity of a panel of 16 BTOs in initial studies (Hicks et al 2006) and has subsequently been used to drive lead optimisation studies. This has resulted in the identification of SN30000 as the lead candidate that outperforms tirapazamine in preclinical studies (Hicks et al 2010) and has been selected for clinical development (Denny et al personal communication).

Conclusions

Targeting hypoxic cells as a means to improve therapeutic outcome in cancer has been recognised for a number of years. The "holy grail" is an agent that exhibits excellent hypoxic selectivity, potency, and pharmacokinetic and pharmacodynamic properties allowing specific clearance of hypoxic cells within the tumour microenvironment. Many agents have shown significant promise in preclinical models, but have failed clinically due to unforeseen side effects, pharmacological barriers and/or apparently poor efficacy. Further late stage clinical trials have been hampered by the fact that bioreductive agents are most likely to be beneficial in combination with standard treatments. If the standard treatment is poorly administered it becomes impossible to interpret the efficacy of the hypoxia-selective agent. An additional confounding factor is that although hypoxia is almost universally observed in solid tumours, the extent varies significantly. Identifying those patients who have tumours most likely to respond to bioreductives (and that are coincidentally those most likely to be refractory to standard treatments that predominantly target oxygenated cells) is imperative to better interpret trial data. Without this, effective agents may fail as their benefits in specific patients will be masked by a potential lack of effectiveness against the population as a whole. Increasingly early phase trials incorporate significant translational research and there have been many recent advances in developing biomarkers for hypoxia, from bioreductive tracers for non-invasive imaging (including ^{18}F-MISO PET) or histological assessment (for example pimonidazole), through endogenous tissue markers (GLUT-1, carbonic anhydrase IX) to highly predictive gene signatures (Buffa et al 2010) and microRNAs (Gee et al 2010). The agents that have most recently entered, or are about to enter clinical trial have been developed on the back of a wealth of understanding gained from trials and pitfalls of their predecessors. One can only hope that this tortuous path has resulted in agents that will soon be used routinely in clinical practice to yield step-change improvements in therapeutic outcome.

References

Albertella MR, Loadman PM, Jones PH, et al. Hypoxia-selective targeting by the bioreductive prodrug AQ4N in patients with solid tumours: results of a phase I study.
Clin Cancer Res 2008;14:1096–104.

Bailey SM, Lewis AD, Patterson LH, Fisher GR, Knox RJ, Workman P. Involvement
of NADPH: cytochrome P450 reductase in the activation of indoloquinone EO9
to free radical and DNA damaging species. Biochem Pharmacol 2001; 62:461-468.

Belcourt MF, Hodnick WF, Rockwell S, Sartorelli AC. Differential toxicity of mitomycin C and porfiromycin to aerobic and hypoxic Chinese hamster ovary cells overexpressing human NADPH:cytochrome c (P-450) reductase. Proc Natl Acad Sci U
S A 1996; 93:456-460.

Bendell JC, Weiss GJ, Infante JR, Chiorean EG, Borad M, Tibes R, Jones SF, Langmuir
VK, Kroll S, Burris HA. Final results of a phase I study of TH-302, a hypoxia-activated cytotoxic prodrug (HAP). J Clin Oncol 2009; 27 15S 2573.

Breider MA, Pilcher GD, Graziano MJ, Gough AW. Retinal degeneration in rats
induced by Cl-1010, a 2-nitroimidazole radiosensitizer. Toxicol Pathol 1998; 234-239.

Brown JM Tumour microenvironment and the response to anticancer therapy. Cancer Biol Ther. 2002;1:453-8.

Buffa FM, Harris AL, West CM, Miller CJ. Large meta-analysis of multiple cancers
reveals a common, compact and highly prognostic hypoxia metagene. Br J Cancer. 2010; 102:428-35.

Chinje EC, Cowen RL, Feng J, Sharma SP, Wind NS, Harris AL, Stratford IJ. Non-
nuclear localized human NOSII enhances the bioactivation and toxicity of tirapazamine (SR4233) in vitro. Mol Pharmacol 2003; 63:1248-1255.

Cowen RL, Patterson AV, Telfer BA, Airley RE, Hobbs S, Phillips RM, Jaffar M, Stratford IJ, Williams KJ. Viral delivery of P450 reductase recapitulates the ability of
constitutive overexpression of reductase enzymes to potentiate the activity of
mitomycin C in human breast cancer xenografts. Mol Cancer Ther 2003; 2:901-909.

Cowen RL, Williams KJ, Chinje EC, Jaffar M, Sheppard FC, Telfer BA, Wind NS, Stratford IJ. Hypoxia targeted gene therapy to increase the efficacy of tirapazamine
as an adjuvant to radiotherapy: reversing tumour radioresistance and effecting
cure. Cancer Res 2004; 64:1396-1402.

Danson S, Johnson P, Ward T, Dawson M, Denneny O, Watson A, Jowle D, Sharpe P,
Dive C, Ranson M. Final results of a phase I clinical trial of the bioreductive drug
RH1. J Clin Oncol 2007; 25, 18S: 2514.

Denny WA. Hypoxia-activated prodrugs in cancer therapy: progress towards the
clinic. Future Oncol 2010; 6: 419-28.

Dirix LYF, Tonnesen J, Cassidy R, et al. EO9 phase II study in advanced breast, gastric,
pancreatic and colorectal carcinoma by the EORTC early clinical studies group.
Eur J Cancer 1996; 32A:2019-2022.

Duan JX, Jiao H, Kaizerman J, Stanton T, Evans JW, Lan L, Lorente G, Banica M, Jung
D, Wang J, Ma H, Li X, Yang Z, Hoffman RM, Ammons WS, Hart CP, Matteucci M.

Potent and highly selective hypoxia-activated achiral phosphoramidate mustards as anticancer drugs. J Med Chem. 2008; 51:2412-20.

Fitzpatrick B, Mehibel M, Cowen RL, Stratford IJ. iNOS as a therapeutic target for treatment of human tumours. Nitric Oxide. 2008;19:217-24.

Fracasso PM, Sartorelli AC. Cytotoxicity and DNA lesions produced by mitomycin C and porfiromycin in hypoxic and aerobic EMT6 and Chinese hamster ovary cells. Cancer Res 1986; 46:3939-3944.

Friery OP, Gallagher R, Murray MM, Hughes CM, Galligan ES, McIntyre IA, Patterson LH, Hirst DG, McKeown SR. Enhancement of the anti-tumour effect of cyclophosphamide by the bioreductive drugs AQ4N and tirapazamine. Br J Cancer 2000; 82:1469-1473.

Gallagher R, Hughes CM, Murray MM, Friery OP, Patterson LH, Hirst DG, McKeown SR. The chemopotentiation of cisplatin by the novel bioreductive drug AQ4N. Br J Cancer 2001; 85:625-629. Erratum in: Br J Cancer 2002; 87:1339.

Gan Y, Mo Y, Kalns JE, Lu J, Danenberg K, Danenberg P, Wientjes MG, Au JL Expression of DT-diaphorase and cytochrome P450 reductase correlates with mitomycin C activity in human bladder tumours. Clin Cancer Res 2001; 7:1313-1319.

Gee HE, Camps C, Buffa FM, Patiar S, Winter SC, Betts G, Homer J, Corbridge R, Cox G, West CM, Ragoussis J, Harris AL. hsa-mir-210 is a marker of tumour hypoxia and a prognostic factor in head and neck cancer. Cancer. 2010; 116:2148-58.

Gray LH, Conger AD, Ebert M, Hornsey S, Scott OC. The concentration of oxygen dissolved in tissues at the time of irradiation as a factor in radiotherapy.Br J Radiol 1953; 26:638-648.

Guise CP, Wang AT, Theil A, Bridewell DJ, Wilson WR, Patterson AV. Identification of human reductases that activate the dinitrobenzamide mustard prodrug PR-104A: a role for NADPH:cytochrome P450 oxidoreductase under hypoxia. Biochem Pharmacol. 2007; 74:810-20.

Guise CP, Abbattista MR, Singleton RS, Holford SD, Connolly J, Dachs GU, Fox SB, Pollock R, Harvey J, Guilford P, Doñate F, Wilson WR, Patterson AV. The bioreductive prodrug PR-104A is activated under aerobic conditions by human aldo-keto reductase 1C3. Cancer Res. 2010; 70:1573-84.

Haffty BG, Wilson LD, Son YH, et al. Concurrent chemoradiotherapy with mitomycin C compared with porfiromycin in squamous cell cancer of the head and neck: final results of a randomized clinical trial. Int J Radiat Oncol Biol Phys 2005; 61:119-128.

Hicks KO, Pruijn FB, Secomb TW, Hay MP, Hsu R, Brown JM, Denny WA, Dewhirst MW, Wilson WR. Use of three-dimensional tissue cultures to model extravascular transport and predict in vivo activity of hypoxia-targeted anticancer drugs. J Natl Cancer Inst. 2006; 98:1118-28.

Hicks KO, Siim BG, Jaiswal JK, Pruijn FB, Fraser AM, Patel R, Hogg A, Liyanage HD, Dorie MJ, Brown JM, Denny WA, Hay MP, Wilson WR. Pharmacokinetic/pharmacodynamic modeling identifies SN30000 and SN29751 as tirapazamine analogues with improved tissue penetration and hypoxic cell killing in tumours. Clin Cancer Res. 2010;16:4946-57.

Horwich A, Holliday SB, Deacon JM, Peckham MJ. A toxicity and pharmacokinetic study in man of the hypoxic-cell radiosensitiser RSU-1069. Br J Radiol 1986; 59: 1238-1240.

Hu J, Handisides DR, Van Valckenborgh E, De Raeve H, Menu E, Vande Broek I, Liu Q, Sun JD, Van Camp B, Hart CP, Vanderkerken K. Targeting the multiple myeloma hypoxic niche with TH-302, a hypoxia-activated prodrug. Blood. 2010;116:1524-7.

Hussein D, Holt SV, Brookes KE, Klymenko T, Adamski JK, Hogg A, Estlin EJ, Ward T, Dive C, Makin GWJ. Preclinical efficacy of the bioreductive alkylating agent RH1 against paediatric tumours. British J Cancer 2009; 101: 55–63.

Jameson MB, Rischin D, Pegram M, Gutheil J, Patterson AV, Denny WA, Wilson WR. A phase I trial of PR-104, a nitrogen mustard prodrug activated by both hypoxia and aldo-keto reductase 1C3, in patients with solid tumours. Cancer Chemother Pharmacol. 2010;65:791-801.

Kennedy KA, Teicher BA, Rockwell S, Sartorelli AC The hypoxic tumour cell: a target for selective cancer chemotherapy. Biochem Pharmacol 1980; 29:1-8.

Keyes SR, Rockwell S, Sartorelli AC. Correlation between drug uptake and selective toxicity of porfiromycin to hypoxic EMT6 cells. Cancer Res 1987; 47:5654-5657.

Koch CJ. Unusual oxygen concentration dependence of toxicity of SR-4233, a hypoxic cell toxin. Cancer Res 1993; 53:3992-3997.

Lalani AS, Alters SE, Wong A, Albertella MR, Cleland JL, Henner WD. Selective tumour targeting by the hypoxia-activated prodrug AQ4N blocks tumour growth and metastasis in preclinical models of pancreatic cancer. Clin Cancer Res. 2007; 13:2216-25.

Le QT, Moon J, Redman M, Williamson SK, Lara PN Jr, Goldberg Z, Gaspar LE, Crowley JJ, Moore DF Jr, Gandara DRPhase II study of tirapazamine, cisplatin, and etoposide and concurrent thoracic radiotherapy for limited-stage small-cell lung cancer: SWOG 0222. J Clin Oncol. 2009; 27:3014-9.

Li D, Gan Y, Wientjes MG, Badalament RA, Au JL. Distribution of DT-diaphorase and reduced nicotinamide adenine dinucleotide phosphate: cytochrome p450 oxidoreductase in bladder tissues and tumours. J Urol 2001; 166: 2500-2505.

Lin AJ, Cosby LA, Shansky CW, Sartorelli AC. Potential bioreductive alkylating agents. 1. Benzoquinone derivatives. J. Med. Chem. 1973: 15; 1247–1252.

Loadman PM, Phillips RM, Lim LE, Bibby MC Pharmacological properties of a new aziridinylbenzoquinone, RH1 (2,5-diaziridinyl-3-(hydroxymethyl)-6-methyl-1,4-benzoquinone), in mice. Biochem Pharmacol. 2000; 59:831-7.

Loadman PM, Bibby MC, Phillips RM. Pharmacological approach towards the development of indolequinone bioreductive drugs based on the clinically inactive agent EO9. Br J Pharmacol 2002;137:701-709.

Lunt SJ, Telfer BA, Fitzmaurice RJ, Stratford IJ & Williams KJ, Selective killing of hypoxic cells in primary tumours using tirapazamine reduces metastatic dissemination. Clin Cancer Res 2005; 11:4212-4216.

Lunt SJ, Chaudary N, Hill RP. The tumour microenvironment and metastatic disease. Clin Exp Metastasis. 2009; 26:19-34.

Lunt SJ, Cawthorne C, Ali M, Telfer BA, Babur M, Smigova A, Julyan PJ, Price PM,

Stratford IJ, Bloomer WD, Papadopoulou MV, Williams KJ. The hypoxia-selective cytotoxin NLCQ-1 (NSC 709257) controls metastatic disease when used as an adjuvant to radiotherapy. Br J Cancer. 2010;103:201-8.

Malkinson, AM, Siegel D, Forrest GL, Gazdar AF, Oie HK, Chan DC, Bunn PA, Mabry M, Dykes DJ, Harrison SD, et al. Elevated DT-diaphorase activity and messenger RNA content in human non-small cell lung carcinoma: relationship to the response of lung tumour xenografts to mitomycin C. Cancer Res 1992; 52: 4752-4757.

Marin A, Lopez de Cerain A, Hamilton E, Lewis AD, Martinez-Penuela JM, Idoate MA, Bello J. DT-diaphorase and cytochrome B5 reductase in human lung and breast tumours. Br J Cancer 1997; 76: 923-929.

McLeod HL, Graham MA, Aamdal S, Setanoians A, Groot Y, Lund B. Phase I pharmacokinetics and limited sampling strategies for the bioreductive alkylating drug EO9. Eur J Cancer 1996;32A:1518-1522.

McKeown SR, Hejmadi MV, McIntyre IA, McAleer JJ, Patterson LH. AQ4N: an alkylaminoanthraquinone N-oxide showing bioreductive potential and positive interaction with radiation in vivo. Br J Cancer 1995; 72:76-81.

McKeown SR, Friery OP, McIntyre IA, Hejmadi MV, Patterson LH and Hirst DG. Evidence for a therapeutic gain when AQ4N or tirapazamine is combined with radiation. Br J Cancer 1996; 74: S39-S42

McKeown SR, Cowen RL & Williams KJ. Bioreductive drugs: from concept to clinic. Clinical Oncology 2007; 19: 427-442.

Mehibel M, Singh S, Chinje EC, Cowen RL, Stratford IJ. Effects of cytokine-induced macrophages on the response of tumour cells to banoxantrone (AQ4N). Mol Cancer Ther. 2009; 8:1261–9

Moeller BJ, Dreher MR, Rabbani ZN, Schroeder T, Cao Y, Li CY, Dewhirst MW. Pleiotropic effects of HIF-1 blockade on tumour radiosensitivity. Cancer Cell. 2005; 8: 99-110.

Nishida CR, Ortiz de Montellano PR. Reductive heme-dependent activation of the n-oxide prodrug AQ4N by nitric oxide synthase. J Med Chem. 2008; 51:5118-20.

Papadopoulou MV, Ji M, Rao MK, Bloomer WD. 4-[3-(2-Nitro-1-imidazolyl)propylamino]-7-chloroquinoline hydrochloride (NLCQ-1), a novel bioreductive compound as a hypoxia-selective cytotoxin. Oncol Res 2000;12:185-192.

Papadopoulou MV, Ji M, Bloomer WD. Schedule-dependent potentiation of chemotherapeutic drugs by the bioreductive compounds NLCQ-1 and tirapazamine against EMT6 tumours in mice. Cancer Chemother Pharmacol 2001a; 48:160-168.

Papadopoulou MV, Ji M, Rao MK, Bloomer WD. 4-[3-(2-Nitro-1-imidazolyl)propylamino]-7-chloroquinoline hydrochloride (NLCQ-1), a novel bioreductive agent as radiosensitizer in vitro and in vivo: comparison with tirapazamine. Oncol Res 2001b; 12:325-333.

Papadopoulou MV, Ji M, Ji X, Bloomer WD. Therapeutic advantage from combining 5-fluorouracil with the hypoxia-selective cytotoxin NLCQ-1 in vivo; comparison with tirapazamine. Cancer Chemother Pharmacol 2002a; 50:291-298.

Papadopoulou MV, Ji M, Bloomer WD. Synergistic enhancement of the antitumour effect of taxol by the bioreductive compound NLCQ-1, in vivo: comparison with tirapazamine. Oncol Res 2002b;13:47-54.

Papadopoulou MV, Bloomer WD. NLCQ-1 (NSC 709257): exploiting hypoxia with a weak DNA-intercalating bioreductive drug. Clin Cancer Res 2003; 9:5714-5720.

Papadopoulou MV, Ji X, Bloomer WD. Potentiation of alkylating agents by NLCQ-1 or TPZ in vitro and in vivo. J Exp Ther Oncol 2006; 5:261-272.

Papadopoulos KP, Goel S, Beeram M, Wong A, Desai K, Haigentz M, Milian ML, Mani S, Tolcher A, Lalani AS, Sarantopoulos J. A Phase 1 open-label, accelerated dose-escalation study of the hypoxia-activated prodrug AQ4N in patients with advanced malignancies. Clin Cancer Res 2008;14: 7110-7115.

Patterson AV, Saunders MP, Chinje EC, Talbot DC, Harris AL, Strafford IJ. Overexpression of human NADPH:cytochrome c (P450) reductase confers enhanced sensitivity to both tirapazamine (SR 4233) and RSU 1069. Br J Cancer 1997; 76:1338-1334.

Patterson AV, Saunders MP, Chinje EC, Patterson LH, Stratford IJ. Enzymology of tirapazamine metabolism: a review. Anticancer Drug Des 1998; 13:541-573.

Patterson LH, McKeown SR, Robson T, Gallagher R, Raleigh SM, Orr S. Antitumour prodrug development using cytochrome P450 (CYP) mediated activation. Anti-Cancer Drug Des 1999; 14:473-486.

Patterson LH, McKeown SR, Ruparelia K, Double JA, Bibby MC, Cole S, Stratford IJ. Enhancement of chemotherapy and radiotherapy of murine tumours by AQ4N, a bioreductively activated anti-tumour agent. Br J Cancer 2000; 82:1984-1990.

Patterson LH, McKeown SR. AQ4N: a new approach to hypoxia-activated cancer chemotherapy. Br J Cancer 2000; 83:1589-1593.

Patterson AV, Williams KJ, Cowen RL, Jaffar M, Telfer BA, Saunders M, Airley R, Honess D, van der Kogel AJ, Wolf CR, Stratford IJ. Oxygen-sensitive enzyme-prodrug gene therapy for the eradication of radiation-resistant solid tumours. Gene Ther. 2002; 9: 946-54.

Patterson AV, Ferry DM, Edmunds SJ, Gu Y, Singleton RS, Patel K, Pullen SM, Hicks KO, Syddall SP, Atwell GJ, Yang S, Denny WA, Wilson WR. Mechanism of action and preclinical antitumour activity of the novel hypoxia-activated DNA cross-linking agent PR-104. Clin Cancer Res. 2007;13:3922-32.

Pavlidis N, Hanauske AR, Gamucci T, et al. A randomized phase II study with two schedules of the novel indoloquinone EO9 in non-small-cell lung cancer: a study of the EORTC Early Clinical Studies Group (ECSG). Ann Oncol 1996;7:529-531.

Peters LJ, O'Sullivan B, Giralt J, Fitzgerald TJ, Trotti A, Bernier J, Bourhis J, Yuen K, Fisher R, Rischin D. Critical impact of radiotherapy protocol compliance and quality in the treatment of advanced head and neck cancer: results from TROG 02.02. J Clin Oncol. 2010; 28 :2996-3001.

Plumb JA, Gerritsen M, Milroy R, Thomson P, Workman P. Relative importance of DT-diaphorase and hypoxia in the bioactivation of EO9 by human lung tumour cell lines. Int J Radiat Oncol Biol Phys 1994; 29:295-299.

Puri R, Palit V, Loadman PM, et al. Phase I/II pilot study of intravesical apaziquone (EO9) for superficial bladder cancer. J Urol 2006;176:1344-1348.

Raleigh JA, Liu SF. Reductive fragmentation of 2-nitroimidazoles: amines and aldehydes. Int J Radiat Oncol Biol Phys. 1984; 108:1337-40.

Raleigh SM, Wanogho E, Burke MD, Mckeown SR, Patterson LH. Involvement of human cytochrome P450(CYP)in the reductive metabolism of AQ4N,a hypoxia activated anthraquinone di-n-oxide prodrug. Int J Radiation Oncology Biol Phys. 1998; 42:763-767.

Rischin D, Peters L, Fisher R, et al. Tirapazamine, cisplatin, and radiation versus fluorouracil, cisplatin, and radiation in patients with locally advanced head and neck cancer: a randomized phase II trial of the Trans-Tasman Radiation Oncology Group (TROG 98.02). J Clin Oncol 2005; 23:79-87.

Rischin D, Hicks RJ, Fisher R, et al. Prognostic significance of [18F]-misonidazole positron emission tomography-detected tumour hypoxia in patients with advanced head and neck cancer randomly assigned to chemoradiation with or without tirapazamine: a substudy of Trans-Tasman Radiation Oncology Group study 98.02. J Clin Oncol 2006; 24:2098-2104.

Rischin D, Peters LJ, O'Sullivan B, Giralt J, Fisher R, Yuen K, Trotti A, Bernier J, Bourhis J, Ringash J, Henke M, Kenny L. Tirapazamine, cisplatin, and radiation versus cisplatin and radiation for advanced squamous cell carcinoma of the head and neck (TROG 02.02, HeadSTART): a phase III trial of the Trans-Tasman Radiation Oncology Group. J Clin Oncol. 2010; 28:2989-95.

Robertson N, Haigh A, Adams GE, Stratford IJ. Factors affecting sensitivity to EO9 in rodent and human tumour cells in vitro: DT-diaphorase activity and hypoxia. Eur J Cancer 1994; 30A:1013-1019.

Rockwell S. Effect of some proliferative and environmental factors on the toxicity of mitomycin C to tumour cells in vitro. Int J Cancer 1986; 38:229-235.

Rockwell S, Keyes SR, Sartorelli AC. Preclinical studies of porfiromycin as an adjunct to radiotherapy. Radiat Res 1988; 116:100-113.

Saunders MP, Jaffar M, Patterson AV, Nolan J, Naylor MA, Phillips RM, Harris AL, Stratford IJ. The relative importance of NADPH: cytochrome c (P450) reductase for determining the sensitivity of human tumour cells to the indolequinone EO9 and related analogues lacking functionality at the C-2 and C-3 positions. Biochem Pharmacol 2000; 59:993-996.

Saunders MP, Patterson AV, Chinje EC, Harris AL, Stratford IJ. NADPH:cytochrome c (P450) reductase activates tirapazamine (SR4233) to restore hypoxic and oxic cytotoxicity in an aerobic resistant derivative of the A549 lung cancer cell line. Br J Cancer 2000b; 82:651-656.

Schellens JHM, Planting AST, Van Acker BAC, et al. Phase I and pharmacologic study of the novel indoloquinone bioreductive alkylating cytotoxic drug EO9. J Natl Cancer Inst 1994; 86: 906-912.

Sharp SY, Kelland LR, Valenti MR, Brunton LA, Hobbs S, Workman P. Establishment of an isogenic human colon tumour model for NQO1 gene expression: application to investigate the role of DT-diaphorase in bioreductive drug activation in vitro and in vivo. Mol Pharmacol. 2000; 58:1146-55.

Shinde SS, Anderson RF, Hay MP, Gamage SA, Denny WA. Oxidation of 2-deoxyribose by benzotriazinyl radicals of antitumour 3-amino-1,2,4-benzotriazine 1,4-dioxides. J Am Chem Soc. 2004; 126:7865-74.

Singleton RS, Guise CP, Ferry DM, Pullen SM, Dorie MJ, Brown JM, Patterson AV, Wilson WR. DNA cross-links in human tumour cells exposed to the prodrug PR-104A: relationships to hypoxia, bioreductive metabolism, and cytotoxicity. Cancer Res. 2009;69:3884-91.

Smitskamp-Wilms E, Giaccone G, Pinedo HM, van der Laan BF, Peters GJ. DT-diaphorase activity in normal and neoplastic human tissues; an indicator for sensitivity to bioreductive agents? Br J Cancer 1995; 72: 917-921.

Steward WP, Middleton M, Benghiat A, et al. The use of pharmacokinetic and pharmacodynamic end points to determine the dose of AQ4N, a novel hypoxic cell cytotoxin, given with fractionated radiotherapy in a phase I study. Ann Oncol 2007;18:1098-103.

Stratford IJ, O'Neill P, Sheldon PW, Silver AR, Walling JM, Adams GE. RSU 1069, a nitroimidazole containing an aziridine group. Bioreduction greatly increases cytotoxicity under hypoxic conditions. Biochem Pharmacol 1986; 35:105-109.

Stratford IJ, Stephens MA. The differential hypoxic cytotoxicity of bioreductive agents determined in vitro by the MTT assay. Int J Radiat Oncol Biol Phys 1989; 16:973-976.

Stratford IJ, Adams GE, Godden J, Howells N. Induction of tumour hypoxia post-irradiation: a method for increasing the sensitizing efficiency of misonidazole and RSU 1069 in vivo. Int J Radiat Biol 1989b; 55:411-422.

Stratford IJ, Williams KJ, Cowen RL, Jaffar M. Combining bioreductive drugs and radiation for the treatment of solid tumours. Semin Radiat Oncol 2003; 13:42-52.

Teicher BA. Hypoxia and drug resistance. Cancer Metas Rev 1994; 13:139-168.

Thomlinson RH, Gray LH. The histological structure of some human lung cancers and the possible implications for radiotherapy. Br J Cancer 1955; 9:539-549.

Traver RD, Horikoshi T, Danenberg KD, Stadlbauer TH, Danenberg PV, Ross D, Gibson NW. NAD(P)H:quinone oxidoreductase gene expression in human colon carcinoma cells: characterization of a mutation which modulates DT-diaphorase activity and mitomycin sensitivity. Cancer Res 1992; 52:797-802.

Tre'dan O, Garbens AB, Lalani AS, Tannock IF. The hypoxia-activated prodrug AQ4N penetrates deeply in tumour tissues and complements the limited distribution of mitoxantrone. Cancer Res 2009; 69 :940-7

Tudor G, Alley M, Nelson CM, Huang R, Covell DG, Gutierrez P, Sausville EA. Cytotoxicity of RH1: NAD(P)H:quinone acceptor oxidoreductase (NQO1)-independent oxidative stress and apoptosis induction. Anticancer Drugs. 2005;16:381-91.

van der Heijden AG, Moonen PM, Cornel EB, et al. Phase II marker lesion study with intravesical instillation of apaziquone for superficial bladder cancer: toxicity and marker response. J Urol 2006;176:1349-1353.

Walton MI, Smith PJ, Workman P. The role of NAD(P)H: quinone reductase (EC 1.6.99.2, DT-diaphorase) in the reductive bioactivation of the novel indoloquinone antitumour agent EO9. Cancer Commun. 1991; 3:199-206.

Weber RW, Weiss GJ, Chiorean EG, Senzer NN, Borad MJ, Markovic S, Molina JR, Langmuir VK, Lee H, Infante JR. Safety and activity of TH-302, a hypoxia-activated cytotoxic prodrug (HAP), in patients with metastatic melanoma and lung cancer. J Clin Oncol 2010 28, 15S 19009

Williams KJ, Telfer BA, Xenaki D, Sheridan MR, Desbaillets I, Peters HJ, Honess D, Harris AL, Dachs GU, van der Kogel A, Stratford IJ. Enhanced response to radiotherapy in tumours deficient in the function of hypoxia-inducible factor-1. Radiother Oncol. 2005;75: 89-98.

Williams KJ, Albertella MR, Fitzpatrick B, Loadman PM, Shnyder SD, Chinje EC, Telfer BA, Dunk CR, Harris PA, Stratford IJ. In vivo activation of the hypoxia-targeted cytotoxin AQ4N in human tumour xenografts. Mol Cancer Ther. 2009; 8:3266-75.

Williamson SK, Crowley JJ, Lara PN Jr, et al. Phase III trial of paclitaxel plus carboplatin with or without tirapazamine in advanced non-small-cell lung cancer: Southwest Oncology Group Trial S0003. J Clin Oncol 2005;23:9097-9104.

Wilson WR, Pullen SM, Degenkolbe A, et al. Water-soluble dinitrobenzamide mustard phosphate pre-prodrugs as hypoxic cytotoxins. Eur J Cancer 2004;Suppl. 2:151.

Yan C, Kepa JK, Siegel D, Stratford IJ, Ross D. Dissecting the role of multiple reductases in bioactivation and cytotoxicity of the antitumour agent 2,5-diaziridinyl-3-(hydroxymethyl)-6-methyl-1,4-benzoquinone (RH1). Mol Pharmacol. 2008;74:1657-65.

Zeman EM, Brown JM, Lemmon MJ, Hirst VK, Lee WW. SR-4233: a new bioreductive agent with high selective toxicity for hypoxic mammalian cells.Int J Radiat Oncol Biol Phys 1986;12:1239-1242.

Chapter 18

Targeting the hypoxic tumour microenvironment: a unique role for HIF-1 inhibitors

Annamaria Rapisarda[1], Nicole Fer[1] and Giovanni Melillo[2*]

*Author for correspondence:
[1] SAIC Frederick, Inc., Developmental Therapeutics Program, Tumour Hypoxia Laboratory, National Cancer Institute at Frederick, Frederick, MD 21702
[2] Director, Discovery Medicine and Clinical Pharmacology, Oncology/Immunology, Bristol-Myers Squibb, Princeton, NJ 08540, Email: giovanni.melillo@bms.com

Contents

Key points

— The hypoxic microenvironment is a key feature of solid tumours and HIF is the main signalling pathway that drives adaptation to hypoxia.

— Increasing evidence highlights the functional difference between HIF-1α and HIF-2α in cancer and their contrasting effects on tumour growth.

— The majority of HIF inhibitors identified are not specific for the HIF pathway; this feature might might impact of their development for cancer therapy.

— HIF inhibitors described hitherto are either targeting HIF-1α or both HIF-1α and HIF-2α. No selective HIF-2α inhibitors have been identified thus far.

— HIF-1 inhibitors should be tested in carefully designed clinical trials, primarily in combination studies to fully exploit their potential.

Summary

Within solid tumours, an imbalance between increased oxygen consumption by proliferating tumour cells and decreased delivery from an aberrant vasculature creates areas of low oxygen concentration (hypoxia). Intratumour hypoxia is an independent indicator of unfavourable patient prognosis and adaptation to hypoxia is an important contributing factor to a more aggressive tumour phenotype. The discovery of hypoxia inducible factors (HIF-1α and HIF-2α) as the main mediators of hypoxia dependent responses has provided identifiable molecular targets associated with hypoxia and has lead to the discovery and development of targeted therapies exploiting the hypoxic tumour microenvironment. Indeed, a fairly large number of small molecules that inhibit HIF in cell lines and have anti-tumour activity in animal models have been identified; however, whether and how these agents might be exploited in the clinical setting remains poorly defined. Interestingly, despite their high homology, HIF-1α and HIF-2α have been shown to have different roles in tumourigenesis depending on specific tumour types and genetic backgrounds, making the discovery of small molecules that would selectively inhibit one or the other an attractive possibility; nevertheless most of the inhibitors described hitherto may indeed block both HIF-1α and HIF-2α. In this chapter we will review the role of HIF-1α and HIF-2α in cancer, HIF inhibitors in clinical trials and those for which validation in animal models has been provided and we will discuss how to best exploit HIF targeted agents for cancer therapy.

HIF-α: molecular target of the tumour microenvironment

Solid tumours are characterized by areas of very steep oxygen concentration gradients, as well as by temporal fluctuations in oxygenation, that are not present in normal tissues (Brown, 2004; Dewhirst, 2008). Of the many survival pathways co-opted by cancer cells, adaptation to low oxygen concentration (hypoxia) is an important driving force in the clonal selection that leads to invasive and metastatic disease as well as to resistance to treatment (Semenza, 2007).

Adaptation to hypoxia is predominantly regulated by Hypoxia Inducible Factor 1 (HIF-1), a heterodimeric transcription factor consisting of a constitutively expressed β-subunit (HIF-1β) and of an oxygen regulated α-subunit (HIF-1α or HIF-2α) that activates transcription of numerous target genes involved in key steps of tumourigenesis, including angiogenesis, metabolism, proliferation, metastasis, differentiation and resistance to therapy (Semenza, 2008; Qing, 2009). Indeed, HIF-1α and/or HIF-2α expression has been shown in the majority of human cancers and their metastases, where they are associated with patient mortality and poor response to treatment (Table 18.1). Increased HIF-α expression is also associated with a variety of genetic alterations that inactivate tumour suppressor genes or activate oncogenic pathways, as well as with activation of Receptor Tyrosine Kinase-dependent signalling pathways (Semenza, 2003).

HIF1α and HIF-2α: similar but distinct

Under normal oxygen conditions, HIF-α subunits are subjected to oxygen dependent hydroxylation by prolyl hydroxylases (PHDs) and to von Hippel-Lindau (VHL)-dependent proteasomal degradation (Kaelin, Jr., 2008). Furthermore, HIF-α subunits are hydroxylated on asparagine residues by Factor inhibiting HIF-1 (FIH), which blocks HIF-1-dependent transcriptional activation under normoxia (Mahon, 2001). Hypoxia inhibits HIF-α hydroxylation, allowing HIF-α to dimerize with HIF-1β, translocate to the nucleus and, upon recruitment of p300, induce expression of HIF-1 dependent genes.

HIF-1α and HIF-2α are thought to be regulated in a similar fashion; however, accumulating evidence highlights clear differences amid the signalling that controls the two subunits. Indeed, it has been reported that iron regulatory protein (IRP) controls HIF-2α, but not HIF-1α, translation in response to cellular iron availability (Sanchez, 2007). In addition, HIF-1α protein levels have been shown to be dependent on both mTORC1 and mTORC2 in renal cell carcinomas, while HIF-2α accumulation was dependent only on the expression of the mTORC2 (Toschi, 2008). Moreover, it has been recently suggested that mutant KRAS induces HIF-1α protein translation in a PI3K-dependent manner in colon cancer cells, while HIF-2α translation is up-regulated in cells with mutant BRAF in a MEK-dependent fashion, indicating that genetic alterations may play different roles in the regulation of HIF-1α and HIF-2α (Kikuchi, 2009). Interestingly, HIF-2α appears to be less sensitive than HIF-1α to inhibition by FIH (Koivunen, 2004) and to PHD-dependent degradation at near-physiological oxygen tension (5%) (Holmquist-Mengelbier, 2006), suggesting that HIF-2α plays a major role in mediating mild hypoxia-dependent responses. In addition, HIF-2α, but not HIF-1α, has been shown to interact with the NFκB essential modulator (NEMO) resulting in an enhanced HIF-2α transcriptional activity (Bracken, 2005). Furthermore, redox-sensitive class III histone deacetylase sirtuin proteins (Sirt1 and Sirt6) have been shown to affect HIF responses by inhibiting HIF-1α transcriptional activity while increasing HIF-2α dependent gene expression (Dioum, 2009; Lim, 2010; Zhong, 2010b). Notably, Sirt1 expression and activity has been reported to gradually decrease during hypoxia, suggesting that HIF-1α may determine hypoxia-dependent responses during its early phases, and HIF-2α may then take over the hypoxic signalling during protracted hypoxia.

It is important to point out that HIF-2α has an extensive sequence similarity with HIF-1α, although it regulates a set of genes that overlap with, but are distinct from, those regulated by HIF-1α in several cell types (Lau, 2007). For instance, HIF-1α is responsible for the regulation of transcription of genes encoding enzymes involved in the glycolytic pathway, while Oct4, a crucial transcription factor regulating stem cell self-renewal, is a specific target of HIF-2α (Qing, 2009; Semenza, 2010). In addition, HIF-1α induces cell cycle arrest during hypoxia, which is attributed to its interaction with MAX and subsequent inhibition of c-Myc-dependent responses, while HIF-2α has been shown to promote tumour growth and proliferation, partially by interacting and stabilizing c-Myc/MAX complex (Gordan, 2007). Moreover, it has been recently reported that HIF-2α enhances the transcriptional activity of β-catenin in renal cell carcinomas (Choi, 2010), while HIF-1α down-regulates β-catenin-dependent responses (Kaidi, 2007). Furthermore, HIF-2α, but not HIF-1α, has been shown to up-regulate EGFR protein synthesis in several cancer cell types and to mediate tumour cell proliferation (Franovic, 2007). Hence, there is increasing evidence for the functional non-equivalence of HIF-1α and HIF-2α in cancer and for their contrasting effects on tumour growth in certain models. Nevertheless, the relative contribution of HIF-1α and/or HIF-2α to tumour progression is still poorly understood and may be tumour type dependent.

HIF inhibitors

Despite the challenges associated with targeting transcription factors, several attempts have been made to identify HIF-1 inhibitors based, for the most part, on high throughput screening assays designed to identify small molecules affecting HIF-1 expression and/or transcriptional activity (Rapisarda, 2002; Melillo, 2007). This strategy allows the identification of compounds that affect HIF-1 through several pathways adding, on the one hand, knowledge on the signalling involved in HIF-1 regulation and, on the other hand, challenges associated with elucidation of the molecular mechanism of the hits identified. Furthermore, the majority of HIF-1 inhibitors discovered so far target signalling pathways that are not only involved in HIF-1 regulation but also affect distinct cellular functions. It should also be noted that many of the HIF inhibitors described hitherto may indeed block both HIF-1α and HIF-2α, making pharmacological validation of their relative contribution to tumourigenesis very complicated. The effects on HIF-2α expression and/or activity has not been reported for many of the agents identified to this point and high throughput screening aimed at identifying selective HIF-2α inhibitors did not yield selective hits (Woldemichael, 2006). Interestingly, only one example of a putative HIF-2α selective inhibitor has been described (Zimmer, 2008), however, this molecule has been recently used as a HIF-1α inhibitor as well (Zhong, 2010a).

Table 18.1 _ Studies in which over-expression of HIF-1α (or HIF-2α) protein in tumour biopies was demonstrated.

Cancer Type	Reference
Astrocytoma (diffuse)	(Theodoropoulos, 2004)
Bladder (superficial urothelial)[1]	(Theodoropoulos, 2005)
Bladder (transitional cells)	(Vleugel, 2005)
Breast	(Dales, 2005; Generali, 2006)
Breast (estrogen receptor positive)	(Giatromanolaki, 2007)
Breast (c-Erb2 positive)	(Schindl, 2002)
Breast (positive linfonode)	(Bos, 2003)
Breast (negative linfonode)	(Birner, 2000)
Cervix (early stage)	(Burri, 2003)
Cervix (radiation therapy)	(Bachtiary, 2003)

Cancer Type	Reference
Cervix (grade IB-IIIB, radiation therapy)	(Rajaganeshan, 2008; Schmitz, 2009)
Colorectal	(Cleven, 2007)
Colorectal[2]	(Sivridis, 2002)
Endometrial	(Tzao, 2008)
Esophageal squamous cell carcinoma	(Griffiths, 2007)
Gastric	(Takahashi, 2003)
Gastrointestinal stromal tumour (stomach)	(Koukourakis, 2002)
Head and Neck squamous cell carcinoma[3]	(Schrijvers, 2008)
Laryngeal	(Swinson, 2004)
Lung (non small cell lung carcinoma)	(Giatromanolaki, 2001)
Lung (non small cell lung carcinoma)[4]	(Giatromanolaki, 2003)
Melanoma (malignant)[4]	(Holmquist-Mengelbier, 2006)
Neuroblastoma[4]	(Birner, 2001a)
Oligodendrioglioma	(Aebersold, 2001)
Oropharynx-squamous cell carcinoma	(Birner, 2001b)
Ovarian[1]	(Daponte, 2008)
Ovarian (serous)	(Sun, 2007)
Pancreatic	(Nanni, 2009)
Prostate[5]	(Rasheed, 2009)
Rectal	(Raval, 2005; Kondo, 2002; Kondo, 2003)
Renal clear cell carcinoma4	(Mandriota, 2002)

[1] Combination of HIF-1α over-expression and mutant p53 was associated with mortality.

[2] HIF2α expression in stromal, but not cancer, cells was associated with mortality.

[3] High HIF-1α and high HIF-2α expression were associated with mortality.

[4] High HIF-2α, but not HIF-1α, expression was associated with mortality.

[5] A combination of high HIF-2α expression and nuclear localisation of endothelial nitric oxide synthase was associated with mortality.

Mechanisms of HIF-1 inhibition

The mechanism of action of HIF inhibitors reported varies from an effect on HIF-α protein levels (by either decreasing HIF-α mRNA levels, protein translation, or by increasing HIF-α protein degradation) to an inhibition of HIF-1 transcriptional activity, HIF-1α HIF-1β dimerization or HIF-1 DNA binding.

We will review HIF-1 inhibitors below, which are in pre-clinical or clinical development, based on their proposed mechanism of action.

Inhibitors of HIF-α mRNA expression

Antisense oligonucleotides

Modulation of HIF-1α mRNA levels using antisense oligonucleotides (EZN-2968) has been proposed as a "specific" avenue to inhibit HIF-1α activity (Greenberger, 2008). EZN-2968 is a locked nucleic acid RNA antagonist that specifically binds to and inhibits the expression of HIF-1α mRNA. In vitro and *in vivo* experiments confirmed that EZN-2968 induced a potent, selective, and durable inhibition of HIF-1α mRNA and protein expression associated with inhibition of HIF-1-dependent gene expression. Ongoing phase I studies of EZN-2968 in patients with advanced malignancies have shown durable stable disease in two patients with soft tissues sarcomas (angiosarcoma, leiomyosarcoma), in one patient with renal cell carcinoma, and in one patient with ovarian cancer. However, delivery of this therapeutic agent to cancer cells remains a main practical challenge of this approach.

Aminoflavone

Aminoflavone (AF), the active component of the novel anticancer agent AFP464, is a ligand of the aryl-hydrocarbon receptor (AhR). Based on the notion that AhR dimerizes with HIF-1β, it was hypothesized that pharmacological activation of the AhR pathway using AF might affect HIF-α levels and/or activity. Results of these studies have shown that AF does indeed inhibit HIF-1α accumulation, although in an AhR-independent fashion. The proposed mechanism of HIF-1 inhibition by AF is modulation of HIF-1α mRNA expression, although the exact mechanism remains to be fully elucidated (Terzuoli, 2010). Interestingly, AF inhibits HIF-2α protein expression in clear cell renal carcinoma, although its effect on HIF-2α mRNA and translation were not investigated. AFP464 is currently in phase I clinical trials in patients with metastatic cancer.

Inhibitors of HIF-α protein accumulation

PI3K/AKT/mTOR inhibitors

HIF-α expression is largely controlled at the level of protein degradation; however, since HIF-α is degraded under normoxic conditions, ongoing protein translation is essential for its accumulation. HIF-α protein synthesis is controlled, at least in part, by the PI3K/AKT/mTOR pathway (Semenza, 2003). It is then conceivable that mTOR inhibitors currently in clinical development might inhibit HIF-1 and impact on downstream pathways including angiogenesis. Indeed, inhibitors of mTOR have been shown to inhibit HIF-1α protein accumulation (temsirolimus/CCI-779 and everolimus/RAD001) (Thomas, 2006). Notably, loss of VHL sensitized kidney cancer cells to the mTOR inhibitor temsirolimus both in vitro and in mouse models (Narita, 2009). HIF-1α might be a determinant of response in cancers in which the mTOR pathway is deregulated and may also represent an attractive biomarker of activity of mTOR inhibitors; however, this possibility has yet to be validated in the clinical setting. Interestingly, a differential sensitivity of HIF-1α and HIF-2α to rapamycin has been reported; yet, both HIF-1α and HIF-2α expression have been shown to be dependent upon mTOR (Toschi, 2008; Bhatt, 2008). This observation is explained by a dependence of HIF-2α expression on the rapamycin-resistant mTORC2, whereas there is a dependence of HIF-1α expression on both mTORC1 and mTORC2 (Toschi, 2008). Considering that HIF-2α has been suggested as the primary HIF-α subunit accounting for renal cell carcinomas aggressiveness, it is likely that available mTOR inhibitors might function through HIF-α-independent mechanism in clear cell renal carcinoma patients. Notably, NVP-BEZ235, a novel, orally bioavailable imidazoquinoline that potently and reversibly inhibits class 1 PI3K activity as well as both mTORC1 and mTORC2, has been shown to inhibit HIF-2α expression and function in renal cell carcinomas in vitro and in vivo (Cho, 2010), providing a new tool to down-regulate HIF-dependent responses in renal carcinomas.

RTKs inhibitors

HIF-α protein accumulation can be induced by a variety of growth factor-mediated Receptors Tyrosine Kinase (RTKs)-dependent signalling pathways in a cell type dependent fashion. Indeed, EGFR inhibitors, such as gefitinib (Iressa), erlotinib (Tarceva) and cetuximab, have been shown to inhibit HIF-1α protein expression (Luwor, 2005; Pore, 2006). Likewise, it has been suggested that trastuzumab (herceptin), a humanized monoclonal antibody approved for the treatment of patients with Her2/Neu positive breast cancer, may exert its antiangiogenic effects, at least in part, by inhibiting HIF-1α-dependent induction of VEGF (Koukourakis, 2003). In addition, imatinib, a small molecule inhibitor of BCR/ABL (an oncoprotein present in chronic myelogenous leukemia) has also been suggested to down-regulate HIF-1α expression in small cell lung cancer cell lines, presumably by inhibiting c-Kit-dependent induction of the PI3K pathway (Litz, 2006).

Recently, it has been shown that HIF-1α and HIF-2α are differentially regulated by RTKs in neuroblastoma (Nilsson, 2010). In particular, normoxic accumulation of HIF-1α was induced by EGFR, RET, PDGFR-β and VEGFR-1 dependent signalling, while HIF-2α accumulation was observed only following VEGFR-1 activation. Indeed, hypoxic accumulation of HIF-1α was inhibited by sorafenib, sunitinib and imatinib, while HIF-2α was affected by sunitinib and imatinib, but not by sorafenib. Interestingly, sunitinib down-regulates HIF-α subunits by a mechanism involving both modulation of mRNA levels and decreased protein stability. These findings suggest that multikinase inhibitors may exert antiangiogenic effects also by blocking compensatory hypoxia- and ligand-induced changes in HIF-1α and HIF-2α.

Topoisomerase inhibitors

Topotecan (TPT), an FDA approved topoisomerase I (Top 1) poison, was one of the first small molecule inhibitors of HIF-1α identified in a cell-based HTS at the NCI in Frederick (Rapisarda, 2002). TPT inhibits HIF-1α expression by a Top 1-dependent pathway, independent from DNA replication and DNA damage, yet requires ongoing RNA transcription. Notably, inhibition of HIF-1α protein translation by TPT does not require AKT-mTOR signalling pathway (Rapisarda, 2004a). Interestingly, TPT also inhibits HIF-2α protein accumulation; although to a lesser extent than HIF-1α in certain cell types (Rapisarda A and Melillo G unpublished observation). Daily administration of low doses of topotecan (1 mg/Kg) inhibited tumour growth, angiogenesis and expression of HIF-1-target genes in a human glioma xenograft model, suggesting a potential association between HIF-1 inhibition and a beneficial therapeutic effect (Rapisarda, 2004b). However, a limitation of these studies is that topotecan may also exert cytostatic/cytotoxic effects, which precludes from conclusively relating HIF-1 inhibition to tumour growth delay. A pilot study to address whether oral administration of "metronomic" topotecan modulates HIF-1 expression in tumour tissue has just been completed at NCI (http://clinicaltrials.gov/ct2/show/NCT00182676).

The ability to inhibit HIF-1α protein translation appears to be shared by all Top1 poisons (Rapisarda A, Shoemaker RH and Melillo G unpublished observation). Recently, EZN-2208, a PEGylated form of SN38 (the active component of CPT-11 or Irinotecan), has been shown to have improved pharmacokinetics and remarkable antitumour activity in preclinical models of solid tumours, lymphomas and neuroblastomas, including CPT-11-resistant tumours (Sapra, 2008; Pastorino, 2010). The demonstrated activity of EZN-2208 in CPT-11 refractory tumours could be explained by its increased stability that would allow a more persistent inhibition of HIF-1α and HIF-2α accumulation, thus exerting a more profound effect on the tumour microenvironment rather than only on cancer cells (Sapra, 2008; Pastorino, 2010). EZN-2208 is currently in phase I and phase II clinical trials. Based on the increased therapeutic advantage observed combining TPT with anti-angiogenic agents (Rapisarda, 2009a; Rapisarda, 2009b), a clinical trial, combining EZN-2208 and bevacizumab in solid tumours, is currently ongoing at NCI (http://clinicaltrials.gov/ct2/show/NCT01251926).

Microtubule inhibitors

Microtubule stabilizing and destabilizing agents have been reported to inhibit HIF-α expression (Escuin, 2005). In particular 2ME2, a naturally occurring estrogen metabolite, and its analog ENMD-1198, inhibit HIF-1α and HIF-2α protein accumulation, downstream of microtubules disruption (Mabjeesh, 2003; Moser, 2008). Conversely, another study showed that microtubules depolymerizing agents induce the accumulation of a transcriptionally active HIF-1 through the induction of NF-κB (Jung, 2003), emphasizing a potential pathway specific regulation of HIF-1 in different cell types.

Cardiac glycosides

Recently, cardiac glycosides, including digoxin, have been shown to inhibit HIF-1α and HIF-2α protein translation by a yet undefined mechanism of action (Zhang, 2008). In addition, glycosides isolated from natural products have also been identified in a HIF-1 cell-based assay (Klausmeyer, 2009). However, the potential clinical application of this class of compounds as HIF-1 inhibitors remains to be established, based on concerns of potential toxicity.

PX478

PX-478 is a small molecule that inhibits HIF-1α, but not HIF-2α, expression and has pronounced anti-tumour activity in a number of xenograft models (Welsh, 2004). Studies on the mechanism of action of PX-478 have shown that this compound decreases the levels of HIF-1α mRNA and inhibits its translation. In addition, treatment with this agent also results, although to a lesser extent, in inhibition of HIF-1α de-ubiquitination, therefore enhancing HIF-1α degradation (Koh, 2008). PX478 is currently in a phase I clinical trial in patients with metastatic cancer and results should become available in the near future.

HSP90 and HDAC inhibitors

The chaperon protein Hsp90 is pivotal for HIF-1α correct folding after translation, a necessary step to prevent its degradation. Accordingly, Hsp90 inhibitors (17-AAG, 17-DMAG) have been shown to increase HIF-1α protein degradation (Isaacs, 2002; Mabjeesh, 2002). Inhibition of Hsp90 has been implicated in the mechanism of action of a variety of other small molecules, including histone deacetylase inhibitors. Interestingly, HDAC inhibitors (vorinostat, LAQ824, FK228) may affect HIF-1α protein levels by several mechanisms, including: increased HIF-1α degradation and inhibition of HIF-1α transcriptional activity by direct acetylation of the co-factor p300 and inhibition of its binding to HIF-1α (Ellis, 2008). The effect of these molecules on HIF-2α still needs to be determined.

NSAIDs

Nonsteroidal anti-inflammatory drugs (NSAIDs), both nonselective (indomethacin, ibuprofen) and COX-2 selective (NS-398) (Jones, 2002; Palayoor, 2003), as well as NO-sulindac (Stewart, 2009), have been shown to down-regulate HIF-1α and HIF-2α protein accumulation and angiogenesis. Interestingly, NO-sulindac has been shown to do so by inhibiting AKT-dependent HIF-1α translation (Stewart, 2009).

Inhibitors that affect HIF-1α dimerization

HIF-1 dimerization and DNA binding are mediated by the basic-helix-loop-helix and PAS domains, PAS-A and PAS-B, present in the N-terminal end of HIF-α and HIF-1β. Protein domains that mediate dimerization of HIF-1 are attractive, yet elusive, targets for development of selective small molecule inhibitors. A screen of chemical libraries using recombinant fragments containing the HIF-1α and HIF-1β PAS-A identified NSC50352 as a potentially specific inhibitor of HIF-1α and HIF-1β dimerization mediated by PAS-A containing fragments, but it did not inhibit the interaction mediated by unrelated domains. However NSC50352 was inactive in cell-based assays (Park, 2006); analogs of this compound are being generated and tested to address whether they may retain activity in intact cells.

Acriflavine

Acriflavine is a mixture of 3,6-diamino-10-methylacridinium chloride (trypaflavin) and 3,6-diaminoacridine (proflavine), which has trypanocidal, antibacterial and antiviral activities. It was recently identified as a HIF inhibitor by screening a library of FDA approved drugs using a cell-based split-luciferase assay. Acriflavine inhibits HIF-1 dimerization by binding to the PAS-B sub-domain of HIF-1α and HIF-2α. Interestingly, it does not affect MYC dependent gene expression, showing a certain degree of selectivity for the HIF-1 pathway. Consistent with inhibition of HIF-1 dimerization, acriflavine inhibited HIF-1 transcriptional activity, leading to inhibition of tumour growth and vascularization (Lee, 2009b).

Inhibitors of HIF-1 binding to DNA

In an attempt to identify small molecule inhibitors with a higher degree of selectivity for HIF-1, assays have been developed to target HIF-1-DNA binding. Indeed, several small molecules that inhibit HIF-1 DNA binding have been identified, including echinomycin (Kong, 2005) and anthracyclines (Lee, 2009a). Interestingly, these molecules bind DNA and therefore inhibit both HIF-1α and HIF-2α transcriptional activity.

Echinomycin

Echinomycin (NSC-13502), a cyclic peptide of the family of quinoxaline antibiotics known to bind DNA in a sequence-specific fashion, was identified as a potent inhibitor of HIF-1 DNA binding in a 96-well plate DNA binding ELISA, and was further confirmed by EMSA and chromatin immunoprecipitation experiments (Kong, 2005). Notably, it inhibited the binding of Myc to the E-box sequence (5'-CACGTG-3'), which shares sequence homology with the core HIF-1 DNA binding site, but not of AP-1 or NF-κB. Echinomycin was extensively tested as an anticancer agent in phase I/II clinical trials in the late 1980s and found to be fairly inactive. It remains to be determined if schedules aimed to modulate HIF-1 activity may increase its therapeutic efficacy.

Anthracyclines

Anthracyclines (daunorubicin, epirubicin, idarubicin and doxorubicin) were recently identified as inhibitors of HIF-1 DNA binding in a recent screen of a library of FDA approved agents (Lee, 2009a). Anthracyclines have been shown to inhibit HIF-1 binding to DNA and HIF-1-dependent gene expression and angiogenesis in tumour bearing mice. Anthracyclines have also been reported to inhibit AP-1, GATA4, and Sp-1 (Kim, 2003; Szulawska, 2005; Mansilla, 2008), indicating that they may have multiple effects on transcription.

Inhibitors of HIF1 transcriptional activity

HIF-1 transcriptional activity is largely mediated by two functional domains of HIF-α, N-TAD and C-TAD. Hydroxylation by FIH-1 prevents HIF-α binding to the co-activator p300/CBP and down-regulates its transcriptional activity under normoxic conditions.

Chetomin

Chetomin is a member of the epidithiodiketopiperazine family of natural products previously known to have antimicrobial activity. It was identified as a potential HIF-1 inhibitor in a high-throughput screen aimed to dis-cover small molecules capable of disrupting the interaction between HIF-1α and p300. Chetomin binds to the CH1 domain of p300 and prevents its interaction with HIF-1α and HIF-2α (Kung, 2004; Cook, 2009). Systemic adminis-tration of chetomin inhibited HIF-1-dependent gene expression in tumours, as well as tumour growth in HCT116 and PC3 xenograft models (Kung, 2004). However, toxicity concerns discouraged its further development for clinical application.

Proteasome inhibitors

The proteasome inhibitor bortezomib (Velcade®) has the paradoxical effect of inducing accumulation of HIF-1α protein by inhibiting its protea-somal degradation while, at the same time, interfering with the function of the carboxyl-terminal transactivation domain (TAD-C) of HIF-1α (Kaluz, 2006). TAD-C is a domain essential for the recruitment of co-factors such as p300/CBP. A potential mechanism of inhibition of HIF-1 by bortezomib implicates increased HIF-1α hydroxylation on asparagine 803, which pre-vents binding of p300/CBP to HIF-1 (Shin, 2008), although additional mecha-nisms have been suggested (Kaluz, 2008). Its effect on HIF-2α was not tested; however, the high homology between HIF-1α and HIF-2α TAD-C suggests that HIF-2α could be affected in a similar fashion.

HIF-1 inhibitors: single agents or combination strategies?

The potential therapeutic benefit of HIF-1 inhibition has been extensively documented in preclinical models using both genetic and pharmacological tools (Semenza, 2003; Melillo, 2006). However, even conceptually, inhibition of HIF-1 expressing cells, as single agent strategy in the clinical setting, may not be particularly effective for a number of reasons, including the focal and heterogeneous expression of HIF-α in solid tumours, the reliance of cancer cells on HIF-1-independent pathways in oxygenated areas of the tumour, and the overall well established redundancy of oncogenic signalling path-ways that may be hardly affected by single agent strategies. Indeed, HIF inhibitors may be more effective in a context in which survival of tumour cells may be largely and more consistently relying on HIF-1-dependent mechanisms. An example may be vascular regression caused by administration of the antiangiogenic agent bevacizumab, which has been shown to be associated with a concomitant increase in intratumour hypoxia, creating a therapy-induced hypoxic stress of the tumour microenvironment that allows to fully exploit HIF-1 inhibition (Rapisarda, 2009a; Rapisarda, 2009b). Indeed, the broad involvement of HIF-α in a number of biological pathways that are relevant for tumourigenesis, as well as for resistance to current therapeutic strategies, provides unique opportunities for combination therapies (Rapisarda, 2010). Notably, the potential synergistic activity of HIF-1 inhibition in combination with chemotherapy has been formally tested in a glioma xenograft model in which HIF-1α expression was down-regulated by an inducible shRNA system (Li, 2006). In addition, it has been shown that HIF-1α and HIF-2α inhibition improves tumour response to treatment with the targeted agent sunitinib in colon cancer cell (Burkitt, 2009) and combination of low doses of rapamycin, in combination with the camptothecin analog irinotecan (a topoisomerase I inhibitor), showed a marked increase of anti-tumour activity associated with a profound inhibition of HIF-1α protein accumulation that was not observed with either agent alone (Pencreach, 2009), providing supporting evidence for this approach. Nevertheless, the relative contribution of HIF-1α and/or HIF-2α to cancer progression of different tumour types needs to be fully elucidated to be able to exploit HIF inhibitors correctly. Indeed, it has been suggested that HIF-2α, and not HIF-1α, inhibition might be beneficial in several tumour types (Raval, 2005; Franovic, 2009). Alas, the lack of selective HIF-2α inhibitors, to date, hinders the possibility to selectively target this subunit in those tumours where HIF-2α plays a major role.

Conclusions

In the complex biology of human cancers, the role of HIF-1 in resistance to therapy and tumour progression has been extensively validated. Hence, HIF-1 inhibition appears as a logical therapeutic strategy and many small molecule inhibitors of HIF-1 have been described, several of which have been validated in pre-clinical models and have entered early clinical development. However, we still have limited understanding of when, and to what extent, inhibition of HIF-1 in cancer patients may be effective. Single agent studies are required to have a better appreciation of the biological consequence associated with HIF-1 inhibition in human cancers, yet the lack of selective pharmacological inhibitors of HIF-1 significantly hinders this task. On the other hand, we have learned over the last few years that targeting multiple signalling pathways deregulated in cancer cells may be a more effective therapeutic strategy. The broad involvement of HIF-1 in many biological processes associated with, and required for, tumour progression provides unique opportunities for the development of combination therapies.

Acknowledgements – The authors would like to thank Robert H Shoemaker for helpful discussion. This project has been funded in whole or in part with federal funds from the National Cancer Institute, National Institutes of Health, under Contract No. HHSN261200800001E. The content of this publication does not necessarily reflect the views or policies of the Department of Health and Human Services, nor does mention of trade names, commercial products, or organizations imply endorsement by the U.S. Government. This research was supported [in part] by the Developmental Therapeutics Program in the Division of Cancer Treatment and Diagnosis of the National Cancer Institute.

References

Aebersold DM, Burri P, Beer KT et al (2001) Expression of hypoxia-inducible factor-1alpha: a novel predictive and prognostic parameter in the radiotherapy of oropharyngeal cancer. Cancer Res 61: 2911-2916

Bachtiary B, Schindl M, Potter R et al (2003) Overexpression of hypoxia-inducible factor 1alpha indicates diminished response to radiotherapy and unfavourable prognosis in patients receiving radical radiotherapy for cervical cancer. Clin Cancer Res 9: 2234-2240

Bhatt RS, Landis DM, Zimmer M et al (2008) Hypoxia-inducible factor-2alpha: effect on radiation sensitivity and differential regulation by an mTOR inhibitor. BJU Int 102: 358-363

Birner P, Gatterbauer B, Oberhuber G et al (2001a) Expression of hypoxia-inducible factor-1 alpha in oligodendrogliomas: its impact on prognosis and on neoangiogenesis. Cancer 92: 165-171

Birner P, Schindl M, Obermair A et al (2001b) Expression of hypoxia-inducible factor 1alpha in epithelial ovarian tumours: its impact on prognosis and on response to chemotherapy. Clin Cancer Res 7: 1661-1668

Birner P, Schindl M, Obermair A et al (2000) Overexpression of hypoxia-inducible factor 1alpha is a marker for an unfavourable prognosis in early-stage invasive cervical cancer. Cancer Res 60: 4693-4696

Bos R, van der GP, Greijer AE et al (2003) Levels of hypoxia-inducible factor-1alpha independently predict prognosis in patients with lymph node negative breast carcinoma. Cancer 97: 1573-1581

Bracken CP, Whitelaw ML, and Peet DJ (2005) Activity of hypoxia-inducible factor 2alpha is regulated by association with the NF-kappaB essential modulator. J Biol Chem 280: 14240-14251

Brown JM and Wilson WR (2004) Exploiting tumour hypoxia in cancer treatment. Nat Rev Cancer 4: 437-447

Burkitt K, Chun SY, Dang DT et al (2009) Targeting both HIF-1 and HIF-2 in human colon cancer cells improves tumour response to sunitinib treatment. Mol Cancer Ther

Burri P, Djonov V, Aebersold DM et al (2003) Significant correlation of hypoxia-inducible factor-1alpha with treatment outcome in cervical cancer treated with radical radiotherapy. Int J Radiat Oncol Biol Phys 56: 494-501

Cho DC, Cohen MB, Panka DJ et al (2010) The efficacy of the novel dual PI3-kinase/mTOR inhibitor NVP-BEZ235 compared with rapamycin in renal cell carcinoma. Clin Cancer Res 16: 3628-3638

Choi H, Chun YS, Kim TY et al (2010) HIF-2{alpha} Enhances {beta}-Catenin/TCF-Driven Transcription by Interacting with {beta}-Catenin. Cancer Res 70: 10101-10111

Cleven AH, van EM, Wouters BG et al (2007) Stromal expression of hypoxia regulated proteins is an adverse prognostic factor in colorectal carcinomas. Cell Oncol 29: 229-240

Cook KM, Hilton ST, Mecinovic J et al (2009) Epidithiodiketopiperazines block the interaction between hypoxia-inducible factor-1alpha (HIF-1alpha) and p300 by a zinc ejection mechanism. J Biol Chem 284: 26831-26838

Dales JP, Garcia S, Meunier-Carpentier S et al (2005) Overexpression of hypoxia-inducible factor HIF-1alpha predicts early relapse in breast cancer: retrospective study in a series of 745 patients. Int J Cancer 116: 734-739

Daponte A, Ioannou M, Mylonis I et al (2008) Prognostic significance of Hypoxia-Inducible Factor 1 alpha(HIF-1 alpha) expression in serous ovarian cancer: an immunohistochemical study. BMC Cancer 8: 335

Dewhirst MW, Cao Y, and Moeller B (2008) Cycling hypoxia and free radicals regulate angiogenesis and radiotherapy response. Nat Rev Cancer 8: 425-437

Dioum EM, Chen R, Alexander MS et al (2009) Regulation of hypoxia-inducible factor 2alpha signalling by the stress-responsive deacetylase sirtuin 1. Science 324: 1289-1293

Ellis L, Hammers H, and Pili R (2008) Targeting tumour angiogenesis with histone deacetylase inhibitors. Cancer Lett 282(2):145-53.

Escuin D, Kline ER, and Giannakakou P (2005) Both microtubule-stabilizing and microtubule-destabilizing drugs inhibit hypoxia-inducible factor-1alpha accumulation and activity by disrupting microtubule function. Cancer Res 65: 9021-9028

Franovic A, Gunaratnam L, Smith K et al (2007) Translational up-regulation of the EGFR by tumour hypoxia provides a nonmutational explanation for its overexpression in human cancer. Proc Natl Acad Sci U S A 104: 13092-13097

Franovic A, Holterman CE, Payette J et al (2009) Human cancers converge at the HIF-2alpha oncogenic axis. Proc Natl Acad Sci U S A 106: 21306-21311

Generali D, Berruti A, Brizzi MP et al (2006) Hypoxia-inducible factor-1alpha expression predicts a poor response to primary chemoendocrine therapy and disease-free survival in primary human breast cancer. Clin Cancer Res 12: 4562-4568

Giatromanolaki A, Koukourakis MI, Simopoulos C et al (2007) Metastatic cancer cells from c-erbB-2 negative primary breast cancer maintain the original c-erbB-2/HIF1alpha phenotype. Cancer Biol Ther 6: 153-155

Giatromanolaki A, Koukourakis MI, Sivridis E et al (2001) Relation of hypoxia inducible factor 1 alpha and 2 alpha in operable non-small cell lung cancer to angiogenic/molecular profile of tumours and survival. Br J Cancer 85: 881-890

Giatromanolaki A, Sivridis E, Kouskoukis C et al (2003) Hypoxia-inducible factors 1alpha and 2alpha are related to vascular endothelial growth factor expression and a poorer prognosis in nodular malignant melanomas of the skin. Melanoma Res 13: 493-501

Gordan JD, Thompson CB, and Simon MC (2007) HIF and c-Myc: sibling rivals for control of cancer cell metabolism and proliferation. Cancer Cell 12: 108-113

Greenberger LM, Horak ID, Filpula D et al (2008) A RNA antagonist of hypoxia-inducible factor-1alpha, EZN-2968, inhibits tumour cell growth. Mol Cancer Ther 7: 3598-3608

Griffiths EA, Pritchard SA, Valentine HR et al (2007) Hypoxia-inducible factor-1alpha expression in the gastric carcinogenesis sequence and its prognostic role in gastric and gastro-oesophageal adenocarcinomas. Br J Cancer 96: 95-103

Holmquist-Mengelbier L, Fredlund E, Lofstedt T et al (2006) Recruitment of HIF-1alpha and HIF-2alpha to common target genes is differentially regulated in neuroblastoma: HIF-2alpha promotes an aggressive phenotype. Cancer Cell 10: 413-423

Isaacs JS, Jung YJ, Mimnaugh EG et al (2002) Hsp90 regulates a von Hippel Lindau-independent hypoxia-inducible factor-1 alpha-degradative pathway. J Biol Chem 277: 29936-29944

Jones MK, Szabo IL, Kawanaka H et al (2002) von Hippel Lindau tumour suppressor and HIF-1alpha: new targets of NSAIDs inhibition of hypoxia-induced angiogenesis. FASEB J 16: 264-266

Jung YJ, Isaacs JS, Lee S et al (2003) Microtubule disruption utilizes an NFkappa B-dependent pathway to stabilize HIF-1alpha protein. J Biol Chem 278: 7445-7452

Kaelin WG, Jr. and Ratcliffe PJ (2008) Oxygen sensing by metazoans: the central role of the HIF hydroxylase pathway. Mol Cell 30: 393-402

Kaidi A, Williams AC, and Paraskeva C (2007) Interaction between beta-catenin and HIF-1 promotes cellular adaptation to hypoxia. Nat Cell Biol 9: 210-217

Kaluz S, Kaluzova M, and Stanbridge EJ (2006) Proteasomal inhibition attenuates transcriptional activity of hypoxia-inducible factor 1 (HIF-1) via specific effect on the HIF-1alpha C-terminal activation domain. Mol Cell Biol 26: 5895-5907

Kaluz S, Kaluzova M, and Stanbridge EJ (2008) Comment on the role of FIH in the inhibitory effect of bortezomib on hypoxia-inducible factor-1. Blood 111: 5258-5259

Kikuchi H, Pino MS, Zeng M et al (2009) Oncogenic KRAS and BRAF differentially regulate hypoxia-inducible factor-1alpha and -2alpha in colon cancer. Cancer Res 69: 8499-8506

Kim Y, Ma AG, Kitta K et al (2003) Anthracycline-induced suppression of GATA-4 transcription factor: implication in the regulation of cardiac myocyte apoptosis. Mol Pharmacol 63: 368-377

Klausmeyer P, Zhou Q, Scudiero DA et al (2009) Cytotoxic and HIF-1alpha Inhibitory Compounds from Crossosoma bigelovii. J Nat Prod 72(5): 805-812.

Koh MY, Spivak-Kroizman T, Venturini S et al (2008) Molecular mechanisms for the activity of PX-478, an antitumour inhibitor of the hypoxia-inducible factor-1alpha. Mol Cancer Ther 7: 90-100

Koivunen P, Hirsila M, Gunzler V et al (2004) Catalytic properties of the asparaginyl hydroxylase (FIH) in the oxygen sensing pathway are distinct from those of its prolyl 4-hydroxylases. J Biol Chem 279: 9899-9904

Kondo K, Kim WY, Lechpammer M et al (2003) Inhibition of HIF2alpha is sufficient to suppress pVHL-defective tumour growth. PLoS Biol 1: E83

Kondo K, Klco J, Nakamura E et al (2002) Inhibition of HIF is necessary for tumour suppression by the von Hippel-Lindau protein. Cancer Cell 1: 237-246

Kong D, Park EJ, Stephen AG et al (2005) Echinomycin, a small-molecule inhibitor of hypoxia-inducible factor-1 DNA-binding activity. Cancer Res 65: 9047-9055

Koukourakis MI, Giatromanolaki A, Sivridis E et al (2002) Hypoxia-inducible factor (HIF1A and HIF2A), angiogenesis, and chemoradiotherapy outcome of squamous cell head-and-neck cancer. Int J Radiat Oncol Biol Phys 53: 1192-1202

Koukourakis MI, Simopoulos C, Polychronidis A et al (2003) The effect of trastuzumab/ docatexel combination on breast cancer angiogenesis: dichotomus effect predictable by the HIFI alpha/VEGF pre-treatment status? Anticancer Res 23: 1673-1680

Kung AL, Zabludoff SD, France DS et al (2004) Small molecule blockade of transcriptional coactivation of the hypoxia-inducible factor pathway. Cancer Cell 6: 33-43

Lau KW, Tian YM, Raval RR et al (2007) Target gene selectivity of hypoxia-inducible factor-alpha in renal cancer cells is conveyed by post-DNA-binding mechanisms. Br J Cancer 96: 1284-1292

Lee K, Qian DZ, Rey S et al (2009a) Anthracycline chemotherapy inhibits HIF-1 transcriptional activity and tumour-induced mobilization of circulating angiogenic cells. Proc Natl Acad Sci U S A 106: 2353-2358

Lee K, Zhang H, Qian DZ et al (2009b) Acriflavine inhibits HIF-1 dimerization, tumour growth, and vascularization. Proc Natl Acad Sci U S A 106: 17910-17915

Li L, Lin X, Shoemaker AR et al (2006) Hypoxia-inducible factor-1 inhibition in combination with temozolomide treatment exhibits robust antitumour efficacy in vivo. Clin Cancer Res 12: 4747-4754

Lim JH, Lee YM, Chun YS et al (2010) Sirtuin 1 modulates cellular responses to hypoxia by deacetylating hypoxia-inducible factor 1alpha. Mol Cell 38: 864-878

Litz J and Krystal GW (2006) Imatinib inhibits c-Kit-induced hypoxia-inducible factor-1alpha activity and vascular endothelial growth factor expression in small cell lung cancer cells. Mol Cancer Ther 5: 1415-1422

Luwor RB, Lu Y, Li X et al (2005) The antiepidermal growth factor receptor monoclonal antibody cetuximab/C225 reduces hypoxia-inducible factor-1 alpha, leading to transcriptional inhibition of vascular endothelial growth factor expression. Oncogene 24: 4433-4441

Mabjeesh NJ, Escuin D, LaVallee TM et al (2003) 2ME2 inhibits tumour growth and angiogenesis by disrupting microtubules and dysregulating HIF. Cancer Cell 3: 363-375

Mabjeesh NJ, Post DE, Willard MT et al (2002) Geldanamycin induces degradation of hypoxia-inducible factor 1alpha protein via the proteosome pathway in prostate cancer cells. Cancer Res 62: 2478-2482

Mahon PC, Hirota K, and Semenza GL (2001) FIH-1: a novel protein that interacts with HIF-1alpha and VHL to mediate repression of HIF-1 transcriptional activity. Genes Dev 15: 2675-2686

Mandriota SJ, Turner KJ, Davies DR et al (2002) HIF activation identifies early lesions in VHL kidneys: evidence for site-specific tumour suppressor function in the nephron. Cancer Cell 1: 459-468

Mansilla S and Portugal J (2008) Sp1 transcription factor as a target for anthracyclines: effects on gene transcription. Biochimie 90: 976-987

Melillo G (2006) Inhibiting hypoxia-inducible factor 1 for cancer therapy. Mol Cancer Res 4: 601-605

Melillo G (2007) Hypoxia-inducible factor 1 inhibitors. Methods Enzymol 435: 385-402

Moser C, Lang SA, Mori A et al (2008) ENMD-1198, a novel tubulin-binding agent reduces HIF-1alpha and STAT3 activity in human hepatocellular carcinoma(HCC) cells, and inhibits growth and vascularization in vivo. BMC Cancer 8: 206

Nanni S, Benvenuti V, Grasselli A et al (2009) Endothelial NOS, estrogen receptor beta, and HIFs cooperate in the activation of a prognostic transcriptional pattern in aggressive human prostate cancer. J Clin Invest 119: 1093-1108

Narita T, Yin S, Gelin CF et al (2009) Identification of a novel small molecule HIF-1alpha translation inhibitor. Clin Cancer Res 15: 6128-6136

Nilsson MB, Zage PE, Zeng L et al (2010) Multiple receptor tyrosine kinases regulate HIF-1alpha and HIF-2alpha in normoxia and hypoxia in neuroblastoma: implications for antiangiogenic mechanisms of multikinase inhibitors. Oncogene 29: 2938-2949

Palayoor ST, Tofilon PJ, and Coleman CN (2003) Ibuprofen-mediated reduction of hypoxia-inducible factors HIF-1alpha and HIF-2alpha in prostate cancer cells. Clin Cancer Res 9: 3150-3157

Park EJ, Kong D, Fisher R et al (2006) Targeting the PAS-A domain of HIF-1alpha for development of small molecule inhibitors of HIF-1. Cell Cycle 5: 1847-1853

Pastorino F, Loi M, Sapra P et al (2010) Tumour regression and curability of preclinical neuroblastoma models by PEGylated SN38 (EZN-2208), a novel topoisomerase I inhibitor. Clin Cancer Res 16: 4809-4821

Pencreach E, Guerin E, Nicolet C et al (2009) Marked activity of irinotecan and rapamycin combination toward colon cancer cells in vivo and in vitro is mediated through cooperative modulation of the mammalian target of rapamycin/hypoxia-inducible factor-1alpha axis. Clin Cancer Res 15: 1297-1307

Pore N, Jiang Z, Gupta A et al (2006) EGFR tyrosine kinase inhibitors decrease VEGF expression by both hypoxia-inducible factor (HIF)-1-independent and HIF-1-dependent mechanisms. Cancer Res 66: 3197-3204

Qing G and Simon MC (2009) Hypoxia inducible factor-2alpha: a critical mediator of aggressive tumour phenotypes. Curr Opin Genet Dev 19: 60-66

Rajaganeshan R, Prasad R, Guillou PJ et al (2008) The role of hypoxia in recurrence following resection of Dukes' B colorectal cancer. Int J Colorectal Dis 23: 1049-1055

Rapisarda A, Hollingshead M, Uranchimeg B et al (2009a) Increased antitumour activity of bevacizumab in combination with hypoxia inducible factor-1 inhibition. Mol Cancer Ther 8: 1867-1877

Rapisarda A and Melillo G (2009b) Role of the hypoxic tumour microenvironment in the resistance to anti-angiogenic therapies. Drug Resist Updat 12: 74-80

Rapisarda,A. and Melillo,G. (2010). Combination strategies targeting Hypoxia Inducible Factor 1 (HIF-1) for cancer therapy. In The Tumour Microenvironment, Rebecca G.Bagley, ed. Springer Science+Business Media, LLC). pp 3-21

Rapisarda A, Uranchimeg B, Scudiero DA et al (2002) Identification of small molecule inhibitors of hypoxia-inducible factor 1 transcriptional activation pathway. Cancer Res 62: 4316-4324

Rapisarda A, Uranchimeg B, Sordet O et al (2004a) Topoisomerase I-mediated inhibition of hypoxia-inducible factor 1: mechanism and therapeutic implications. Cancer Res 64: 1475-1482

Rapisarda A, Zalek J, Hollingshead M et al (2004b) Schedule-dependent inhibition of hypoxia-inducible factor-1alpha protein accumulation, angiogenesis, and tumour growth by topotecan in U251-HRE glioblastoma xenografts. Cancer Res 64: 6845-6848

Rasheed S, Harris AL, Tekkis PP et al (2009) Hypoxia-inducible factor-1alpha and -2alpha are expressed in most rectal cancers but only hypoxia-inducible factor-1alpha is associated with prognosis. Br J Cancer 100: 1666-1673

Raval RR, Lau KW, Tran MG et al (2005) Contrasting properties of hypoxia-inducible factor 1 (HIF-1) and HIF-2 in von Hippel-Lindau-associated renal cell carcinoma. Mol Cell Biol 25: 5675-5686

Sanchez M, Galy B, Muckenthaler MU et al (2007) Iron-regulatory proteins limit hypoxia-inducible factor-2alpha expression in iron deficiency. Nat Struct Mol Biol 14: 420-426

Sapra P, Zhao H, Mehlig M et al (2008) Novel delivery of SN38 markedly inhibits tumour growth in xenografts, including a camptothecin-11-refractory model. Clin Cancer Res 14: 1888-1896

Schindl M, Schoppmann SF, Samonigg H et al (2002) Overexpression of hypoxia-inducible factor 1alpha is associated with an unfavourable prognosis in lymph node-positive breast cancer. Clin Cancer Res 8: 1831-1837

Schmitz KJ, Muller CI, Reis H et al (2009) Combined analysis of hypoxia-inducible factor 1 alpha and metallothionein indicates an aggressive subtype of colorectal carcinoma. Int J Colorectal Dis 24: 1287-1296

Schrijvers ML, van der Laan BF, de Bock GH et al (2008) Overexpression of intrinsic hypoxia markers HIF1alpha and CA-IX predict for local recurrence in stage T1-T2 glottic laryngeal carcinoma treated with radiotherapy. Int J Radiat Oncol Biol Phys 72: 161-169

Semenza GL (2007) Hypoxia and cancer. Cancer Metastasis Rev 26: 223-224

Semenza GL (2003) Targeting HIF-1 for cancer therapy. Nat Rev Cancer 3: 721-732

Semenza GL (2010) HIF-1: upstream and downstream of cancer metabolism. Curr Opin Genet Dev 20: 51-56

Semenza GL (2008) Hypoxia-inducible factor 1 and cancer pathogenesis. IUBMB Life 60: 591-597

Shin DH, Chun YS, Lee DS et al (2008) Bortezomib inhibits tumour adaptation to hypoxia by stimulating the FIH-mediated repression of hypoxia-inducible factor-1. Blood 111: 3131-3136

Sivridis E, Giatromanolaki A, Gatter KC et al (2002) Association of hypoxia-inducible factors 1alpha and 2alpha with activated angiogenic pathways and prognosis in patients with endometrial carcinoma. Cancer 95: 1055-1063

Stewart GD, Nanda J, Brown DJ et al (2009) NO-sulindac inhibits the hypoxia response of PC-3 prostate cancer cells via the Akt signalling pathway. Int J Cancer 124: 223-232

Sun HC, Qiu ZJ, Liu J et al (2007) Expression of hypoxia-inducible factor-1 alpha and associated proteins in pancreatic ductal adenocarcinoma and their impact on prognosis. Int J Oncol 30: 1359-1367

Swinson DE, Jones JL, Cox G et al (2004) Hypoxia-inducible factor-1 alpha in non small cell lung cancer: relation to growth factor, protease and apoptosis pathways. Int J Cancer 111: 43-50

Szulawska A, Gniazdowski M, and Czyz M (2005) Sequence specificity of formaldehyde-mediated covalent binding of anthracycline derivatives to DNA. Biochem Pharmacol 69: 7-18

Takahashi R, Tanaka S, Hiyama T et al (2003) Hypoxia-inducible factor-1alpha expression and angiogenesis in gastrointestinal stromal tumour of the stomach. Oncol Rep 10: 797-802

Terzuoli E, Puppo M, Rapisarda A et al (2010) Aminoflavone, a ligand of the aryl hydrocarbon receptor, inhibits HIF-1alpha expression in an AhR-independent fashion. Cancer Res 70: 6837-6848

Theodoropoulos VE, Lazaris AC, Kastriotis I et al (2005) Evaluation of hypoxia-inducible factor 1alpha overexpression as a predictor of tumour recurrence and progression in superficial urothelial bladder carcinoma. BJU Int 95: 425-431

Theodoropoulos VE, Lazaris AC, Sofras F et al (2004) Hypoxia-inducible factor 1 alpha expression correlates with angiogenesis and unfavorable prognosis in bladder cancer. Eur Urol 46: 200-208

Thomas GV, Tran C, Mellinghoff IK et al (2006) Hypoxia-inducible factor determines sensitivity to inhibitors of mTOR in kidney cancer. Nat Med 12: 122-127

Toschi A, Lee E, Gadir N et al (2008) Differential dependence of hypoxia-inducible factors 1 alpha and 2 alpha on mTORC1 and mTORC2. J Biol Chem 283: 34495-34499

Tzao C, Lee SC, Tung HJ et al (2008) Expression of hypoxia-inducible factor (HIF)-1alpha and vascular endothelial growth factor (VEGF)-D as outcome predictors in resected esophageal squamous cell carcinoma. Dis Markers 25: 141-148

Vleugel MM, Greijer AE, Shvarts A et al (2005) Differential prognostic impact of hypoxia induced and diffuse HIF-1alpha expression in invasive breast cancer. J Clin Pathol 58: 172-177

Welsh S, Williams R, Kirkpatrick L et al (2004) Antitumour activity and pharmacodynamic properties of PX-478, an inhibitor of hypoxia-inducible factor-1alpha. Mol Cancer Ther 3: 233-244

Woldemichael GM, Vasselli JR, Gardella RS et al (2006) Development of a cell-based reporter assay for screening of inhibitors of hypoxia-inducible factor 2-induced gene expression. J Biomol Screen 11: 678-687

Zhang H, Qian DZ, Tan YS et al (2008) Digoxin and other cardiac glycosides inhibit HIF-1alpha synthesis and block tumour growth. Proc Natl Acad Sci U S A 105: 19579-19586

Zhong L, D'Urso A, Toiber D et al (2008) The histone deacetylase Sirt6 regulates glucose homeostasis via Hif1alpha. Cell 140: 280-293

Zimmer M, Ebert BL, Neil C et al (2008) Small-molecule inhibitors of HIF-2a translation link its 5'UTR iron-responsive element to oxygen sensing. Mol Cell 32: 838-848

Chapter 19

New Drugs Interfering with pH Regulation in Tumours

Claudiu T. Supuran[*]

[*]Address for correspondence:
University of Florence, Dipartimento di Chimica, Laboratorio di Chimica Bioinorganica,
Via della Lastruccia, 3, Rm. 188, Polo Scientifico, 50019 –Sesto Fiorentino (Firenze), Italy,
Phone: +39-055-4573005, Fax: +39-055-4573385, E-mail: Claudiu.Supuran@unifi.it

Contents

Key points

—   The regulation of pH in tumours involves the interplay of several
     proteins which include carbonic anhydrases (CAs, EC 4.2.1.1) IX and
     XII; aquaporins AQP1-5; anion exchangers AE1-3; sodium bicarbonate
     co-transporters (NBCs), the sodium-dependent chloride-bicarbonate
     exchangers (NDCBE); monocarboxylate transporters MCT1-4, the
     sodium-proton exchanger NHE1, and the vacuolar H+-ATPase (V-ATPase)
     among others. Some of them are overexpressed in tumours through the
     HIF-1 pathway.

—   The concerted action of these proteins assures a slightly alkaline internal
     pH (pHi) and an acidic external pH (pHe) within the tumours, which
     favors proliferation of the primary tumour and its spread, leading to the
     formation of metastases.

—   Inhibition of one or more of them with specific inhibitors leads to the
     return of both pHi and pHe towards normal values with the consequent
     impairment of the tumour growth. This constitutes an antitumour
     mechanism not exploited by the classical anticancer drugs.

—   CA IX/XII inhibition with sulfonamide or coumarin inhibitors reverses
     the effect of tumour acidification, leading to inhibition of the cancer
     cell growth, both for primary tumours and metastases. This effect can
     be exploited for the imaging and treatment of tumours overexpressing
     them.

—   There are few specific, non toxic and effective compounds interfering
     with other proteins mentioned above than the CAs, but some
     sulfonamides seem to also inhibit AQPs and AEs, whereas proton pump
     inhibitors of the omeprazole type show antitumour effects by inhibiting
     V-ATPase. Potent, specific and non-toxic compounds inhibiting one or
     more of these proteins may represent valuable new antitumour drugs.

Introduction

pH homeostasis in any cell type is a complicated process in which many proteins and buffer systems are involved (Boron, 2004). For tumours, these processes are even more complex due to the specific features of the tumour microenvironment, characterized by hypoxia, acidosis (with acidic extracellular pH) resulting from enhanced glucose uptake and metabolism to lactic acid, and impaired removal of metabolic acids (carbonic and lactic acid) (Chiche et al, 2010; Huber et al, 2010; Parks et al, 2010; Swietach et al, 2008a,b). Both the internal pH (pHi) and the external pH (pHe) within the tumour are deregulated compared to their values in normal cells, with the internal compartment slightly more alkaline (pH 7.4 or more) and the external one more acidic (pH values of up to 6.5) than the physiological pH values (Parks et al, 2010; Swietach et al, 2008a,b).

Since a variation in pHi/pHe as low as 0.1 units may disrupt important biochemical/biological processes, such as ATP synthesis, enzyme function, proliferation, migration, invasion and metastasis of tumour cells (Chiche et al, 2010), it is obvious that a tight regulation of these processes has evolved (Chiche et al, 2010; Huber et al, 2010; Parks et al, 2010; Swietach et al, 2008a,b). Several highly sophisticated molecular mechanisms are thus responsible for maintaining the alkaline pHi and the acidic pHe in tumour cells, which allow them to survive and proliferate in hypoxia, but also favoring metastasis (Wykoff et al., 2000; Swietach et al., 2008a,b; Parks et al., 2010; Huber et al., 2010). They include both proteins which import weak bases (such as bicarbonate) within the cells, or others which extrude the weak acids generated during metabolism, such as CO_2/carbonic acid or lactic acid (Boron, 2004). The principal metabolic acids are indeed carbonic acid, formed by the hydration of CO_2 which is the final product of all oxidative processes, and lactic acid which is formed through the glycolytic transformation of glucose in hypoxic conditions (glucose has an increased uptake in tumour cells, the so-called Warburg effect, not fully explained even 80 years after its discovery (Huber et al., 2010)). In addition, there are also molecular mechanisms by which the H^+ ions are directly extruded from the cells, either in exchange for other cations (such as Na^+) or through the energy furnished by the hydrolysis of ATP, by means of the vacuolar ATPase V-ATPase (Chiche et al, 2010; Huber et al, 2010; Parks et al, 2010; Swietach et al, 2008a,b; Kremer and Pouyssegur, 2008; Pouysségur et al, 2006).

In Figure 19.1, some of the main players involved in the regulation of tumour pH are presented and they include: carbonic anhydrases (CAs, EC

4.2.1.1) IX and XII (Pastorek et al, 1994; Supuran, 2008, 2010); acquaporins AQP1-5 (Endeward et al, 2006); anion exchangers AE1-3 (Sterling et al, 2002; Morgan et al, 2004); sodium bicarbonate co-transporters (NBCs) (Pouyssegur et al, 2006), the sodium-dependent chloride-bicarbonate exchangers (NDCBE) (Pouyssegur et al, 2006); monocarboxylate transporters MCT1-4 (Halestrap and Price, 1999; Enerson and Drewes, 2003), the sodium-proton exchanger NHE1 (Pouyssegur et al, 2006), and the vacuolar V-ATPase (Perez-Sayans et al, 2009). It may be observed that many of these proteins exist as many isoforms, which may represent a complication from the medicinal chemistry viewpoint, since a good drug

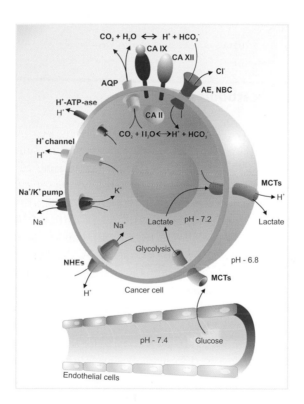

Figure 19.1 _ Proteins involved in pH regulation within a tumour cell: monocarboxylate transporters (MCTs), which extrude lactic acid and other monocarboxylates formed by the glycolytic degradation of glucose; Na^+/ H^+ antiporter (NHE); ATP-dependent Na^+/K^+ antiporter; H^+ channels; plasma membrane proton pump H+–ATP-ase (V-ATP-ase); CA IX and/or CA XII, which catalyze CO_2 hydration to bicarbonate and protons; anion exchangers (AE1-AE3 isoforms) and acquaporins (AQP) (adapted from Supuran, 2008).

should target just the desired isoform, without affecting the activity of the house-keeping ones. This is particularly true for the CAs (for which 15 isoforms are present in humans, Supuran 2008, 2010), but also the AEs, the AQPs and the MCTs have several isoforms, not all of them being normally associated with tumours. There are various approaches nowadays to target one or more of these proteins in order to restore both pHi and pHe in cancer cells towards normal values, with the consequent impairment of the tumour growth. This constitutes in fact an antitumour mechanism not yet fully exploited by any of the classical anticancer drugs. However, the last several years saw the proof-of-concept studies which validated some of these proteins as new anticancer drug targets. This chapter will present the state of the art in the field of such drugs wich interfere with the pH regulation in tumours.

Tumour-associated carbonic anhydrases

α-Carbonic anhydrases (CAs, EC 4.2.1.1) are widespread metalloenzymes in higher vertebrates, including humans (Supuran, 2008, 2010). 16 isozymes have been characterized to date in mammals, which differ in their subcellular localization, catalytic activity, and susceptibility to different classes of inhibitors. There are cytosolic isozymes (CA I, CA II, CA III, CA VII and CA XIII), membrane bound ones (CA IV, CA IX, CA XII, CA XIV and CA XV), mitochondrial (CA VA and CA VB) and secreted (CA VI) isoforms. Three acatalytic forms, called CA-related proteins (CARPs), CARP VIII, CARP X and CARP XI, are also known (Scozzafava et al, 2004, 2006). Most CAs are very efficient catalysts for the reversible hydration of carbon dioxide to bicarbonate and protons ($CO_2 + H_2O \leftrightarrow HCO_3^- + H^+$), which is the only physiological reaction in which they are involved (Supuran, 2008,2010; Supuran et al, 2003).

Most CA isoforms are involved in critical physiologic processes such as respiration and acid-base regulation, electrolyte secretion, bone resorption, calcification and biosynthetic reactions which require bicarbonate as a substrate (lipogenesis, gluconeogenesis, and ureagenesis) (Supuran, 2008; 2010). Two CA isozymes (CA IX and CA XII) are predominantly associated with and overexpressed in many tumours, being involved in critical processes connected with cancer progression and response to therapy (Pastorek et al, 1994; Tureci et al., 1998; Svastova et al, 2004; Supuran, 2008; 2010). CA IX is confined to few normal tissues (stomach and body cavity lining), but it is ectopically induced and highly overexpressed in many solid tumour types, through the strong transcriptional activation by hypoxia, accomplished via the hypoxia inducible factor 1 (HIF-1) transcription factor (Pastorek et al, 1994; Wykoff et al, 2000; Svastova et al, 2004; Supuran, 2008; 2010; Hilvo et al., 2008). Interestingly, CA IX is the most strongly overexpressed gene in response to hypoxia in human cancer cells (Svastova et al, 2004) and it is also the most active CA isoform for the CO_2 hydration reaction (Hilvo et al., 2008; Innocenti et al., 2009). Its X-ray crystal structure has recently been reported (Alterio et al., 2009) evidencing a dimeric enzyme, unique among all CAs known so far. CA XII is also a transmembrane isoform with an extracellular active site, similar to CA IX (Tureci et al, 1998) but its catalytic activity is lower compared to CA IX (Vullo et al., 2005; Supuran, 2008). Similar to CA IX, CA XII is expressed in many tumours but it is also more diffuse in normal tissues (Tureci et al, 1998). Since CO_2 is the main byproduct of all oxidative processes, being thus generated in large amounts in metabolically active tissues, and as its spontaneous hydration is a very slow process, the CAs play a fundamental role in acid-base equilibria in all systems, including tumours (Supuran 2008, 2010; Swietach et al, 2008a,b). Considering the fact that these are relatively simple enzymes, rather well characterized biochemically, with a multitude of known inhibitors (Supuran, 2008, 2010), it appeared of great interest to investigate whether their inhibition may lead to an antitumour effect.

Many sulfonamide/sulfamate/sulfamide act as CA inhibitors (CAIs) (Supuran, 2008, 2010). Some have also been reported as inhibitors of both CA IX and XII in recent years (Supuran, 2008, 2010; Pastorekova et al, 2004a,b; Cecchi et al, 2005; Thiry et al, 2006; Vullo et al., 2005). In fact, in recent years, a large number of such compounds have been specifically designed for targeting the tumour-associated CA isoforms (Guler et al, 2010). The main approaches for obtaining such compounds include:

(i) fluorescent sulfonamides, used for imaging purposes and for determining the role of CA IX in tumour acidification (Svastova et al, 2004; Alterio et al, 2006);

(ii) positively or negatively-charged compounds, which cannot cross plasma membranes due to their charged character and thus inhibit selectively only extracellular CAs, among which are CA IX and XII (Supuran and Scozzafava, 2007);

(iii) hypoxia-activatable compounds, which exploit the reducing conditions of hypoxic tumours to convert an inactive prodrug into an active CAI (Supuran and Scozzafava, 2007);

(iv) sugar-containing sulfonamides/sulfamates/sulfamides, which due to their highly hydrophilic character do not easily cross membranes and thus possess an enhanced affinity for extracellular CAs such as CA IX and XII (Supuran and Scozzafava, 2007; Supuran, 2010);

(v) more diverse chemotypes than the sulfonamides and their bioisosteres, such as the phenols, coumarins and other compounds recently investigated as alternative CAIs to the classical sulfonamide inhibitors (Maresca et al., 2009, 2010).

Some of the most interesting CA IX inhibitors available at this time are the compounds investigated by Svastova et al (2004) (possessing structures **1** and **2**, see Figure 19.2) for their *in vivo* role in tumour acidification. These compounds present a special interest because derivative **1** is a fluorescent sulfonamide with high affinity for CA IX and XII (K_Is of 5-24 nM) (Cecchi et al, 2005), which was shown to be useful as a fluorescent probe for hypoxic tumours (Svstova et al, 2004; Dubois et al 2007, 2009). This inhibitor binds to CA IX only under hypoxia *in vivo*, in cell cultures or animals with transplanted tumours. Although the biochemical rationale for this phenomenon is not yet understood, these properties may be exploited for designing diagnostic tools for the imaging of hypoxic tumours. Compound **2** on the other hand, belongs to type (ii) mentioned above, of permanently charged, membrane-impermeant derivatives, and is also a very strong CA IX/XII inhibitor ((K_Is of 7-14 nM) (Pastorekova et al, 2004a). It belongs to the class of positively charged, membrane-impermeant compounds which are highly attractive for targeting CA IX with its extracellular active site, since such compounds do not inhibit intracellular CAs, and may thus lead to drugs with less side effects as compared to the presently, clinically available compounds such as acetazolamide **3** (Figure 19.2), which indiscriminately inhibit all CAs (Supuran, 2008; 2010). It is interesting to note that tumour cell cultures treated with compounds **1** or **2** showed a reversing of the acidic pHe towards more normal pH values, undoubtedly due to the inhibition of the tumour-associated CAs (Svastova et al., 2004; Dubois et al., 2007, 2009). The fluorescent sulfonamide **1** with a high affinity for CA IX has been shown to bind to cells only when CA IX protein was expressed and while cells were hypoxic, in an *in vivo* cancer model too (Dubois et al, 2009). NMRI-nu mice subcutaneously transplanted with HT-29 colorectal tumours were treated with 7% oxygen or with nicotinamide and carbogen and were compared with control animals. Accumulation of CAI compound **1** was monitored by non-invasive fluorescent imaging. Specific accumulation of **1** could be observed in delineated tumour areas as compared with a structurally similar non-sulfonamide analogue incorporating the same scaffold (i.e., a derivative with the same structure as compound 1 but without the SO_2NH_2 moiety). Administration of nicotinamide and carbogen, decreasing acute and chronic hypoxia, respectively prevented accumulation of **1** in the tumour. When treated with 7% oxygen breathing, a 3-fold higher accumulation of **1** was observed. Furthermore, the bound inhibitor fraction was rapidly reduced upon tumour reoxygenation. Such *in vivo* imaging results confirm previous *in vitro* data demonstrating that CAI binding and retention require exposure to hypoxia. Fluorescent labelled sulfonamides may thus provide a powerful tool to visualize hypoxia response in solid tumours. An important step was thus made towards clinical applicability, indicating the potential of patient selection for CA IX-directed therapies (Dubois et al, 2009).

Chiche et al (2009) showed recently that in hypoxic LS174Tr tumour cells expressing either CA IX or both CA IX and XII isoforms, in response to a CO_2 load, both enzymes contribute to extracellular acidification and to maintaining a more alkaline resting intracellular pH (pHi), an action that preserves ATP levels and cell survival in a range of acidic outside pH (6.0-6.8) and low bicarbonate medium. *In vivo* experiments showed that silencing of CA IX alone leads to a 40% reduction in xenograft tumour volume, with up-regulation of the second gene, and encoding for CA XII. Silencing of both CAIX and CAXII gave an impressive 85% reduction of tumour growth. Thus, hypoxia-induced CA IX and CA XII are major tumour prosurvival pH-regulating enzymes, and their combined targeting (i.e., inhibition) held potential for the design of anticancer drugs with a novel mechanism of action (Chiche et al, 2009).

However the *in vivo* proof-of-concept study showing that sulfonamide CA IX inhibitors may indeed have significant antitumour effects, has been only recently published by Neri's group (Ahlskog et al, 2009). By using the membrane-impermeant derivatives **4** and **5** (Figure 19.2), based on the acetazolamide scaffold to which either fluorescein-carboxylic acid or albumin-binding moieties were attached, this group demonstrated a strong tumour growth retardation (in mice with xenografts of a renal clear cell carcinoma line, SK-RC-52) in animals treated for one month with these CAIs (alone or in combination with other anticancer drugs). This preliminary data demonstrated the great promise of tumour growth inhibition with sulfonamides acting as CA IX/XII or related agents, making thus possible the development of alternative anticancer drugs (Supuran, 2008). Very recently, the same group used DNA-encoded chemical libraries to identify potent CA IX inhibitors from a library of one million DNA-encoded compounds (Buller et al., 2011). Some potent bis-sulfonamide CA IX inhibitors have been detected, one of which also showed accumulation in colorectal adenocarcinoma LS174T xenografted tumour sections in mice (Buller et al, 2011).

More recently, a series of ureido-substituted benzenesulfonamides were reported which showed a very interesting profile for the inhibition

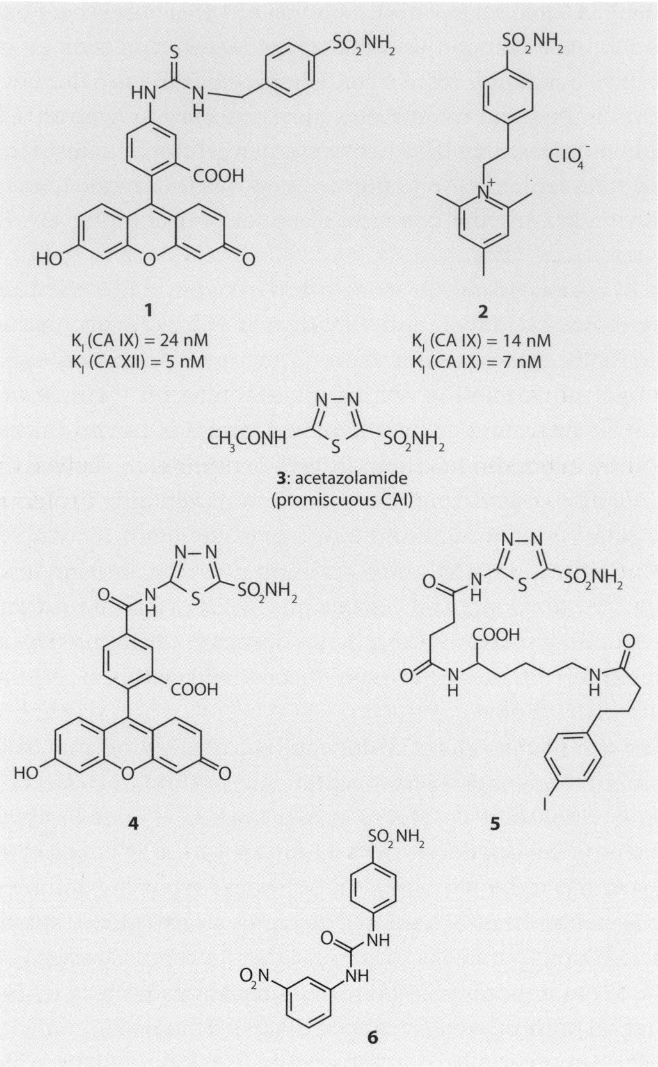

Figure 19.2 _ Compounds 1-6.

of several CAs (Pacchiano et al., 2011). CA IX and XII were highly inhibited by some members of the series, depending on the substitution pattern at the urea moiety. Several low nanomolar CA IX/XII inhibitors also showed good selectivity for the transmembrane over the cytosolic isoforms. One of them, 4-{[(3'-nitrophenyl)carbamoyl]amino} benzenesulfonamide **6**, completely inhibited the formation of metastases by the highly aggressive 4T1 mammary tumour cells at pharmacologic concentrations of 45 mg/kg (Figure 19.2), thus constituting an interesting candidate for the development of conceptually novel antimetastatic drugs (Pacchiano et al, 2011). The compound **6**, similar to **1**, also inhibited the growth of the primary tumours (Lou et al, 2011).

Coumarin and thiocoumarins were only recently discovered to act as CAIs, and their inhibition mechanism was deciphered in detail by one of our groups (Maresca et al., 2009; 2010). We demonstrated recently that the natural product 6-(1S-hydroxy-3-methylbutyl)-7-methoxy-2H-chromen-2-one **7** as well as the simple, unsubstituted coumarin **8** are hydrolyzed within the CA active site with formation of the 2-hydroxy-cinnamic acids **9** and **10** (Figure 19.3), respectively, which represent the *de facto* enzyme inhibitors. At least two other interesting facts emerged during these studies: (i) this new class of CAIs, the coumarins/thiocoumarins, binds in hydrolyzed form at the entrance of the CA active site and does not interact with the metal ion, constituting thus an entirely new category of mechanism-based inhibitors; and (ii) for the specific case of compound **7**, the formed substituted-cinnamic acid **9** was observed bound within the CA active site as the *cis* isomer, although these derivatives are stable in solution as *trans* isomers. However, for the simpler coumarin **8**, the *trans*-2-hydroxycinnamic acid **10** has been evidenced bound within the enzyme active site, by means of X-ray crystallography (Maresca et al., 2009; 2010). The tentative explanation for the unusual geometry of inhibitor **9** within the enzyme active site was that **9** would be too bulky as *trans*-isomer in the restricted space of the CA active site, while the unstable in solution *cis*-isomer would be stabilized when bound within the enzyme cavity. It should be also mentioned that coumarins **7** and **8** were potent inhibitors against some investigated human CA isoforms, which makes this entire class of derivatives of paramount interest for designing novel applications for the CAIs.

In order to understand in greater detail the CA inhibition mechanism with the (thio)coumarins, which might be useful for the design of new pharmacological applications, we investigated thereafter a series of derivatives possessing various moieties substituting the (thio)coumarin ring in the 3-, 6-, 7-, 3,6-, 4,7 and 3,8- positions, of types **11-20** (Figure 19.3) (Maresca et al., 2010). The most significant finding of this second study was that some coumarins are truly isoform-selective CAIs, inhibiting efficiently only one isoform of the 13 catalytically active ones found in humans. For example, thiocoumarin **15** and several coumarins (**13**, **14**, **16** and **17**) showed low nanomolar affinity for CA IX, with inhibition constants in the range of 45 – 98 nM (Maresca et al., 2010).

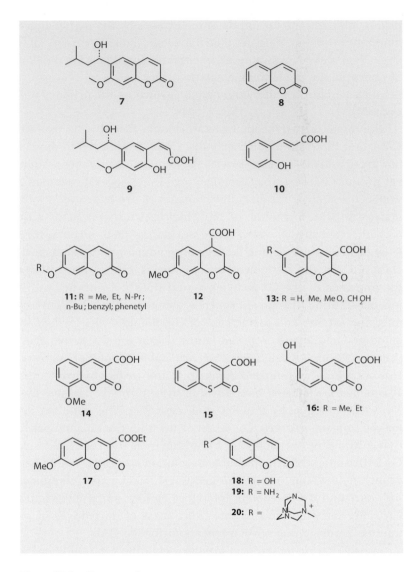

Figure 19.3 _ Compounds 7-20.

The monosubstituted derivatives **18** and **20** on the other hand contained either a compact (CH$_2$OH) or a rather bulky (hexamethylenetetramine) group in position 6 of the coumarin ring, which render our findings quite important, as it is clear that for effective CA IX inhibition, a large variation of structural motifs are allowed in the 3- and 6-positions of the (thio)coumarin ring. Compound **20** (which is membrane impermeant) was shown to be a low nanomolar inhibitor of only CA IX (K_I of 48 nM) whereas it inhibited in the micromolar range all other 12 CAs, a feature never evidenced before for a sulfonamide CAI. Thus, this is the first CA IX-selective inhibitor ever reported up to now (Maresca et al., 2010). hCA XII, the other transmembrane isoform present in tumours, was poorly inhibited by **8**, whereas the natural product coumarin **7** was slightly more inhibitory (K_I of 48.6 µM) (Maresca et al., 2009).

However, most of the investigated (thio)coumarins **11-20** were effective, low micromolar hCA XII inhibitors, with K_Is in the range of 3.2 – 9.0 µM. Thus, a lot of substitution patterns present in compounds **11-20** investigated up to now lead to effective hCA XII inhibitors, although compounds with nanomolar affinity for this isozyme have not been evidenced so far. Very recently, a glycosyl-coumarin derivative with potent hCA IX/XII inhibitory effects was shown to have very strong antimetastatic effects in the very aggressive 4T1 mammary tumour cells at pharmacologic concentrations of 15 –30 mg/kg (Lou et al., 2011).

All this data clearly demonstrates that at least CA IX and XII are validated targets for developing novel antitumour drugs which interfere with the pH regulation in cancer cells.

Aquaporins targeting

The aquaporins (AQPs) are a family of water channel proteins of which at least 13 isoforms have been identified so far (Ding et al, 2010; Endeward et al, 2006). Most of these isoforms transport water but some of them were reported to transport glycerol and possibly other small solutes/molecules, including CO_2 (Endeward et al, 2006). As CO_2 contributes significantly to the regulation of the acid-base equilibrium in the tumour cells (as also outlined above for the CAs discussion) it is reasonable to predict that AQPs may also participate in such processes (Parks et al, 2010). The expression of some AQPs, such as AQP1, 4 and 5 seems to be induced by hypoxia (Ding et al, 2010). For example, Ding et al. (2010) reported a strong overexpression of AQP4 in glioblastoma multiforme, suggesting that it may be involved in brain tumour malignancy.

To make things even more complicated, it has been recently reported that some sulfonamides also acting as CAIs (e.g., acetazolamide **3**), act as inhibitors of some AQPs (e.g., AQP4) but not of other isoforms, such as AQP1 (Tanimur et al, 2009). Huber et al (2007) on the other hand showed that acetazolamide and structurally related compounds (ethoxzolamide or 4-acetamidobenzenesulfonamide) are low micromolar inhibitors of AQP4. Thus, compounds showing antitumour activity due to their CA IX/XII inhibitory action, may have additional anticancer mechanisms due to their interaction with some AQP isoforms. Further studies to find specific inhibitors just for these proteins (and not for the CAs) may help to better understand the role, if any, of AQPs in tumourigenesis and pH regulation.

Interference with the anion exchangers AE1-AE3

Bicarbonate transport proteins facilitate the movement of the membrane-impermeant bicarbonate ion across biological membranes (Johnson and Casey, 2009). They cluster phylogenetically into three classes: (i) electroneutral Cl^-/HCO_3^- exchangers of the SLC4A family (solute carrier 4A) – the AEs; (ii) Na^+-coupled HCO_3^- co-transporters (SLC4A family), and (iii) anion transporters of the SLC26 family (Johnson and Casey, 2009).

The anion exchanger (AE) family is composed of three isoforms (AE1, AE2 and AE3). In humans, AE1 is formed of a 43 kDa amino-terminal cytoplasmic domain that interacts with cytoskeletal proteins and glycolytic enzymes, a 55 kDa membrane spanning domain, responsible for Cl^-/HCO_3^- exchange activity, and a short 33 amino acid cytoplasmic carboxyl-terminal domain that contains the binding site for CA II (Johnson and Casey, 2009). AE2 is the most widely expressed isoform and is found in the basolateral membrane of many epithelial cells whereas AE3 is expressed predominantly in excitable tissues, including brain, heart and retina, and throughout the gastrointestinal tract (Johnson and Casey, 2009). Casey proposed the concept of bicarbonate transport metabolon, composed of a bicarbonate transporter (AE1-3) and a CA protein, based on the physical and functional interactions between the transporters and the enzyme (reviewed in Johnson and Casey, 2009). The linked physiological function (catalysis and transport of HCO_3^-) and the widespread tissue distribution of both AEs and CAs (as multiple isoforms of both proteins) suggests indeed that they could form a complex. CAs both supply the HCO_3^- substrate for transport and remove HCO_3^- following transport, whereas the transporter translocates the membrane-impermeant bicarbonate in or out of the cell (Johnson and Casey, 2009). The tumour-associated enzyme CA IX has been demonstrated to form such a metabolon with AE2 (Morgan et al., 2007).

4,4'-Diisothiocyano-2,2'-stilbenedisulfonic acid (DIDS) **21** and structurally related stilbenes are AE inhibitors, but they also inhibit other bicarbonate transporters indiscriminately (Jessen et al., 1986; Parks et al, 2010). These compounds initially block the AEs and the BTs reversibly and later irreversibly (Jessen et al., 1986). It has been shown recently that DIDS induces apoptosis in hepatocellular carcinoma cells HA22T overexpressing AE2, thus having antitumour activity (Liu et al., 2008).

Morgan et al (2004) showed that celecoxib **22** (which is also a strong CA IX/XII inhibitor, Supuran, 2008) and several other potent sulfonamide CAIs (of type **23**) significantly inhibited AE1 Cl^-/NO_3^- exchange activity with EC_{50} values in the range 0.22- 2.8 µM. It was evident that bulkier compounds of type **23** showed greater AE1 inhibitory potency compared to sulfonamides incorporating less bulky moieties (Figure 19.4). Maximum inhibition using 40 µM of each compound was of only 22- 53% of the AE1 transport activity, possibly because the assays were performed in the presence of competing substrate. In the Cl^-/HCO_3^- exchange assays, which depend on functional CA to produce the transport substrate, 40 µM celecoxib inhibited AE1 by 62 %. It was concluded that some sulfonamide CAIs, including the clinically used pain-killer celecoxib, inhibit bicarbonate transport mediated by AE1 at clinically-significant concentrations (Morgan et al., 2004). Celecoxib shows significant antitumour activity, possibly due to its COX2 and CA IX/XII inhibitory properties, although other mechanisms of action are probable (Supuran et al, 2004). It would be thus highly important to design specific ligands for the AEs, which do not interfere with other enzymes or transport proteins, but such compounds are not available so far.

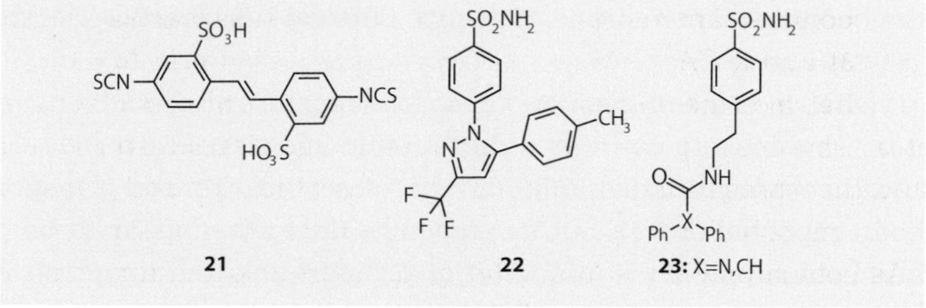

Figure 19.4 _ Compounds 21-23.

Other bicarbonate transporters

A second family of bicarbonate transporters are the Na^+/HCO_3^- co-transporters (NBCs) that facilitate the co-transport of Na^+ and HCO_3^- across the plasma membrane with either an electroneutral (NBC3/NBCn1) or electrogenic (2/3 HCO_3^-:1 Na^+) (NBCe1, NBCe2/ NBC4) mechanism (Johnson and Casey, 2009). The sodium-coupled HCO_3^- transporter family is on the other hand composed of NBCe1, NBCe2, NBCn1, NDCBE and NCBE. NBCs have a widespread tissue distribution, including pancreas, kidney and heart (Johnson and Casey, 2009). NBC3 is an electroneutral Na^+/HCO_3^- transporter that is involved in intracellular pH regulation in heart, skeletal muscle and kidney. Like other bicarbonate transporters, a region in the C-terminus of NBC3 (D1135-D1136) was shown to bind CA II, and this interaction was essential for maximal HCO_3^- transport (Johnson and Casey, 2009). NBCe1 is an electrogenic Na^+/HCO_3^- co-transporter, which operates with either a 3:1 or 2:1 HCO_3^-:Na^+ stoichiometry. Splicing variant NBCe1a (kNBCe1) plays the central role in HCO_3^- reabsorption in the basolateral membranes of the proximal tubule in conjunction with the luminal Na^+/H^+ exchanger, NHE3, and a H^+-ATPase, which secrete acid (Johnson and Casey, 2009). NBCe1a thus mediates HCO_3^- efflux from the cell to the blood, and normally works with a stoichiometry of 3 HCO_3^- per Na^+. NBCe1b (pNBCe1) is expressed in the basolateral membranes of pancreatic duct cells where it transports HCO_3^- into the cell and functions with a 2 HCO_3^- per Na^+ stoichiometry. CA IV and NBCe1 were shown to co-localise in mammalian kidney, pancreas and heart (Sterling et al., 2002). Four members of the SLC26a SLC26A4 (pendrin) are insensitive to intra- and extracellular pH, while SLC26A3 (DRA) is inhibited by intracellular acidification and activated by intracellular alkalinization, ammonium and hyper-tonicity. SLC26A6 carries out both Cl/HCO_3^- and Cl/OH^- exchange and is the predominant anion exchanger in the heart. SLC26A7 is a Cl/HCO_3^- exchanger localised predominantly in the basolateral membrane of gastric parietal cells (Sterling et al., 2002; Johnson and Casey, 2009).

DIDS **21** is an inhibitor for these transporters also, but being quite toxic, it is impossible to use it as a therapeutic agent (Yamagata and Tannock, 1996). More recently another inhibitor of these bicarbonate transporters has been reported (S3705, but its structure does not appear to be disclosed) and evaluated for the inhibition of proliferation and apoptosis of human cholangiocarcinoma cells HUH-28 and Mz-ChA-1 cells (Di Sario et al, 2007). The intracellular pH of the treated cells was shown to drop. Incubation of

HUH-28 cells with cariporide and/or S3705 was also able to reduce proliferation, and to induce apoptosis (Di Sario et al, 2007). The same two agents (cariporide and S3705) were investigated for their effects on the toxicity of the anticancer drug melphalan against two human breast cancer cell lines (MDA-MB231 and MCF7) by Wong et al (2005). These authors concluded that the effects on pHe of the two drugs were rather small and irrelevant to warrant clinical studies.

However the lack of selective ligands for all these multiple transport proteins should be stressed once again (cariporide is an NHE1 inhibitor, see the next paragraph).

The Na⁺/H⁺ exchanger NHE1

NHE1 is expressed in most cells all over the body, being one of the crucial proteins involved in pH regulation (Pouyssegur et al, 2006; Parks et al 2010). NHE1 is involved in tumourigenesis, as demonstrated by Pouyssegur's group, who showed a drastic reduction of tumour growth for cells lacking this protein (Lagarde et al, 1988). The same effects have been observed by using pharmacological inhibitors (Parks et al, 2010; Harley et al, 2010), such as amiloride **24** or cariporide **25** (Figure 19.5), two of the most investigated compounds acting as inhibitors of this protein (Masereel et al, 2003). There are numerous NHE1 inhibitors structurally related to amiloride/cariporide, all of them possessing the pyrazine-acylguanidine scaffold present in **24**, but various other substituents to the pyrazine ring (Masereel et al, 2003).

Inhibition of NHE1 has been proposed to be effective not only for the management of tumours, but also for obtaining cardioprotective and cer-

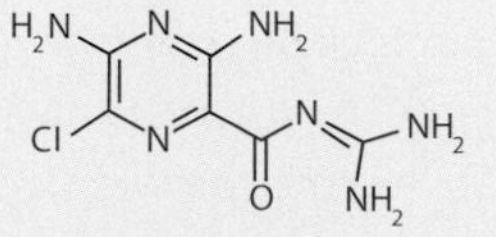

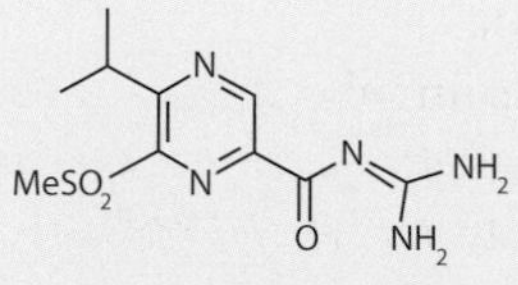

Figure 19.5 _ Compounds 24-25.

ebroprotective agents, or for the treatment of acute renal failure (Masereel et al, 2003). However the diffuse presence of NHE1 in many tissues and its fundamental role in crucial physiological processes, warns as a potential risk of life-threatening side effects for this class of agents. In fact the clinical development of cariporide by Sanofi-Aventis has been stopped in Phase III (Chin and Lip, 2000). It would be crucial to develop agents targeting NHE1 only in tumours, thus leaving the enzyme present in other tissues unaffected, but such a goal has not been explored so far.

Monocarboxylate transporter inhibitors

There are at least nine different isoforms of proteins involved in the transport of monocarboxylates (e.g., lactate, pyruvate, etc) out of the cells, but the first four of them, the monocarboxylate transporters (MCT)1-4, seem to play crucial physiological roles (Halestrap and Price, 1999). Indeed, tumour cells fuel their metabolism with glucose and glutamine to meet the bioenergetic and biosynthetic demands of increased proliferation typical of cancers (Feron, 2009). Hypoxia and oncogenic mutations favor glycolysis, with the pyruvate to lactate conversion being promoted by increased expression of lactate dehydrogenase A and inactivation of pyruvate dehydrogenase, with the overall effect of high amounts of lactic acid being produced (Feron, 2009). The preferential use of lactate for oxidative metabolism spares glucose which may in turn reach hypoxic tumour cells (Feron, 2009).

MCTs (mostly MCT1) regulate the entry of lactate into oxidative tumour cells (Feron, 2009) and its inhibition favors the switch from lactate-fuelled respiration to glycolysis, which consecutively kills hypoxic tumour cells through glucose starvation. On the other hand, MCT4 mediates lactate export from

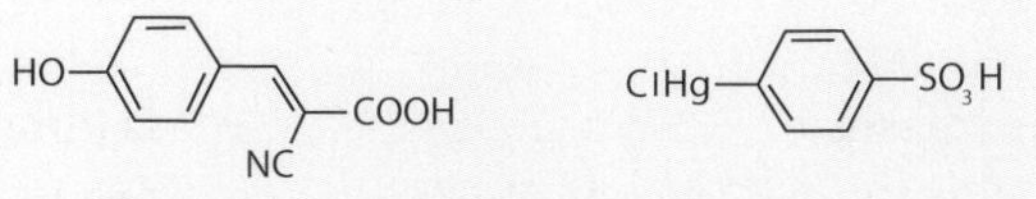

Figure 19.6 _ Compounds 26-27.

hypoxic tumour cells. MCT overexpression is indeed high in many tumours, with MCT4 also being induced by hypoxia through the HIF-1 cascade (Ullah et al, 2006). Thus, MCTs inhibitors might prove useful as antitumour agents. There are in fact various classes of such inhibitors, among which are DIDS **22**, α-cyano-4-hydroxycynnamic acid **26** or 4-chloromercuribenzenesulfonic acid **27** (Enerson and Drewes, 2003). Their efficacy on the different MCTs is very different as well as their mechanisms of action (**27** is a thiol reagent which inactivates many other enzymes and not only MCTs, whereas the mechanisms of inhibition with DIDS and **26** are less well understood, Enerson and Drewes, 2003) see Figure 19.6.

Although the involvement of MCTs in tumours is well established, as far as we know, there are no studies in which pharmacological inhibitors (at least **26** which should be much less toxic compared to the mercury derivative **27**) were used to investigate their role in the growth of the tumours. Thus, additional studies for developing potent, non-toxic, isoform-selective MCT inhibitors and their potential applications as antitumour agents, are stringently needed.

V-ATPase inhibitors and proton pump inhibitors

The vacuolar ATPase (V-ATPase) is an ATP-dependent proton pump involved in the acidification of intracellular compartments and the extrusion of protons through the cell cytoplasmic membrane (Fais, 2010; Perez-Syans et al, 2009; Spugnini et al, 2010). This enzyme plays a crucial role in the pH regulation of normal and tumour cells being formed of multiple subunits including both cytosolic and transmembrane domains, each of them being in turn formed from several multisubunit proteins (Fais, 2010; Perez-Syans et al, 2009; Spugnini et al, 2010). V-ATPase is involved in a host of physiological and pathological processes, such as endocytosis, intracellular trafficking and acidification of endosomes, creation of the microenvironment for proper protein transport, in addition to proton transfer processes (Perez-Syans et al, 2009).

There are various classes of V-ATPse inhibitors, such as (among others) the macrocyclic antibiotics bafilomycin A and concanamycin A, a large series of benzolactone enmides incorporating a salicylic acid scaffold, the macrocyclic antibiotic archazolid, some free radical indolyls, etc (reviewed in Perez-Sayans et al, 2009), but all of them show rather high toxicity and are difficult to be used as tools for understanding the role of this enzyme in tumourigenesis. However, at least one study suggests that one of these inhibitors, bafilomycin A, retards the growth of pancreatic xenograft tumours (Ohta et al., 1998).

Recently, considering the possible similarity between V-ATPase and H$^+$,K$^+$-ATPase, the enzyme involved in proton secretion in the stomach, Fais' group proposed a revolutionary new approach for the management of tumours: the use of the proton pump inhibitors (PPIs) of the omeprazole type for inhibiting V-ATPase (Fais, 2010, De Milito et al, 2010).

Such compounds (omeprazole **28**, pantoprazole **29**, lnsoprazole **30** and rabeprazole **31** among others) (Figure 19.7) are widely used clinically as ant-acids and are pro-drugs requiring acidity to be activated (Horn, 2000; Fais, 2010, De Milito et al, 2010). Indeed, in acidic environment they undergo a trans-formation which leads to the formation of a sulfenamide which reacts with Cys residues from the protein leading to its inactivation (Mulin et al., 2009). PPIs may also target the acidic (hypoxic) tumour mass, where they are metabolized as in the stomach, thus blocking the formation and traffic of protons (Fais, 2010; Huber et al, 2010). Proton pump inhibition was shown to trig-ger a rapid cell death as a result of the intracellular acidification, caspase activation and early accumulation of reactive oxygen species in tumour cells, by the same group (Fais, 2010). As a whole, the devastating effect of PPIs on tumour cell growth suggest the triggering of a fatal cell toxification pro-cess (Fais, 2010). Many human tumours, including melanoma, osteosarcoma, lymphomas and various adenocarcinomas were shown to be responsive to PPIs (Fais, 2010; Huber et al, 2010). Metastatic tumours appeared to be even

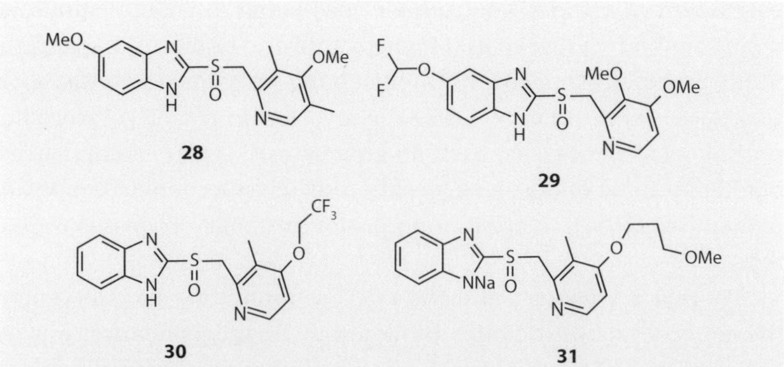

Figure 19.7 _ Compounds 28-31.

more responsive to PPIs, as they are generally more acidic than the majority of primary tumours (Fais, 2010; De Milito et al, 2010). Presently, two clinical trials are testing the effectiveness of PPIs in chemosensitizing melanoma and osteosarcoma patients (Fais, 2010). Indeed, tumour acidity represents a very potent mechanism of chemoresistance, and the majority of cytotoxic agents are weak bases, being thus quickly protonated outside the cell and not entering within them, and preventing the drugs from reaching specific cellular targets. Future clinical data will provide the proof of concept regarding the use of PPIs as a new class of antitumour agent with a low level of systemic toxicity as compared with standard chemotherapeutic agents, but we also estimate that combination therapy of some of these agents with other compounds involved in the regulation of tumour pH may lead to even better antitumour responses.

Conclusions

The regulation of pH in tumours involves the interplay of many proteins, among which are several carbonic anhydrases (CA IX and XII); some acquaporins AQP1-5; many anion exchangers AE1-3 and sodium bicarbonate (co-)transporters (NBCs), the sodium-dependent chloride-bicarbonate exchangers (NDCBE), monocarboxylate transporters MCT1-4, the sodium-proton exchanger NHE1, and the vacuolar H^+-ATPA (V-ATPase). Some of them are overexpressed in tumours through to the HIF-1 pathway, but the particular contribution of most of them is currently poorly understood. The concerted action of these proteins assures a slightly alkaline internal pH (pHi) and an acidic external pH (pHe) within the tumours, which favors proliferation of the primary tumour and formation of metastases. Inhibition studies of one or more of them with specific inhibitors was shown in some cases to lead to the return of both pHi and pHe towards normal values with the consequent impairment of the tumour growth. This constitutes an antitumour mechanism not exploited by the classical anticancer drugs. Among these new possible antitumour targets, the CA IX/XII inhibition with sulfonamide or coumarin inhibitors was undoubtedly proven to reverse the effect of tumour acidification, leading to the inhibition of the cancer cell growth, both for primary tumours and metastases. This approach may be useful for both imaging and treatment purposes of tumours overexpressing these two enzymes.

There are however few specific, non toxic and effective compounds interfering with other proteins mentioned above than the CAs, but some sulfonamides seem to also inhibit AQPs and AEs, whereas proton pump inhibitors of the omeprazole type show antitumour effects possibly by inhibiting V-ATPase. Potent, specific and non toxic compounds inhibiting one or more of these proteins may represent valuable new antitumour drugs.

A c k n o w l e d g m e n t s _ Research from my laboratory is financed by an EU grant of the 7th framework programme (Metoxia).

References

Ahlskog JKJ, Dumelin CE, Trüssel S, Marlind J, Neri D (2009) In vivo targeting of tumour-associated carbonic anhydrases using acetazolamide derivatives. Bioorg Med Chem Lett 19: 4851-4856.

Alterio V, Hilvo M, Di Fiore A, Supuran CT, Pan P, Parkkila S, Scaloni A, Pastorek J, Pastorekova S, Pedone C, Scozzafava A, Monti SM, De Simone G (2009) Crystal structure of the extracellular catalytic domain of the tumour-associated human carbonic anhydrase IX. Proc Natl Acad Sci USA 106: 16233 – 16238.

Alterio V, Vitale RM, Monti SM, Pedone C, Scozzafava A, Cecchi A, De Simone G, Supuran CT (2006) Carbonic anhydrase inhibitors: X-ray and molecular modeling study for the interaction of a fluorescent antitumour sulfonamide with isozyme II and IX. J Am Chem Soc 128: 8329-8335.

Boron WF (2004) Regulation of intracellular pH. Adv Physiol Educ 28: 160-179.

Brahimi-Horn MC, Pouysségur J (2007) Hypoxia in cancer cell metabolism and pH regulation. Essays Biochem 43: 165-178.

Buller F, Steiner M, Frey K, Mircsof D, Scheuermann J, Kalisch M, Bühlmann P, Supuran CT, Neri D. (2011) Selection of carbonic anhydrase IX inhibitors from one million DNA-encoded compounds. ACS Chem Biol 6(4):336-344..

Cecchi A, Hulikova A, Pastorek J, Pastoreková S, Scozzafava A, Winum J-Y, Montero J-L, Supuran CT (2005) Carbonic anhydrase inhibitors. Sulfonamides inhibit isozyme IX mediated acidification of hypoxic tumours. Fluorescent sulfonamides design as probes of membrane-bound carbonic anhydrase isozymes involvement in tumourigenesis. J Med Chem 48: 4834-4841.

Chiche J, Ilc K, Brahimi-Horn MC, Pouysségur J (2010) Membrane-bound carbonic anhydrases are key regulators controlling tumour growth and cell migration. Adv Enz regul 50: 20-33.

Chiche J, Ilc K, Laferrière J, Trottier E, Dayan F, Mazure NM, Brahimi-Horn MC, Pouysségur J (2009) Hypoxia-inducible carbonic anhydrase IX and XII promote tumour cell growth by counteracting acidosis through the regulation of the intracellular pH. *Cancer Res* 69: 358-368.

Chin B, Lip GY (2000) Cariporide Aventis. Curr Opin Investig Drugs 1: 340-6.

De Milito A, Canese R, Marino ML, Borghi M, Iero M, Villa A, Venturi G, Lozupone F, Iessi E, Logozzi M, Della Mina P, Santinami M, Rodolfo M, Podo F, Rivoltini L, Fais S (2010) pH-dependent antitumour activity of proton pump inhibitors against human melanoma is mediated by inhibition of tumour acidity. Int J Cancer 127: 207-219.

Di Sario A, Bendia E, Omenetti A, De Minicis S, Marzioni M, Kleemann HW, Candelaresi C, Saccomanno S, Alpini G, Benedetti A (2007) Selective inhibition of ion transport mechanisms regulating intracellular pH reduces proliferation and induces apoptosis in cholangiocarcinoma cells. Dig Liv Dis 39: 60-69.

Ding T, Gu F, Fu L, Ma YJ (2010) Aquaporin-4 in glioma invasion and an analysis of molecular mechanisms. J Clin Neurosci 17: 1359-61.

Dubois L, Douma K, Supuran CT, Chiu RK, van Zandvoort MAMJ, Pastoreková S, Scozzafava A, Wouters BG, Lambin P (2007) Imaging the hypoxia surrogate marker CA IX requires expression and catalytic activity for binding fluorescent sulfonamide inhibitors. Radiother Oncol 83: 367–373.

Dubois L, Lieuwes NG, Maresca A, Thiry A, Supuran CT, Scozzafava A, Wouters BG, Lambin P (2009) Imaging of CA IX with fluorescent labelled sulfonamides distinguishes hypoxic and (re)-oxygenated cells in a xenograft tumour model. Radiother Oncol 92: 423-428

Endevard V, Musa-Aziz R, Cooper GJ, Chen LM, Pelletier MF, Virkki LK, Supuran CT, King LS, Boron WF, Gros G (2006) Evidence that aquaporin 1 is a major pathway for CO_2 transport across the human erythrocyte membrane. FASEB J 20: 1974-1981

Enerson BE, Drewes LR (2003) Molecular features, regulation, and function of monocarboxylate transporters: implications for drug delivery. J Pharm Sci 92:1531-44.

Fais S (2010) Proton pump inhibitor-induced tumour cell death by inhibition of a detoxification mechanism. J Intern Med 267. 515-25.

Feron O (2009) Pyruvte into lactate and back. Form Warburg effect to symbiotic energy fuel exchange in cancer cells. Radiother Oncol 92: 329-33.

Guler OO, De Simone G, Supuran CT (2010) Drug design studies of the novel antitumour targets carbonic anhydrase IX and XII. Curr Med Chem. 17: 1516-26.

Halestrap AP, Price NT (1999) The proton-linked monocarboxylate transporter (MCT) family: structure, function and regulation. Biochem J 343: 281-99.

Harley W, Floyd C, Dunn T, Zhang XD, Chen TY, Hegde M, Palandoken H, Nantz MH, Leon L, Carraway KL 3rd, Lyeth B, Gorin FA (2010) Dual inhibition of sodium-mediated proton and calcium efflux triggers non-apoptotic cell death in malignant gliomas. Brain Res 1363:159-69.

Hilvo M, Baranauskiene L, Salzano AM, Scaloni A, Matulis D, Innocenti A, Scozzafava A, Monti SM, Di Fiore A, De Simone G, Lindfors M, Janis J, Valjakka J, Pastorekova S, Pastorek J, Kulomaa MS, Nordlund HR, Supuran CT. Parkkila S (2008) Biochemical characterization of CA IX: one of the most active carbonic anhydrase isozymes. J Biol Chem 283: 27799-27809.

Horn J (2000) The proton-pump inhibitors: Similarities and differences. Clin Ther 22: 266-80.

Huber V, De Milito A, Harguindey S, Reshkin SJ, Wahl ML, Rauch C, Chiesi A, Pouysségur J, Gatenby RA, Rivoltini L, Fais S (2010) Proton dynamics in cncer. J Transl Med 8: 57.

Huber VJ, Tsujita M, Yamazaki M, Sakimura K, Nakada T (2007) Identification of arylsulfonamides as aquaporin 4 inhibitors. Bioorg Med Chem Lett 17: 1270-3.

Jessen F, Sjøholm C, Hoffmann EK (1986) Identification of the anion exchange protein of ehrlich cells: A kinetic analysis of the inhibitory effects of 4,4´-diisothiocyano-2,2´-stilbene-disulfonic acid (DIDS) and labelling of membrane proteins with3H-DIDS. J Membr Biol 92: 195 – 205.

Johnson DE, Casey JR (2009) Bicarbonate transport metabolons. In *Drug Design of Zinc-Enzyme Inhibitors: Functional, Structural, and Disease Applications*, Supuran CT, Winum JY Eds., Wiley, Hoboken, pp. 415 – 437.

Kremer G, Pouysségur J (2008) Tumour cell metabolism: Cncer's Achilles' heel. Cancer Cell 13: 472-482.

Innocenti A, Pastorekova S, Pastorek J, Scozzafava A, De Simone G, Supuran CT (2009) The proteoglycan region of the tumour-associated carbonic anhydrase isoform IX acts as an intrinsic buffer optimizing CO_2 hydration at acidic pH values characteristic of solid tumours. Bioorg Med Chem Lett 19: 5825-5828.

Lagarde AE, Franchi AJ, Paris S, Pouysségur JM (1988) Effect of mutations affecting Na+: H+ antiport activity on tumourigenic potential of hamster lung fibroblasts. J Cell Biochem 36: 249-60.

Liu CJ, Hwang JM, Wu TT, Hsieh YH, Wu CC, Hsieh YS, Tsai CH, Wu HC, Huang CY, Liu JY (2008) Anion exchanger inhibitor DIDS induces human poorly-differentiated malignant hepatocellular carcinoma HA22T cell apoptosis. Mol Cell Biochem 308: 117-25.

Lou Y, McDonald PC, Oloumi A, Chia S, Oslund C, Ahmadi A, Kyle A, auf dem Keller U, Leung S, Huntsman D, Clarke B, Sutherland BW, Waterhouse AD, Bally M, Roskelley C, Overall CM, Minchinton A, Pacchiano F, Carta F, Winum JY, Supuran CT, Dedhar S (2011) Targeting tumour hypoxia: suppression of breast tumour growth and metastasis by novel carbonic anhydrase IX inhibitors. Cancer Res 71(9):3364-3376.

Maresca A, Temperini C, Vu H, Pham NB, Poulsen SA, Scozzafava A, Quinn RJ, Supuran CT (2009) Non-zinc mediated inhibition of carbonic anhydrases: coumarins are a new class of suicide inhibitors. J Am Chem Soc 131: 3057-3062.

Maresca A, Temperini C, Pochet L, Masereel B, Scozzafava A, Supuran CT (2010) Deciphering the mechanism of carbonic anhydrase inhibition with coumarins and thiocoumarins. J Med Chem 53: 335-344.

Msereel B, Pochet L, Laeckmann D (2003) An overview of inhibitors of Na^+/H^+ exchanger. Eur J Med Chem 38: 547-54.

Morgan PE, Pastorekova S, Stuart-Tilley AK, Alper SL, Casey JR (2007) Interactions of transmembrane carbonic anhydrase, CAIX, with bicarbonate transporters. Am J Physiol Cell Physiol 293: C738-748

Morgan PE, Supuran CT, Casey JR (2004) Carbonic anhydrase inhibitors that directly inhibit anion transport by the human Cl/HCO_3^- exchanger, AE1. Mol Membr Biol 21: 423-433.

Mullin JM, Gabello M, Murray LJ, Farrell CP, Bellows J, Wolov KR, Kearney KR, Rudolph D, Thornton JJ (2009) Proton pump inhibitors: actions and reactions. Drug Discov Today 14: 647-60.

Ohta T, Arakawa H, Futagami F, Fushida S, Kitagawa H, Kayahara M, Nagakawa T, Miwa K, Kurashima K, Numata M, Kitamura Y, Terada T, Ohkuma S (1998) Bafilomycin A1 induces apoptosis in the human pancreatic cancer cell line Capan-1. J Pathol 185: 324-30.

Pacchiano F, Carta F, McDonald PC, Lou Y, Vullo D, Scozzafava A, Dedhar S, Supuran CT (2011) Ureido-substituted benzenesulfonamides potently inhibit carbonic anhydrase IX and show antimetastatic activity in a model of breast cancer metastasis. J Med Chem 54(6):1896-902..

Parks SK, Chiche J, Pouysségur J (2010) pH control mechanisms of tumour survival and growth. J Cell Physiol 226: 299-308.

Pastorek J, Pastorekova S, Callebaut I, Mornon JP, Zelnik V, Opavsky R, Zatovicova M, Liao S, Portetelle D, Stanbridge EJ, Zavada J, Burny A, Kettmann R (1994) Cloning and characterization of MN, a human tumour-associated protein with a domain homologous to carbonic anhydrase and putative helix-loop-helix DNA binding segment. Oncogene 9: 2877-2888.

Pastorekova S, Casini A, Scozzafava A, Vullo D, Pastorek J, Supuran CT (2004a) Carbonic anhydrase inhibitors: The first selective, membrane-impermeant inhibitors targeting the tumour-associated isozyme IX. Bioorg Med Chem Lett 14: 869-873.

Pastorekova S, Parkkila S, Pastorek J, Supuran CT (2004b) Carbonic anhydrases: current state of the art, therapeutic applications and future prospects. J Enz Inhib Med Chem 19: 199-229.

Pérez-Sayáns M, Somoza-Martín JM, Barros-Angueira F, Rey JM, García-García A (2009) V-ATPase inhibitors and implication in cancer treatment. Cancer Treat Rev 35: 707-13.

Pouysségur J, Dayan F, Mazure NM (2006) Hypoxia signalling in cancer and approaches to enforce tumoour regression. Nature 441: 437-43.

Scozzafava A, Mastrolorenzo A, Supuran CT (2004) Modulation of carbonic anhydrase activity and its applications in therapy. javascript:popRef('A3')Expert Opin Ther Pat 14: 667-702.

Scozzafava A, Mastrolorenzo A, Supuran CT (2006) Carbonic anhydrase inhibitors and activators and their use in therapy. Expert Opin Ther Pat 16: 1627 –1664.

Spugnini E, Citro G, Fais S (2010) Proton pump inhibitors as anti vacuolar-ATPases drugs: a novel anticancer strategy. J Exp Clin Cancer Res 29:44.

Supuran CT (2008) Carbonic anhydrases: novel therapeutic applications for inhibitors and activators.Nat Rev Drug Discov 7: 168-181.

Supuran CT (2010) Carbonic anhydrase inhibitors Bioorg Med Chem Lett 20: 3467-74.

Supuran CT, Casini A, Mastrolorenzo A, Scozzafava A (2004) COX-2 selective inhibitors, carbonic anhydrase inhibition and anticancer properties of sulfonamides belonging to this class of pharmacological agents. Mini-Rev Med Chem 4: 625-632.

Supuran CT, Scozzafava A (2007) Carbonic anhydrases as targets for medicinal chemistry. Bioorg Med Chem 15: 4336-4350.

Supuran CT, Scozzafava A, Casini A (2003) Carbonic anhydrase inhibitors. Med Res-Rev 23: 146-189.

Sterling D, Brown NJD, Supuran CT, Casey JR (2002) The functional and physical relationship between the DRA bicarbonate transporter and carbonic anhydrase II. Am J Physiol Cell Physiol 283: C1522-C1529.

Swietach P, Wigfield S, Supuran CT, Harris AL, Vaughan-Jones RD (2008a) Cancer-associated, hypoxia-inducible carbonic anhydrase IX facilitates CO_2 diffusion. BJU In, 101 Suppl 4: 22-24.

Swietach P, Wigfield S, Cobden P, Supuran CT, Harris AL, Vaughan-Jones RD (2008b) Tumour-associated carbonic anhydrase 9 spatially coordinates intracellular pH in three-dimensional multicellular growth. J Biol Chem 283: 20473-20483.

Švastová E, Hulíková A, Rafajová M, Zat'ovičová M, Gibadulinová A, Casini A, Cecchi A, Scozzafava A, Supuran CT, Pastorek J (2004) Hypoxia activates the capacity of tumour-associated carbonic anhydrase IX to acidify extracellular pH. *FEBS Letters* 577: 439-445.

Tanimura Y, Hiroaki Y, Fujiyoshi Y (2009) Acetazolamide reversibly inhibits water conduction by aquaporin 4. J Struct Biol 166: 16-21.

Thiry A, Dogné J-M, Masereel B, Supuran CT (2006) Targeting tumour-associated carbonic anhydrase IX in cancer therapy. Trends Pharmacol Sci 27: 566–573.

Tureci O, Sahin U, Vollmar E, Siemer S, Gottert E, Seitz G, Parkkila S, Sly WS (1998) Human carbonic anhydrase XII: cDNA cloning, expression, and chromosomal localization of a carbonic anhydrase gene that is overexpressed in some renal cell cancers. Proc Natl Acad Sci USA 95: 7608-13.

Ullah MS, Davies AJ, Halestrap AP (2006) The plasma membrane lactate transporter MCT4, but not MCT1, is up-regulated by hypoxia through a HIF-1alpha-dependent mechanism. J Biol Chem 281: 9030-7.

Vullo D, Innocenti A, Nishimori I, Pastorek J, Scozzafava A, Pastorekova S, Supuran CT (2005) Carbonic anhydrase inhibitors. Inhibition of the transmembrane isozyme XII with sulfonamides – A new target for the design of antitumour and antiglaucoma drugs ? Bioorg Med Chem Lett 15: 963-969.

Wong P, Lee C, Tannock IF (2005) Reduction of intracellular pH as a strategy to enhance the pH-dependent cytotoxic effects of melphalan for human breast cancer cells. Clin Cancer Res 11: 3553-7.

Wykoff CC, Beasley NJ, Watson PH, Turner KJ, Pastorek J Sibtain A, Wilson GD, Turley H, Talks KL, Maxwell PH, Pugh CW, Ratcliffe PJ, Harris AL (2000) Hypoxia-inducible expression of tumour-associated carbonic anhydrases. Cancer Res 60: 7075-7083.

Yamagata M, Tannock IF (1996) The chronic administration of drugs that inhibit the regulation of intracellular pH: in vitro and anti-tumour effects. Br J Cancer 73: 1328-34.

Abbreviations and acronyms

AC — Adenylyl cyclase
AC — Adenocarcinoma
ADAM — A desintegrin and metallo-proteases
AE2 — Anion exchanger 2
AF — Aminoflavone
AhR — Aryl-hydrocarbon receptor
AIDS — Acquired Immune Deficiency Syndrome
AKAP — A-kinase anchoring protein
Akt — Protein kinase B
ALD — Aldolase
AMF — Autocrine motility factor
AMFR — Autocrine motility factor receptor
AMPK — AMP-activated protein kinase
Ang — Angiopoietin
AP1 — Activator protein 1
Apaf — Apoptotic peptidase activating factor
APC — Adenomatous polyposis coli
aPKC — Atypical protein kinase C
AQ4 — Cytotoxin, analogue of mitoxantrone
AQP — Aquaporin
ARD — Ankyrin repeat domain
ARD1 — Arrest-defective protein 1
ARDS — Mountain sickness and acute respiratory distress syndrome
ARNT — Aryl hydrocarbon receptor nuclear translocator

ASC — Alanine, serine, cysteine preferring transport system
ATF — Activating transcription factor
ATL — Adult T-cell leukaemia
ATM — Ataxia-telangiectasia mutated
ATP — Adenosine-5'-triphosphate
ATPase — Adenosine triphosphatase
ATR — Serine/threonine-protein kinase
BAFFR — B-cell activating factor receptor
Bax — Bcl2-associated X protein
bHLH — Basic helix-loop-helix
β2-AR — Beta 2 adrenergic receptor
Bcl-2 — B cell leukemia/lymphoma 2
BCR — B-cell receptor
BCSS — Breast cancer specific survival
bFGF — Basic fibroblast growth factor
BMS-181321 — [^{99m}Tc] labelled 2-nitroimidazole
BNIP3 — Bcl-2/adenovirus E1B 19-kD interacting protein
BOLD MRI — Blood oxygen level dependent magnetic resonance imaging
BPH — Benign prostatic hyperplasia
BRAF — B-Raf oncoprotein

BRCA	Breast cancer type 1 susceptibility protein	c-Src	non-receptor tyrosine kinase
BT	Bicarbonate transporter	CSS	Cancer-specific survival
BTO	Benzotriazine di-N-oxide	CT	Computer tomography
BZLF1	EBV immediate-early gene	C-TAD	C-terminal transactivation domain
15C5	Perfluoro-15-crown-5-ether	Cu-ATSM	Diacetyl-2,3-bis(N(4)-methyl-3-thiosemicarbazone
CA	Carbonic anhydrase		
CAI	Carbonic anhydrase inhibitor	Cul2	Cullin2
		CYP	Cytochrome P
CAD	C-terminal activation domain	DAG	Diacylglycerol
		DHA	Dehydroascorbate
CAMK	Calcium/calmodulin-dependent kinase	DHPR	Dihydropyridine receptor
		DF	Distant failure
CARD9	NF-κB agonist	DFS	Disease-free survival
CBP	CREB binding protein	DFX	Deferoxamine
CCRCC	Clear cell renal cell carcinoma	DKG	Diketogulonate
		DLT	Dose limiting toxicities
CD	Cell differentiation marker	DMFS	Distant metastases-free survival
CDK	Cyclin-dependent kinase		
CHIP	Chaperone interacting protein	DMNQ	Redox cycler
		DMOG	Dimethyloxalylglycine
Chk	Serine/threonine-protein kinase	DNA-PK	DNA-dependent protein kinase
CKI	Cyclin-dependent kinase inhibitor	DNBMs	Dinitrobenzamide mustards
CKII	Casein kinase II	DSB	Double-strand brakes
c-MET	HGF receptor	DSS	Disease-specific survival
c-Myc	v-myc myelocytomatosis viral oncogene homolog	DTD	DT-diaphorase
		E09	Apaziquone
CODD	C-terminal oxygen degradation domain	E2F	Transcription factor
		EBV	Epstein-Barr virus
COX	Cyclooxygenase	EBNA3A/3C	EBV nuclear antigens 3A/3C
C-P4H	Collagen prolyl-4-hydroxylase		
		EF	Fluorinated etanidazole
CREB	cAMP response element-binding protein	EGF	Epidermal growth factor
c-RET	Receptor for glial-derived neurotrophic factor	EGFR	Epidermal growth factor receptor
CSDA	Cold shock domain protein A	EGLN	Egg-laying defective like
		eiF2	Eukaryotic translation initiation factor 2
CSN5	5th component of the constitutive photomorphogenic-9 signalozome	ELISA	Enzyme-linked immunosorbent assay

EMSA	Electrophoretic mobility shift assay	GFR	Growth factor receptor
EMT	Epithelial-mesenchymal transition	GLUT	Glucose transporter
		GOG	Gynecologic Oncology Group
ENO	Enolase	GPX	Glutathione peroxidases
eNOS	Endothelial NO synthase	GSH	Glutathione reduced form
Env	Retrovirus envelope glyco-protein	GSK3	Glycogen synthase kinase 3
		GSSG	Oxidized glutathione dimer
EPAS	Endothelial PAS protein	HAP	Hypoxia activated prodrug
EPC	Endothelial progenitor cells	HBV	Hepatitis B virus
EPO	Erythropoietin	HBx	HBV X-protein
ER	Endoplasmic reticulum	HBx Enh1	HBx enhancer 1
ERK	Extracellular signal-regu-lated kinase	HCC	Human hepatocellular car-cinoma
ERM	ERM protein family	HCR	Hypoxia cytotoxicity ratio
$F(ab')_2$	Antigen-binding fragment	HCV	Hepatitis C virus
FAD	Flavin adenine dinucleotide	HDAC	Histone deacetylase
FAK	Focal adhesion kinase	HDM2	Mouse double minute 2 homologue
Fas	Tumour necrosis factor receptor superfamily mem-ber 6	HER2	Human EGF receptor 2
		HFB	Hexafluorobenzene
FAZA	Fluoroazomycin arabino-side	HHV-4	Human Herpesvirus 4
		HHV-8	Human Herpesvirus 8
FDA	Food and Drug Administra-tion	HGF	Hepatocyte growth factor
		2-HG	2-hydroxyglutarate
FDG	Fluorodeoxyglucose	HIF	Hypoxia inducible factor
FETNIM	Fluoroerythronitroimida-zole	HK	Hexokinase
		HNSCC	Head and neck squamous cell carcinoma
FH	Fumarate hydratase	HPV	Human papillomavirus
$[^{18}F]$-HX4	3-$[^{18}F]$Fluoro-2-(4-((2-ni-tro-1H-imidazol-1-yl)methyl)-1H-1,2,3triazol-1-yl)propan-1-ol	HPV16	Human papillomavirus type 16
		HPV18	Human papillomavirus type 18
FIGO	Federation of Gynecology and Obstetrics	HRE	Hypoxia responsive ele-ment
FIH	Factor inhibiting HIF	HSF	Heat shock factor
FISH	Fluorescence in situ hybrid-ization	HSP	Heat shock protein
		HSV1-TKeGFP	Herpes simplex virus type 1 thymidine kinase and enhanced green fluo-rescence protein
FLT	Fms-related tyrosine kinase		
FMISO	Fluoromisonidazole		
FZD	Frizzled		
Gag	Retrovirus capsid protein		
GAPDH	Glyceraldehyde phosphate dehydrogenase	HTLV-1	Human T-cell leukemia vi-rus type 1

HTS	High-Throughput Screen
([^{123}I]-IAZA)	Iodine-123 labelled iodoazomycin arabinoside
IAZP	Iodoazomycin pyranoside
IAZGP	Beta-D-iodinated azomycin galactopyranoside
IAZXP	Iodoazomycin xylopyranoside
ICAM	Intracellular adhesion molecule
IGF	Insulin growth factor
IKK	IκB kinase
IκB	Inhibitor of NF-κB
IL	Interleukin
ING4	Inhibitor of growth protein 4
iNOS	Inducible nitric oxide synthase
IP$_3$-R	Inositol 1,4,5-triphosphate receptor
IPAS	Inhibitory PAS protein
IRES	Internal ribosomal entry site
IRF	Interferon regulatory factor
IRP	Iron regulatory protein
IQGAP1	Ras GTPase-activating-like protein 1
JmjC	Jumonji family of the Culpin superfamily
JNK	Jun N-terminal kinase
KGF	Keratinocyte growth factor
Ki-67	Cellular marker for proliferation
KRAS	Kirsten rat sarcoma viral oncogene homolog
KRT	Keratin
KS	Kaposi sarcoma
KSHV	Kaposi's sarcoma-associated herpesvirus
LANA	Latency associated nuclear antigen
LC	Local control
LDH	Lactate dehydrogenase

LEF	Lymphoid enhancer-binding factor
LC	Local control
LMP1	Latent membrane protein 1
LN	Lymph nodes
LOX	Lysyl oxidase
LPS	Lipopolysaccharide
LRC	Loco-regional control
LTβR	Lymphotoxin receptor
LTR	Retrovitus 5' and 3' end terminal repetition regions
MAPK	Mitogen-activated protein kinase
MAX	MYC associated factor X
MCP	Monocyte chemotactic protein
MCT	Monocarboxylate cotransporter
MDCK	Madin-Darby canine kidney
MDR	Multidrug resistance
Mdm2	Mouse double minute 2 protein
MEK	Mitogen-activated protein kinase/extracellular signal-regulated kinase
MetAP	Methionine aminopeptidase
MFS	Metastasis-free survival
MHC	Major histocompatibility complex
miR	Micro-RNA
MLPA	Multiplex ligation-dependent probe amplification
MMC	Mitomycin C
MMP	Matrix metalloproteinase
Mn-SOD	Manganese-superoxide dismutase
MRI	Magnetic resonance imaging
MRS	Magnetic resonance spectroscopy
MTD	Maximum tolerated dose
MTIF	Microphtalmia-associated transcription factor

mTOR	Mammalian target of rapamycin	NSCLC	Non-small-cell lung cancer
mTORC	mTOR Complex	OCT4	Octamer-binding transcription factor 4
MUC1	Mucin 1	ODDD	Oxygen-dependent degradation domain
MVD	Microvessel density		
MYND	Myeloid, Nervy and DEAF-type Zn+ finger domain p21	2-OG	2-oxoglutarate
		OPN	Osteopontin
NAC	N-acetyl cysteine	ORFs	Open reading frames
NAD	N-terminal activation domain	OS	Overall survival
		p300	E1A binding protein p300
NADH	Nicotinamide adenine dinucleotide	p14ARF	p14 alternate reading frame product of the CDKN2A locus
NADPH	Nicotinamid adenine dinucleotide phosphate		
		PARP	Poly(ADP-ribose)polymerase
NBCe1	Sodium-bicarbonate cotransporter	PAS	Per/Arnt/Sim
NCI	National Cancer Institute	PCK1	Phosphoenolpyruvate carboxykinase 1
NCX	Sodium-calcium exchanger		
ND6	NADH dehydrogenase subunit 6	PCR	Polymerase chain reaction
NDCBE	Sodium-dependent chloride-bicarbonate exchanger	PD-ECGF	Platelet-derived endothelial cell growth factor
NEDD8	Neural precursor cell expressed, developmentally down-regulated 8	PDGF	Platelet-derived growth factor
		PDGFR	Platelet-derived growth factor receptor
NEMO	NF-kappa-B essential modulator	PDH	Pyruvate dehydrogenase
NF1	Neurofibromatosis type 1	PDK	Pyruvate dehydrogenase kinase
NF-κB	Nuclear factor kappa-light-chain-enhancer of activated B cells	PEL	Primary effusion lymphoma
		PET	Positron emission tomography
NGF	Nerve growth factor		
NHE	Sodium-hydrogen exchanger	PFC	Perfluorocarbon
		PFKFB	6-phosphofructo-2-kinase/fructose-2,6-bihosphatase
NICD	Notch intracellular domain		
NODD	N-terminal oxygen-dependent degradation domain	PFKL	Phosphofructokinase L
		PFS	Progression-free survival
NOS	Nitric oxide synthase	PGI	Phosphoglucose isomerase
NOX	NADPH oxidase	PGK	Phosphoglycerate kinase
NQO1	Quinone oxidoreductase	PGM	Phosphoglycerate mutase
Nrf2	Nuclear factor (erythroid-derived 2)-like 2	pHi	Intracellular pH
		pHe	Extracellular pH
NSAID	Nonsteroidal anti-inflammatory drug	PHD	Prolyl hydroxylase

PI3K	Phosphatidyl inositol 3-kinase	ROC	Receptor operated channel
PIASy	SUMO E3 ligase	ROK	Rho-kinase
PKA	Protein kinase A	ROS	Reactive oxygen species
PKC	Protein kinase C	RSV	Respiratory syncytial virus
PLB	Phospholamban	RSV	Rous sarcoma virus
PLC	Phospholipase C	RT	Radiotherapy
PI3K	Phosphatidyl-3 inositol kinase	RTA	Replication and transcription activator
PlGF	Placental growth factor	RTK	Receptor tyrosine kinase
PKM	Pyruvate kinase M	RyR	Ryanodine receptor
PMCA	Plasma membrane Ca^{2+}-ATPase	SCC	Squamous cell carcinoma
v-pol	Retrovitus RNA polymerase	SCF	Skp1-Cdc53/Cul2-F box ubiquitin ligase
PPI	Proton pump inhibitor	SCO2	Synthesis of cytochrome oxidase 2
pRB	Retinoblastoma protein	SDF	Stromal cell-derived factor
PTB	Polypyrimidine tract binding protein	SDH	Succinate dehydrogenase
PTEN	Phophatase and tensin homolog	SENP3	Sentrin/SUMO-specific protease 3
PTP	Permeability transition pore	SERCA	Sarco/endoplasmic reticulum Ca^{2+}-ATPase
R2	Transverse relaxation time	shRNA	Small hairpin RNA
RACK1	Receptor for activated protein kinase C	Siah	Seven in absentia homologue
pRb	Retinoblastoma tumour suppressor	siRNAs	Small interfering RNAs
		SIRT1	Sirtuin 1 deacetylase
Rbp1	Large subunit of RNA polymerase	SLC4	Solute carrier family 4
Rbx1	RING-box protein 1	SMAD	Homologs of mothers against decapentaplegic
RcGshT	Rat canalicular GSH transporter	Snail	Snail homolog 1 (Drosophila)
RCT	Radiochemotherapy	SOD	Superoxide dismutase
REDD	Transcriptional regulator	SPECT	Single photon emission computed tomography
Ref1	Redox factor 1	Src	Proto-oncogene tyrosine-protein kinase
RET	Proto-oncoprotein		
RH1	Aziridinylbenzoquinone alkylating agent	SRE	Serum response element
		SR-PKPD	Spatially resolved pharmacokinetic /pharmacodynamic
RFS	Relapse-free survival		
Rheb	Ras homolog enriched in brain	SSB	Single-strand brakes
RNI	Reactive nitrogen intermediates	STAT	Signal transducer and activator of transcription

SUMO	Small ubiquitin related modifier	UPR	Unfolded protein response
SUV	Standardized uptake value	VBC	E3 ligase complex pVHL/Elongin B/C
SV40	Simian virus 40	VDCC	Voltage-dependent calcium channel
SVCT	Sodium-dependent vitamin C transporter	VEGF	Vascular endothelial growth factor
TA	Transactivation	VEGFR	Vascular endothelial growth factor receptor
TAD	Transactivation domain	vGPCR	Viral G-protein coupled receptor
TAK	Transforming growth factor-b-activated kinase	VHL	Von Hippel-Lindau
Tax	Human T-cell Receptor viral peptide	VIM	Vimentin
TCA	Tricarboxylic acid	vIFR	Viral interferon regulatory factor
TCF4	Transcription factor 4	VM	Vasculogenic mimicry
TCR	T-cell receptor	v-src	Sarcoma (Schmidt-Ruppin A-2) viral oncogene homolog (avian)
TEM	Tumour endothelial marker	VSV	Vesicular stomatitis virus
TG	Transglutaminase	Wnt	Wg (wingless) and Int
TGF	Transforming growth factor	XBP-1	X-box binding protein 1
Tie	Angiopoietin receptor	ZEB1	Transcriptional repressor
TIGAR	TP53-induced glycolysis and apoptosis regulator		
TLR	Toll-like receptor		
TNF	Tumour necrosis factor		
Top 1	Topoisomerase I		
TPA	12-0-tetradecanyolphorbol-13-acetate		
TPO	Thrombopoietin		
TPT	Topotecan		
TPZ	Tirapazamino		
TRK	Tropomyosin-receptor-kinase		
TROG	Trans-Tasman Radiation Oncology Group		
TRPC	Transient receptor potential channel		
Trx	Thioredoxin		
TSA	Trichostatin A		
TSC	Tuberous sclerosis complex		
Ubc	Ubiquitin conjugating enzyme		
uPA	Plasminogen activator, urokinase		
uPAR	Plasminogen activator, urokinase receptor		

Index